Fertility Cryopreservation

Fertility Cryopreservation

Ri-Cheng Chian
McGill University, Montreal, Canada

Patrick Quinn
Sage IVF, Redmond, OR, USA

CAMBRIDGE
UNIVERSITY PRESS

CAMBRIDGE UNIVERSITY PRESS
Cambridge, New York, Melbourne, Madrid, Cape Town, Singapore,
São Paulo, Delhi, Dubai, Tokyo

Cambridge University Press
The Edinburgh Building, Cambridge CB2 8RU, UK

Published in the United States of America by Cambridge University Press, New York

www.cambridge.org
Information on this title: www.cambridge.org/9780521517782

First published 2010

Printed in the United Kingdom at the University Press, Cambridge

A catalogue record for this publication is available from the British Library

Library of Congress Cataloguing in Publication data
Fertility cryopreservation / [edited by] Ri-Cheng Chian, Patrick Quinn.
p. ; cm.
Includes bibliographical references and index.
ISBN 978-0-521-51778-2 (hardback)
1. Infertility–Prevention. 2. Generative organs–Cryopreservation. I. Chian, Ri-Cheng.
II. Quinn, Patrick, 1946– III. Title.
[DNLM: 1. Infertility–therapy. 2. Antineoplastic Agents–adverse effects. 3. Cryopreservation–methods.
4. Fertility–radiation effects. 5. Infertility–etiology. 6. Neoplasms–complications. WP 570 F4115 2010]
RC889.F43 2010
362.196′692–dc22 2010003022

ISBN 978-0-521-51778-2 Hardback

Contents

List of Contributors *page* vii
Preface xi
Acknowledgements xiii

Section 1: Cryobiology

1 **Cryobiology: an overview 1**
Ri-Cheng Chian

2 **Suppression of ice in aqueous solutions and its application to vitrification in assisted reproductive technology 10**
Patrick Quinn

3 **Movement of water and cryoprotectants in mouse oocytes and embryos at different stages: relevance to cryopreservation 16**
Magosaburo Kasai and Keisuke Edashige

4 **Cryoprotectants 24**
Jason E. Swain and Gary D. Smith

Section 2: Cryopreservation of sperm and testicular tissue

5 **Cryopreservation of sperm: an overview 39**
Fady Shehata and Ri-Cheng Chian

6 **Sperm cryopreservation for a donor program 46**
Zheng Li and Peng Xu

7 **Cryopreservation of surgically retrieved sperm 51**
Peter T. K. Chan

8 **Testicular tissue cryopreservation 57**
Ariel Revel and Javier Mejia

Section 3: Cryopreservation of embryos

9 **Cryopreservation of embryos: an overview 67**
David H. Edgar and Debra A. Gook

10 **Cryopreservation of pronuclear stage human embryos 76**
Barry Behr and Yimin Shu

11 **Cryopreservation of day two and day three embryos 89**
Yunxia Cao and Zhiguo Zhang

12 **Cryopreservation of blastocysts 95**
Yoshiharu Morimoto

13 **Aseptic vitrification of human blastocysts: protocol development and clinical application 106**
Pierre Vanderzwalmen, Luc Grobet, Yannis Prapas, Patricia Frias, and Nicolas Zech

Section 4: Cryopreservation of oocytes

14 **Cryopreservation of human oocytes: an overview 114**
Ri-Cheng Chian

15 **Cryopreservation of oocytes by slow cooling 120**
Andrea Borini and Giovanni Coticchio

16 **Vitrification of human oocytes with different tools 131**
Patrick Quinn

17 **Vitrification of human oocytes using the McGill Cryoleaf protocol 144**
Jack Yu Jen Huang, Seang Lin Tan, and Ri-Cheng Chian

18 **Cryopreservation of human oocytes and embryos either by direct plunging into liquid nitrogen or by using an aseptic approach 157**
Evgenia Isachenko, Vladimir Isachenko, Jurgen M. Weiss, and Rolf Kreienberg

19 **Vitrification of human oocytes for a donor program 169**
Elkin Lucena, Carolina Lucena, and Sandra Mojica

20 **Obstetric and perinatal outcomes in pregnancies conceived following oocyte cryopreservation 178**
William Buckett and Ri-Cheng Chian

Section 5: Cryopreservation of ovarian tissue

21 **Cryopreservation of ovarian tissue: an overview 189**
Jacques Donnez, Pascale Jadoul, Olivier Donnez, Anne-Sophie van Eyck, Jean Squifflet, and Marie-Madeleine Dolmans

22 **In vitro culture of human primordial follicles 200**
Benoit Schubert and Johan Smitz

23 **Concept of human ovarian tissue cryobanking 213**
Vladimir Isachenko, Friedrich Gagsteiger, Evgenia Isachenko, Juergen Weiss, and Rolf Kreienberg

24 **Transplantation of cryopreserved ovarian tissues 218**
Dror Meirow

25 **Whole ovary cryopreservation 233**
Jason G. Bromer and Pasquale Patrizio

26 **Transplantation of whole frozen–thawed ovaries 241**
Amir Arav and Yehudit Natan

Section 6: Ethical considerations

27 **Ethical considerations in fertility cryopreservation in young cancer patients 248**
Edwin C. Hui

Appendix 1 Autotransplantation of cryopreserved thawed human ovarian tissue 257

Index 260

Contributors

Amir Arav
Institute of Animal Science
Agricultural Research Organization
Bet Dagan, Israel

Barry Behr
Department of Obstetrics and Gynecology
University of Stanford School of Medicine
Stanford, CA, USA

Andrea Borini
Tecnobios Procreazione
Centre for Reproductive Health
Bologna, Italy

Jason G. Bromer
Department of Obstetrics, Gynecology, and Reproductive Sciences
Yale University School of Medicine
New Haven, CT, USA

William Buckett
Department of Obstetrics and Gynecology
McGill University
Montréal, Québec, Canada

Yunxia Cao
Reproduction Medicine Centre
Department of Obstetrics and Gynecology
The First Affiliated Hospital of Anhui Medical University
Hefei, China

Peter T. K. Chan
Department of Urology
McGill University
Montréal, Québec, Canada

Ri-Cheng Chian
Department of Obstetrics and Gynecology
McGill University
Montréal, Québec, Canada

Giovanni Coticchio
Tecnobios Procreazione
Centre for Reproductive Health
Bologna, Italy

Marie-Madeleine Dolmans
Department of Gynecology
Université Catholique de Louvain
Brussels, Belgium

Jacques Donnez
Department of Gynecology
Université Catholique de Louvain
Brussels, Belgium

Olivier Donnez
Department of Gynecology
Université Catholique de Louvain
Brussels, Belgium

Keisuke Edashige
Laboratory of Animal Science
College of Agriculture
Kochi University
Kochi, Japan

David H. Edgar
Reproductive Services
Royal Women's Hospital
Melbourne, Australia

Patricia Frias
Fertility and Sterility National Centre
Cochabamba, Bolivia

Friedrich Gagsteiger
2IVF Zentrum Ulm
Ulm, Germany

Debra A. Gook
Reproductive Services
Royal Women's Hospital
Carlton, Victoria, Australia

Luc Grobet
GIGA-Research, University of Liège
Liège, Belgium

Jack Yu Jen Huang
Department of Obstetrics and Gynecology
McGill University
Montréal, Québec, Canada

Edwin C. Hui
Faculty of Medicine
The University of Hong Kong
Hong Kong

Evgenia Isachenko
Section of Reproductive Medicine
Department of Obstetrics and Gynecology
University of Ulm
Ulm, Germany

Vladimir Isachenko
Section of Reproductive Medicine
Department of Obstetrics and Gynecology
University of Ulm
Ulm, Germany

Pascale Jadoul
Department of Gynecology
Université Catholique de Louvain
Brussels, Belgium

Magosaburo Kasai
Laboratory of Animal Science
College of Agriculture
Kochi University
Kochi, Japan

Rolf Kreienberg
Section of Reproductive Medicine
Department of Obstetrics and Gynecology
University of Ulm
Ulm, Germany

Zheng Li
Shanghai Human Sperm Bank
Shanghai Institute of Andrology
Department of Urology
Shanghai Jiaotong University
School of Medicine
Shanghai, China

Carolina Lucena
CECOLFES Bogota, Colombia

Elkin Lucena
CECOLFES Bogota, Colombia

Dror Meirow
IVF Unit, Department of Obstetrics and Gynecology
Sheba Medical Center
Tel Hashomer, Israel

Javier Mejia
Department of Obstetrics and Gynecology
Hadassah Medical Center
Hebrew University-Hadassah Medical School
Jerusalem, Israel

Sandra Mojica
CECOLFES Bogota, Colombia

Yoshiharu Morimoto
IVF Namba Clinic Osaka, Japan

Yehudit Natan
Institute of Animal Science
Agricultural Research Organization
Bet Dagan, Israel

Pasquale Patrizio
Yale University Fertility Center
New Haven, CT, USA

Yannis Prapas
Iakentro IVF Centre, Thessaloniki, Greece

Patrick Quinn
Sage IVF, A Cooper Surgical Company,
Redmond, Oregon, USA

Ariel Revel
Department of Obstetrics and Gynecology
Hadassah Medical Center
Hebrew University-Hadassah Medical School
Jerusalem, Israel

Benoit Schubert
Hôpitaux de Paris Unit of Biology of Reproduction
Groupe Hospitalier Pitié-Salpétrière
Paris, France

Fady Shehata
Department of Obstetrics and Gynecology
McGill University
Montréal, Québec, Canada

Yimin Shu
IVF Program Division of Reproductive Endocrinology and Infertiltiy
Stanford University Medical Center
Stanford, CA, USA

Gary D. Smith
Department of Obstetrics and Gynecology
University of Michigan
Ann Arbor, MI, USA

Johan Smitz
Follicle Biology Laboratory
Center for Reproductive Medicine
Free University Brussels,
Brussels, Belgium

Jean Squifflet
Department of Gynecology
Université Catholique de Louvain
Cliniques Universitaires St Luc
Brussels, Belgium

Jason E. Swain
Center for Reproductive Medicine
University of Michigan
Ann Arbor, MI, USA

Seang Lin Tan
Department of Obstetrics and Gynecology
McGill University
Montréal, Québec,
Canada

Pierre Vanderzwalmen
IVF Centers Prof. Zech
Bregenz, Austria

Anne-Sophie van Eyck
Department of Gynecology
Université Catholique de Louvain
Cliniques Universitaires St Luc
Brussels, Belgium

Jurgen M. Weiss
Department of Obstetrics and Gynecology,
University of Ulm,
Ulm, Germany

Peng Xu
Department of Andrology
Center for Reproductive Medicine
Shenyang Jinhua Hospital
Shenyang, China

Nicolas Zech
IVF Centers Prof. Zech Bregenz, Austria

Zhiguo Zhang
Reproduction Medicine Centre
Department of Obstetrics and Gynecology
The First Affiliated Hospital of Anhui Medical University
Hefei, China

Preface

An introduction to fertility cryopreservation

Infertility or impaired fertility may be caused by a wide range of reasons, including reproductive disorders, gonadal toxic therapy (chemotherapy, radiation therapy), surgery, genetic predisposition, or exposure to environmental toxins. Among these, a large group of potential infertility patients will include survivors of childhood and adult cancer. Since the late 1970s, the incidence of cancer in children has increased by up to 20% while mortality rates have declined remarkably as a result of progress in cancer treatment [1].

Each year, more than half a million young adult men and women living in the USA have been diagnosed with some form of invasive cancer [2,3]. With earlier diagnosis and aggressive chemotherapy and/or radiotherapy coupled with bone marrow transplantation, more than 90% of teenage boys and girls as well as young adults affected by some malignancies will survive [4]. It has been estimated that approximately 1 in 250 young adults will be long-term survivors of cancer [5]. However, there is often a loss of both endocrine and reproductive function because of the sensitivity of the ovaries to cytotoxic treatment and ionizing radiation, and one of the major concerns is whether these patients will be able to have healthy children after cancer cure treatment [6,7]. Therefore, it has been suggested that providing options for preservation of fertility for men and women is not only an important issue for reproductive health but also a quality-of-life consideration [8].

Currently, there are a number of options available to try to preserve fertility. Adult males have the option of cryopreserving their sperm for later use, but this is not the case for prepubertal boys and and for some post-adolescent boys [7,9,10]. Adult females have an option for embryo cryopreservation, but this is feasible only if a male partner is available and is not suitable for prepubertal girls [11]. Furthermore, this option requires time for the preparation and stimulation of the ovaries, which delays the treatment of cancer, and the ovarian stimulation may be deleterious in the context of certain types of cancer. Therefore, attempts have been made to preserve fertility with gametes (sperm and oocytes) and gonadal tissues (testicular and ovarian tissues) as well as with whole gonadal organs (ovary). Apart from sperm and embryo cryopreservation, other technologies are still considered to be largely experimental by the American Society for Reproductive Medicine (ASRM) [3] even though tremendous developments have been achieved recently, especially with cryopreservation of oocytes and ovarian tissues. In fact, it is important to be aware that developing new technologies for preserving or restoring fertility should be considered in relation to the long-term effects of such technologies, healthy babies.

It has become apparent as fertility cryopreservation is increasingly practiced throughout the world that there is a real need for a comprehensive book for fertility cryopreservation. We have endeavored to collect contributors with international expertise in all aspects of fertility cryopreservation, from gametes (sperm and oocytes) and embryos to gonadal tissues as well as whole gonadal organs and who cover all areas from basic science to clinical application. The book is divided into five sections.

Section 1 covers the scientific rationale for cryobiology by outlining aqueous solutions, mechanism of cell cryopreservation, and cryoprotectants as well as the pathway for the movement of water and cryoprotectants during cryopreservation. Here we have to mention that cryobiology is a complicated area and not all the details can be covered in these chapters.

Section 2 covers cryopreservation of human sperm and testicular tissue. It gives brief information about historical aspects of sperm cryopreservation and the protocols developed. It also covers donor program and freezing of surgically retrieved sperm.

Section 3 covers human embryo cryopreservation from pronuclear stage to cleavage stage to blastocyst stage, using slow-freezing or rapid cooling (vitrification) methods. It also covers the recent development of blastocyst cryopreservation with the vitrification method.

Section 4 covers human oocyte cryopreservation either with slow freezing or vitrification. It briefly introduces the use of different tools to vitrify the oocytes, and the efficiency of donor programs with frozen–thawed oocytes. It also covers the initial information available about prenatal development and live births using vitrified oocytes.

Finally, Section 5 covers different technologies for the cryopreservation of ovarian tissue. It describes briefly the technologies for in vitro culture of primordial follicles isolated from ovarian tissue. It also covers transplantation of cryopreserved ovarian tissue and whole ovaries. Section 6 considers ethical issues involved in fertility cryopreservation with gametes, embryos, and gonadal tissues.

Although it is still considered a relatively new procedure for oocyte cryopreservation, ovarian tissue freezing can be followed by ovarian tissue transplantation. We hope that this book will be a helpful overview in the field of fertility cryopreservation and its development and will contribute towards its increased availability. We believe that fertility cryopreservation offers an option for people who need it urgently in order to have a possibility of having their own biological children in the near future.

References

1. Jemal A, Murray T, Samuels A, *et al.* Cancer statistics, 2003. *CA Cancer J Clin* 2003; **53**: 5–26.
2. American Cancer Society. *Cancer Facts and Figures – 2001*. Atlanta, GA: American Cancer Society, 2001.
3. Lamar CA, DeCherney AH. Fertility preservation: state of the science and future research direction. *Fertil Steril* 2009; **91**: 316–319.
4. Ries LAG, Percy CL, Bunin GR. Introduction. In Ries LAG, Smith MA, Gurney JG, *et al.* eds. *Cancer Incidence and Survival among Children and Adolescents: United States SEER Program* 1975–1995. [NIH Pub. No. 99-4649.] Bethesda, MD: National Cancer Institute, 1999, pp. 1–15.
5. Bleyer WA. The impact of childhood cancer on the United States and the world. *Cancer* 1990; **40**: 355–367.
6. Apperley JF, Reddy N. Mechanism and management of treatment-related gonadal failure in recipients of high dose chemoradiotherapy. *Blood Rev* 1995; **9**: 93–116.
7. Revel A, Revel-Vilk S. Pediatric fertility preservation: is it time to offer testicular tissue cryopreservation? *Mol Cell Endocrinol* 2008; **282**: 143–149.
8. Garner E, Goldstein DP, Berkowitz RS, Wenzel L. Psychosocial and reproductive outcomes of gestational trophoblastic diseases. *Best Pract Res Clin Obstet Gynecol* 2003; **17**: 959–968.
9. Sanger WG, Olson JH, Sherman JK. Semen cryobanking for men with cancer: criteria change. *Fertil Steril* 1992; **58**: 1024–1027.
10. Oehninger S. Strategies for fertility preservation in female and male cancer survivors. *J Soc Gynecol Invest* 2005; **12**: 222–231.
11. Su HI, Lin K, Gracia CR. Early menopause in cancer survivors: fertility options. *Menopausal Med* 2008; **16**: 51–56.

Acknowledgements

To my mother, Dr. Hui-Shu Jin (D.V.M.), who showed me for the first time liquid nitrogen (LN_2) and frozen–thawed bull sperm under a microscope when I was a child at primary (elementary) school.

Ri-Cheng Chian

To my loving wife Kay, and family, who make all of this worthwhile.

Patrick Quinn

Section 1 Chapter 1

Cryobiology

Cryobiology: an overview

Ri-Cheng Chian

Introduction

Cryobiology deals with life at low temperature [1,2]. The word cryobiology is relatively new. Literature search indicates that cryobiology was first used in the early 1950s to describe the newly developing field of low temperature biology [3–9]. Living things must be able to adapt to the changing surface environment of the earth in order to preserve the existence of life itself. The principal effects of cold on living tissue are destruction of life and preservation of life at a reduced level of activity. Both of these effects are demonstrated in nature. Death by freezing is a relatively common occurrence in severe winter storms. Among cold-blooded animals, winter weather usually results in a coma-like sleep that may last for a considerable length of time. Therefore, the definition of cryobiology is to study living organisms at low temperature. In other words, cryobiology is the branch of biology involving the study of the effects of low temperatures on organisms (most often for the purpose of achieving cryopreservation).

In cryobiological applications, much lower temperatures are used are present in natural environments. Liquid nitrogen (at −196°C or −320°F) can either destroy living tissue in a matter of seconds or it can preserve it for years, and possibly for centuries, with essentially no detectable biochemical activity. The end result when heat is withdrawn from living tissue depends on processes occurring in the individual cells. Basic knowledge of the causes of cell death, especially during the process of freezing, and the discovery of methods which prevented these causes, have led to practical applications for long-term storage of both living cells and living tissues. In the industrial food area, the microorganisms used in cheese production can be frozen, stored, and transported without loss of lactic acid-producing activity. In the medical field, it is commonly known that whole blood or separated blood cells can be cryopreserved and stored for their valuable applications.

Water is the fundamental molecule of life. The biochemical constituents of a cell are either dissolved or suspended in water. Water is essential for the survival of all known forms of life; without an environment of water, life would not exist. Water has many distinct properties that are critical for the proliferation of life and these set it apart from other substances. It enables the proliferation of life by allowing organic compounds to react in ways that ultimately allow replication. Water is vital both as a solvent for many of the body's solutes and as an essential part of many metabolic processes within the body. Water is essential and central to these metabolic processes. Metabolic processes are affected by temperature. When the temperature falls, cells may slow down or stop all metabolic processes, and extremely low temperature may cause cell death.

During the physical process of freezing, water tends to crystallize in pure form, while the dissolved or suspended materials concentrate in the remaining liquid. In the living cell, this process is quite destructive. In a relatively slow-freezing process, ice first begins to form in the fluid surrounding the cells, and the concentration of dissolved materials in the remaining liquid increases. A concentration gradient is established across the cell wall, and water moves out of the cell in response to the osmotic force. As freezing continues, the cell becomes relatively dehydrated. Salts may concentrate to extremely high levels. In a similar manner, the acid–base ratio of the solution may be altered during the concentration process.

Dehydration can affect the gross organization of the cell and also molecular relationships, some of which depend on the presence of water at particular sites. Cellular collapse resulting from loss of water may bring into contact intracellular components that are normally separated to prevent any destructive interaction. Finally, as the ice crystals grow in size, the cell walls may be ruptured by the crystals themselves or

Fertility Cryopreservation ed. Ri-Cheng Chian and Patrick Quinn. Published by Cambridge University Press.

by the high concentration gradients that are imposed upon the walls. To prevent dehydration, steps must be taken to stop the separation of water in the form of pure ice so that all of the cell fluids can solidify together.

Cryobiology is the core of fertility cryopreservation. The earliest application of fertility cryopreservation was in the storage of animal sperm cells for use in artificial insemination. The principal application for human fertility cryopreservation was also begun with sperm freezing, and then with embryo and oocyte as well as gonadal cryopreservation. Knowledge and medical achievement have steadily advanced in the field of fertility cryopreservation, especially with recent oocyte and ovarian tissue cryopreservation. These historic accomplishments in the application of the scientific method can provide overwhelming support for continuing on this path. This chapter will try to set out briefly the scientific background and our current basic knowledge of cryobiology.

Basic science of cryobiology

Nature of water

Water appears in nature in all three common states of matter: vapor, liquid, and solid. Water is a tasteless, odorless liquid at standard temperature and pressure. The color of water and ice is, intrinsically, a very light blue, although water appears colorless in small quantities. Ice also appears colorless, and water vapor is essentially invisible as a gas. The maximum density of water occurs at 3.98°C (39.16°F). Water becomes even less dense upon freezing, expanding 9%. This causes an unusual phenomenon: ice floats upon water, and so organisms can live inside a partly frozen pond because the water on the bottom has a temperature of around 4°C (39°F). The boiling point of water is 100°C (212°F) at sea level and one atmosphere pressure. The freezing point of water is very close to 0°C (32°F) in the presence of nucleating substances, but in their absence it can be supercooled to −42°C (−43.6°F) before freezing. For most substances, freezing and melting points are approximately equal. Therefore, the melting point of ice at one atmosphere pressure is very close to 0°C (32°F). The melting point of water is relatively insensitive to change in pressure because the solid–liquid transition represents only a small change in volume.

The transition between liquid water and solid ice is one of the most commonly observed events in nature. As mentioned above, when water is cooled, it often is taken substantially below the freezing point before ice begins to form. This is because of the need for nucleation to occur before an ice crystal can begin to grow. Nucleation refers to the process by which a minimum crystal is formed, which can then expand. The continued expansion of the crystal is a process known as growth. When an ice nucleus begins to grow, any solutes that are present in the liquid will be excluded from this growing ice front. If the rate of crystal growth is faster than the rate at which diffusion of the particular solutes can carry them away from the ice front, then a concentration gradient will very quickly form in the liquid that surrounds the ice crystal. The concentrated solute will then lower the freezing point of the solution. When a certain amount of ice has formed, the solution at the interface will have a freezing point equal to the temperature of the interface. At this point, ice growth will be limited by diffusion of the solute away from the crystal. If the temperature is reduced to far below the melting point with supercooling speed, the solution may be prevented from reaching this situation of ice crystal nucleation and growth. If water is cooled sufficiently fast enough so that nucleation cannot occur, it is possible to avoid ice crystal formation [10]; this process is known as vitrification.

Temperature measurement

Thermometers measure temperature by using materials that change in some way when they are heated or cooled. In a mercury or alcohol thermometer, the liquid expands as it is heated and contracts when it is cooled, so the length of the liquid column is longer or shorter depending on the temperature. Modern thermometers are calibrated in standard temperature units such as Fahrenheit (F), Celsius (C), or kelvin (K).

Celsius is converted to Fahrenheit by multiplying by 1.8 (or 9/5) and add 32, and to Kelvin by adding 273 (e.g. 37°C is equivalent to 98.6°F and 310K).

Glass transition temperature

The glass transition temperature (T_g) is the temperature at which an amorphous solid becomes brittle on cooling or soft on heating. Glass transition is a pseudo-second phase transition in which a supercooling melt yields on cooling a glassy structure with properties similar to those of crystalline materials. Below T_g, amorphous solids in a glassy state, and most of their joining bonds are intact. It is important to note that T_g is a kinetic parameter and, therefore, parametrically depends on the melt cooling rate. Consequently, the slower the melt cooling rate, the lower the value of T_g. In addition, T_g depends on the measurement conditions, which are not universally defined.

At a certain temperature, the average kinetic energy of molecules no longer exceeds the binding energy between neighboring molecules, and growth of an organized solid crystal begins. Formation of an ordered system takes a certain amount of time since the molecules must move from their current location to energetically preferred points at crystal nodes. As the temperature falls, molecular motion slows down further and if the cooling rate is fast enough, molecules never reach their destination: the substance enters into dynamic arrest and a disordered glassy solid form. A full discussion of T_g requires an understanding of mechanical loss mechanisms of specific functional groups and molecular arrangements. The value of T_g is somewhat dependent on the time-scale of the imposed change in contrast to the melting point temperatures of crystalline materials. Time and temperature are interchangeable quantities when dealing with glasses, a fact often expressed in the time–temperature superposition principle. An alternative way to discuss the same issue is to say that a T_g is only a point on the temperature scale if the change is imposed at one particular frequency. Since T_g is dependent on the cooling rate as the glass is formed, the glass transition is not considered a true thermodynamic phase transition by many in the field.

The viscosity at T_g depends on the sample preparation (especially the cooling curve), the heating or cooling curve during measurement, and the chemical composition. Proteins possess a T_g value below which both anharmonic motions and long-range correlated motion within a single molecule are quenched. The origin of this transition is primarily a consequence of caging by glassy water, but it can also be modeled in the absence of explicit water molecules, suggesting that part of the transition reflects internal protein dynamics. Glass formation of water below the melting point can occur, usually through very rapid cooling or the introduction of agents that suppress the formation of ice crystals.

Vitrification

Vitrification is defined as the process of glass solidification of a liquid. The liquid is in a metastable state until it gets below a characteristic temperature, T_g, which is indicated by a sharp exothermic event. This heat loss occurs because of the loss of metastable clusters. Those clusters that have more energy than can be held by the bonds which they are able to form will oscillate for a short time and then disintegrate. Upon reaching T_g, the excess energy will be lost, thereby stabilizing the clusters. Once below T_g, the system is not merely a viscous liquid but is also a solid that is in a stable thermodynamic state. Achieving vitrification with pure water requires very small amounts and incredibly fast cooling. However, it is important to mention that vitrification can also occur in aqueous solution during slow freezing.

Aqueous solutions

A solution is a mixture containing at least two kinds of pure substance. In most solutions, one material predominates and this is called the solvent, with the other compounds being called solutes. When the components of a solution are in different states of matter, the solvent is considered to be the one that does not undergo a change of state upon mixing. Aqueous solutions are important for cryobiology since the freezing of biological systems always involves solutions containing substances such as electrolytes, non-electrolytes, polymers, and so on. During the phase change that occurs with vitrification, the concentration and distribution of the solutions are altered, sometimes accompanied by irreversible chemical reactions.

Molarity and molality

The composition of a solution is described by the concentration of its constitutions. There are two primary ways of expressing concentration: molarity and molality. Molarity is another term for concentration (M) and is the number of moles of solute in 1 liter of solution. Molality (m) is the number of moles of solute associated with 1000 g of solvent. Therefore, molarity is based on the volume of solution whereas molality is based on the weight of solvent. The difference becomes most noticeable when temperature effects are considered. Because the volume of liquids can expand or contract with changes in temperature, molarity can change with change of temperature. By comparison, the weight of solvent is constant with temperature, so molality gives a measure of concentration that is independent of temperature.

Solubility

A property of any particular combination of solute and solvent is the solubility of the solute in the solvent. This is the amount of solute that can be associated with a given amount of solvent in the context of a solution. Most solids show a well-defined saturation point in liquid when no more solid can be dissolved. The ratio of solute to solvent at this point defines the solubility. In general, solubility in liquids increases with temperature. Therefore, the solubility is a temperature-dependent property, although there are some exceptions. If a saturated solution is made at a certain temperature and then the temperature of the solution decreases, the solubility of the solution will be exceeded. The solution becomes supersaturated and exists in a metastable state. The solute will precipitate out of solution, usually forming crystals in the liquid. Even in crystalline form, solute molecules continually leave and join the crystal surface, going back and forth from solution to the solid phase. This has the effect of increasing the average crystal size, since small crystals have a high surface energy while large crystals have a small surface energy. The constant movement between crystal and solution tends to minimize the total surface energy of all the crystals present in the solution. The solubility is important for cryobiology because the solubility of solutes in extracellular and intracellular water will be changed following the change of temperature. Therefore, changes in solubility during freezing may induce ice crystal formation and cause cell death.

Colligative properties

The properties that solutions exhibit that arise from the behavior of the collection rather than from the behavior of individual components are called colligative properties. Vapor pressure, boiling point elevation, and freezing point depression are three such properties, depending upon the concentration of the solutions rather than the chemical properties of the constituents.

Osmosis

Water can be transported across semipermeable membranes separating compartments containing different concentrations of solutes. The membrane must be impermeable to the solute but permeable for water. This process is called osmosis and has enormous significance for living organisms. The most important and most widely occurring process for water transfer in and out of living cells is osmosis.

Cell permeability

Changes in the extracellular osmotic pressure will create a situation in which a cell will attempt to attain equilibration by either gaining or losing water until there is no osmotic gradient across the plasma membrane. If the cell volume is measured as a function of time, then it can be seen that equilibrium is only achieved after a certain amount of time has elapsed. The kinetics of water movement out of the cell is determined by the physical structure of the membrane. With biological membranes, the phenomenological permeability is complicated. Since freezing and thawing introduce opportunities for osmotic swelling and shrinkage of cells, it may be important to know the tolerance of each type of cell for the osmotic pressure during a given cell type's response to exposure to low temperatures.

Cryoinjury

Some of the classic papers in the field of cryobiology describe the theories and the mechanisms of cryoinjury during cell freezing and thawing [11–14]. These theories have made great contributions to developments and understanding in cryobiology [15–19]. Cryoinjury has been successfully simulated by changing the concentration of solutes surrounding cells in suspension so as to simulate the changes in concentration that take place upon freezing and thawing when water is subtracted or added back to yield the original pre-freezing concentrations [20–29]. Many theories and mechanisms have been proposed for cryoinjury, but none may exactly explain the nature of the phenomenon. For example, it is not surprising that survival rates can vary from cell type to cell type for the same cooling rate and freezing solution. Although there are mathematical models describing how to calculate appropriate cooling rates for avoiding intracellular ice formation [30–41], the theoretical predictions may not apply for all types of cell, particularly for aqueous solutions supplemented with cryoprotective additives. Some cryoprotectants reduce the injury of cells during freezing and thawing. Cryoprotectants are usually divided into two broad classes based on their ability to diffuse across cell membranes. Penetrating cryoprotectants are able to move across cell membranes whereas non-penetrating agents cannot. Since Chapter 4 specifically deals with cryoprotectants, this chapter will describe the penetrating cryoprotectants and will touch briefly on the potential mechanisms involved in cell cryopreservation.

Cryoprotectants

Discovery of cryoprotectant properties

Although a good survival rate of deep-frozen cells has occasionally been observed without a protective agent, a suitable cryoprotectant usually increases the survival rate. Usually the literature indicates that Polge *et al.* [3] first reported that glycerol has cryoprotective function to improve survival rate of frozen–thawed cells (chicken spermatozoa). However, the cryoprotective effect of glycerol was discovered much earlier than is usually stated [42–45]. Although survived cells have been occasionally without a cryoprotectant, the presence of a suitable cryoprotectant usually increases the cell survival rates considerably. The discovery that glycerol, first, and later dimethyl sulfoxide protect eukaryotic cells against freezing damage marked the beginning of modern cryobiology [9].

Today, the most commonly used cryoprotectants in the field are glycerol, dimethyl sulfoxide, ethylene glycol, and propylene glycol. The cryoprotective action of each type of cryoprotective agent must be similar, but although many hypotheses have been proposed to explain their mechanism of action, it is still unclear what role they do actually play in the freezing or vitrification solutions. For example, Lovelock [4] proposed that glycerol acted colligatively (altering the phase diagram of the solution) to reduce the high salt concentration that occurs during freezing. Later, phase diagrams were produced that described the mechanism of action of cryoprotectants, especially dimethyl sulfoxide [15]. Phase diagrams are used to describe equilibrium situations in which two or more phases of matter exist together as pure substances or in solutions. In the freezing system, the primary component is water, and the entire system is a collection of compartments filled with an aqueous solution. As aqueous solutions are cooled, the water forms a crystalline solid that has almost no solubility for the solutes that were in the aqueous solution. As ice forms, the solutes will be confined to the remaining liquid phase, becoming more concentrated. Because this lowers the freezing point of the aqueous phase, the system can remain in equilibrium with a substantial unfrozen fraction. As cooling continues, the solubility limit of the solution will also be reached, leading to the precipitation of solutes. The ternary systems of glycerol–NaCl–water and dimethylsulfoxide–NaCl–water have been described [15,26,27]. From these diagrams, it is clear that the solubility and eutectic behavior of a single solute can be altered significantly by the amount and type of additional solutes introduced into the system. It is also clear that the equilibrium between solids and liquid becomes increasingly complex as the number of components is increased. Therefore, the action of cryoprotectants can be described as lowering the freezing point and reducing/preventing ice crystal formation of aqueous (freezing) solutions.

The following compounds are commonly used cryoprotectants in field of cryobiology. Since Chapter 4 will deal with more details about the cryoprotectants, here we just briefly introduce these classic permeable cryoprotectants.

Glycerol

Glycerol, also known as glycerin or glycerine, is a sugar alcohol. It is a colorless, odorless, viscous, sweet-tasting liquid that is soluble in water and low in toxicity. Each glycerol molecule has a three-carbon chain, with a hydroxyl group (OH) attached to each carbon atom (Figure 1.1a). The hydroxyl groups are responsible for making the substance highly soluble in water and hygroscopic. A hygroscopic substance is one that attracts water molecules from the surrounding environment. It has only slight solubility in organic solvents such as ethyl acetate and diethyl ether, and it does not dissolve in hydrocarbons. Its melting point is 18°C (64.4°F), and its boiling point is 290°C (554°F). Its surface tension is 64.00 mN/m at 20°C, and it has a temperature coefficient of −0.0598 mN/(m K). The glycerol substructure is a central component of many lipids. Glycerol is useful for numerous applications. It is a common component of solvents for enzymatic reagents stored at temperatures below 0°C as the presence of glycerol depresses the freezing temperature of the solution. Glycerol is compatible with other biochemical materials in living cells and is frequently used in cell preservation to reduce damage caused by ice crystal formation.

Dimethyl sulfoxide

Dimethyl sulfoxide, also known as methyl sulfoxide or methylsulfinylmethane, is a clear and colorless liquid. The sulfur center in dimethyl sulfoxide is nucleophilic toward soft electrophiles and the oxygen is nucleophilic toward hard electrophiles (Figure 1.1b). The methyl groups are somewhat acidic in character ($pK_a = 35$) because of the stabilization of the resultant carbanion by the S(O)R group, and so are deprotonated with strong bases such as lithium diisopropylamide and sodium hydride. Dimethyl sulfoxide is an important polar aprotic solvent that dissolves both polar and non-polar compounds and it is miscible in a wide range of organic solvents as well as water.

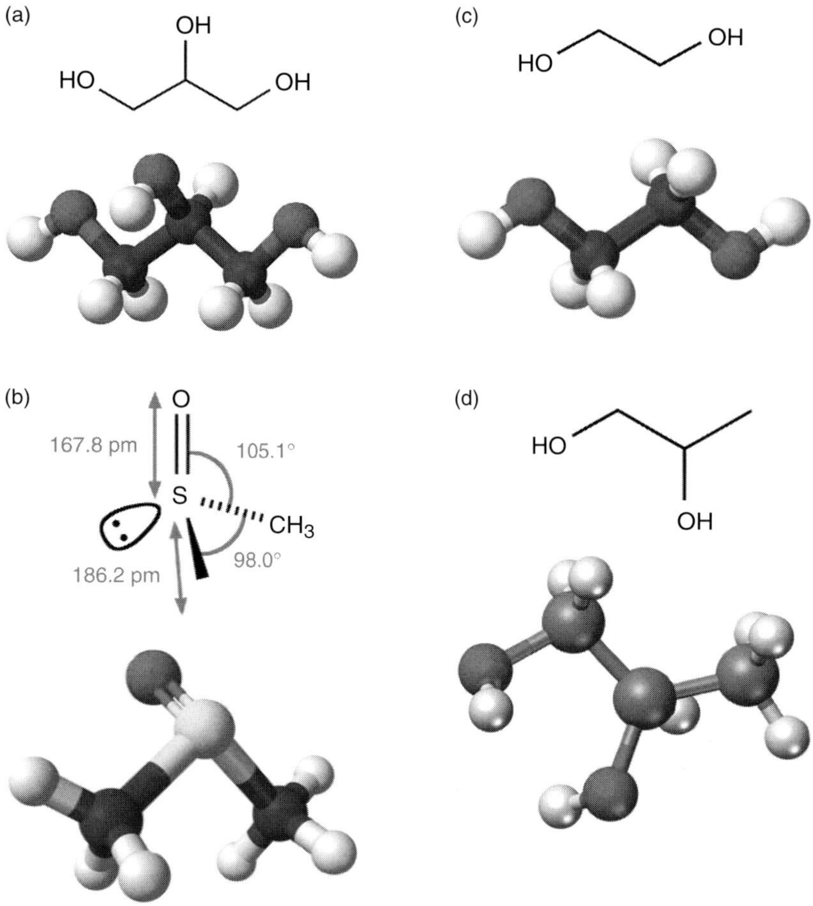

Figure 1.1. The structure of cryoprotectants commonly used in cryobiology: (a) glycerol; (b), dimethyl sulfoxide; (c) ethylene glycol; (d) propylene glycol (1,2-propanediol). (Adapted from Wikipedia.)

It dissolves a variety of organic substances, including carbohydrates, polymers, and peptides, as well as many inorganic salts and gases. Its melting point is 18.5°C (65.3°F), and its boiling point is 189°C (372.2°F). It has a distinctive property of penetrating the skin very readily. Its taste has been described as oyster- or garlic-like. Other reported side effects include stomach upset, sensitivity to light, visual disturbances, and headache. Skin irritation can develop at the site where dimethyl sulfoxide is applied topically. Loading levels of 50–60 wt% are often observed compared with 10–20 wt% with typical solvents. For this reason, dimethyl sulfoxide plays a role in sample management and high-throughput screening operations in drug design [46]. In cryobiology, dimethyl sulfoxide has been used as a cryoprotectant and it is still an important cryoprotectant for vitrification used to preserve organs, tissues, and cell suspensions.

Ethylene glycol

Ethylene glycol, also known as monoethylene glycol or 1,2-ethanediol, is an alcohol with two hydroxyl groups (a diol) (Figure 1.1c). It may also be used as a protecting group for carbonyl groups in organic synthesis and it is widely used as an antifreeze in vehicles. In its pure form, it is an odorless, colorless, syrupy, sweet-tasting, toxic liquid. Its melting point is −12.9°C (8.8°F), and its boiling point is 197.3°C (387.1°F). The major use of ethylene glycol is as a medium for convective heat transfer in, for example, automobiles and liquid-cooled computers. Because of its low freezing point, it is used as a de-icing fluid for windshields and aircraft. It is also commonly used in chilled water air conditioning systems that place either the chiller or the air handler outside, or systems that must cool below the freezing temperature of water. Ethylene glycol is also used in the manufacture of some vaccines, but it is not itself present in the vaccines. The major toxicity from ethylene glycol is through ingestion, where it is oxidized to glycolic acid and then oxalic acid, which is toxic. Ethylene glycol and its toxic byproducts first affect the central nervous system, then the heart, and finally the kidneys. Ingestion of sufficient amounts can be fatal. Ethylene glycol is used widely for vitrification, especially oocyte and embryo vitrification.

Propylene glycol

Propylene glycol, known also by its systematic name 1,2-propanediol and as 1,2-dihydroxypropane, methylethyl glycol, methylethylene glycol, Sirlene or Dowfrost, is an organic compound (a diol alcohol) (Figure 1.1d). Propylene glycol is usually a faintly sweet and colorless, clear viscous liquid that is hygroscopic and miscible with water, acetone, and chloroform. It contains an asymmetrical carbon atom, so it exists in two stereoisomers. Propylene glycol has properties similar to those of ethylene glycol. Pure optical isomers can be obtained by hydration of optically pure propylene oxide. Its melting point is −59°C (−74.2°F), and its boiling point is 188.2°C (370.8°F). Propylene glycol usually is used in antifreeze solutions, in hydraulic fluids, and as a solvent. It has numerous applications, for example as a solvent in many pharmaceuticals and as a less-toxic antifreeze, especially for human embryo cryopreservation.

Toxicity of cryoprotectants

The toxicity of cryoprotectants refers to at least two effects. The first is the chemical reacting with cells before cryopreservation, and the second is the chemical causing the change of osmosis of freezing solutions. Relatively low concentrations of cryoprotectants are usually used in cryobiology and, therefore, the chemicals themselves may not be a major concern for toxicity, although the concentration of cryoprotectants used in rapid cooling is relatively high. For assessment of the toxicity of cryoprotectants, it seems necessary to consider the colligative property of the aqueous (freezing) solution, which may be related directly to the cell permeability of each cryoprotectant and may cause osmotic stress in the cells before freezing and thawing procedures. The permeating speed of cryoprotectants is related directly to temperature. Consequently, major factors to be considered in assessing the toxicity of cryoprotectants are their concentration, the exposure temperature, and the time in aqueous (freezing) solution.

Cryoprotectants can interact with each other in a mixture, or with crucial cell molecules, thereby producing effects other than those that would occur with an individual cryoprotectant [47]. It has been observed that the protective effect of combinations of cryoprotectants can be greater than would be expected if the action of each agent were simply additive [48]. Whether the toxicity of cryoprotectants can be reduced, or not, by mixing two or more cryoprotectants (in a system where there is a reduction in the concentration of each cryoprotectant) in the aqueous (freezing) solution needs to be further investigated.

Equilibration

It is common practice to suspend cells in aqueous (freezing) solution containing permeable cryoprotectants for the time that is required to equilibrate intracellular solutes before freezing [49]. Many cells, especially eukaryotic cells, are sensitive to osmotic stress. Therefore, the permeating cryoprotectants are added gradually to the freezing solution in order to minimize osmotic stress as well as to allow removal of the cryoprotectants from the suspensions gradually. It means that the cells need time to balance and to adapt to osmotic shock. Different cell types require different equilibration times. Based on the permeating speed of the cryoprotectants and the cell types, different equilibration times will be required. Normally, lower temperature requires a longer period of equilibration, and higher temperature needs a shorter period.

The success of cryopreservation is determined by whether or not the cell undergoes intracellular ice formation during freezing. As mentioned above, vitrification can occur by either a slow-freezing or a rapid-cooling procedure. In the slow freezing procedure, intracellular ice formation is avoided by sufficiently slow cooling that osmotic dehydration results in the water remaining in near chemical potential equilibrium with the outside solution and ice. In the rapid cooling procedure, the cooling rate needed for vitrification is approaching T_g. Different freezing solutions with different concentrations of cryoprotectants need different cooling rates for vitrification. These rates are derived primarily from calculations using mathematical models of ice crystallization in very dilute solutions [20,50–53]. However, the actual situation may differ from the theoretical rate in the different cell types.

Conclusions

Cryobiology is the branch of biology involving the study of the effects of low temperatures on organisms and is most often used for the purpose of achieving cryopreservation. Cryobiology is the core of fertility cryopreservation. The principal application for human fertility cryopreservation began with sperm freezing, and then developed to include embryo and oocyte as well as gonadal cryopreservation. Although knowledge and medical achievements have advanced in fertility cryopreservation, especially with the recent development of oocyte and ovarian tissue cryopreservation, cryobiology can still be considered as a relatively new branch of biology.

Many factors affect successful cryopreservation of cells. First, it may depend on the cell type, cell size, cell growth phase, cell water content, cell lipid content, and the composition of the cells, as well as cell density. Second, it may depend on the composition of the freezing or vitrification medium, the cooling rate, the storage temperature, the duration of storage, and the warming rate and recovery medium. Third, it may be important to add cryoprotectants(s) into aqueous (freezing) solutions for freezing.

The mechanism of action of cryoprotectants can be considered as lowering the freezing point and preventing ice crystal formation in intracellular and extracellular solvents. It has been considered that there may be minor or severe cryoprotectant toxicity. This toxicity is related directly to the concentration used, and the cell exposure temperature and time. Although some mathematical theories have been developed in cryobiology [54], these theories may not be applicable to all types of cell. Further theoretical considerations are needed for developments in the field of cryobiology.

References

1. Luyet B. Working hypotheses on the nature of life. *Biodynamics* 1934; **1:** 1–7.
2. Luyet B. The vitrification of organic colloids and of protoplasm. *Biodynamica* 1937; **1:** 1–14.
3. Polge C, Smith AU, Parkes, AS. Revival os spermatozoa after vitrification and dehydration at low temperatures. *Nature* 1949; **164:** 666.
4. Lovelock JE. The haemolysis of human red blood cells by freezing and thawing. *Biochim Biophys Acta* 1953; **10:** 414–426.
5. Lovelock JE. The mechanism of the protective action of glycerol against haemolysis by freezing and thawing. *Biochim Biophys Acta* 1953; **11:** 28–36.
6. Luyet B, Gonzales F. Growth of nerve tissue after freezing in liquid nitrogen. *Biodynamica* 1953; **7:** 171–174.
7. Lovelock JE, Polge C. The immobilization of spermatozoa by freezing and thawing and protective action of glycerol. *Biochem J* 1954; **58:** 618–622.
8. Luyet B, Rapatz G. Patterns of ice formation in some aqueous solutions. *Biodynamica* 1958; **8:** 1–68.
9. Lovelock JE, Bishop MWH. Prevention of freezing damage to living cells by dimethylsulphoxide. *Nature* 1959; **183:** 1394–1395.
10. Zachariassen KE, Kristiansen E. Ice nucleation and antinucleation in nature. *Cryobiology* 2000; **41:** 257–279.
11. Mazure P. The kinetics of water loss from cells at subzero temperature and the likelihood of intracellular freezing. *J Gen Physiol* 1963; **47:** 347–369.
12. Mazur P. Cryobiology: the freezing of biological systems. *Science* 1970; **168:** 939–949.
13. Mazur P. Freezing of living cells: mechanisms and implications. *Am J Physiol* 1984; **247**:C125–142.
14. Luyet B, Rasmussen D. Study by differential thermal analysis of the temperatures of instability of rapidly cooled solutions of glycerol, ethylene glycol, sucrose, and glucose. *Biodynamica* 1968; **10:** 167–191.
15. Cocks FH, Brower WE. Phase diagram relationships in cryobiology. *Cryobiology* 1974; **11:** 340–358.
16. McGann LE. Differing action of penetrating and nonpenetrating cryoprotective agents. *Cryobiology* 1978; **15:** 382–390.
17. Meryman HT. Modified model for the mechanism of freezing injury in erythrocytes. *Nature* 1968; **218:** 333–336.
18. Meryman HT. Osmotic stress as a mechanism of freezing injury. *Cryobiology* 1971; **8:** 489–500.
19. Pegg DE, Diaper MP. On the mechanism of injury to slowly frozen erythrocytes. *Biophys J* 1988; **54:** 471–488.
20. Boutron P, Kaufmann A. Stability of the amorphous state in the system water–glycerol–dimethylsulfoxide. *Cryobiology* 1978; **15:** 93–108.
21. Boutron P, Kaufmann A. Stability of the amorphous state in the system water-glycerol–ethylene glycol. *Cryobiology* 1979; **16:** 83–89.
22. Boutron P. Stability of the amorphous state in the system water–1,2-propanediol. *Cryobiology* 1979; **16:** 557–568.
23. McGann LE. Optimal temperature ranges for control of cooling rate. *Cryobiology* 1979; **16:** 211–216.
24. Meryman HT, Williams RJ, Douglas MSJ. Freezing injury from 'solution effects' and its prevention by natural or artificial cryoprotection. *Cryobiology* 1977; **14:** 287–302.
25. Rall WF, Reid DS, Farrant J . Innocuous biological freezing during warming. *Nature* 1980; **286:** 511–514.
26. Pegg DE. Simple equation for obtaining melting points and eutectic temperatures for the ternary system glycerol/sodium chloride/water. *Cryo Letters* 1983; **4:** 259–268.
27. Pegg DE. Equations for obtaining melting points and eutectic temperatures for the ternary system dimethyl sulphoxide/sodium chloride/water. *Cryo Letters* 1986; **7:** 387–394.

28. Pegg DE, Arnaud FG . Equations for obtaining melting points in the quaternary system propane-1,2-diol/glycerol/sodium chloride/water. *Cryo Letters* 1988; **9:** 404–417.
29. Boutron P, Arnaud F. Comparison of the cryoprotection of red blood cells by 1,2-propanediol and glycerol. *Cryobiology* 1984; **21:** 348–358.
30. Fahy GM. Analysis of 'solution effects' injury: equations for calculating phase diagram information for the ternary systems NaCl–dimethylsulfoxide–water and NaCl–glycerol–water. *Biophys J* 1980; **32:** 837–850.
31. Fahy GM. Simplified calculation of cell water content during freezing and thawing in nonideal solutions of cryoprotective agents and its possible application to the study of 'solution effects' injury. *Crybiology* 1981; **18:** 473–482.
32. Fahy GM. Cryoprotectant toxicity neutralizers reduce freezing damage. *Cryo Letters* 1983; **4:** 309–314.
33. Fahy GM. Cryoprotectant toxicity reduction: specific or nonspecific? *Cryo Letters* 1984; **5:** 287–294.
34. Fahy GM. The relevance of cryoprotectant 'toxicity' to cryobiology. *Cryobiology* 1986; **23:** 1–13.
35. Rall WF, Mazur P, Souzu H. Physical–chemical basis of the protection of slowly frozen human erythrocytes by glycerol. *Biophys J* 1978; **23:** 101–120.
36. Fahy GM, Karow AM, Jr. Ultrastructure-function correlative studies for cardiac cryopreservation. V. Absence of a correlation between electrolyte toxocity and cryoinjury in the slowly frozen, cryoprotected rat heart. *Cryobiology* 1977; **14:** 418–427.
37. Fahy GM, MacFarlane DR, Angell CA, *et al.* Vitrification as an approach to cryopreservation. *Cryobiology* 1984; **21:** 407–426.
38. Fahy GM, Lilley TH, Linsdell H, *et al.* Cryoprotectant toxicity and cryoprotectant toxicity reduction: in search of molecular mechanism. *Cryobiology* 1990; **27:** 247–268.
39. Fahy GM, Wowk B, Wu J, *et al.* Improved vitrification solutions based on predictability of vitrification solution toxicity. *Cryobiology* 2004; **48:** 22–35.
40. Fahy GM, Wowk B, Wu J, *et al.* Cryopreservation of organs by vitrification: perspectives and recent advances. *Crybiology* 2004; **48:** 157–178.
41. Rall WF, Fahy GM. Ice-free cryopreservation of mouse embryos at −196°C by vitrification. *Nature* 1985; **313:** 573–575.
42. Keith SC. Factors influencing the survival of bacteria at temperatures in the vicinity of the freezing point of water. *Science* 1913; **37:** 877–879.
43. Spencer RR, Parker RR. Rocky mountain spotted fever. *Public Health Rep* 1924; **39:** 3027–3040.
44. Francis E. Duration of viability of Pasteurella pestis. *Public Health Rep* 1932; **47:** 1287–1294.
45. Pabst AM. Use of below freezing temperatures for maintenance of meningococcus cultures (Neisseria intracellularis). *Public Health Rep* 1935; **50:** 732–737.
46. Balakin KV, Savchuk NP, Tetko IV. In silico approaches to prediction of aqueous and DMSO solubility of drug-like compounds: trends, problems and solutions. *Curr Med Chem* 2006; **13:** 223–241.
47. Ruwart MJ, Holland JF, Haug A. Fluorimetric evidence of interactions involving cryoprotectants and biomolecules. *Cryobiology* 1975; **12:** 26–33.
48. Chian R-C, Kuwayama M, Tan L, *et al.* High survival rate of bovine oocytes matured in vitro following vitrification. *J Reprod Dev* 2004; **50:** 685–696.
49. Mazur P, Seki S, Pinn IL, Kleinhans FW, Edashige K. Extra- and intracellular ice formation in mouse oocytes. *Cryobiology* 2005; **51:** 29–53.
50. Bruggeller P, Mayer E. Complete vitrification in pure liquid water and dilute aqueous solutions. *Nature* 1980; **288:** 569–571.
51. Boutron P. Comparison with the theory of the kinetics and extent of ice crystallization and of the glass-forming tendency in aqueous cryoprotective solutions. *Cryobiology* 1986; **23:** 88–102.
52. Toner M, Cravalho EG, Chiang YM. Vitrification of biological cell suspensions: the importance of ultrarapid cooling and warming. *Cryobiology* 1988; **25:** 551.
53. Baudot A, Odagescu V. Thermal properties of ethylene glycol and aqueous solutions. *Cryobiology* 2004; **48:** 283–294.
54. Fahy GM. Theoretical considerations for oocyte cryopreservation by freezing. *Reprod Biomed Online* 2007; **14:** 709–714.

Chapter 2

Suppression of ice in aqueous solutions and its application to vitrification in assisted reproductive technology

Patrick Quinn

Introduction

This chapter draws on several sources that have comprehensively reviewed this topic and here I want to especially acknowledge Dr. Helmy Selman, who organized a conference in Perugia, Italy on cryopreservation in 2006. Other sources are the classic work by Fahy and colleagues [1], which gives a thorough and in-depth look at the theoretical and biophysical aspects of this topic. This review is structured so that the more practical aspects are considered first followed by some of the more theoretical components involved. This approach will allow first an analysis of what works in a clinical setting and then a return to consider what is happening at the physical and molecular level. I believe this approach will allow a better understanding of the process.

Background

Slow cooling cryopreservation of mammalian oocytes and embryos has been extensively discussed and reviewed both in the chapters of this book and in other literature in the area for more than four decades and will not be further discussed in detail in this chapter. A concise description can be found in Wikipedia [2].

Although cryopreservation of human embryos and zygotes has become a well-established procedure in assisted reproductive technology (ART), oocyte freezing has proved to be technically challenging and until recently remained experimental. For several decades, attempts to cryopreserve human oocytes have been performed in many in vitro fertilization (IVF) centers worldwide, with variable results. When the slow freezing method traditionally used for embryos or zygotes was initially applied to oocytes, there were poor success rates. A major factor contributing to the poor results was that much of the cryobiology carried out by embryologists was empirical, based on "rules of thumb" rather than basic principles and knowledge.

Increasing knowledge of cryobiological mechanisms gave major insights to improve freezing–thawing protocols (Chapter 1). As one of the major components in any cell, including oocytes and embryos, is water, great care has to be taken that lethal ice crystal formation does not take place. Other critical factors during slow cooling include solution effects, osmotic stress, and intracellular dehydration. A summary of some of these factors and how they are handled with vitrification are given in Tables 2.1 and 2.2 [3].

Membrane permeability to water and solutes

The oocyte is the largest human cell (130 μm diameter). Large cells have a low surface-to-volume ratio and hence they are less efficient at taking up cryoprotectants (CPAs) and at losing water. The overall effect is that oocytes are more likely to retain water during cryopreservation and thus can be damaged by intracellular ice formation and growth. Also, oocytes can be seriously damaged even before freezing by excessive osmotic stress resulting from the addition or dilution of CPAs. The flow of water across each unit of the cell surface as a function of time is called the hydraulic conductivity or hydraulic coefficient (LP). Hydraulic conductivity is related to the volume of the cell. There is great variability between cell types and even species among mammals. In fact, membrane permeability changes with the developmental stages of oocyte, zygote, and embryo [4–6]. An example with human oocytes that caused some confusion initially is that freshly collected human oocytes are more prone to cryoinjuries than ones that are 1 day old, such as oocytes that fail to fertilize. Subsequently, it was found that methods established with "old" oocytes were often not suitable for the more sensitive freshly collected oocytes with full developmental potential [7], and it was suggested that this

Fertility Cryopreservation, ed. Ri-Cheng Chian and Patrick Quinn. Published by Cambridge University Press.

Table 2.1. Primary benefits of vitrification[a]

1.	Direct contact between cells/tissue and liquid nitrogen (see item 9 in Table 2.2 and Chapter 16)
2.	No ice crystallization
3.	Utilizes a higher concentration of CPA, which allows shorter exposure times to the CPA (but shorter exposure times are necessary because of toxicity of the CPAs)
4.	Rapid vitrification/warming
5.	Small volume used provides a significant increase in the cooling rate
6.	Cooling rates from ~15 000 to 30 000°C/min
7.	Minimizes osmotic injuries
8.	Reduces the time of cryopreservation procedure: duration from 2 to 10 min
9.	Very simple protocols
10.	Eliminates the cost of expensive programmable freezing equipment, and their service and maintenance

CPA, cryoprotectant.
[a] Comments in parentheses added by P. Quinn.
Source: Liebermann et al. 2002 [3].

Table 2.2. Variables of vitrification that can profoundly influence its effectiveness

1.	Type and concentration of cryoprotectant (almost all cryoprotectants are toxic)
2.	Media used as base medium (holding media)
3.	Temperature of the vitrification solution at exposure
4.	Length of time cells/tissue are exposed to the final cryoprotectant before plunging into liquid nitrogen
5.	Variability in the volume of cryoprotectant solution surrounding the cells/tissue
6.	Device used for vitrification (size of the vapor coat and cooling rate)
7.	Technical proficiency of the embryologist
8.	Quality and development stage of the tested cells/tissue
9.	Direct contact of the liquid nitrogen and the vitrification solution containing the biological material can be a source of contamination; to eliminate this danger, using sterile liquid nitrogen for cooling and storage is essential

Source: Liebermann et al. 2002 [3].

could be because of changes in membrane composition between the two types of oocyte [8].

Temperature

During handling of oocytes and embryos, it is important to choose a suitable temperature. Elevated temperature could increase the CPA toxicity. Very slow and very high cooling rates can damage cells through osmotic effect and pH changes. Very slow cooling rates tend to encourage extracellular ice formation, while the very high cooling rates tend to promote intracellular ice formation: both could be lethal to cells. With vitrification, however, the cooling and warming rate are sufficiently fast to never allow ice crystal formation either upon cooling or upon warming. Most other physiological changes that occur with slow cooling cryopreservation, such as osmotic effect, solution effects, and dehydration, are also eliminated by vitrification as during the process the entire solution remains unchanged except for the transition of water from a liquid to a glassy phase [3]. With warming, the rate is sufficient that devitrification, the formation of ice crystals from vitrified water, does not occur.

Vitrification

"Ice formation is not compatible with the survival of living system and ought to be avoided during freezing" (Luyet, 1937 [9]), and "good vitrification is not injurious, there being no molecular disturbance, while an incomplete vitrification or devitrification and, a fortiori, crystallization, are injurious to the extent that they disrupt the living structure" (Luyet and Gehenio, 1940 [10]). These two concise statements epitomize the core of vitrification. Ice-free cryopreservation is an attempt to circumvent the hazards of water crystallization as ice. The vitreous state is essentially a solidified, amorphous liquid state obtained by specific conditions of cooling and solute concentration that inhibit ice nucleation and growth. During cooling, the molecular motions within a liquid are slowed and eventually arrested with extreme viscosity. The arrested liquid state is a glass. So, vitrification is the direct conversion of a liquid state into glass, bypassing or rapidly passing through the critical temperature of ice formation (no phase transition). A striking illustration of vitrification is shown in Figure 2.1. More details of vitrification will be given below in the discussion of the phase diagram.

Probability of vitrification

Three key factors influence the probability of successful vitrification: cooling and warming rates, the composition of the CPA solution, and the sample volume [12]. Increasing CPA concentration and decreasing sample volume will each increase the probability of vitrification. Pressure is another factor that increases the chance of vitrification [1] but this has had very little, if any, application in the clinical ART arena.

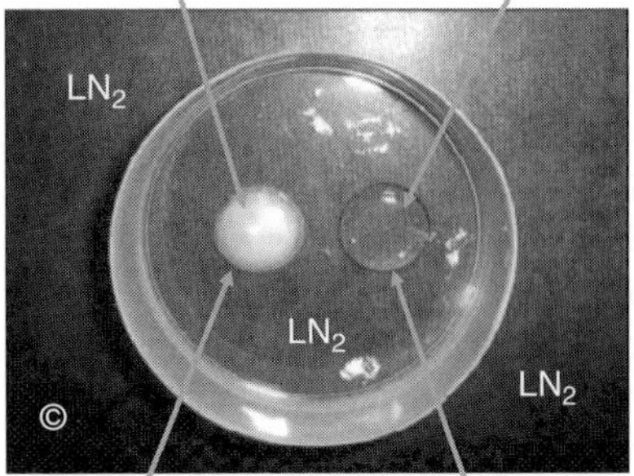

Figure 2.1. Optical difference between ice crystals and vitrification [18]. DPBS, Dulbecco's phosphate-buffered saline; EG, ethylene glycol; DMSO, dimethyl sulfoxide; LN_2, liquid nitrogen. (Courtesy of Juergen Liebermann [11].)

Application of cryoprotectants for assisted reproductive technology

Calculating the permeability of the cell to a CPA is necessary because some CPAs have less permeability than others. Permeability of a CPA is also temperature dependent. The toxicity of a CPA is correlated to its concentration, the time of exposure, and the temperature. Using CPAs at room temperature or lower rather than 37°C may decrease their toxicity. In summary, when choosing a CPA, the temperature and time of exposure to be used and the permeability of the CPA must be known as prerequisites for cryopreservation protocols [13].

The osmotic stress during removal of CPAs was initially reduced in slow cooling by a stepwise dilution (using reduced concentration of CPAs progressively), allowing enough time for the cell to return to an equilibrium volume [14]. However, the initial use of dilution in the presence of sucrose [15] soon became widespread and is now used in most dilution protocols after removal of specimens from liquid nitrogen (LN_2) in both slow-cooling and vitrification protocols. The presence of this impermeable solute in the extracellular solution maintains the volume excursion and osmotic stress on the cells within tolerable limits by counteracting the influx of water that occurs during the removal of intracellular CPAs.

Finally, it should be noted that during slow cooling, with the increasing concentration of solutes as more and more extracellular ice forms, the conditions are such that when the sample is plunged into LN_2 at the subzero temperature often used (e.g. −30 to −35°C), the conditions in the microenvironment are such (high CPA concentration, rapid cooling rate, and small volume) that in all likelihood the cell(s) will be vitrified during this final part of the process [7,14].

Phase diagram

Two of the dangers of cryopreservation are solution effects and intracellular ice formation. Other factors causing damage are extracellular ice and intracellular dehydration. Solution effects are caused by the increasing concentration of solutes during freezing as these solutes are excluded from the crystals of ice that form as the temperature reduces. As water leaves the cell during slow cooling and contributes to the formation of extracellular ice, more water will leave the cell up an osmotic gradient as the solute concentration in the remaining extracellular water increases with extracellular ice formation. This can cause excessive and damaging dehydration to the cell. High concentrations of solutes can be damaging. Intracellular ice is almost always fatal to cells but it does not necessarily form in the presence of extracellular ice. Studies have shown that embryos can survive some extracellular ice but the mechanical stress on the cells can cause damage directly if there is too much.

Cellular material that can be vitrified can escape solution effects, the dangers of intracellular injury, and the other damaging effects of slow cooling. This is because with vitrification, in contrast to slow-freezing protocols, the entire solution remains unchanged; water does not form ice crystals but is converted directly to a glassy, solid state, both intra- and extracellularly [1]. In practical terms, as has been discussed above, the current parameters that affect this from an ART perspective are first the rates of cooling and warming, which are influenced by both the volume of the specimen undergoing cooling and warming and the temperature gradient in use (e.g. LN_2 at −196°C, liquid nitrogen slush at −210°C, or warming solution at ambient room temperature or 37°C) and, second, the type and concentration of CPA used.

To understand what is going on during the processes of slow cooling and vitrification it is helpful to look at a phase diagram for a typical CPA. Before that is done, however, Figure 2.2 compares cooling rates and the so-called dangerous zones [7] when cells are taken from ambient room temperature to the temperature of LN_2 (−196°C) by either slow cooling or by vitrification. With slow cooling, there are critical events that, if not optimized, can cause cell death at all

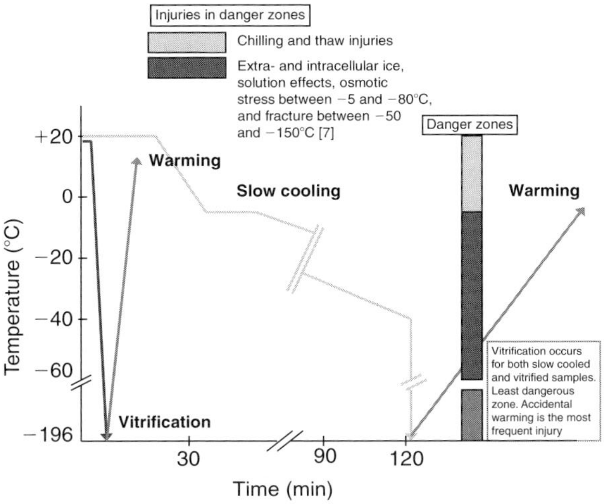

Figure 2.2. Cooling rates and dangerous zones during cryopreservation.

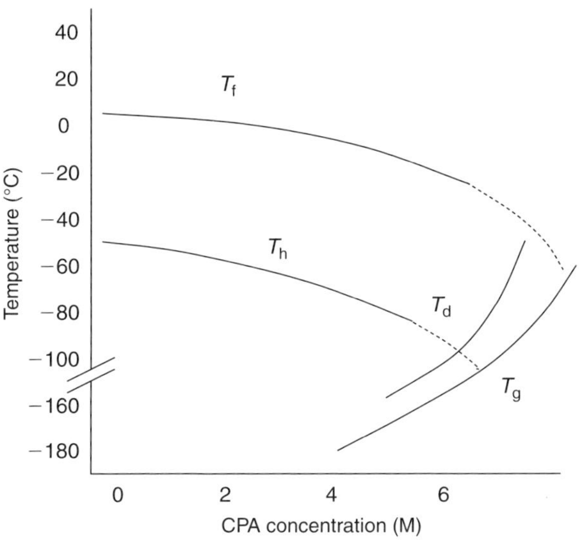

Figure 2.3. Phase diagram of hypothetical aqueous solution of cryoprotectants.

stages from room temperature to −196°C; however, with vitrification, these events are basically eliminated, giving vitrification a huge advantage over slow cooling, at least in the field of ART and in most other areas where it is used.

A phase diagram shows conditions at which thermodynamically distinct phases can occur in equilibrium [16]. Examples of different phases of water that can occur in cryopreservation are liquid, ice, and glass. In a phase diagram, lines of equilibrium, also called phase boundaries, are shown that mark conditions under which multiple phases can exist in equilibrium, for example water changing to and from a liquid phase into an ice phase. A typical phase diagram for a CPA solution is shown in Figure 2.3.

In this figure, T_f (also called T_m) is the equilibrium freezing temperature of the melting point curve, T_h is the homogeneous nucleation temperature before the solution actually nucleates (i.e. begins to freeze), T_g is the glass transition temperature at which supercooled liquid vitrifies, and T_d is the temperature at which devitrification occurs. Solutions normally supercool to some point between T_f and T_h.

Crystallization of the solvent (e.g. water) is possible in the region between T_f and T_h. At some temperature, the water solidifies as glass and any previously formed ice crystals are embedded in the glass. The opportunity for vitrification depends on CPA concentration and temperature and lies along T_g, the glass transition curve. To make a glass with a minimum of embedded ice crystals, high concentrations of CPA must be used and one must also cool as quickly as possible to a temperature below Tg. Devitrification (T_d), crystallization in vitrified system, occurs when the glass warms above T_g through the growing of embedded ice crystals. This means that thawing should also be as quickly as possible.

There are a number of ways to reduce the concentration of CPA required for vitrification [1].

Apply a high hydrostatic pressure. Increasing the pressure lowers T_h and increases T_g, thus shifting the point of intersection of these two curves to a lower CPA concentration. Once the temperature is below T_g, the pressure can be released without danger of crystallization (ice formation). The application of this strategy in clinical ART has not occurred, probably because the major factors of low volumes, high rates of cooling/warming, and sufficient CPA to vitrify but minimize toxicity have been invoked.

Add a non-permeating polymer or agent. This strategy, for example adding polyvinylpyrrolidone or Ficoll, is used in some protocols.

Combine CPAs. The mixture of dimethyl sulfoxide and EG appears to be one of the most popular combinations currently. Another combination is ethylene glycol and 1,2-propanediol. Measuring the glass-forming efficacy of the CPAs that compose the vitrification solution has revealed that an excellent vitrification solution can be formed by a combination of a balanced concentration of a strong glass former such as dimethyl sulfoxide and a weak glass former such as ethylene glycol, acetamide, or formamide. This favors cell viability [17,18]. It has been reported that a combination of dimethyl sulfoxide and ethylene glycol gave superior results for human oocyte vitrification compared with dimethyl sulfoxide and 1,2-propanediol, [11] and a combination of ethylene glycol and 1,2-propanediol has also been reported to give good results (Chapter 17).

Other strategies have been used in specific circumstances but none has found any application in clinical ART.

Conclusions

The requirements and relationships for conditions to achieve satisfactory vitrification in the area of mammalian ART are well displayed in the pseudo-equation of Yavin and Arav [12]:

$$\text{Probability of vitrification} = \frac{\text{Cooling and warming rates} \times \text{Viscosity (CPA concentration)}}{\text{Volume}}$$

The main points to be gathered from this relationship are that the smaller the volume of the vitrification solution, in which the cellular material is placed for the vitrification process, the faster the cooling and warming rates that can be achieved and the lower the concentrations of CPAs that can be used. In association with these requirements, the elegant studies of Kasai and collaborators (Chapter 3) suggest time and temperature requirements for vitrification and warming protocols based on the permeation mechanisms for water and the CPAs used in early and later stage mammalian preimplantation embryos and oocytes. Taking all of this into consideration, it seems that perhaps the protocols for vitrification of human oocytes and preimplantation embryos have been maximized, but there are still avenues that require attention. The primary one at the moment appears to be a regulatory one to ensure the safety of the process to avoid microbial contamination. Here, it is mainly the cooling rates that are impacted by the imposition of some sort of protective covering around the primary carrier tool to prevent direct exposure to LN_2. Developing knowledge in the areas described above should assist in dealing with this problem. It is also likely that the whole vitrification process from loading CPAs into the oocytes and embryos, optimizing cooling and warming rates, and then diluting the intracellular CPAs out of the cells will be optimized so that this process will become a major technology available in all ART programs worldwide.

References

1. Fahy GM, MacFarlane DR, Angell CA, *et al.* Vitrification as an approach to cryopreservation. *Cryobiology* 1984; **21:** 407–426.
2. Wikipedia. *Controlled-rate and slow freezing in cryopreservation.* 2009. http://en.wikipedia.org/wiki/Controlled-Rate_and_Slow_Freezing_in_Cryopreservation (accessed July 28, 2009.).
3. Liebermann J, Nawroth F, Isachenko V, *et al.* Potential importance of vitrification in reproductive medicine. *Biol Reprod* 2002; **67:** 1671–1680.
4. Le Gal F, Gasqui P, Renard JP. Differential osmotic behavior of mammalian oocytes before and after maturation: a quantitative analysis using goat oocytes as a model. *Cryobiology* 1994; **31:** 154–170.
5. Younis AI, Toner M, Albertini DF, *et al.* Cryobiology of non-human primate oocytes. *Hum Reprod* 1996; **11:** 156–165.
6. Agca Y, Liu J, Peter AT, *et al.* Effect of developmental stage on bovine oocyte plasma membrane water and cryoprotectant permeability characteristics. *Mol Reprod Dev* 1998; **49:** 408–415.
7. Vajta G, Nagy ZP. Are programmable freezers still needed in the embryo laboratory? Review on vitrification. *Reprod Biomed Online* 2006; **12:** 779–796.
8. Stachecki JJ, Cohen J. An overview of oocyte cryopreservation. *Reprod Biomed Online* 2004; **9:** 152–163.
9. Luyet BJ. The vitrification of organic colloids and of protoplasm. *Biodynamica* 1937; **1**: 1–14.
10. Luyet BJ, Gehenio PM. *Life and Death at Low Temperatures.* Normandy, MO: Biodynamica, 1940.
11. Liebermann J, Tucker MJ. Vitrification: a successful technique for cryopreserving human cells in ART. *Alpha Scientists Reprod Med* 2005; **32:** 4–9.
12. Yavin S, Arav A. Measurement of essential physical properties of vitrification solutions. *Theriogenology* 2007; **67:** 81–89.
13. Mazur P. Equilibrium, quasi-equilibrium, and nonequilibrium freezing of mammalian embryos. *Cell Biophys* 1990; **17:** 53–92.
14. Quinn P. Cryopreservation of embryos and oocytes. In Keye WR, Chang RJ, Rebar RW, Soules MR, eds. *Infertility. Evaluation and Treatment.* Philadelphia, PA: Saunders, 1995, pp. 821–840.
15. Leibo SP, Mazur P. Methods for the preservation of mammalian embryos by freezing. In Daniel JC, ed. *Methods in Mammalian Reproduction.* New York: Academic Press, 1978, pp. 179–201.

16. Wikipedia . *Phase Diagram*. 2009. http://en.wikipedia.org/wiki/Phase_diagram (accessed July 30, 2009.).
17. Fahy GM. Biological effects of vitrification and devitrification. In Pegg DE, Karow AM, eds. *The Biophysics of Organ Cryopreservation*. New York: Plenum, 1987, pp. 265–297.
18. Fahy GM, Wowk B, Wu J, Paynter S. Improved vitrification solutions based on the predictability of vitrification solution toxicity. *Cryobiology* 2004; **48:** 22–35.

Chapter 3

Movement of water and cryoprotectants in mouse oocytes and embryos at different stages: relevance to cryopreservation

Magosaburo Kasai and Keisuke Edashige

Introduction

During cryopreservation, mammalian oocytes and embryos can be damaged by chilling, the toxicity of the cryoprotectant, the formation of extracellular ice, the formation of intracellular ice, fracturing, osmotic swelling, and osmotic shrinkage [1]. Such damage needs to be avoided to maintain the survival of oocytes/embryos after cryopreservation. Most of these injuries are closely related to the cryobiological properties of oocytes/embryos, such as sensitivity to chilling, the permeability of the plasma membrane to water and cryoprotectants, sensitivity to the chemical toxicity of the cryoprotectant, and tolerance of osmotic swelling and shrinkage.

The most suitable procedure for the cryopreservation of oocytes/embryos differs among maturational/developmental stages even in the same species. For example, mouse morulae can be vitrified without an appreciable loss of viability by a simple one-step method using ethylene glycol as the permeating cryoprotectant [2], whereas pretreatment with a low concentration of ethylene glycol is preferable when vitrifying 2-cell embryos [3,4]. In the mouse, therefore, morulae appear to survive cryopreservation more easily than 2-cell embryos. In general, differences in cryobiological properties among oocytes/embryos at different maturational/developmental stages will be closely related to the difference in the most suitable procedure for cryopreservation.

Among these cryobiological properties, the permeability of the plasma membrane to water and cryoprotectants would be most important, because it is closely related to major types of cell injury during cryopreservation: damage caused by the toxicity of the cryoprotectant, by the formation of intracellular ice, and by osmotic swelling during removal of the cell-permeating cryoprotectant.

There are two pathways for the movement of water and cryoprotectants across the plasma membrane of oocytes/embryos. One is simple diffusion through the lipid bilayer, in which case permeability is low and temperature dependency is high. The other is facilitated diffusion via channels, in which case permeability is markedly high and temperature dependency is low. Therefore, low permeability with high temperature dependency is suggestive of the movement of water and cryoprotectants across the plasma membrane by simple diffusion, whereas high permeability with low temperature dependency is suggestive of movement via channels.

Specifying the principal pathway for the movement of water and cryoprotectants in oocytes/embryos at various stages will help in the selection of suitable cryoprotectant(s) and optimal conditions for cryopreservation, for example the time, temperature, and number of steps (one or multiple) for exposure of oocytes/embryos to the cryoprotectant solution before cooling, and the procedure for removal of the cryoprotectant after warming.

Measurement of the permeability of the plasma membrane to water and cryoprotectants

The permeability to water and cryoprotectants of mammalian oocytes/embryos can be measured as changes in volume in hypertonic solutions containing sucrose or cryoprotectant [5]. Figure 3.1 shows the method that we have developed for measuring changes in volume [6,7]. An oocyte or embryo is placed in a drop of PB1 medium [8] covered with paraffin oil in a Petri dish (90 mm × 10 mm). It is held by a holding pipette connected to a micromanipulator on an inverted microscope. The inner diameter of the mouth of the pipette is small enough not to distort the oocyte/

Fertility Cryopreservation, ed. Ri-Cheng Chian and Patrick Quinn. Published by Cambridge University Press.

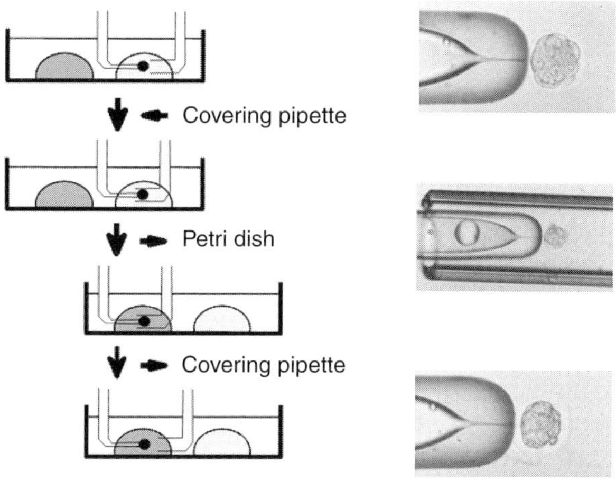

Figure 3.1. The method for abrupt exposure of an oocyte/embryo to a hypertonic solution containing sucrose or cryoprotectant for accurate measurement of the change in volume.

embryo. The oocyte/embryo held by the holding pipette is covered with a covering pipette having a large diameter (~200 μm) connected to another manipulator. By sliding the dish, the oocyte/embryo is introduced into a drop of a hypertonic solution containing sucrose or cryoprotectant. By removing the covering pipette, the oocyte/embryo is abruptly exposed to the hypertonic solution. The temperature of the paraffin oil covering the solution is considered to be the temperature of the solution, and this is adjusted by controlling room temperature. Microscopic images are recorded by a time-lapse video recorder, and relative cross sectional area (S) measured at various points in time after the exposure is converted into relative volume (V) with the equation $V = S^{3/2}$. This method allows accurate measurements of changes in the volume of oocytes/embryos upon exposure to various solutions. Water permeability (L_p) and cryoprotectant permeability are determined by fitting water and cryoprotectant movement with experimental data by a permeability model, for example the two-parameter formalism [6,9].

Pathway for water movement in mouse oocytes and embryos

It has been suggested that a low L_p value with temperature dependency (Arrhenius activation energy, E_a) for permeability higher than 10 kcal/mol is suggestive of movement of water across the plasma membrane principally by simple diffusion through the lipid bilayer, whereas an L_p value higher than 4.5 μm/min-atm with an E_a for permeability lower than 6 kcal/mol is suggestive of movement principally by facilitated diffusion through channels [10]. This criterion may be a rough estimate but is useful for deducing the principal pathway for the movement of water in the cell.

If this criterion is applied to metaphase II (MII) mouse oocytes, water is assumed to move predominantly by simple diffusion through the lipid bilayer and not via channels, because studies have shown that the L_p of oocytes at 20–25°C is low (0.41–0.70 μm/min-atm [11–17] and the E_a for permeability is high (10–13 kcal/mol) [11–13,17,18]. Although the mRNAs for several types of water channel are expressed in MII mouse oocytes [19,20], most water molecules appear to move across the plasma membrane by simple diffusion (Figure 3.2a), probably because expression levels of channel proteins are quite low.

Similarly, mouse 1-, 2-, and 4-cell embryos have low permeability to water at 24°C (0.49–0.80 μm/min-atm) [16]. We have also examined the L_p and the E_a for that L_p for 4-cell embryos and reported that the L_p at 25°C is low (0.63 μm/min-atm) and the E_a is high (12 kcal/mol) [17], as in the case of oocytes. In MII oocytes and 1- to 4-cell embryos, therefore, water appears to move across the plasma membrane predominantly by simple diffusion (Figure 3.2a).

In morulae and blastocysts, by comparison, the L_p at 25°C is quite high (3.6–4.5 μm/min-atm) and the E_a for permeability is low (5–6 kcal/mol) [17]. If the criterion for deducing the pathway for the movement of water is applied, water movement is considered to be dependent on channel processes. However, the L_p of morulae at 25°C varies widely, from 2.0 to 9.4 μm/min-atm [17]. This may be because there are differences in the expression levels of water channels among morulae, because the L_p of oocytes, in which virtually no water channel is expressed, is not as variable. In mouse morulae/blastocysts, therefore, most water molecules appear to move across the plasma membrane via channels.

Several intrinsic membrane proteins, such as aquaporins [21], glucose transporters [22], a urea transporter (UTB1) [23], and multiple sodium cotransporters [24], can transport water across the plasma membrane. Among the channels, however, only aquaporins would contribute to the movement of water substantially when expressed at a physiological level [25]. Therefore, aquaporins may be the major contributor to the transport of water in mouse morulae/blastocysts.

Mouse oocytes/embryos express mRNAs of various aquaporins, including aquaporins 3, 7, 8, 9, and 11 [19, 20 , 26]. In blastocysts, the mRNA of aquaporin 3 is

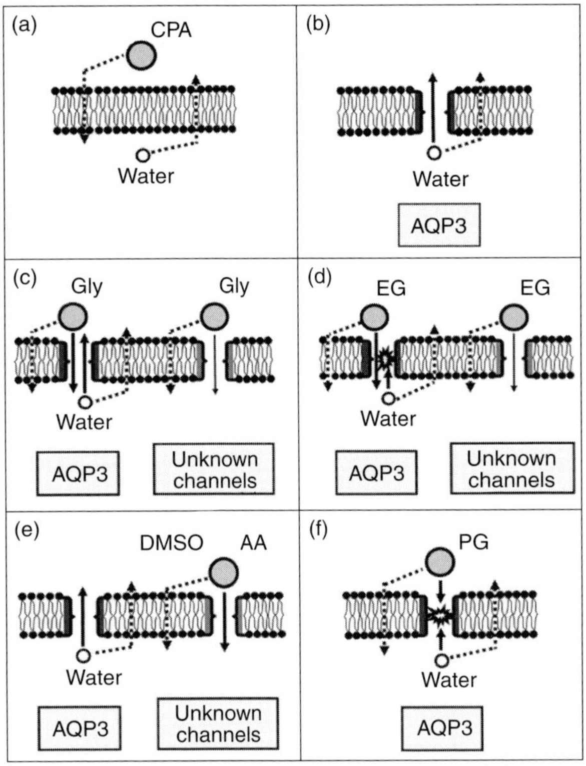

Figure 3.2. Schematic presentation of the pathway for the movement of water and cryoprotectants across the plasma membrane of mouse oocytes at the metaphase II stage and morulae. Solid lines indicate the movement of water and cryoprotectants by facilitated diffusion through channels and dotted lines indicate movement by simple diffusion through the lipid bilayer. (a) Movement of water and cryoprotectants (CPA) in oocytes; (b) movement of water in morulae in the absence of cryoprotectant; (c) movement of glycerol (Gly) and water in the presence of Gly in morulae; (d) movement of ethylene glycol (EG) and water in the presence of EG in morulae; (e) movement of dimethyl sulfoxide (DMSO), acetamide (AA), and water in the presence of DMSO or AA in morulae; (f) movement of propylene glycol (PG) and water in the presence of PG in morulae. AQP3, aquaporin 3.

much more abundant than that of any other aquaporin [26]. Moreover, morulae and blastocysts have substantial production of aquaporin 3 protein [17,27]. We have shown that the exogenous expression of aquaporin 3 in MII oocytes achieved by injecting complementary RNA of mouse aquaporin 3 at the germinal vesicle stage markedly increases the permeability of the oocytes to water [28]. In addition, the suppression of aquaporin 3 in morulae, achieved by injecting double-stranded RNA of mouse aquaporin 3 markedly decreases permeability to water to a similar level to that of MII oocytes [28]. Therefore, aquaporin 3 appears to be a major pathway for the movement of water in mouse morulae (and probably blastocysts), at least in the absence of cryoprotectant (Figure 3.2b).

Pathway for the movement of cryoprotectants and water in the presence of cryoprotectant in mouse oocytes and embryos

A criterion for deducing the pathway for the movement of cryoprotectants in cells has not been established. Considering the permeability to water, however, it would be reasonable to assume that low permeability to cryoprotectants with a high E_a value for the permeability is suggestive of the movement of cryoprotectants across the plasma membrane predominantly by simple diffusion through the lipid bilayer, whereas high permeability to cryoprotectants with a low E_a value is suggestive of movement predominantly by facilitated diffusion through channels.

Permeability differs among the maturational/developmental stages of oocytes/embryos but can be classified into two types; that typical in MII oocytes and early cleavage stage embryos, in which case, permeability to cryoprotectants is low, and that typical in morulae and blastocysts, in which case, permeability is high [7]. Aquaporin 3 is a major channel for the transportation of water across the plasma membrane in mouse morulae/blastocysts. Aquaporins can be classified into two subgroups: those that transport only water and those that transport not only water but also neutral solutes of low molecular weight. It has been shown that aquaporin 3 exogenously expressed in *Xenopus* oocytes efficiently transports five major cryoprotectants: glycerol, ethylene glycol, dimethyl sulfoxide (DMSO), acetamide, and propylene glycol [29–33]. Therefore, mouse morulae/blastocysts may transport not only water but also cryoprotectants through aquaporin 3. Among oocytes/embryos, MII oocytes and morulae would be especially suitable for measuring changes in volume, because they are a single mass and thus shrink and re-swell with less distortion.

Glycerol

Mazur and colleagues [5,34] have shown that is quite low in MII mouse oocytes (0.01×10^{-3} cm/min). We have also shown low glycerol permeability in MII oocytes (0.02×10^{-3} cm/min) and that the E_a for the permeability to glycerol is markedly high (42 kcal/mol) [17]. In MII mouse oocytes, therefore, glycerol appears to move across the plasma membrane predominantly by simple diffusion (Figure 3.2a). The pathway for the movement of water may be affected by the presence of cryoprotectant. The permeability to water of MII oocytes in the presence of glycerol at 25°C is quite low (0.6 μm/min-atm) and the E_a for this permeability is high (14 kcal/mol) [17,28]. In MII oocytes, therefore, water would move across the plasma membrane predominantly by simple diffusion also in the presence of glycerol (Figure 3.2a).

In morulae, by comparison, permeability to glycerol is remarkably high (4.7×10^{-3} cm/min) [7, 17] and the E_a for the permeability (10 kcal/mol) is much lower than that in oocytes (42 kcal/mol) [17], suggesting that glycerol moves across the plasma membrane predominantly by facilitated diffusion through channels. The permeability to water of morulae in the presence of glycerol is also high (2.2 μm/min-atm) and the E_a for the permeability (9 kcal/mol) is lower than that of oocytes (14 kcal/mol) [28]. In morulae, therefore, most glycerol molecules and many water molecules (in the presence of glycerol) appear to move across the plasma membrane predominantly by facilitated diffusion through channels.

Aquaporin 3 may play an important role as the channel, because water appears to move through it in the absence of cryoprotectant, and aquaporin 3 is known to transport various cryoprotectants, as described above. This notion is supported by the results of an experiment in which aquaporin 3 was expressed exogenously in MII oocytes and of another experiment in which the expression of aquaporin 3 was suppressed in morulae [28]. In the aquaporin 3-expressing oocytes, the permeability to glycerol and water (in the presence of glycerol) increased markedly, while in aquaporin 3-suppressed morulae, the permeability to glycerol and water decreased markedly [28]. Therefore, aquaporin 3 appears to play an essential role in the transportation process (Figure 3.2c). However, since the permeability to glycerol of aquaporin 3-suppressed morulae was significantly higher than that of oocytes, channels other than aquaporin 3 might play a role in the movement of glycerol in morulae (Figure 3.2c).

Ethylene glycol

The permeating properties of ethylene glycol in oocytes/embryos appear to be similar to those of glycerol. However, the permeating properties of water in the presence of ethylene glycol are different in morulae. In MII mouse oocytes, permeability to ethylene glycol at 25°C is low (0.6×10^{-3} cm/min-atm) and the E_a for the permeability is high (17 kcal/mol) [28]. The permeability to water of oocytes in the presence of ethylene glycol at 25°C is also low (0.4 μm/min-atm) and the E_a is high (10 kcal/mol) [28]. In MII oocytes, therefore, ethylene glycol and water (in the presence of ethylene glycol) appear to move across the plasma membrane predominantly by simple diffusion (Figure 3.2a). In morulae, by comparison, the permeability to ethylene glycol at 25°C is extremely high (10.0×10^{-3} cm/min-atm) [7, 28], and the E_a for the permeability (9 kcal/mol) is lower than that in oocytes (17 kcal/mol) [28]. In morulae, therefore, ethylene glycol appears to move across the plasma membrane predominantly via channels.

Aquaporin 3 appears to play an important role, because its exogenous expression in MII oocytes greatly increased permeability to ethylene glycol [28]. In addition, the suppression of aquaporin 3 expression in morulae markedly decreased permeability to ethylene glycol [28]. However, since the permeability to ethylene glycol of aquaporin 3-suppressed morulae was significantly higher than that of oocytes, channels other than aquaporin 3 could play a role in the movement of ethylene glycol (Figure 3.2d).

The permeability to water of morulae in the presence of ethylene glycol is quite low (0.5 μm/min-atm) and the E_a for the permeability is quite high (14 kcal/mol) [28]. In the presence of ethylene glycol, therefore, most water molecules appear to move across the plasma membrane of morulae by simple diffusion, in spite of an abundance of water channels.

This speculation is supported by the finding that the exogenous expression of aquaporin 3 in MII oocytes did not increase permeability to water at all in the presence of ethylene glycol [28]. In addition, the suppression of aquaporin 3 expression in morulae did not affect permeability to water [28]. The movement of ethylene glycol probably hinders that of water in aquaporin 3 as a result of strong interaction between ethylene glycol and water (Figure 3.2d).

Dimethyl sulfoxide and acetamide

We have shown that the permeating properties of DMSO are similar to those of acetamide in mouse oocytes/embryos [7]. The permeability to water in the presence of DMSO is also similar to that in the presence of acetamide [28]. In MII oocytes, permeability to DMSO and to acetamide is low (1.0×10^{-3} and 0.9×10^{-3} cm/min, respectively) and the E_a values for permeability are high (18 and 23 kcal/mol, respectively) [28]. Therefore, DMSO and acetamide appear to move slowly across the plasma membrane of oocytes predominantly by simple diffusion (Figure 3.2a). The permeability to water of oocytes in the presence of DMSO or acetamide is also low (0.5 and 0.5 μm/min-atm) and the E_a values are high (12 and 15 kcal/mol, respectively). Therefore, water appears to move across the plasma membrane of oocytes by simple diffusion in the presence of DMSO or acetamide (Figure 3.2a).

In morulae, permeability to DMSO and acetamide is high (3.0×10^{-3} and 4.1×10^{-3} cm/min-atm, respectively) and the E_a values (12 and 12 kcal/mol) are lower than those in oocytes (18 and 23 kcal/mol, respectively) [28]. Therefore, DMSO and acetamide appear to move rapidly across the plasma membrane of morulae predominantly through channels (Figure 3.2e). However, aquaporin 3 would not be involved in the movement through channels, because its exogenous expression in oocytes did not increase permeability to DMSO or acetamide, and the suppression of aquaporin 3 expression in morulae did not affect permeability [28].

The permeability to water of morulae in the presence of DMSO or acetamide is high (2.3 and 2.0 μm/min-atm, respectively) and the E_a values for the permeability are relatively low (7 and 9 kcal/mol, respectively). Therefore, many water molecules (in the presence of DMSO or acetamide) would also move across the plasma membrane of morulae via channels (Figure 3.2e). Aquaporin 3 would be responsible for this movement (Figure 3.2e), because its exogenous expression in oocytes increased permeability to water without increasing permeability to DMSO and acetamide, and the suppression of aquaporin 3 expression markedly decreased the permeability to water of morulae in the presence of DMSO or acetamide [28].

Propylene glycol

Propylene glycol appears to permeate MII mouse oocy tes [7], but the permeability is low (1.7×10^{-3} cm/min) and the E_a for the permeability is high (20 kcal/mol) [28]. The permeability to water of oocytes in the presence of propylene glycol is low (0.5 μm/min-atm) and the E_a for the permeability is high (13 kcal/mol). In oocytes, therefore, propylene glycol and water (in the presence of propylene glycol) would move slowly across the plasma membrane predominantly by simple diffusion (Figure 3.2a).

In morulae, permeability to propylene glycol is not low (3.8×10^{-3} cm/min) but the E_a for this permeability is clearly high (20 kcal/mol) [28]. The permeability of morulae to water in the presence of propylene glycol is low (1.0 μm/min-atm) and the E_a for this permeability is high (15 kcal/mol). The exogenous expression of aquaporin 3 in oocytes does not increase permeability to propylene glycol and water (in the presence of propylene glycol), and the suppression of aquaporin 3 in morulae does not affect permeability to propylene glycol and water [28]. Therefore, propylene glycol would move across the plasma membrane predominantly by simple diffusion, as in oocytes, in spite of the abundant expression of aquaporin 3 in morulae. It is probable, in morulae, that propylene glycol and water interact to hinder each other's movements through aquaporin 3 (Figure 3.2f).

Embryos other than mouse morulae

The permeability of 2-cell mouse embryos to cryoprotectants and of 4-cell embryos to water are quite similar to that of MII oocytes, whereas the permeability of blastocysts appears to be essentially similar to that of morulae [7,17], as in the case of permeability to water in the absence of cryoprotectant described above. Therefore, the pathway for the movement of cryoprotectants and water (in the presence of cryoprotectant) in MII oocytes and morulae would provide useful information on the permeability of embryos at other stages.

In oocytes and early embryos, cryoprotectants and water (in the presence of cryoprotectant) would move slowly across the plasma membrane predominantly by simple diffusion. In morulae and blastocysts, by contrast, they would move rapidly across the plasma membrane predominantly through channels in most cases. However, the extent of the contribution of channels depends on the cryoprotectant. Moreover, the transporting characteristics of aquaporin 3 expressed in morulae [28] differ from those of aquaporin 3 expressed in *Xenopus* oocytes [33]. Further studies are necessary to clarify this discrepancy.

The permeability of oocytes/embryos appears to differ more among maturational/developmental stages than among species in mammals [7,35]. Therefore, the membrane-related properties of mouse oocytes/embryos described here might provide useful information on the cryobiological properties of oocytes/embryos in other mammalian species, which would contribute to designing optimal protocols for cryopreservation.

Movement of water and cryoprotectants and its relevance to cryopreservation

In mammalian oocytes/early embryos, water and cryoprotectants appear to move across the plasma membrane slowly by simple diffusion. Therefore, a longer exposure to the cryoprotectant solution(s) would be necessary to dehydrate the cells and allow the cryoprotectant(s) to permeate sufficiently. In addition, the suitable period of exposure to the cryoprotectant would vary depending on the temperature. When oocytes/embryos are cryopreserved by vitrification, length of time and temperature are critical, because vitrification solutions contain a high concentration of cryoprotectant(s) and toxicity is dependent on the period of exposure and temperature [36].

For vitrification of oocytes/early embryos, a two-step treatment would be effective, in which oocytes/embryos are first pretreated in a solution containing a low concentration of cryoprotectant for permeation in less toxic conditions, and then in the vitrification solution for a short time to cause the embryos to shrink by rapid dehydration. After warming, it would be preferable to remove permeated cryoprotectant(s) from oocytes/early embryos at a higher temperature to prevent osmotic over-swelling, because the movement of water and cryoprotectants by simple diffusion is largely affected by temperature.

In morulae, by comparison, a one-step treatment would be effective even for vitrification, because water and cryoprotectants permeate rapidly via channels. However, the period of exposure to the vitrification solution needs to be limited to prevent damage. The temperature at which morulae are exposed to the cryoprotectant before cooling and at which the permeated cryoprotectant is removed from morulae after warming may not be very important in terms of permeability, because facilitated diffusion through channels is less affected by temperature. For considerations of the toxicity of cryoprotectants, however, exposure to the cryoprotectant at high temperature should be avoided, because cryoprotectants are more toxic at higher temperature.

In blastocysts, cells would be highly permeable to water and cryoprotectants, as in morulae. However, blastocysts have a large amount of water in the blastocoele, within which ice is likely to form during cryopreservation. Therefore, it is preferable that most of the water in the blastocoele diffuses out before cryopreservation. An effective way to reduce the chance of intracellular ice forming is ultrarapid vitrification, in which oocytes/embryos suspended in a minimal amount of vitrification solution are cooled and warmed extremely rapidly [37,38]. In addition, the inner cell mass faces not the outside of the blastocyst but the blastocoele or trophoectoderm, indicating that water and cryoprotectants do not move across the plasma membrane of the inner cell mass directly from/to the solution in which the blastocyst is suspended but through the trophoectodermal cells or the blastocoele solution. Furthermore, it has been reported that the distribution of aquaporins is not homogeneous among the apical and basolateral sides of the trophoectoderm [27], suggesting that the blastocyst has compartments differing in permeability to water and cryoprotectants. When blastocysts are cryopreserved by vitrification, therefore, they are usually exposed to the cryoprotectant(s) in two steps to promote permeation under less toxic conditions [3,39].

Conclusions

The permeability of oocytes and embryos varies among maturational/developmental stages because the pathway by which water and cryoprotectants move across the plasma membrane is different. Therefore, the survival of oocytes/embryos after cryopreservation differs among maturational/developmental stages when the same cryopreservation protocol is used. In MII oocytes (and probably 2- to 4-cell embryos), water and cryoprotectants would move across the plasma membrane slowly by simple diffusion through the lipid bilayer. In morulae (and probably blastocysts), glycerol, ethylene glycol, DMSO, and acetamide would move rapidly by facilitated diffusion through channels, but propylene glycol would move by simple diffusion. Water appears to move in morulae via channels in the presence of glycerol, DMSO, or acetamide, but by simple diffusion in the presence of ethylene glycol or propylene glycol. In order to design protocols suitable for the cryopreservation of oocytes/embryos, it is necessary to consider the pathway for the movement of cryoprotectants and water at each stage of development.

Conditions suitable for the cryopreservation of mammalian oocytes and embryos differ among maturational/developmental stages even in the same species. Differences in cryobiological properties would be responsible for the variation. The permeability of the plasma membrane to water and cryoprotectants is the most important of these properties because it is closely related to major types of cellular injury during cryopreservation, such as the damage caused by the toxicity of cryoprotectants, by the formation of intracellular ice, and by osmotic swelling during removal of the cell-permeating cryoprotectant.

In mouse oocytes at the MII stage and embryos at early cleavage stages (early embryos), water and cryoprotectants appear to move slowly across the plasma membrane predominantly by simple diffusion, because permeability is low and temperature dependency is high. In morulae and blastocysts, on the other hand, water appears to move rapidly across the plasma membrane predominantly by facilitated diffusion through channels, because permeability is high and temperature dependency is low. Accordingly, morulae and blastocysts are highly permeable to cryoprotectants, such as glycerol, ethylene glycol, DMSO, and acetamide, and tolerate cryopreservation better than oocytes and early embryos.

As a channel, aquaporin 3, which is permeable to water and many cryoprotectants, is expressed abundantly in mouse morulae but not in oocytes. It has been shown in morulae that aquaporin 3 plays an important role in the movement of water, glycerol, and ethylene glycol, although not in the movement of DMSO and acetamide. In addition, water also moves across the plasma membrane of morulae by simple diffusion in the presence of ethylene glycol or propylene glycol. As an exception, propylene glycol appears to permeate morulae predominantly by simple diffusion concomitant with the slow movement of water by simple diffusion. It has been shown that the permeability characteristics of mouse oocytes/embryos at various stages are similar to those of bovine oocytes/embryos. This suggests that the permeability of oocytes/embryos will be similar among species in mammals. Information on the pathway for the movement of cryoprotectants and water would be useful as a basis for the selection of a suitable cryoprotectant(s) and for the design of suitable protocols for the cryopreservation of oocytes/embryos at various stages.

References

1. Kasai M, Ito K, Edashige K. Morphological appearance of the cryopreserved mouse blastocyst as a tool to identify the type of cryoinjury. *Hum Reprod* 2002; **17**: 1863–1874.
2. Kasai M, Komi JH, Takakamo A, *et al.* A simple method for mouse embryo cryopreservation in a low toxicity vitrification solution, without appreciable loss of viability. *J Reprod Fertil* 1990; **89**: 91–97.
3. Kasai M. Cryopreservation of mammalian embryos. *Mol Biotech* 1997; **7**: 173–179.
4. Edashige K, Asano A, An TZ, *et al.* Restoration of resistance to osmotic swelling of vitrified mouse embryos by short-term culture. *Cryobiology* 1999; **38**: 273–280.
5. Jackowski S, Leibo SP, Mazur P. Glycerol permeability of fertilized and unfertilized mouse ova. *J Exp Zool* 1980; **212**: 329–341.
6. Edashige K, Yamaji Y, Kleinhans FW, *et al.* Artificial expression of aquaporin-3 improves the survival of mouse oocytes after cryopreservation. *Biol Reprod* 2003; **68**: 87–94.
7. Pedro PB, Yokoyama E, Zhu SE, *et al.* Permeability of mouse oocytes and embryos at various developmental stages to five cryoprotectants. *J Reprod Dev* 2005; **51**: 235–246.
8. Whittingham DG. Survival of mouse embryos after freezing and thawing. *Nature* 1971; **233**: 125–126.
9. Kleinhans FW. Membrane permeability modeling: Kedem–Katchalsky vs a two-parameter formalism. *Cryobiology* 1998; **37**: 271–289.
10. Verkman AS, van Hoek AN, Ma T, *et al.* Water transport across mammalian cell membranes. *Am J Physiol* 1996; **270**: C12–C30.
11. Leibo SP. Water permeability and its activation energy of fertilized and unfertilized mouse ova. *J Membr Biol* 1980; **53**: 179–188.
12. Hunter J, Bernard A, Fuller B, *et al.* Measurements of the membrane water permeability (L_p) and its temperature dependence (activation energy) in human fresh and failed-to-fertilize oocytes and mouse oocytes. *Cryobiology* 1992; **29**: 240–249.
13. Benson CT, Critser JK. Variation of water permeability (LP) and its activation energy (Ea) among unfertilized golden hamster and ICR murine oocytes. *Cryobiology* 1994; **31**: 215–223.
14. Gao DY, Benson CT, Liu C, *et al.* Development of a novel microperfusion chamber for determination of cell membrane transport properties. *Biophys J* 1996; **71**: 443–450.
15. Litkouhi B, Marlow D, McGrath JJ, *et al.* The influence of cryopreservation on murine oocyte water permeability and osmotically inactive volume. *Cryobiology* 1997; **34**: 23–35.
16. Pfaff RT, Liu J, Gao D, *et al.* Water and DMSO membrane permeability characteristics of in-vivo and in-vitro derived and cultured murine oocytes and embryos. *Mol Hum Reprod* 1998; **4**: 51–59.
17. Edashige K, Tanaka M, Ichimaru N, *et al.* Channel-dependent permeation of water and glycerol in mouse morulae. *Biol Reprod* 2006; **74**: 625–632.
18. Toner M, Cravalho EG, Armant DR. Water transport and estimated transmembrane potential during freezing of mouse oocytes. *J Membr Biol* 1990; **115**: 261–272.
19. Edashige K, Sakamoto M, Kasai M. Expression of mRNAs of the aquaporin family in mouse oocytes and embryos. *Cryobiology* 2000; **40**: 171–175.
20. Offenberg H, Barcroft LC, Caveney A, *et al.* mRNAs encoding aquaporins are present during murine

preimplantation development. *Mol Reprod Dev* 2000; **57**: 323–330.

21. King LS, Kozono D, Agre P. From structure to disease: the evolving tale of aquaporin biology. *Nat Rev Mol Cell Biol* 2004; **5**: 687–698.
22. Fischbarg J, Kuang KY, Vera JC, *et al.* Glucose transporters serve as water channels. *Proc Natl Acad Sci USA* 1990; **87**: 3244–3247.
23. Yang B, Verkman AS. Urea transporter UT3 functions as an efficient water channel: direct evidence for a common water/urea pathway. *J Biol Chem* 1998; **273**: 9369–9372.
24. Loo DDF, Hirayama BA, Meinild AK, *et al.* Passive water and ion transport by cotransporters. *J Physiol* 1999; **518:** 195–202.
25. Verkman AS, Mitra AK. Structure and function of aquaporin water channels. *Am J Physiol Renal Physiol* 2000; **278**: F13–F28.
26. Offenberg H, Thomsen PD. Functional challenge affects aquaporin mRNA abundance in mouse blastocysts. *Mol Reprod Dev* 2005; **71**: 422–430.
27. Barcroft LC, Offenberg H, Thomsen P, *et al.* Aquaporin proteins in murine trophectoderm mediate transepithelial water movements during cavitation. *Dev Biol* 2003; **256**: 342–354.
28. Edashige K, Ohta S, Tanaka M, *et al.* The role of aquaporin 3 in the movement of water and cryoprotectants in mouse morulae. *Biol Reprod* 2007; **77**: 365–375.
29. Ishibashi K, Sasaki S, Fushimi K, *et al.* Molecular cloning and expression of a member of the aquaporin family with permeability to glycerol and urea in addition to water expressed at the basolateral membrane of kidney collecting duct cells. *Proc Natl Acad Sci USA* 1994; **91**: 6269–6273.
30. Meinild AK, Klaerke DA, Zeuthen T. Bidirectional water fluxes and specificity for small hydrophilic molecules in aquaporins 1–5. *J Biol Chem* 1998; **273**: 32446–32451.
31. Tsukaguchi H, Shayakul C, Berger UV, *et al.* Molecular characterization of a broad selectivity neutral solute channel. *J Biol Chem* 1998; **273**: 24737–24743.
32. Zeuthen T, Klaerke DA. Transport of water and glycerol in aquaporin 3 is gated by H^+. *J Biol Chem* 1999; **274**: 21631–21636.
33. Yamaji Y, Valdez DM, Seki S, *et al.* Cryoprotectant permeability of aquaporin-3 expressed in *Xenopus* oocytes. *Cryobiology* 2006; **53**: 258–267.
34. Mazur P, Rigopoulos N, Jackowski SC, *et al.* Preliminary estimates of the permeability of mouse ova and early embryos to glycerol. *Biophys J* 1976; **16**: 232a.
35. Pedro PB, Kasai M, Mammaru Y, *et al.* Change in the permeability to different cryoprotectants of bovine oocytes and embryos during maturation and development. *Proc 13th Int Congr Anim Reprod* 1996; **3**: P15–P19.
36. Kasai M, Nishimori M, Zhu SE, *et al.* Survival of mouse morulae vitrified in an ethylene glycol-based solution after exposure to the solution at various temperatures. *Biol Reprod* 1992; **47**: 1134–1139.
37. Martino A, Songsasen N, Leibo SP. Development into blastocysts of bovine oocytes cryopreserved by ultra-rapid cooling. *Biol Reprod* 1996; **54:** 1059–1069.
38. Kasai M. Advances in the cryopreservation of mammalian oocytes and embryos: development of ultrarapid vitrification. *Reprod Med Biol* 2002; **1**: 1–9.
39. Zhu SE, Kasai, M, Otoge, H, *et al.* Cryopreservation of expanded mouse blastocysts by vitrification in ethylene glycol-based solutions. *J Reprod Fertil* 1993; **98**: 139–145.

Chapter 4

Cryoprotectants

Jason E. Swain and Gary D. Smith

Introduction

Cryopreservation has been a very important factor in the progress and advancement of clinical in vitro fertilization (IVF), allowing for long-term storage of sperm, embryos, and, more recently, oocytes for future use. This is not only helpful for preserving fertility in patients who may be undergoing treatment for cancer or other life-threatening illnesses but also allows for storage of these cells to permit genetic screening, as well as the ability to test samples for communicable diseases prior to use. Furthermore, methods to store, rather than discard, embryos provide alternatives to alleviate various ethical concerns. As a result, cryopreservation has become the standard of care in infertility treatment.

Though it may now be considered a routine procedure, cryobiology itself is a complex discipline and multiple variables must be accounted for in developing successful protocols. Many of these considerations are discussed in the accompanying chapters and include cell- and tissue-specific sensitivities, which are influenced by cell size, membrane permeability, lipid content, and other factors. Regardless of these variables, a primary consideration, and one of the most basic components of a successful cryopreservation protocol, is selection of an effective cryoprotectant additive. Cryoprotectants function as their name implies, guarding cells from damage during cryopreservation by either freezing or vitrification. Protective effects of these agents are conveyed primarily through interactions with, and manipulation of, intracellular and extracellular water.

The manner in which water interacts within and around the cell, as well as its behavior during cooling/freezing, is a key determinant in maintaining cellular viability during cryopreservation. Consequently, an understanding of the physicochemical properties of water is required for a truly complete understanding of the theoretical and functional basis of cryobiology and the functioning of cryoprotectants. Factors such as hydrogen bonding, water's interactions with ions and macromolecules, dielectric constants, thermodynamic equilibrium, and osmosis all provide information on the underlying biophysical and biochemical mechanisms by which cryopreservation and cryoprotectants operate. Though brief mention of these factors may be insightful in certain instances, a detailed discussion is beyond the scope of this chapter, and more in-depth analysis can be found in accompanying chapters or other reviews [1,2].

Several substances convey cryoprotective activity, with up to 56 individual compounds reported to convey a protective effect in various cellular systems [3,4]. For purposes of this chapter, we will focus on various cryoprotectants and their application in preserving gametes and embryos (Table 4.1). In general, although cryoprotectants defend against cellular damage by regulating dynamics of water during cooling, the actual manner by which they convey their protection depends largely on whether the particular compounds permeate the cell or whether they remain in the extracellular space (Figure 4.1). Therefore, cryoprotectants are grouped into two major categories: penetrating and non-penetrating agents.

Penetrating cryoprotectants

Penetrating cryoprotectants are generally small, nonionic compounds with a high solubility in water at low temperatures. Given time, these chemical compounds can diffuse through cellular membranes, permeating the cell and equilibrating within the cytoplasm, replacing the bulk of intracellular water without over-dehydrating the cell. Permeating cryoprotectants solidify at lower temperatures than water and thus subsequently reduce the amount of intracellular ice formation at a given temperature. This decreased amount of intracellular ice-crystal formation mitigates

Fertility Cryopreservation, ed. Ri-Cheng Chian and Patrick Quinn. Published by Cambridge University Press.

Table 4.1. List of various cryoprotective agents used in assisted reproductive technologies

Cryoprotectant	Cell type	Example species
Penetrating agents		
Dimethyl sulfoxide	Oocyte, embryo, sperm	Mouse, human, cow
Amides and imides		
Formamide	Sperm	Horse, goose, dog, mouse
Acetamide	Oocyte, embryo	Mouse, rabbit, pig, rat
Propionamide	Sperm	Rabbit
Lactamide	Sperm	Rabbit
Butyramide	Sperm	Rabbit
Malonamide	Sperm	Rabbit
Alcohols		
Methanol	Sperm	Horse
Propylene glycol	Oocyte, embryo, sperm	Mouse, human, cow
Ethylene glycol	Oocyte, embryo, sperm	Mouse, human, cow
Butylene glycol	Oocyte, embryo	Mouse, cow, sheep
Glycerol	Oocyte, embryo, sperm	Mouse, human, cow
Adonitol	Embryo, sperm	Mouse, sheep, human, rat
Erythritol	Embryo	Rat
Arabitol	Embryo	Rat
Perseitol	Embryo	Rat
Xylitol	Embryo	Rat
Non-penetrating agents		
Monosaccharide sugars		
Glucose	Sperm	Cat
Galactose	Sperm	Horse
Arabinose	Sperm	Horse
Mannose	Sperm	Deer
Fructose	Sperm	Deer
Xylose	Sperm	Deer
Disaccharide sugars		
Sucrose	Oocyte, embryo, sperm	Mouse, human, cow
Trehalose	Oocyte, embryo, sperm	Mouse, human, horse, cow
Lactose	Sperm	Mouse, cow
Maltose	Sperm	Mouse, deer, rabbit
Polysaccharides		
Raffinose	Oocyte, sperm	Mouse, horse
Dextran	Embryo	Cat, mouse
Macromolecules		
Ficoll	Oocyte, embryo	Mouse, human, cow
Polyethylene glycol	Oocyte, embryo	Mouse, human, cow
Polyvinylpyrrolidone	Embryo	Mouse
Polyvinyl alcohol	Oocyte, embryo	Mouse, cow, sheep,
Hyaluronan	Embryo, sperm	Mouse, cow, sheep, pig

damage resulting from physical perturbations to cellular organelles and membranes. Additionally, penetrating cryoprotectants provide buffering against salt-induced stress by acting as solvent, reducing the solute concentration in the remaining water fraction inside the cell until the system is cooled to a low enough temperature.

Various penetrating cryoprotectants have been used successfully in IVF to preserve sperm, embryos, and oocytes. Success using each type of permeating cryoprotectant depends in part on the speed at which they can cross cellular membranes, and this rate is dictated by various factors, such as viscosity. However, permeation is dependent not only upon the cryoprotectant itself but also upon the membrane properties of the cell, which vary between cell types as well as cell stages. As one may expect with decreasing blastomere size, it appears as though permeability to various cryoprotectants increases as embryos progress in development [5]. As further examples of stage-specific permeability, immature and mature monkey [6], bovine [7], frog [8], and fish [9] oocytes all have different permeabilities to cryoprotectants. Furthermore, membrane permeability of sperm and oocytes can vary between individuals of certain species, such as cow and mouse [10,11]. Common groups of permeating cryoprotectants are discussed below, the most common of which include dimethyl sulfoxide (DMSO), propylene glycol (1,2 propanediol, propylene diol, PROH), ethylene glycol (1,2-ethandiol), and glycerol, though other agents have received attention on a more limited basis.

Sulfoxides

Dimethyl sulfoxide (Me_2SO_4) is an amphipathic molecule soluble in both aqueous and organic media and is commonly used as a solvent. However, DMSO has also received widespread use as a cryoprotectant [12].

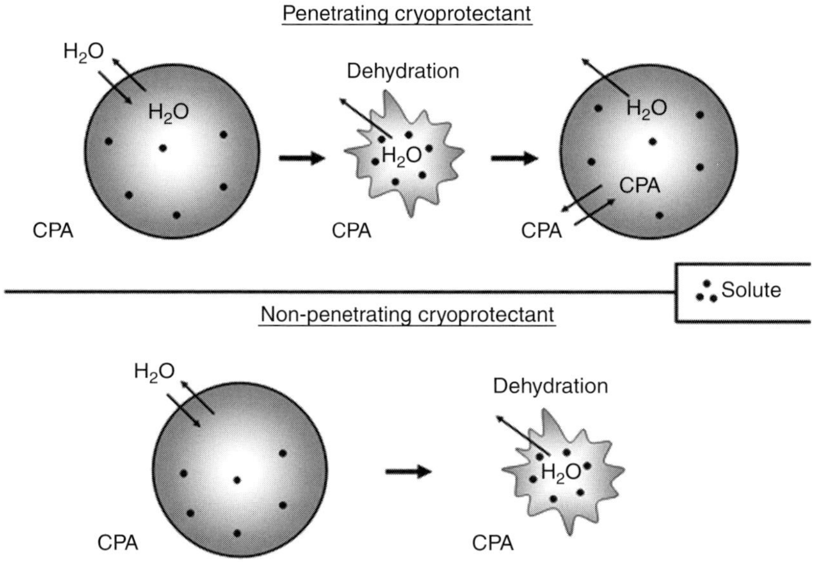

Figure 4.1. Schematic representation of the manner by which penetrating and non-penetrating cryoprotectants (CPAs) exert their actions upon cells, both of which result in reduced intracellular water.

In addition to glycerol, DMSO was the first permeating cryoprotectant used to successfully freeze rodent cleavage-stage embryos to result in subsequent live births [13]. This same protocol was later used to freeze the first human embryos that established successful pregnancies [14,15]. Dimethyl sulfoxide was also the cryoprotectant used to freeze the first human oocytes that resulted in live birth following thaw [16]. This sulfoxide is now included in several successful published vitrification protocols. An added benefit of DMSO may be its ability to scavenge reactive oxygen species [12]. However, as discussed later in this chapter, there are concerns with use of DMSO as a cryoprotective agent in reproductive tissues [17–25].

Amides and imides

Formamide

Formamide (methanamide) is used sporadically as a cryoprotectant and has received the most attention for use with sperm, most notably that from the stallion (reviewed by Alvarenga [26]). These compounds offer an alternative to more conventional cryoprotectants, such as glycerol, and may create less osmotic stress for sensitive species/cells through their low molecular weight and low viscosity. Both methyl formamide and dimethyl formamide are reported as adequate alternative cryoprotectants for use with stallion sperm, yielding equivalent or better survival to that seen with glycerol [27,28]. Dimethyl formamide has also been used to successfully preserve goose sperm [29]. Interestingly, methyl formamide, but not dimethyl formamide, provided adequate protection to canine sperm during freezing, similar to glycerol [30]. It should be mentioned that at least one report indicates that methyl formamide is not efficient in preserving mouse sperm [31], and neither methyl formamide nor dimethyl formamide provided efficient cryoprotection for rabbit sperm compared with other amides tested [32].

Acetamide

Acetamide (acetic acid amide, ethanamide) was a component of the cryoprotecant solution utilized by Rall and Fahy in their pioneering report of embryo vitrification [33]. Permeability for acetamide in relation to other cryoprotectants has been examined in mouse oocytes and various stages of mouse embryos, where it was shown that its permeability increased sharply after the 8-cell stage [5]. However, mode of entry into cells is unknown, as in mouse morulae acetamide does not appear to utilize aquaporin 3 for intracellular diffusion [34]. Use of acetamide did not yield high cryosurvival following freezing of stallion sperm [27]. However, the compound has been used in conjunction with several other cryoprotectants to successfully vitrify 2-cell mouse embryos [35], mouse ovarian tissue [36], rabbit pronuclear zygotes [37], pig and rat blastocysts [38,39], as well as mouse oocytes [40]. Caution should be used with application of acetamide as a cryoprotectant. A solution of

30–40% acetamide provided very poor cryosurvival following vitrification of mouse 8-cell embryos compared with other cryoprotectants at similar concentrations, as these embryos had abnormal morphology and could not develop to blastocysts upon warming [41]. Furthermore, it was shown that short exposure to acetamide at 1.5 mol/l was best to avoid toxicity to mouse oocytes and embryos [5].

Other amides

Additional amides that have been tested as cryoprotectants for use with sperm are propionamide, lactamide, butryamide, and maloamide [32], but each has met with limited success. Other amides that have been used as cryoprotective agents in microbiology, but have not received widespread use in assisted reproduction therapy (ART), include methyl acetamide, demethylacetamide, and succinimide [3].

Alcohols (monhydric, diols, triols, polyols)

Methanol

Methanol as a cryoprotectant is used more commonly for preservation of various microorganisms (reviewed by Hubalek [3]). There are several reports in the literature using methanol to freeze gametes and embryos from various marine species [42–45], but very little mention of methanol for use in mammalian reproductive tissues. At least one report indicates that methanol can be used to successfully cryopreserve equine embryos and has similar efficiency to glycerol [46].

Propylene glycol

Propylene glycol is a solvent, commonly used in various lotions and creams, and sometimes as a food additive in ice cream. It is, therefore, generally considered non-toxic at low levels. Bovine blastocysts exposed for up to 30 minutes to 1.6 mol/l PROH showed no apparent adverse effects on continued development [47,48]. Propylene glycol was one of the first permeating cryoprotectants used to successfully cryopreserve mammalian sperm [49] as well as human pronuclear embryos [50]. It continues to be used successfully in a variety of both slow-rate and vitrification protocols found throughout the reproductive scientific literature.

Ethylene glycol

Ethylene glycol is most widely known for its use as an antifreeze in vehicles, which makes it a logical choice for use as an "antifreeze" cryoprotectant. Ethylene glycol seems to have minimal effects on mouse oocyte morphology or cytoskeletal structure [51], and exposure of bovine blastocysts for up to 30 minutes to 1.6 mol/l ethylene glycol had no apparent adverse effects on development [47,48]. Mouse epididymal sperm is extremely permeable to ethylene glycol [52], which appears to utilize aquaporin 3 channels for cell entry [34]. There are numerous protocols throughout the literature utilizing ethylene glycol as a cryoprotectant additive for sperm, oocytes, and embryos from a variety of species.

Butylene glycol

Butylene glycol (1,3-butanediol) is not a widely used cryoprotectant additive in reproductive tissues. One report indicates the compound was not effective in freezing bovine blastocysts when used alone at 1.1 mol/l [53] but was able to provide adequate cryosurvival following vitrification of bovine [54] and mouse [55] blastocysts when used in a complex formulation of multiple cryoprotectants. Compared with nine other cryoprotectants, butylene glycol was the most toxic to mouse and sheep embryos [56], and a similar compound, 2,3-butanediol, also caused membrane abnormal blebbing in mouse oocytes [57].

Glycerol

Glycerol is a triol, or sugar alcohol, and is arguably the most used/studied cryoprotectant. Though several studies examined the effects of cooling/freezing on the male gamete from several species in the 1930s and 1940s, glycerol was the first permeating cryoprotectant used to successfully cryopreserve mammalian sperm [49,58,59], including that from humans [60]. Additionally, glycerol has been used to successfully freeze the first mouse oocyte [61,62] and was also the penetrating cryoprotectant used to obtain the first live birth following freezing of various stage mouse embryos [13]. It is proposed that glycerol acts primarily by adding to the colligative properties of a solution and reducing the salt concentration during freezing [63]. Although permeability of glycerol is low compared with that of other cryoprotectants, several successful cryopreservation protocols still utilize glycerol. It appears that aquaporin 3 plays an instrumental role in the facilitated diffusion of glycerol into oocytes and embryos [34,64,65].

Adonitol

Adonitol belongs to a group known as polyols or sugar alcohols, and it is postulated that these compounds may offer cryoprotection through interactions of their many hydroxyl groups, forming hydrogen bonds with the cellular membrane as well as water [66]. It appears that the cryoprotective nature of these compounds increases with increases in the number of hydroxyl groups, provided that the compounds are still able to permeate the cell [66]. This is important because increasing numbers of hydroxyl groups seemed to lower membrane permeability. Adonitol was used as a cryoprotectant with mouse sperm but did not offer superior protection when compared with more traditional cryoprotectants, such as DMSO [31]. Additionally, adonitol, along with several other polyols, was used to successfully freeze ram [67] and human [68] sperm though none of the treatments was superior to glycerol alone. Finally, adonitol was used in the fast-rate freezing of rat embryos and gave the highest cryosurvival (88% survival) when compared with DMSO and various other polyol compounds tested at 1 mol/l [66]. It should be noted, however, that adonitol, along with DMSO, did facilitate fusing of blastomere membranes [66] and, therefore, requires careful use.

Other alcohols

Ethanol, though used to cryopreserve some microorganisms, has not been widely used for reproductive cells or tissues. Other alcohols and their derivatives that have been used as cryoprotectants in other scientific disciplines include trimethylene glycol, diethylene glycol, polyethylene oxide, and polypropylene glycol [3]. Additional polyols studied for embryo cryopreservation include erythritol, sorbitol, and xythyritol [66].

Non-penetrating cryoprotectants

Non-penetrating cryoprotectants are generally long-chain polymers too large to diffuse into cells. These compounds act to increase osmolarity of the extracellular space, which results in cellular dehydration and thus reduces the chance of intracellular ice crystal formation. It is also postulated that some non-permeating cryoprotectants may absorb on membrane surfaces, inhibiting ice crystal formation in the immediate vicinity of the cell by keeping ice in the amorphous state. Additionally, non-penetrating cryoprotectants are often included in media used for warming/thawing of cells to help to avoid osmotic shock. Osmotic shock describes the phenomenon that occurs when the osmotic pressure of the intracellular compartment is greater than the extracellular compartment, which occurs as a result of cellular dehydration. Upon thawing, traumatic cell expansion and lysis can occur following the accompanying water influx.

Sugars

Non-permeating cryoprotectants are commonly mono-, oligo-, and polysaccharides. Some of these sugars are used by various plant and animal species in nature as a means of protection from cold climate (reviewed by Fuller *et al.* [69]). Consequently, their application in laboratory cryobiology seems logical. Monosaccharides dissolve in solution more readily than disaccharides and vitrify at lower temperatures [70]. However, because monosaccharides are prone to non-enzymatic glycosylation, which can result in protein interactions, many cryopreservation protocols utilize di- and polysaccharides. Though studies indicate that several sugars are non-toxic to oocytes and embryos at concentrations up to 7 mmol/l for 10 minutes [70], other sugars at higher concentrations or for extended time periods can impact cell morphology and functionality [70,71]. It is important to note that different sugars provide different levels of protection during cryopreservation [70,72–75], and this can vary depending on media composition and cooling conditions. These differences may depend, in part, on the differential effects of specific sugars on raising the glass transition temperature of vitrification solutions [70].

Monosaccharides

Glucose

Glucose is a hexose sugar (six carbon atoms). This sugar is used as an energy source by gametes and embryos and is, therefore, included in most culture media in millimolar concentrations. As a result, glucose is present in most cryopreservation media as part of the base solution, though not commonly mentioned as a specific cryoprotective agent. Interestingly, glucose is one of the sugars that appears to be used by organisms in nature to protect themselves from cold, harsh climates (reviewed by Fuller *et al.* [69]) but has not received widespread attention in reproductive methodology. One study mentions the use of glucose for successful freezing of cat sperm [76].

Galactose

Galactose is another hexose sugar that has received limited attention as a non-permeating cryoprotectant. Galactose has been shown to be detrimental to stallion sperm motility when included in freeze extender media, compared with use of non-glycolysable disaccharide sugars [74].

Arabinose

Arabinose is a pentose sugar that has also been shown to be detrimental to stallion sperm motility when included in freezing solution [74].

Other monosaccharides

Other monosaccharides, such as fructose, xylose, and mannose, have been tested on a limited basis as cryoprotective agents for deer sperm [75], and mannose was actually one of the two least effective sugars at preserving mouse embryos for short-term storage at 0°C [77].

Disaccharides

Sucrose

Sucrose is a naturally occurring sugar used by various plants and animals to avoid damage during freezing (reviewed by Fuller *et al.* [69]). Consequently, it makes the compound an obvious choice as a non-permeating cryoprotectant. In regard to gametes and embryos, sucrose was first used to vitrify frog sperm [78], and 1–2 mol/l concentrations were also used, in conjunction with PROH, in the first protocol that resulted in successful cryopreservation of human pronuclear stage embryos [50]. As an additive in conjunction with permeating cryoprotectants, sucrose is now used in numerous freeze–thaw protocols in a variety of reproductive tissues across a wide range of species. It should be noted that exposure to concentrations of 1 mol/l sucrose for 10 minutes resulted in lack of fertilization in mouse oocytes [70], possibly through premature cortical granule exocytosis [71].

Trehalose

Trehalose is another naturally occurring sugar found in systems able to tolerate freezing in nature and, as a result, the sugar has received great attention in cryobiology and has been used extensively in other cell systems because of its apparent unique properties. For example, the hydration radius of trehalose is approximately 2.5 times greater than that of other sugars [79], which may result in its exclusion from the hydration shells of proteins, thereby increasing protein stability [80]. Trehalose has been used as a component of various embryo vitrification protocols [55,81–84] but was no better than sucrose or raffinose in vitrifying/warming of mouse pronuclear stage embryos [85]. Additionally, because trehalose is a non-permeating cryoprotectant unable to cross cellular membranes, the sugar has been microinjected into oocytes and this benefited both human and mouse cryosurvival [86–88]. Trehalose has been shown to be beneficial as an additive for freezing sperm [89], though its superiority over other sugars in protecting mouse, bull, and stallion sperm is debatable [27,31,90].

Lactose

Lactose is the disaccharide commonly found in milk and made up of one molecule of glucose and one of galactose. Lactose has been used as a cryoprotecting agent for bovine sperm and proved no different to other disaccharides tested (sucrose or rabinose), though all were better than the monosaccharides tested [74]. Lactose was also used as a cryoprotectant with hybrid mouse sperm; although it did not preserve motility post-thaw as well as sucrose or trehalose, it did produce sperm with high fertilization capability [31].

Maltose

Maltose is malt sugar comprising two units of glucose. In contrast to other reports indicating superiority of di- and polysaccharides as cryoprotectants, maltose was not as effective as various monosaccharides in preserving red deer sperm following freezing [75]. Additionally, maltose was not as effective as sucrose in preserving rabbit semen [91]. Of seven sugars examined, maltose was one of the two least effective in preserving mouse embryos during short-term storage at 0°C [77]. Therefore, not all disaccharides function equally as cryoprotectants.

Polysaccharides

Raffinose

Raffinose is a trisaccharide composed of galactose, fructose, and glucose units and is commonly found in various vegetables. This sugar has been used as a cryoprotectant primarily for mouse sperm: 18% raffinose proved effective in protecting mouse sperm, both alone and in conjunction with glycerol [92]. A similar combination of raffinose and glycerol was later used to freeze epididymal mouse sperm [93], and its functionality was confirmed via IVF and birth of live pups [94]. When compared with disaccharides, raffinose gave comparable results to sucrose and trehalose in preserving mouse sperm [31] and provided similar protection as glucose and fructose with stallion sperm [27]. Raffinose has also been used to preserve sperm from a variety of other species [74,95]. Interestingly, raffinose was shown to change the vitrification properties of solutions containing ethylene glycol, raising the glass transition temperature more than either sucrose or trehalose [70], and so it may be an important component in optimizing vitrification solutions. Pre-exposure of mouse oocytes to raffinose prior to vitrification in an ethylene glycol/raffinose vitrification solution was non-toxic and improved viability [96]. This sugar has also been used in vitrification solutions for mouse preantral follicles, which resulted in live birth [96]. One report did indicate that inclusion of raffinose as a cryoprotectant for mouse follicles increased vacuolization of granulosa cells, though this was likely to have resulted from excessive exposure and cellular dehydration [97].

Dextran

Dextran is a complex branched polysaccharide made of repeating glucose molecules. Dextran 10% has been used in conjunction with other permeating and non-permeating cryoprotectants to successfully freeze cat [98] and mouse [99] embryos. Inclusion of dextran in media has also been shown to alleviate cracking of mouse zona pellucida following cryopreservation [100]. Interestingly, dextran did little to alter the glass transition temperature of an ethylene glycol vitrification solution [101]. Efficacy of dextran for use with human oocytes or embryos is unknown.

Macromolecules/polymers

Macromolecules or polymers are often included, though not required, as additional protective additives in cryopreservation media. These compounds promote vitrification of a solution [102] and thus may help to reduce toxicity concerns by allowing the concomitant decrease in concentrations of potentially harmful permeating agents. Macromolecules tend to increase viscosity of the cryoprotectant solution and also form interactions through hydrogen bonding with water, thereby decreasing the propensity for ice crystal formation [103]. Protein is a common macromolecule that is added to media used for cryopreservation in ART and while it may play a role as a cryoprotectant, it certainly serves as a surfactant to prevent sticking of cells to cryostraws or other containers. Whether protein sources used in clinical IVF, such as human serum albumin, serum substitute supplement, dextran serum supplement, or other similar products all function similarly, or provide comparable levels of protection during cryopreservation, is not known. Several studies have looked at other suitable macromolecules to be used in conjunction with, or as a replacement for, undefined protein sources. Two large considerations with including such macromolecules as cryoprotectants include solubility and viscosity.

Ficoll

Ficoll is a non-ionic synthetic polymer of sucrose and it could also be grouped as a polysaccharide. Inclusion of Ficoll in cryopreservation media reduced zona pellucida cracking in both human and mouse following freezing [100]. Ficoll is included as one of several ingredients in various vitrification protocols for oocytes from several species including mouse [99,104], cat [105], pig [106], cow [107,108], monkey [109], and others. Ficoll, used at 10 mg/ml, was also one of the protective agents in the vitrification solution used to preserve over 1000 human oocytes [110]. Numerous protocols utilize Ficoll as a macromolecule additive to cryopreservation media used to freeze various stages of preimplantion embryos from a variety of species. Interestingly, in solutions of ethylene glycol, Ficoll at concentrations ranging from 5 to 20% did little to alter the glass transition temperature [101].

Polyethylene glycol

Although polyethylene glycol is also an alcohol derivative, this compound is a non-penetrating cryoprotectant. It has been used to vitrify mouse oocytes [40] and improved mouse oocyte vitrification over DMSO alone [111]. It has also been used in conjunction with other cryoprotectants to successfully freeze human oocytes [110]. Mouse, bovine [112], and rat [38] blastocysts have all also been cryopreserved using polyethylene glycol as a protecting agent.

Polyvinylpyrrolidone

Polyvinylpyrrolidone was the first non-permeating cryoprotectant used as the sole cryoprotectant to successfully cryopreserve 8-cell mouse embryos at −79°C for 30 minutes, which subsequently led to the first birth of a mammal following cryopreservation [113]. However, it should be mentioned that this protocol did not succeed using 2-cell embryos and these results could not be repeated with any great success. In conjunction with other cryoprotectants, polyvinylpyrrolidone has been used at various concentrations to freeze bovine oocytes [108] and was an effective replacement for human serum albumin for vitrifying mouse 8-cell embryos [114]. Although polyvinylpyrrolidone prevented zona pellucida cracking following freezing, it did not result in high efficiency of blastocyst development compared with other macromolecule cryoprotectants following freezing of 2-cell embryos [100].

Polyvinylpyrrolidone has been shown to raise the glass transition temperature of an ethylene glycol vitrification solution [101].

Polyvinyl alcohol

Polyvinyl alcohol is a water-soluble synthetic polymer and can be used as a replacement for fetal calf serum in media used to cryopreserve mouse embryos [115], yielding morphologically normal fetuses and live birth of pups [116]. It has also been used successfully as a macromolecule supplement in bovine oocyte vitrification solution at concentrations ranging from 0.1 to 1% [108,117], and it can be used to freeze various stages of sheep embryos [118,119]. However, with at least some embryo cryopreservation protocols, polyvinyl alcohol can be less effective than serum [120,121].

Hyaluronan

Hyaluronan (hyaluronic acid, hyaluronate) is a major component of the extracellular matrix and is found throughout the expanded cumulus cell mass. This substance has been shown to be a suitable replacement for newborn calf serum in freezing solutions used for murine and bovine embryos [121–124] and ovine blastocysts [125]. Hyaluronan supplementation also improved post-thaw motility and membrane stability in boar sperm [126].

Cryoprotectant toxicity and damage

Though the purpose of cryoprotectants is to prevent damage during cooling/freezing, some of these compounds can themselves result in damage to cells. However, in order to validate whether damage is caused by the cryoprotectant itself, and to determine possible mechanisms of toxicity, certain criteria should be met [127]. These critieria include examining effects of cryoprotectants under conditions in which they may actually be used (concentrations, exposure time, temperature, etc.) and demonstrating that any alterations actually have an effect on function, are irreversible, and result from the cryoprotectant agent itself rather than cooling or the technique involved. For example, the damage induced by ice crystal formation or osmotic stress is often referred to but may be caused by the freeze–thaw process itself rather than actual toxic effects of the cryoprotecting agent. In general, most toxicity concerns exist with penetrating cryoprotectants rather than the non-penetrating cryoprotectants.

In regard to reproductive biology and assessing suitability/toxicity of a cryoprotective agent, certain endpoint measures are commonly assessed. In sperm, these endpoints often include effects on motility, capacitation, and ability to fertilize. In oocytes, assessment of damage from cryoprotectants often focuses on the meiotic spindle, actin cytoskeleton, chromosomal arrangement, and ability to fertilize. In regard to embryos, toxicity studies tend to examine ability to continue embryonic development, or effects on various molecular and biochemical signaling pathways. Unfortunately, the exact mechanisms by which the toxicity of cryoprotective agents arises are unknown. Examples of damage induced by improper exposure to various cryoprotectants range from removal or fusing of cellular membranes to impaired enzyme activity, altered organelle structure/function, and perturbed protein interactions [127–129]. However, potential mechanisms of damage are being identified. In respect to DMSO and membrane fusing, a model system indicates that lipid molecules are desorbed from the membrane followed by disintegration of the bilayer structure [130]. More recently, a new approach to quantify cryoprotectant toxicity has been developed, examining the average water hydrogen bonding of the polar groups [131]. This modeling has been used to design less-toxic cryoprotectant mixtures to enhance survival following freezing in mouse oocytes [131].

The effects of exposure time, concentration, and temperature on toxicity

The conditions under which cryoprotectant exposure occurs can influence their toxicity for reproductive cells. Factors such as time of exposure, concentration of cryoprotectant, as well as temperature of exposure all impact the effect of the particular protecting agent. While cryoprotectants themselves are generally non-toxic when exposed to cells for short periods of time, extended exposure or exposure at elevated concentrations can result in metabolism of the cryoprotecting agents, which can subsequently disrupt cellular function and viability. As an example, increasing concentrations of DMSO, PROH, and glycerol were shown to result in increased non-enzymatic formation of formaldehyde, and this formation was dependent upon the type of base media utilized [17]. Exposure of bovine blastocysts to ethylene glycol concentrations greater than 5.4 mol/l for 10 minutes was detrimental to continued development [120]. Cryoprotectants can also be damaging to oocytes. Compounds such as DMSO and PROH can cause depolymerization of oocyte tubulin and malformation of the meiotic spindle [24,25,132,133]. This is of great concern in regard to chromosomal remodeling, especially when one considers that the oocyte is notorious for high rates of aneuploidy. Additionally, PROH resulted in actin destabilization in rabbit oocytes and zygotes, which was reversible, while no such destabilization was observed with DMSO [25,134,135]. However, the same authors reported that DMSO did disrupt actin filaments in mouse oocytes [20]. In the case of DMSO, deleterious effects on the spindle appear with extended exposure and appear to be irreversible [21]. In the case of PROH, effects appear to be dose dependent [136]. Extended exposure of oocytes to PROH also leads to degeneration and parthenogenetic activation [133,137,138]. As mentioned above, with advances in technology, possible mechanisms for cryotoxicity are emerging. Exposure of MII mouse oocytes to 1.5 mol/l PROH for 10 minutes resulted in alterations to the proteonome [139]. Additionally, DMSO also leads to premature cortical granule release and zona pellucida hardening in oocytes, which can affect fertilization [19,140]. This hardening effect may be caused by the premature release of intracellular calcium ions, as under certain conditions DMSO, PROH, and ethylene glycol all induced premature calcium ion oscillations in mouse oocytes [18].

In addition to concentration and time of exposure, the temperature at which cryoprotectant exposure occurs can also impact cellular damage. It was reported that exposure to 1.5 mol/l DMSO at 37°C perturbed microtubule actin microfilament arrangement in mouse oocytes, which was less apparent when cooled [20]. Similarly, use of DMSO at 4°C did not produce the same negative effects on subsequent fertilization as when used at 37°C [22]. Interestingly, examining another common permeating cryoprotectant, it was shown that lowering the temperature of oocyte exposure to solutions of PROH reduced side effects [133]. In these cases, lowering the temperature of cryoprotectant exposure likely decreased uptake and metabolism of the toxic agents. However, when using a more viscous cryoprotectant, higher temperatures and resulting greater permeation may be advantageous. As an example, exposure of buffalo sperm to glycerol at 37°C yielded better post-thaw survival and motility than seen with exposure at 4°C [141]. Generally, while lowering the temperature of cryoprotectant exposure may alleviate some concerns regarding toxicity of the agent, it also induces depolymerization of tubulin and the oocyte meiotic spindle [142,143]. Interestingly, a more recent report indicates that exposing oocytes to cryoprotectants for fast-rate vitrification at 37°C resulted in maintenance of the mouse oocyte meiotic spindle, compared with cells exposed to cryoprotectant solutions at 24°C [144]. Because exposing gametes and embryos to permeating cryoprotectants at higher temperatures results in faster permeation, this practice likely requires an even shorter exposure time compared with that needed at lower temperatures, and this may be compensating.

Avoiding toxicity and damage

From the above discussion, it is apparent that selection of a suitable cryoprotectant and optimizing its concentration, as well as monitoring the time and temperature of exposure, all influence the potential damage a cryoprotectant may cause to a cell. Therefore, a common approach to reduce toxicity has emerged that entails combining various cryoprotectants, both permeating and non-permeating, thereby reducing individual concentrations and mitigating damage while maintaining the overall protective effects. A very early example of this can be seen in the research of Ian Wilmut, who successfully produced offspring after freezing mouse embryos [145], as well as the first live birth following cryopreservation of bovine embryos [146]. Both of these landmark events utilized a protocol that combined DMSO, sucrose, and polyvinylpyrrolidone. Combining multiple cryoprotectants may also alleviate, or at least lessen, toxicity through one cryoprotectant counteracting the negative effects of another. For example, formamide was shown to mitigate the toxic effects of DMSO [127]. Many successful cryopreservation protocols now utilize a combination of penetrating and non-penetrating cryoprotectants in conjunction with macromolecule supplementation, and this approach is undoubtedly a large reason for continued increases in efficiency.

Methods of introducing and removing cryoprotectants offer another means to reduce toxicity or resulting damage. Stepwise addition of cryoprotective agents, or gradually increasing concentrations, has been useful. Additionally, stepwise removal of these compounds upon warming/thawing helps to minimize osmotic stress. Furthermore, altering the ionic composition of the carrier solution in which the cryoprotectant is dissolved offers another means of mitigating damage. Specifically, replacing sodium with choline attenuates damage from the solute effect and may also benefit from increasing solution viscosity [147].

Conclusions

Cryoprotectants serve to prevent damage induced by the cooling/freezing process, in part by reducing ice crystal formation and by reducing stress resulting from osmotic shock. Consequently, variables such as cell size and membrane permeability are important factors in selecting appropriate cryoprotectants. These two variables are likely large contributors to the historical difficulty of cryopreserving oocytes, but this also reinforces the idea that no one cryoprotectant or cryopreservation protocol can serve as a universal procedure. To achieve success, critical factors include careful selection of cryoprotective agents; close monitoring of their temperature, time, and concentration of exposure; and their stepwise addition and removal from cells. Furthermore, the base media utilized to dissolve cryoprotectants deserves more attention. We often take it for granted, yet this media has varying sugar content and sugar concentration, and these sugars can serve as cryoprotectants themselves. Additionally, a variety of protein supplements are used in ART, and it is unclear if all of these protein sources function similarly or provide comparable protection during cryopreservation. As different media respond differently to the freeze process, some leading to large perturbations in pH, this could be problematic for slow-rate protocols. Lest we forget, base media can also impact the toxic effects of cryoprotectants [17]. When these variables are taken into consideration, efficient cryopreservation of reproductive cells has been achieved. However, there is still room for improvement. Continued evaluation of various and new cryoprotective agents, their concentrations and combination with other compounds, and integration of techniques with developments in emerging biomedical engineering fields such as microfluidics and automated gradual media exchange can still provide opportunities to increase efficiency. Additionally, continued diligence in assessing molecular and biochemical endpoint measures following cryoprotectant exposure is crucial if approaches in ART are to be further refined [18].

References

1. Mazur P. Equilibrium, quasi-equilibrium, and nonequilibrium freezing of mammalian embryos. *Cell Biophys* 1990; **17:** 53–92.
2. Mazur P. Principles of cryobiology. In Fuller B, Lane N, Benson E, eds. *Life in the Frozen State.* Boca Raton, FL: CRC Press, 2004, pp. 3–65.
3. Hubalek Z. Protectants used in the cryopreservation of microorganisms. *Cryobiology* 2003; **46:** 205–229.
4. Karow AM, Jr. Cryoprotectants: a new class of drugs. *J Pharm Pharmacol* 1969; **21:** 209–223.
5. Pedro PB, Yokoyama E, Zhu SE, *et al.* Permeability of mouse oocytes and embryos at various developmental stages to five cryoprotectants. *J Reprod Dev* 2005; **51:** 235–246.
6. Karlsson JO, Younis AI, Chan AW, Gould KG, Eroglu A. Permeability of the rhesus monkey oocyte membrane to water and common cryoprotectants. *Mol Reprod Dev* 2009: **76:** 321–333.
7. Agca Y, Liu J, Peter AT, Critser ES, Critser JK. Effect of developmental stage on bovine oocyte plasma membrane water and cryoprotectant permeability characteristics. *Mol Reprod Dev* 1998; **49:** 408–415.
8. Seki A, Miyauchi S, Hayashi S, *et al.* Heterologous expression of Pharaonis halorhodopsin in *Xenopus laevis* oocytes and electrophysiological characterization of its light-driven Cl– pump activity. *Biophys J* 2007; **92:** 2559–2569.
9. Valdez DM, Jr., Miyamoto A, Hara T, *et al.* Water- and cryoprotectant-permeability of mature and immature oocytes in the medaka (Oryzias latipes). *Cryobiology* 2005; **50:** 93–102.
10. Benson CT, Critser JK. Variation of water permeability (Lp) and its activation energy (Ea) among unfertilized golden hamster and ICR murine oocytes. *Cryobiology* 1994; **31:** 215–223.
11. Chaveiro A, Liu J, Engel B, Critser JK, Woelders H. Significant variability among bulls in the sperm membrane permeability for water and glycerol: possible implications for semen freezing protocols for individual males. *Cryobiology* 2006; **53:** 349–359.
12. Santos NC, Figueira-Coelho J, Martins-Silva J, Saldanha C. Multidisciplinary utilization of dimethyl sulfoxide: pharmacological, cellular, and molecular aspects. *Biochem Pharmacol* 2003; **65:** 1035–1041.
13. Whittingham DG, Leibo SP, Mazur P. Survival of mouse embryos frozen to −196 degrees and −269 degrees C. *Science* 1972; **178:** 411–414.
14. Trounson A, Mohr L. Human pregnancy following cryopreservation, thawing and transfer of an eight-cell embryo. *Nature* 1983; **305**: 707–709.
15. Zeilmaker GH, Alberda AT, van Gent I, Rijkmans CM, Drogendijk AC. Two pregnancies following transfer of intact frozen–thawed embryos. *Fertil Steril* 1984; **42:** 293–296.
16. Chen C. Pregnancy after human oocyte cryopreservation. *Lancet* 1986; **i**: 884–886.
17. Karran G, Legge M. Non-enzymatic formation of formaldehyde in mouse oocyte freezing mixtures. *Hum Reprod* 1996; **11:** 2681–2686.
18. Gardner DK, Rienzi L, Katz-Jaffe M, Larman MG. Analysis of oocyte physiology to improve

cryopreservation procedures. *Theriogenology* 2007; **67:** 64–72.
19. Vincent C, Pickering SJ, Johnson MH. The hardening effect of dimethyl sulphoxide on the mouse zona pellucida requires the presence of an oocyte and is associated with a reduction in the number of cortical granules present. *J Reprod Fertil* 1990; **89:** 253–259.
20. Vincent C, Pickering SJ, Johnson MH, Quick SJ. Dimethyl sulphoxide affects the organisation of microfilaments in the mouse oocyte. *Mol Reprod Dev* 1990; **26:** 227–235.
21. Johnson MH, Pickering SJ. The effect of dimethyl sulphoxide on the microtubular system of the mouse oocyte. *Development* 1987; **100:** 313–324.
22. Pickering SJ, Braude PR, Johnson MH. Cryoprotection of human oocytes: inappropriate exposure to DMSO reduces fertilization rates. *Hum Reprod* 1991; **6:** 142–143.
23. Van der Elst J, Nerinckx S, Van Steirteghem AC. In vitro maturation of mouse germinal vesicle-stage oocytes following cooling, exposure to cryoprotectants and ultrarapid freezing: limited effect on the morphology of the second meiotic spindle. *Hum Reprod* 1992; **7:** 1440–1446.
24. George MA, Pickering SJ, Braude PR, Johnson MH. The distribution of alpha- and gamma-tubulin in fresh and aged human and mouse oocytes exposed to cryoprotectant. *Mol Hum Reprod* 1996; **2:** 445–456.
25. Vincent C, Garnier V, Heyman Y, Renard JP. Solvent effects on cytoskeletal organization and in-vivo survival after freezing of rabbit oocytes. *J Reprod Fertil* 1989; **87:** 809–820.
26. Alvarenga MA, Papa FO, Landim-Alvarenga FC, Medeiros AS. Amides as cryoprotectants for freezing stallion semen: a review. *Anim Reprod Sci* 2005; **89:** 105–113.
27. Squires EL, Keith SL, Graham JK. Evaluation of alternative cryoprotectants for preserving stallion spermatozoa. *Theriogenology* 2004; **62:** 1056–1065.
28. Medeiros A, Gomes G, Carmo M, Papa F, Alvarenga M. Cryopreservation of stallion sperm using different amides. *Theriogenology* 2002; **58:** 273–276.
29. Lukaszewicz E. An effective method for freezing White Italian gander semen. *Theriogenology* 2002; **58:** 19–27.
30. Futino DO, Mendes MCB, Matos WNL, Mondadori RG, Lucci CM. Glycerol, methyl-formamide and dimethyl-formamide in canine semen cryopreservation. *Reprod Domest Anim* 2008; epub.
31. Sztein JM, Noble K, Farley JS, Mobraaten LE. Comparison of permeating and nonpermeating cryoprotectants for mouse sperm cryopreservation. *Cryobiology* 2001; **42:** 28–39.
32. Hanada A, Nagase H. Cryoprotective effects of some amides on rabbit spermatozoa. *J Reprod Fertil* 1980; **60:** 247–252.
33. Rall W, Fahy G. Ice-free cryopreservation of mouse embryos at −196°C by vitrification. *Nature* 1985; **313:** 573–575.
34. Edashige K, Ohta S, Tanaka M, *et al.* The role of aquaporin 3 in the movement of water and cryoprotectants in mouse morulae. *Biol Reprod* 2007; **77:** 365–375.
35. Otsuka J, Takahashi A, Nagaoka M, Funabashi H. Optimal equilibration conditions for practical vitrification of two-cell mouse embryos. *Comp Med* 2002; **52:** 342–346.
36. Migishima F, Suzuki-Migishima R, Song SY, *et al.* Successful cryopreservation of mouse ovaries by vitrification. *Biol Reprod* 2003; **68:** 881–887.
37. Hochi S, Hirabayashi M, Hirao M, *et al.* Effects of cryopreservation of pronuclear-stage rabbit zygotes on the morphological survival, blastocyst formation, and full-term development after DNA microinjection. *Mol Reprod Dev* 2001; **60:** 227–232.
38. Kono T, Suzuki O, Tsunoda Y. Cryopreservation of rat blastocysts by vitrification. *Cryobiology* 1988; **25:** 170–173.
39. Yoshino J, Kojima T, Shimizu M, Tomizuka T. Cryopreservation of porcine blastocysts by vitrification. *Cryobiology* 1993; **30:** 413–422.
40. Nakagata N. High survival rate of unfertilized mouse oocytes after vitrification. *J Reprod Fertil* 1989; **87:** 479–483.
41. Mukaida T, Wada S, Takahashi K, *et al.* Vitrification of human embryos based on the assessment of suitable conditions for 8-cell mouse embryos. *Hum Reprod* 1998; **13:** 2874–2879.
42. Guan M, Rawson DM, Zhang T. Cryopreservation of zebrafish (Danio rerio) oocytes using improved controlled slow cooling protocols. *Cryobiology* 2008; **56:** 204–208.
43. Tervit HR, Adams SL, Roberts RD, *et al.* Successful cryopreservation of Pacific oyster (Crassostrea gigas) oocytes. *Cryobiology* 2005; **51:** 142–151.
44. Nascimento IA, Leite MB, Sampaio de Araujo MM, *et al.* Selection of cryoprotectants based on their toxic effects on oyster gametes and embryos. *Cryobiology* 2005; **51:** 113–117.
45. Zhang YZ, Zhang SC, Liu XZ, *et al.* Toxicity and protective efficiency of cryoprotectants to flounder (Paralichthys olivaceus) embryos. *Theriogenology* 2005; **63:** 763–773.
46. Bass LD, Denniston DJ, MacLellan LJ, *et al.* Methanol as a cryoprotectant for equine embryos. *Theriogenology* 2004; **62:** 1153–1159.
47. Takagi M, Otoi T, Suzuki T. Survival rate of frozen–thawed bovine IVM/IVF embryos in relation to post-thaw exposure time in two cryoprotectants. *Cryobiology* 1993; **30:** 466–469.
48. Takagi M, Boediono A, Saha S, Suzuki T. Survival rate of frozen–thawed bovine IVF embryos in relation

to exposure time using various cryoprotectants. *Cryobiology* 1993; **30:** 306–312.

49. Polge C, Smith AU, Parkes AS. Revival of spermatozoa after vitrification and dehydration at low temperatures. *Nature* 1949; **164**: 666.
50. Testart J, Lassalle B, Belaisch-Allart J, *et al.* High pregnancy rate after early human embryo freezing. *Fertil Steril* 1986; **46:** 268–272.
51. Hotamisligil S, Toner M, Powers RD. Changes in membrane integrity, cytoskeletal structure, and developmental potential of murine oocytes after vitrification in ethylene glycol. *Biol Reprod* 1996; **55:** 161–168.
52. Cooper TG, Barfield JP, Yeung CH. The tonicity of murine epididymal spermatozoa and their permeability towards common cryoprotectants and epididymal osmolytes. *Reproduction* 2008; **135:** 625–633.
53. Suzuki T, Takagi M, Yamamoto M, *et al.* Pregnancy rate and survival in culture of in vitro fertilized bovine embryos frozen in various cryoprotectants and thawed using a one-step system. *Theriogenology* 1993; **40:** 651–659.
54. Pugh PA, Tervit HR, Niemann H. Effects of vitrification medium composition on the survival of bovine in vitro produced embryos, following in straw-dilution, in vitro and in vivo following transfer. *Anim Reprod Sci* 2000; **58**: 9–22.
55. Valdez CA, Abas Mazni O, Takahashi Y, Fujikawa S, Kanagawa H. Successful cryopreservation of mouse blastocysts using a new vitrification solution. *J Reprod Fertil* 1992; **96:** 793–802.
56. Ali J, Shelton JN. Design of vitrification solutions for the cryopreservation of embryos. *J Reprod Fertil* 1993; **99:** 471–477.
57. Todorov I, Berstein A, McGrath J, Fuller B, Shaw R. Studies on 2,3-butanediol as a cryoprotectant for mouse oocytes: use of sucrose to avoid damage during exposure or removal. *Cryo Letters* 1993: **14**: 37–42.
58. Hoagland H, Pincus G. Revival of mammalian sperm after immersion in liquid nitrogen. *J Gen Physiol* 1942: 337–344.
59. Parkes A. Preservation of human spermatozoa at low temperatures. *Br J Med* 1945: **2**: 212–213.
60. Sherman JK, Bunge RG. Effect of glycerol and freezing on some staining reactions of human spermatozoa. *Proc Soc Exp Biol Med* 1953; **84:** 179–180.
61. Lin TP, Sherman JK, Willett EL. Survival of unfertilized mouse eggs in media containing glycerol and glycine. *J Exp Zool* 1957; **134:** 275–291.
62. Sherman JK, Lin TP. Effect of glycerol and low temperature on survival of unfertilized mouse eggs. *Nature* 1958; **181**: 785–786.
63. Lovestock J. The mechanism of the protective effect of glycerol against haemolysis by freezing and thawing. *Biochem Biophys Acta* 1959; **31**: 28–36.
64. Seki S, Kouya T, Hara T, *et al.* Exogenous expression of rat aquaporin-3 enhances permeability to water and cryoprotectants of immature oocytes in the zebrafish (Danio rerio). *J Reprod Dev* 2007; **53:** 597–604.
65. Valdez DM, Jr., Hara T, Miyamoto A, *et al.* Expression of aquaporin-3 improves the permeability to water and cryoprotectants of immature oocytes in the medaka (Oryzias latipes). *Cryobiology* 2006; **53:** 160–168.
66. Utsumi K, Hochi S, Iritani A. Cryoprotective effect of polyols on rat embryos during two-step freezing. *Cryobiology* 1992; **29:** 332–341.
67. Molinia FC, Evans G, Maxwell WM. Effect of polyols on the post-thawing motility of pellet-frozen ram spermatozoa. *Theriogenology* 1994; **42:** 15–23.
68. Alvarez JG, Storey BT. Evidence that membrane stress contributes more than lipid peroxidation to sublethal cryodamage in cryopreserved human sperm: glycerol and other polyols as sole cryoprotectant. *J Androl* 1993; **14:** 199–209.
69. Fuller B, Lane N, Benson E. *Life in the Frozen State*. Boca Raton: CRC Press, 2004, p. 672.
70. Kuleshova L, MacFarlane D, Trounson A, Shaw J. Sugars exert a major influence on the vitrification properties of ethylene glycol-based solutions and have low toxicity to embryos and oocytes. *Cryobiology* 1999; **38:** 119–130.
71. Vincent C, Turner K, Pickering SJ, Johnson MH. Zona pellucida modifications in the mouse in the absence of oocyte activation. *Mol Reprod Dev* 1991; **28:** 394–404.
72. Yildiz C, Kaya A, Aksoy M, Tekeli T. Influence of sugar supplementation of the extender on motility, viability and acrosomal integrity of dog spermatozoa during freezing. *Theriogenology* 2000; **54:** 579–585.
73. McWilliams RB, Gibbons WE, Leibo SP. Osmotic and physiological responses of mouse zygotes and human oocytes to mono- and disaccharides. *Hum Reprod* 1995; **10:** 1163–1171.
74. Arns MJ, Webb GW, Kreider JL, Potter GD, Evans JW. Use of different nonglycolysable sugars to maintain stallion sperm viability when frozen or stored at 37 degrees C and 5 degrees C in a bovine serum albumin medium. *J Reprod Fertil Suppl* 1987; **35**: 135–141.
75. Fernandez-Santos MR, Martinez-Pastor F, Garcia-Macias V, *et al.* Extender osmolality and sugar supplementation exert a complex effect on the cryopreservation of Iberian red deer (Cervus elaphus hispanicus) epididymal spermatozoa. *Theriogenology* 2007; **67:** 738–53.
76. Hay MA, Goodrowe KL. Comparative cryopreservation and capacitation of spermatozoa from epididymides and vasa deferentia of the domestic cat. *J Reprod Fertil Suppl* 1993; **47**: 297–305.
77. Kasai M. Nonfreezing technique for short-term storage of mouse embryos. *J In Vitro Fert Embryo Transf* 1986; **3:** 10–14.

78. Luyet B, Hodapp A. Revival of frog's spermatozoa vitrified in liquid air. *Proc Meet Soc Exp Biol* 1938; **36**: 433–434.
79. Sola-Penna M, Meyer-Fernandes JR. Stabilization against thermal inactivation promoted by sugars on enzyme structure and function: why is trehalose more effective than other sugars? *Arch Biochem Biophys* 1998; **360:** 10–14.
80. Lin TY, Timasheff SN. On the role of surface tension in the stabilization of globular proteins. *Protein Sci* 1996; **5:** 372–381.
81. Honadel TE, Killian GJ. Cryopreservation of murine embryos with trehalose and glycerol. *Cryobiology* 1988; **25:** 331–337.
82. Begin I, Bhatia B, Baldassarre H, Dinnyes A, Keefer CL. Cryopreservation of goat oocytes and in vivo derived 2- to 4-cell embryos using the cryoloop (CLV) and solid-surface vitrification (SSV) methods. *Theriogenology* 2003; **59:** 1839–1850.
83. Isachenko V, Alabart JL, Dattena M, *et al.* New technology for vitrification and field (microscope-free) warming and transfer of small ruminant embryos. *Theriogenology* 2003; **59**: 1209–1218.
84. Saha S, Otoi T, Takagi M, *et al.* Normal calves obtained after direct transfer of vitrified bovine embryos using ethylene glycol, trehalose, and polyvinylpyrrolidone. *Cryobiology* 1996; **33:** 291–299.
85. Bagis H, Sagirkaya H, Mercan HO, Dinnyes A. Vitrification of pronuclear-stage mouse embryos on solid surface (SSV) versus in cryotube: comparison of the effect of equilibration time and different sugars in the vitrification solution. *Mol Reprod Dev* 2004; **67:** 186–192.
86. Eroglu A, Bailey SE, Toner M, Toth TL. Successful cryopreservation of mouse oocytes by using low concentrations of trehalose and dimethylsulfoxide. *Biol Reprod* 2009; **80:** 70–78.
87. Eroglu A, Bailey SE, Toner M, Toth TL. Quantitative microinjection of trehalose into mouse oocytes and zygotes, and its effect on development. *Cryobiology* 2003; **46:** 121–134.
88. Eroglu A, Toner M, Toth TL. Beneficial effect of microinjected trehalose on the cryosurvival of human oocytes. *Fertil Steril* 2002; **77:** 152–158.
89. Storey BT, Noiles EE, Thompson KA. Comparison of glycerol, other polyols, trehalose, and raffinose to provide a defined cryoprotectant medium for mouse sperm cryopreservation. *Cryobiology* 1998; **37:** 46–58.
90. Chen Y, Foote RH, Brockett CC. Effect of sucrose, trehalose, hypotaurine, taurine, and blood serum on survival of frozen bull sperm. *Cryobiology* 1993; **30:** 423–431.
91. Vicente JS, Viudes-de-Castro MP. A sucrose–DMSO extender for freezing rabbit semen. *Reprod Nutr Dev* 1996; **36:** 485–492.
92. Tada N, Sato M, Yamanoi J, *et al.* Cryopreservation of mouse spermatozoa in the presence of raffinose and glycerol. *J Reprod Fertil* 1990; **89:** 511–516.
93. Ostermeier GC, Wiles MV, Farley JS, Taft RA . Conserving, distributing and managing genetically modified mouse lines by sperm cryopreservation. *PLoS ONE*, 2008; **3:** e2792.
94. Songsasen N, Betteridge KJ, Leibo SP. Birth of live mice resulting from oocytes fertilized in vitro with cryopreserved spermatozoa. *Biol Reprod* 1997; **56:** 143–152.
95. Garde JJ, del Olmo A, Soler AJ, *et al.* Effect of egg yolk, cryoprotectant, and various sugars on semen cryopreservation in endangered Cuvier's gazelle (Gazella cuvieri). *Anim Reprod Sci* 2008; **108**: 384–401.
96. de la Pena EC, Takahashi Y, Atabay EC, Katagiri S, Nagano M . Vitrification of mouse oocytes in ethylene glycol–raffinose solution: effects of preexposure to ethylene glycol or raffinose on oocyte viability. *Cryobiology* 2001; **42:** 103–111.
97. Nagano M, Atabay EP, Atabay EC, *et al.* Effects of isolation method and pre-treatment with ethylene glycol or raffinose before vitrification on in vitro viability of mouse preantral follicles. *Biomed Res* 2007; **28:** 153–160.
98. Gomez MC, Pope E, Harris R, Mikota S, Dresser BL. Development of in vitro matured, in vitro fertilized domestic cat embryos following cryopreservation, culture and transfer. *Theriogenology* 2003; **60:** 239–251.
99. Kuleshova LL, Shaw JM, Trounson AO. Studies on replacing most of the penetrating cryoprotectant by polymers for embryo cryopreservation. *Cryobiology* 2001; **43:** 21–31.
100. Dumoulin JC, Bergers-Janssen JM, Pieters MH, *et al.* The protective effects of polymers in the cryopreservation of human and mouse zonae pellucidae and embryos. *Fertil Steril* 1994; **62:** 793–798.
101. Shaw JM, Kuleshova LL, MacFarlane DR, Trounson AO. Vitrification properties of solutions of ethylene glycol in saline containing PVP, Ficoll, or dextran. *Cryobiology* 1997; **35:** 219–229.
102. MacKenzie AP. Non-equilibrium freezing behaviour of aqueous systems. *Philos Trans R Soc Lond B Biol Sci* 1977; **278**: 167–189.
103. Fuller BJ. Cryoprotectants: the essential antifreezes to protect life in the frozen state. *Cryo Letters* 2004; **25:** 375–388.
104. Endoh K, Mochida K, Ogonuki N, *et al.* The developmental ability of vitrified oocytes from different mouse strains assessed by parthenogenetic activation and intracytoplasmic sperm injection. *J Reprod Dev* 2007; **53:** 1199–1206.
105. Merlo B, Iacono E, Regazzini M, Zambelli D. Cat blastocysts produced in vitro from oocytes vitrified using the cryoloop technique and cryopreserved

electroejaculated semen. *Theriogenology* 2008; **70:** 126–130.

106. Huang J, Li Q, Zhao R, *et al.* Effect of sugars on maturation rate of vitrified-thawed immature porcine oocytes. *Anim Reprod Sci* 2008; **106**: 25–35.
107. Hurtt AE, Landim-Alvarenga F, Seidel GE, Jr., Squires EL. Vitrification of immature and mature equine and bovine oocytes in an ethylene glycol, Ficoll and sucrose solution using open-pulled straws. *Theriogenology* 2000; **54:** 119–128.
108. Checura CM, Seidel GE, Jr. Effect of macromolecules in solutions for vitrification of mature bovine oocytes. *Theriogenology* 2007; **67:** 919–930.
109. Yeoman RR, Gerami-Naini B, Mitalipov S, *et al.* Cryoloop vitrification yields superior survival of Rhesus monkey blastocysts. *Hum Reprod* 2001; **16:** 1965–1969.
110. Liebermann J, Tucker MJ, Sills ES. Cryoloop vitrification in assisted reproduction: analysis of survival rates in > 1000 human oocytes after ultra-rapid cooling with polymer augmented cryoprotectants. *Clin Exp Obstet Gynecol* 2003; **30**: 125–129.
111. O ' Neil L, Paynter SJ, Fuller BJ. Vitrification of mature mouse oocytes: improved results following addition of polyethylene glycol to a dimethyl sulfoxide solution. *Cryobiology* 1997; **34:** 295–301.
112. Ohboshi S, Etoh T, Sakamoto K, *et al.* Effects of bovine serum proteins in culture medium on post-warming survival of bovine blastocysts developed in vitro. *Theriogenology* 1997; **47:** 1237–1243.
113. Whittingham D. Survival of mouse embryos after freezing and thawing. *Nature* 1971; **233**: 125–126.
114. Titterington JL, Robinson J, Killick SR, Hay DM. Synthetic and biological macromolecules: protection of mouse embryos during cryopreservation by vitrification. *Hum Reprod* 1995; **10:** 649–653.
115. Gutierrez A, Garde J, Artiga CG, Munoz I, Pintado B. In vitro survival of murine morulae after quick freezing in the presence of chemically defined macromolecules and different cryoprotectants. *Theriogenology* 1993; **39:** 1111–1120.
116. Nowshari MA, Brem G. The protective action of polyvinyl alcohol during rapid-freezing of mouse embryos. *Theriogenology* 2000; **53:** 1157–1166.
117. Asada M, Ishibashi S, Ikumi S, Fukui Y. Effect of polyvinyl alcohol (PVA) concentration during vitrification of in vitro matured bovine oocytes. *Theriogenology* 2002; **58:** 1199–1208.
118. Naitana S, Ledda S, Loi P, *et al.* Polyvinyl alcohol as a defined substitute for serum in vitrification and warming solutions to cryopreserve ovine embryos at different stages of development. *Anim Reprod Sci* 1997; **48**: 247–256.
119. Leoni G, Bogliolo L, Berlinguer F, *et al.* Defined media for vitrification, warming, and rehydration: effects on post-thaw protein synthesis and viability of in vitro derived ovine embryos. *Cryobiology* 2002; **45:** 204–212.
120. Sommerfeld V, Niemann H. Cryopreservation of bovine in vitro produced embryos using ethylene glycol in controlled freezing or vitrification. *Cryobiology* 1999; **38:** 95–105.
121. Palasz A, Alkemade S, Mapletoft RJ. The use of sodium hyaluronate in freezing media for bovine and murine embryos. *Cryobiology* 1993; **30:** 172–178.
122. Palasz AT, Alkemade S, Mapletoft RJ. Development, molecular composition and freeze tolerance of bovine embryos cultured in TCM-199 supplemented with hyaluronan. *Zygote* 2008; **16:** 39–47.
123. Palasz AT, Thundathil J, De La Fuente J, Mapletoft RJ. Effect of reduced concentrations of glycerol and various macromolecules on the cryopreservation of mouse and cattle embryos. *Cryobiology* 2000; **41:** 35–42.
124. Franco M, Hansen PJ. Effects of hyaluronic acid in culture and cytochalasin B treatment before freezing on survival of cryopreserved bovine embryos produced in vitro. *In Vitro Cell Dev Biol Anim* 2006; **42**: 40–44.
125. Jolly T, Nibart M, Thibier C. Hyaluranic acid as a substitute for protein in the deep freezing of embryos for mice and sheep: an in vitro investigation. *Theriogenology* 1992; **37**: 473–480.
126. Pena FJ, Johannisson A, Wallgren M, Rodriguez-Martinez H. Effect of hyaluronan supplementation on boar sperm motility and membrane lipid architecture status after cryopreservation. *Theriogenology* 2004; **61:** 63–70.
127. Fahy GM, Lilley TH, Linsdell H, Douglas MS, Meryman HT. Cryoprotectant toxicity and cryoprotectant toxicity reduction: in search of molecular mechanisms. *Cryobiology* 1990; **27:** 247–268.
128. Fahy G. Vitrification: a new approach to organ cryopreservation. *Prog Clin Biol Res* 1986; **224**: 305–335.
129. Anchordoguy TJ, Rudolph AS, Carpenter JF, Crowe JH. Modes of interaction of cryoprotectants with membrane phospholipids during freezing. *Cryobiology* 1987; **24:** 324–331.
130. Gurtovenko AA, Anwar J. Modulating the structure and properties of cell membranes: the molecular mechanism of action of dimethyl sulfoxide. *J Phys Chem B* 2007; **111:** 10453–10460.
131. Fahy GM, Wowk B, Wu J, Paynter S. Improved vitrification solutions based on the predictability of vitrification solution toxicity. *Cryobiology* 2004; **48:** 22–35.
132. Van der Elst J, Nerinckx S, Van Steirteghem A. In vitro maturation of mouse germinal vesicle-stage oocytes following cooling, exposure to cryoprotectants and ultrarapid freezing: limited effect on the morphology of the second meiotic spindle. *Hum Reprod* 1992; **7**: 1440–1446.

133. Van der Elst J, Van den Abbeel E, Nerinckx S, Van Steirteghem A. Parthenogenetic activation pattern and microtubular organization of the mouse oocyte after exposure to 1,2-propanediol. *Cryobiology* 1992; **29:** 549–562.
134. Vincent C, Johnson M. Cooling cryoprotectants and the cytoskeleton of the mammalian oocyte. *Oxford Rev Reprod Biol* 1992; **14:** 73–100.
135. Vincent C, Pruliere G, Pajot-Augy E, *et al.* Effects of cryoprotectants on actin filaments during the cryopreservation of one-cell rabbit embryos. *Cryobiology* 1990; **27:** 9–23.
136. Joly C, Bchini O, Boulekbache H, Testart J, Maro B. Effects of 1,2-propanediol on the cytoskeletal organization of the mouse oocyte. *Hum Reprod* 1992; **7:** 374–378.
137. Shaw JM, Trounson AO. Parthenogenetic activation of unfertilized mouse oocytes by exposure to 1,2-propanediol is influenced by temperature, oocyte age, and cumulus removal. *Gamete Res* 1989; **24:** 269–279.
138. Gook DA, Osborn SM, Johnston WI. Parthenogenetic activation of human oocytes following cryopreservation using 1,2-propanediol. *Hum Reprod* 1995; **10:** 654–658.
139. Katz-Jaffe MG, Larman MG, Sheehan CB, Gardner DK. Exposure of mouse oocytes to 1,2-propanediol during slow freezing alters the proteome. *Fertil Steril* 2008; **89**(Suppl 5): 1441–1447.
140. Pickering S, Braude P, Johnson M. Cryoprotection of human oocytes: inappropriate exposure to DMSO reduces fertilization rates. *Hum Reprod* 1991; **6:** 142–143.
141. Rasul Z, Ahmed N, Anzar M. Antagonist effect of DMSO on the cryoprotection ability of glycerol during cryopreservation of buffalo sperm. *Theriogenology* 2007; **68:** 813–819.
142. Pickering S, Braude P, Johnson M, Cant A, Currie J. Transient cooling to room temperature can cause irreversible disruption of the meiotic spindle in the human oocyte. *Fertil Steril* 1990; **54:** 102–108.
143. Pickering S, Johnson M. The influence of cooling on the organization of the meiotic spindle of the mouse oocyte. *Hum Reprod* 1987; **2:** 207–216.
144. Larman MG, Katz-Jaffe MG, Sheehan CB, Gardner DK. 1,2-Propanediol and the type of cryopreservation procedure adversely affect mouse oocyte physiology. *Hum Reprod* 2007; **22:** 250–259.
145. Wilmut I. The effect of cooling rate, warming rate, cryoprotective agent and stage of development on survival of mouse embryos during freezing and thawing. *Life Sci II* 1972; **11:** 1071–1079.
146. Wilmut I, Rowson LE. The successful low-temperature preservation of mouse and cow embryos. *J Reprod Fertil* 1973; **33:** 352–353.
147. Stachecki JJ, Cohen J, Willadsen SM. Cryopreservation of unfertilized mouse oocytes: the effect of replacing sodium with choline in the freezing medium. *Cryobiology* 1998; **37:** 346–354.

Section 2 Chapter 5

Cryopreservation of sperm and testicular tissue

Cryopreservation of sperm: an overview

Fady Shehata and Ri-Cheng Chian

Introduction

Although the term cryopreservation may sound as though this is one of the recent advancements in medicine, the concept is not modern. In fact, as early as the eighteenth century, Lazaro Spallanzani, a famous Italian biologist who is known to have performed the first artificial insemination in dogs, had observed the effect of freezing on arresting human sperm motility [1]. Also, the idea of sperm banks was conceived as early as the nineteenth century by Montegazza, who discovered that human sperm can actually survive at temperatures below −15°C and saw this as an opportunity to preserve semen for soldiers going off to a battle in order to avoid depriving them of a legal heir [1,2].

In these early experiments, researchers were keen to observe the effect of varying freezing temperatures on sperm viability, but the studies did not extend beyond mere observations and usually these were simply a part of other research projects for different reasons. At the beginning of the nineteenth century, the ability of a sperm to survive at a temperature reaching −160°C was documented; yet, the majority of these sperm samples could not survive the damaging effect of ice formation inside the sperm (i.e. freezing injury) because cryoprotectants were not known at that time [3,4]. Fortunately, the accidental discovery of cryoprotectants, primarily glycerol, boosted the use and application of cryopreservation techniques in both human and animal models and catalyzed the advance in cryopreservation research [2,5]. Subsequently, the first case report of human pregnancy from a frozen sperm specimen was reported by Bunge and colleagues in the middle of the 20th century [1,6]. By 1973, over 500 babies had been born from use of cryopreserved sperm [7,8]. To date, there are thousands and thousands of infants who were born after fertilization using frozen–thawed human sperm.

Sperm cryopreservation is a widely used and established method in humans, animals, fish, and insects. In animals, it forms a part of breeding techniques in cattle, pigs, and sheep, as well as in domestic pets such as cats or dogs. In humans, sperm cryopreservation is a widely used technique in assisted reproductive technologies (ART) and fertility preservation in patients with cancer.

Initially, sperm cryopreservation was used to preserve bulls' semen for future use to inseminate cows located at distant farms [9]. This was made possible after the discovery of glycerol as a cryoprotectant, an incident that revolutionized cryopreservation methodology [5]. Later on, cryopreservation techniques were used either to increase the production of livestock or to introduce breeding of cattle and sheep in areas of the world that lacked primary meat sources [4]. Sperm cryopreservation in animals is also a primary method used in protecting precious lines during epidemics of foot and mouth diseases, as sperm samples can be stored for years and used to produce healthy stock whenever the epidemic disease has disappeared [4].

Nowadays, cryopreservation plays an important role in conservation biology [10]. Protection of endangered species is an important indication for sperm cryopreservation, and scientists can preserve semen from exotic or endangered species for years to use these samples later in artificial insemination to breed animals [11]. Zoos around the world benefit from this technique to preserve various species, including cheetahs, leopard cats [12], and Eld's deers [13].

In insects, sperm cryopreservation has played an important role in preservation of genetic species and maintenance of stocks, for example in silkworm [14], but the use of frozen sperm in artificial insemination in insects has some specific hurdles because of the unique nature of fertilization in insects [15–17]. However, fertilization using frozen–thawed sperm in

Fertility Cryopreservation, ed. Ri-Cheng Chian and Patrick Quinn. Published by Cambridge University Press.

Athalia rosae (Hymenoptera) has been successfully achieved [18].

Clinical applications of sperm cryopreservation in humans

Sperm cryopreservation describes a complex multi-step process for preserving male gametes. The process involves collecting a sperm sample, then gradually cooling the sample in the presence of a cryoprotective agent, followed by storage of the sample for future use. It ends when the sperm is thawed and used to fertilize oocytes naturally or by intracytoplasmic sperm injection (ICSI) [19]. Today, there are numerous clinical applications for human sperm cryopreservation and sperm banking in a wide range of healthcare services, including primary, curative, and prophylactic medicine. However, the major application of sperm cryopreservation resides in the fields of ART and fertility preservation prior to initiation of cancer therapy.

Assisted reproductive technologies

In ART, the most common use of sperm cryopreservation is in artificial insemination, in vitro fertilization (IVF), or ICSI for various infertile couples [20]. One of the ART options usually offered to infertile couples is intrauterine insemination using fresh or frozen sperm. Although the technique is used preferably with a fresh semen sample, the availability of cryopreserved sperm samples is an option usually offered by infertility clinics in case the male partner cannot produce viable sperm, thus preventing fertilization and potential pregnancy [20]. Anonymous frozen sperm banking has been a fundamental concept of ART for several decades.

Fertility preservation with cancer therapy

Another application of sperm cryopreservation is for cancer patients before initiation of cancer therapy. The option of sperm preservation should be offered to any male undergoing chemotherapy or radiotherapy as these treatments can have long-term or permanent cytotoxic side effects on testicular function. One of the advantages of cryopreservation here is that the frozen sperm can stand multiple freezing–thawing cycles with no effect on the sperm quality; this is beneficial in cases where patients might have testicular cancer and require surgical removal of the whole testis, with no future possibility of obtaining sperm again [21]. For young males before puberty, cryopreservation of testicular tissue may be an option for fertility preservation. In the future, improved chemotherapy regimens may give hope to patients in terms of maintaining their sexual and fertility potential after therapy, but at present all male patients diagnosed with cancer who wish to have children should consider sperm cryopreservation or cryopreservation of testicular tissue for future ART use.

Non-malignancy systemic diseases and other conditions

Cryopreservation of sperm or testicular tissue can also be used in patients prior to cytotoxic therapy for non-malignant conditions, such as autoimmune diseases, kidney diseases, inflammatory bowel diseases, and heart transplant procedures [22]. Most of these conditions are not fatal and the patients should be offered cryopreservation of their sperm or testicular tissue prior to the cytotoxic therapy in order to preserve their fertility for the future.

Surgical procedures involving male genitalia

Sperm cryopreservation can also be used prophylactically before, during, or after certain surgical procedures as these may have serious adverse effects on male genital structure and function. An example is the varicocele ligation procedure [23] or reconstructive surgery (e.g. vasovasectomy or vasoepididmostomy) [24]. Sperm cryopreservation may also be used postoperatively to insure against subsequent loss of patency of the vas deferens.

Social and other reasons

Sperm cryopreservation could be a mean of preserving fertility in men with social reasons to preserve their rights to have children bearing their names, for example soldiers being deployed to combat missions in war. Other reasons for sperm cryopreservation might be immediately pre and postmortem where relatives of a person wish to ensure that that the person can have a legal heir [25–28].

Sperm cryopreservation protocols

Raw techniques in sperm cryopreservation developed as early as the eighteenth century; however, these studies were mere observations of the effect of freezing on arresting sperm motility and speculation about the idea of preserving semen in sperm banks. A cascade of research studies examined the effect of different cooling and thawing temperatures on sperm motility and function. Hoagland and Pincus in 1941 [29] applied an ultrarapid freezing technique for human and rabbit sperms and observed good cryosurvival rates following rapid immersion of sperm samples in liquid nitrogen. Polge and his colleagues [5,30] stored fowl semen samples at −70°C using levulose as a cryoprotectant when they accidentally discovered that adding glycerol instead of levulose to frozen semen actually protected sperm from cryoinjury. This method is now referred to as the classic approach to cryopreservation and is still used basically in some cryopreservation facilities today.

Cryoprotectants such as glycerol revolutionized cryopreservation techniques and paved the way for storing sperm samples for up to several years. As new cryoprotectants were discovered, the main issue was the degree of protection that they could provide for sperm from damage caused by rapid freezing. Nowadays, techniques of sperm cryopreservation are diverse, and each technique is tested for its effect in protecting sperm from damage and for the percentage of sperm surviving following thawing. There is no current gold standard technique, and all techniques are being constantly evaluated and optimized for better results [31–34].

Method of sperm collection

Sperm cryopreservation starts with sperm collection. The most common method of sperm collection used is masturbation followed by analysis of the collected sample [35]. In men with obstructive azoospermia or other cause preventing them from producing a sperm sample by masturbation, surgical approaches are used to retrieve sperm from the epididymis using microsurgical epididymal sperm aspiration [36,37] or percutaneous epididymal sperm aspiration [38]. The majority of studies suggest that the microsurgical approach gives overall better results in terms of sperm count [39,40]. There are several other methods of collecting sperm, but these are not covered here as they feature in other chapters in this section.

The classic technique for sperm cryopreservation

The classic technique is a slow-freezing method. The most classic sperm cryopreservation protocol was developed by Polge *et al.* in the 1950s [5]. After sperm collection, semen is mixed with freezing solution containing cryoprotectant. Although there are various sperm-freezing solutions being used to freeze human sperm, normally 10% glycerol as cryoprotectant in hen's egg yolk–citrate buffer (20% egg yolk) in equal ratios is used at room temperature. This will protect the sperm from cryoinjury and at the same time prevent hyperosmolar stress [41]. Vials or straws are suspended in liquid nitrogen vapor for 15 minutes (cooling speed at average 16–25°C/min) and then rapidly immersed into liquid nitrogen at −196°C for storage.

Vitrification method

Another technique for sperm cryopreservation is called rapid freezing or vitrification. Vitrification means cooling without formation of ice. The instant freezing–instant thawing technique is used for sperm cryopreservation. After sperm collection, the semen is processed as in the slow-freezing method, and the sperm is contained in vials, straws, or special design carriers and then directly plunged into liquid nitrogen for storage. Polge *et al.*(1949) had used the phrase "sperm after vitrification" in their publication; surprisingly, the most advanced cryopreservation technique developed almost half a century later bears the same wording:"sperm vitrification"[5]. In fact, in industrial animal breeding, it has been called the vitrification method for sperm cryopreservation since the early 1970s (Figure 5.1).

Recent sperm vitrification methodology has reached a more advanced stage because cryoprotectant is not used [42–44]; this avoids the potential for osmotic shock in the sperm retrieved caused by the presence of a cryoprotectant. This approach allows the survival of sperm carrying enough fertilization capacity for either IVF or ICSI following vitrification [43].

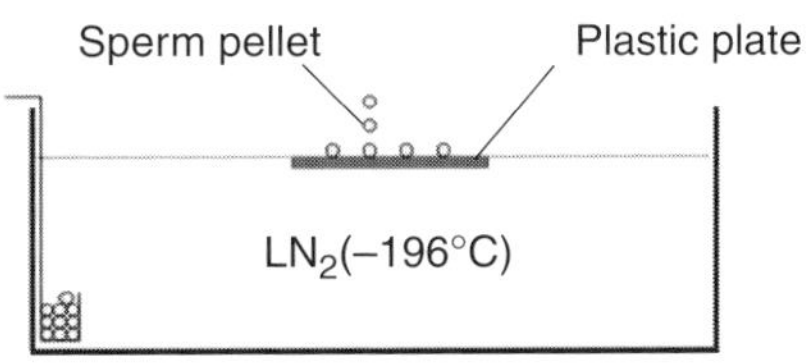

Figure 5.1. Sperm vitrification. After equilibration, bovine sperm pellets are dropped on to a floating plastic plate in liquid nitrogen (LN_2) for vitrification. Following vitrification, the pellets are peeled off for storage. This was the method used in the early days (1960–1970s) in the bovine breeding industry to freeze bull semen by vitrification.

Contraindictions, complications, and adverse effects

Relative contraindications

There are no absolute contraindications for cryopreservation based on current knowledge, but there are a few relative contraindications that could affect the decision to go on with sperm cryopreservation.

Sperm quality and quantity

Sperm quality and quantity are the two main factors that can have an effect on the success of sperm cryopreservation. Sperm analysis results indicating poor quality or low quantity may indicate the potential for significant problems with sperm cryopreservation. Consequently, it is advisable not to proceed with sperm cryopreservation for a sperm donor program whenever there is very poor quality or low quantity sperm. This can be a problem as patients with cancer often show poor sperm analysis even before initiation of chemotherapy [27,29]. Fortunately, with current advanced ART, specifically in ICSI, it is possible now to use only one viable sperm to achieve a healthy pregnancy and live birth.

Infectious diseases

The ability of some viruses to survive liquid nitrogen freezing has been documented. Hence, all men who are undergoing sperm cryopreservation should undergo regular screening for common infectious diseases as hepatitis A, B, C, and the human immunodeficiency virus (HIV) [45,46].

Complications and adverse effects

There are no complications or adverse effects for the patient himself, but there may be effects of freezing, storage, and thawing on sperm motility, viability, and morphology, and these will be discussed in this section.

Motility

When assessing the effect of cryopreservation on sperm motility, the cryopreservation process can be considered as three independent processes: freezing, storage, and thawing. The effects of each of these processes on sperm motility can be considered per se. A considerable decrease in sperm motility is usually noticed, to approximately 45%, after the slow-freezing process [47]. In patients with abnormal sperm, as in oligoasthenoteratozooaspermia, sperm motility may be reduced by up to 75%, suggesting that the sperm sample from fertile males can actually withstand cryoinjury better than samples from infertile patients [48–50]. Other studies have suggested that some agents could be added to the sperm during the thawing process to increase motility, but these agents improve sperm motility not its quality [51]. A further study examining the thawing recovery of cryopreserved sperm suggested that the freezing–thawing process triggers oxidative stress processes, which affect subsequent sperm motility [52]. This study also suggested that adding enzyme enhancers to the medium could improve the post-thawing recovery process [52].

Viability

Viability of sperm after cryopreservation is considered a key point for measuring cryopreservation success, and the ultimate indicator of its usefulness. Obviously, there is no reason to preserve semen samples if freezing, storage, and thawing will severely affect later viability. One study has analyzed how sperm viability is affected by the freezing–thawing process, and whether the freezing or the thawing phase is responsible for the damage. The authors concluded that the freezing process triggers an apoptotic cascade of events that might explain the failure of some sperms to survive after thawing [53].

Morphology

Some studies have looked into the structure of sperm before and after the freezing–thawing process and have shown numerous alterations in the cell membrane, creating severe morphological alterations [34,54–57]. In addition, there are changes in acrosomal structure, nucleus size, chromatin structure, cell organelles, and plasma membrane integrity [58–62], which are not detectable by light microscopy [50] but affect the structural and functional integrity of the sperm [34,57] during the freezing–thawing process. All of these morphological changes will affect the ability of the sperm to fertilize an oocyte successfully, even with the use of ICSI and other ART [49,57,63].

Effect on fertilization and pregnancy rates

It has been reported that there is no difference in terms of fertilization and pregnancy rates using frozen–thawed sperm versus fresh sperm in IVF/ICSI cycles [20]. However, in intrauterine insemination, fresh sperm is three times better than frozen sperm [54,64]. With sperm extracted by microsurgical epididymal sperm aspiration, the fertilization and pregnancy rates are as good as with fresh sperm [23,65], suggesting that sperm extracted from certain sites in the male genital tract might maintain the same quality after cryopreservation.

Legal and ethical aspects of sperm cryopreservation

Although the scientific concept behind sperm cryopreservation might look simple, the procedure itself is very complex, and it requires highly advanced sperm banking and cryopreservation facilities with proper equipment to handle semen collection, freezing, and storage. Surprisingly, when it comes to complexity, the legal aspect of cryopreservation is no different than its scientific aspect in terms of superficial simplicity and underlying complexity. However, in contrast to the firm foundation that currently underlies sperm cryopreservation, the legal considerations are ambiguous, sometimes vague, and still in a premature stage. Few publications in the literature have addressed this issue, and all the current data regarding informed consent and disposition contracts offered by the sperm banking and fertility center facilities around the world are very dependent on emerging litigation and court orders [66]. More details of this issue are given in Chapter 27.

Conclusions

Sperm cryopreservation is an ancient method of preserving male fertility in a way that will maintain sperm viability for a long period of time. Applications of sperm cryopreservation nowadays are diverse and include humans, animals, and insects. Despite the undeniable morphological and functional adverse effects that cryopreservation exerts on sperm, it still remains one of the core methods of fertility preservation for patients and healthy volunteer donors. Future studies are expected to concentrate on advancing technology to achieve the goal of "damage-free" sperm after cryopreservation. Encouragingly, recent advances in ART suggest that it will be possible eventually to achieve a healthy pregnancy and live birth from cryopreservation of a single sperm/sample.

References

1. Mahony MC, Morshedi M, Scott RT, *et al.* Role of spermatozoa cryopreservation in assisted reproduction. *Hum Spermatozoa Assist Reprod* 1990: 310–318.
2. Triana V. Artificial insemination and semen banks in Italy. *Hum Artif Inseminination Semen Preservation* 1980: 51.
3. Matheson GW, Carlborg L, Gemzell C. Frozen human semen for artificial insemination. *Am J Obstet Gynecol* 1969; **104:** 495–501.
4. Pegg DE. The history and principles of cryopreservation. *Semin Reprod Med* 2002; **20:** 5–13.
5. Polge C, Smith AU, Parkes AS. Revival of spermatozoa after vitrification and dehydration at low temperatures. *Nature* 1949; **164:** 666–668.
6. Bunge RG, Sherman JK. Fertilizing capacity of frozen human spermatozoa. *Nature* 1953; **172:** 767–768.
7. Nelson C, Bunge R. Semen analysis: evidence for changing parameters of male fertility potential. *Fertil Steril* 1974; **25:** 503–507.
8. Sherman JK. Synopsis of the use of frozen human semen since 1964: state of the art of human semen banking. *Fertil Steril* 1973; **24:** 397–412.
9. Smith Audrey U. *Biological Effects of Freezing and Supercooling* London: Edward Arnold, 1961.
10. Wildt DE. Genome resource banking for wildlife research, management, and conservation. *ILAR J* 2000; **41:** 228–234.
11. Dinnyes A, Liu J, Nedambale TL. Novel gamete storage. *Reprod Fertil Dev* 2007; **19:** 719–731.
12. Howard JG. Assisted reproductive techniques in nondomestic carnivores. *Zoo Wild Anim Med* IV 1999; **4:** 449–457.
13. Monfort SL, Asher GW, Wildt DE, *et al.* Successful intrauterine insemination of Eld's deer (Cervus eldi thamin) with frozen–thawed spermatozoa. *J Reprod Fertil* 1993; **99:** 459–465.
14. Takemura Y, Kanda T, Horie Y. Artificial insemination using cryopreserved sperm in the silkworm, Bombyx mori. *J Insect Physiol* 2000; **46:** 491–497.
15. Clarke CA. In vitro fertilization: some comparative aspects. *J R Soc Med* 1990; **83:** 214.
16. Sander K. Fertilization and egg cell activation in insects. *Biol Fertilization* 1985; **2:** 409–430.
17. Hatakeyama M, Lee JM, Sawa M, *et al.* Artificial reproduction in a hymenopteran insect, Athalia rosae, using eggs matured with heterospecific yolk proteins and fertilized with cryopreserved sperm. *Arch Insect Biochem Physiol* 2000; **43:** 137–144.
18. Hatakeyama M, Sawa M, Oishi K. Fertilization by micro-injection of cryopreserved sperm in the sawfly, Athalia rosae (Hymenoptera). *J Insect Physiol* 1994; **40:** 909–912.
19. Anger JT, Gilbert BR, Goldstein M. Cryopreservation of sperm: indications, methods and results. *J Urol* 2003; **170:** 1079–1084.
20. Kuczyski W, Dhont M, Grygoruk C, *et al.* The outcome of intracytoplasmic injection of fresh and cryopreserved

ejaculated spermatozoa: a prospective randomized study. *Hum Reprod* 2001; **16:** 2109–2113.

21. Rofeim O, Brown TA, Gilbert BR. Effects of serial thaw-refreeze cycles on human sperm motility and viability. *Fertil Steril* 2001; **75:** 1242–1243.
22. Ranganathan P, Mahran AM, Hallak J, *et al.* Sperm cryopreservation for men with nonmalignant, systemic disease: a descriptive study. *J Androl* 2001; **23:** 71–75.
23. Janzen N, Goldstein M, Schlegel PN, *et al.* Use of electively cryopreserved microsurgically aspirated epididymal sperm with IVF and intracytoplasmic sperm injection for obstructive azoospermia. *Fertil Steril* 2000; **74:** 696–701.
24. Tash JA, Goldstein M. The use of intra-operative sperm cryopreservation in men with obstructive azoospermia. *Fertil Steril* 2002; **76** *Suppl*: 208.
25. Tash JA, Applegarth L, Kerr S, *et al.* Post-mortem sperm procurement: the effect of instituting guidelines. *J Urol* 2003; **170:** 1922–1925.
26. Sherman JK. Cryopreservation of human semen. In Keel BA, Webster BW, eds. *CRC Handbook of the Laboratory Diagnosis and Treatment of Infertility.* Boca Raton, FL: CRC Press, 1990, pp. 229–259.
27. Ohl DA, Park J, Cohen C, *et al.* Procreation after death or mental incompetence: medical advance or technology gone awry? *Fertil Steril* 1996; **66:** 889–895.
28. Ahuja KK, Mamiso J, Emmerson G, *et al.* Pregnancy following intracytoplasmic sperm injection treatment with dead husband's spermatozoa: ethical and policy considerations. *Hum Reprod* 1997; **12:** 1360–1363.
29. Hoagland H, Pincus G. Revival of mammalian sperm after immersion in liquid nitrogen. *J Genet Physiol* 1942; **25:** 337–344.
30. Polge C, Lovelock JE. Preservation of bull sperm at −70°C. *Vet Rec* 1952; **64:** 296–297.
31. Leffler KS, Walters CA. A comparison of time, temperature, and refreezing variables on frozen sperm motility recovery. *Fertil Steril* 1996; **65:** 272–274.
32. Ragni G, Caccamo AM, Dalla Serra A, *et al.* Computerized slow-staged freezing of semen from men with testicular tumors or Hodgkin's disease preserves sperm better than standard vapor freezing. *Fertil Steril* 1990; **53:** 1072–1075.
33. Taylor PJ, Wilson J, Laycock R, *et al.* A comparison of freezing and thawing methods for the cryopreservation of human semen. *Fertil Steril* 1982; **37:** 100–103.
34. Verheyen G, Pletincx I, Van Steirteghem A. Effect of freezing method, thawing temperature and post-thaw dilution/washing on motility (CASA) and morphology characteristics of high-quality human sperm. *Hum Reprod* 1993; **8:** 1678–1684.
35. Hallak J, Hendin BN, Thomas Jr AJ, *et al.* Investigation of fertilizing capacity of cryopreserved spermatozoa from patients with cancer. *J Urol* 1998; **159:** 1217–1220.
36. Patrizio P, Silber S, Ord T, *et al.* Two births after microsurgical sperm aspiration in congenital absence of vas deferens. *Lancet* 1988; **ii:** 1364.
37. Silber SJ, Ord T, Balmaceda J, *et al.* Congenital absence of the vas deferens: the fertilizing capacity of human epididymal sperm. *N Engl J Med* 1990; **323:** 1788–1792.
38. Craft I, Tsirigotis M, Bennett V, *et al.* Percutaneous epididymal sperm aspiration and intracytoplasmic sperm injection in the management of infertility due to obstructive azoospermia. *Fertil Steril* 1995; **63:** 1038–1042.
39. Patrizio P. Cryopreservation of epididymal sperm. *Mol Cell Endocrinol* 2000; **169:** 11–14.
40. Tournaye H, Merdad T, Silber S, *et al.* No differences in outcome after intracytoplasmic sperm injection with fresh or with frozen–thawed epididymal spermatozoa. *Hum Reprod* 1999; **14:** 90–95.
41. Michelmann HW. Sperm and testicular tissue. In Healy, RO, Kovacs DL, McLachlan R, Rodriguez-Armas O, eds. *Reproductive Medicine in the Twenty-first Century: Proceedings of the 17th World Congress on Fertility and Sterility, Melbourne, Australia.* Boca Raton, FL: Parthenon, 2002, pp. 287–294.
42. Nawroth F, Isachenko V, Dessole S, *et al.* Vitrification of human spermatozoa without cryoprotectants. *Cryo Letters* 2002; **23:** 93–102.
43. Isachenko V, Isachenko E, Katkov II, *et al.* Cryoprotectant-free cryopreservation of human spermatozoa by vitrification and freezing in vapor: effect on motility, DNA integrity, and fertilization ability. *Biol Reprod* 2004; **71:** 1167–1173.
44. Isachenko E, Isachenko V, Katkov II, *et al.* Vitrification of mammalian spermatozoa in the absence of cryoprotectants: from past practical difficulties to present success. *Reprod BioMed Online* 2003; **6:** 191–200.
45. Tedder RS, Zuckerman MA, Goldstone AH, *et al.* Hepatitis B transmission from contaminated cryopreservation tank. *Lancet* 1995; **346:** 137–140.
46. Benifla JL, Letur-Konirsch H, Collin G, *et al.* Safety of cryopreservation straws for human gametes or embryos: a preliminary study with human immunodeficiency virus-1. *Hum Reprod* 2000; **15:** 2186–2189.
47. Donnelly ET, Kristine Steele E, McClure N, *et al.* Assessment of DNA integrity and morphology of ejaculated spermatozoa from fertile and infertile men before and after cryopreservation. *Hum Reprod* 2001; **16:** 1191–1199.
48. Esteves SC, Sharma RK, Thomas Jr AJ, *et al.* Improvement in motion characteristics and acrosome status in cryopreserved human spermatozoa by swim-up processing before freezing. *Hum Reprod* 2000; **15:** 2173–2179.

49. Hammadeh ME, Askari AS, Georg T, *et al.* Effect of freeze–thawing procedure on chromatin stability, morphological alteration and membrane integrity of human spermatozoa in fertile and subfertile men. *Int J Androl* 1999; **22:** 155–162.
50. Nijs M, Cox A, Bosmans E, *et al.* Comparison of 3 different cryopreservation methods: are they cryoprotective? In *A Journey from Gamete to Newborn: Proceedings of an International Meeting*, Leuven, Belgium, 2000, pp. 14–25.
51. Sharma RK, Kohn S, Padron OF, *et al.* Effect of artificial stimulants on cryopreserved spermatozoa from cancer patients. *J Urol* 1997; **157:** 521–524.
52. Meseguer M, Garrido N, Simon C, *et al.* Concentration of glutathione and expression of glutathione peroxidases 1 and 4 in fresh sperm provide a forecast of the outcome of cryopreservation of human spermatozoa. *J Androl* 2004; **25:** 773–780.
53. Paasch U, Sharma RK, Gupta AK, *et al.* Cryopreservation and thawing is associated with varying extent of activation of apoptotic machinery in subsets of ejaculated human spermatozoa 1. *Biol Reprod* 2004; **71:** 1828–1837.
54. Richter MA, Haning Jr RV, Shapiro SS. Artificial donor insemination: fresh versus frozen semen – the patient as her own control. *Fertil Steril* 1984; **41:** 277–280.
55. Centola GM, Raubertas RF, Mattox JH. Cryopreservation of human semen: comparison of cryopreservatives, sources of variability, and prediction of post-thaw survival. *J Androl* 1992; **13:** 283–288.
56. Wong AWY, Ho PC, Kwan M, *et al.* Factors affecting the success of artificial insemination by frozen donor semen. *Int J Fertil* 1989; **34:** 25–29.
57. Critser JK, Arneson BW, Aaker DV. Cryopreservation of human spermatozoa. II. Postthaw chronology of motility and of zona-free hamster ova penetration. *Fertil Steril* 1987; **47:** 980–984.
58. Barthelemy C, Royere D, Hammahah S, *et al.* Ultrastructural changes in membranes and acrosome of human sperm during cryopreservation. *Syst Biol Reprod Med* 1990; **25:** 29–40.
59. Henry MA, Noiles EE, Gao D, *et al.* Cryopreservation of human spermatozoa, IV. The effects of cooling rate and warming rate on the maintenance of motility, plasma membrane integrity, and mitochondrial function. *Fertil Steril* 1993; **60:** 911–918.
60. Nogueira D, Bourgain C, Verheyen G, *et al.* Light and electron microscopic analysis of human testicular spermatozoa and spermatids from frozen and thawed testicular biopsies. *Hum Reprod* 1999; **14:** 2041–2049.
61. Holt WV, Head MF, North RD. Freeze-induced membrane damage in ram spermatozoa is manifested after thawing: observations with experimental cryomicroscopy. *Biol Reprod* 1992; **46:** 1086–1094.
62. Mack SR, Zaneveld LJD. Acrosomal enzymes and ultrastructure of unfrozen and cryotreated human spermatozoa. *Gamete Res* 1987; **18:** 375–383.
63. Van Steirteghem A. Freezing of testicular tissue as a minced suspension preserves sperm quality better than whole-biopsy freezing when glycerol is used as cryoprotectant. *Int J Androl* 1999; **22:** 43–48.
64. Sherman JK. Synopsis of the use of frozen human semen since 1964: state of the art of human semen banking. *Fertil Steril* 1973; **24:** 397–412.
65. Oates RD, Lobel SM, Harris DH, *et al.* Efficacy of intracytoplasmic sperm injection using intentionally cryopreserved epididymal spermatozoa. *Hum Reprod* 1996; **11:** 133–138.
66. Schuster TG, Hickner-Cruz K, Ohl DA, *et al.* Legal considerations for cryopreservation of sperm and embryos. *Fertil Steril* 2003; **80:** 61–66.

Chapter 6

Sperm cryopreservation for a donor program

Zheng Li and Peng Xu

Introduction

Human sperm cryopreservation that has produced live births has been available for over 50 years [1]. Over that time, considerable research and clinical trials have contributed to understanding of the mechanisms that occur during semen freezing. Anonymous donor sperm banking has been a fundamental concept of reproductive medicine for several decades. In 1987, more than 170 000 women in the USA were treated for infertility using artificial insemination with donor sperm (AID) [2]. Approximately 3000 couples seek AID treatment and more than 16 000 AID cycles were performed in the UK in 1992 [3]. For many years, the use of donor semen has been the only approach to obtain a successful pregnancy for couples who are affected by severe male problems with fertility. Since the use of intracytoplasmic sperm injection (ICSI) became widespread in 1993, the frequency of AID has been reduced. However AID remains an alternative therapy to produce a healthy baby for infertile couples for several reasons, including where there is no spermatogenesis in non-obstructive azoospermia, where there are repeating failed ICSI cycles, and to avoid any genetic risks for offspring of ICSI fertilization [3]. Use of AID can prove valuable for a number of male dysfunctions, although its success rate is variable. A retrospective analysis of the results of 6139 cycles performed in 1001 women during an 18-year period in Israel showed a pregnancy rate per cycle of 12.6% and a cumulative pregnancy rate after 12 months of treatment of 75%. As infections with the human immunodeficiency virus (HIV) increased, frozen donor semen that has been cryopreserved for at least 6 months was substituted for fresh semen.

A standard protocol for human sperm banking was initiated in 2001 by the Chinese Ministry of Health. In 2008 there were about 10 sperm banks across mainland China that were licensed by the Chinese Government. Cryopreserved donor semen that has been checked for HIV may be used for artificial insemination or for in vitro fertilization (IVF). The improvement in and development of human sperm banking have had an enormous impact on reproductive medicine. The availability of frozen donor sperm has become a mainstay for the treatment of serious male infertility worldwide.

Sperm banking also can be used for men with cancer or who suffer from sexual dysfunction. Contemporary therapy for cancer and/or some non-malignant diseases applies combination chemotherapy and radiotherapy, which can have severe side effects through its cytotoxic effects on the testis [4]. Elective sperm cryopreservation programs have been provided for cancer patients all over the world, including China. Sperm cryopreservation is likely to be a temporary or permanent approach for these patients and could create the opportunity for paternity in the future. The number of patients referred for cryostorage and the number seeking to use cryostored semen have been increasing progressively over recent years in mainland China.

Donor sperm banking program

The program in China

The use of AID or IVF with donor sperm may result in a pregnancy when the male partner has severe problems with fertility. The Chinese Ministry of Health published guidelines for screening and testing anonymous donors for sperm donation. Anonymous sperm donation is acceptable in China, but immediately direct sperm donation is not permitted. The clinical procedures for screening anonymous donors should take into account a number of factors, the most important of which are the age of the sperm donors and then their health status. Most guidelines from the Chinese Ministry of Health have been adapted from or make reference to those of other countries. Of these, the programs in the UK and the USA are significant.

Fertility Cryopreservation, ed. Ri-Cheng Chian and Patrick Quinn. Published by Cambridge University Press.

In 2005, the UK Government instituted the requirement that any sperm donor had to agree to the disclosure of their identity to any offspring reaching the age of 18 years. There was a survey of donor opinions about the cancellation of anonymity. Some donors thought it was problematic, indicating that some donors will be reluctant to donate under conditions of non-anonymity and others would have concerns about the removal of anonymity [5].

The 2006 Guidelines for Gamete and Embryo Donation provide the latest recommendations for evaluation of potential sperm donors in the USA, incorporating recent information about optimal screening and testing for sexually transmitted infections, genetic diseases, and psychological assessments. This revised document from the American Society for Reproductive Medicine Practice Committee incorporates recent information from the US Centers for Disease Control and Prevention, the US Food and Drug Administration, and the American Association of Tissue Banks, with which all programs offering gamete and embryo donation services must be thoroughly familiar [6].

Criteria for selection of anonymous donors in China

The guidelines for selection of anonymous sperm donors in China are as follows. Sperm donors should have a good health status and no known genetic diseases in their family. Sperm donors should be between 22 and 44 years of age, because male aging is associated with a progressive increase in the number of aneuploid sperm. Sperm donor recruitment with confirmed fertility is desirable but not a mandatory requirement. Psychological and genetic evaluation and counseling by professional doctors is recommended strongly for all sperm donors. It is essential for the donors to sign a written consent. It is important that the donor should be well informed about the extent to which information about him might be disclosed and about any procedures that may occur related to a future contact by recipients and/or offspring. Physicians, laboratory staff, or other employees related to the treatment center are prohibited from becoming sperm donors in the donor programs.

Screening and testing program for sperm donors in China

Screening and testing of sperm donors are in accord with the regulations published by the Chinese Ministry of Health. Semen analysis is suggested for several samples (each sample after 2 to 7 days of abstinence) before proceeding with more extensive testing for the donors. The criteria used for judging the semen sample may vary among laboratories. The criteria for semen quality have been applied in China since 2003: (1) liquefaction time less than 60 minutes; (2) sperm concentration more than 60×10^6 sperm/ml; (3) percentage of rapid and slow progressive spermatozoa more than 60%; (4) normal morphology in more than 30% of sperm (see the World Health Organization *Laboratory Manual for the Examination of Human Semen and Sperm–Cervical Mucus Interaction* [7]).

Genetic screening for heritable diseases should be evaluated in potential sperm donors. Chromosomal analyses on all donors are required but cystic fibrosis carrier status is not assessed for all donors because this disorder is rare in the Chinese population. Genetic consulting should be performed after screening family history. Sperm donors should be healthy and have no history of genetic disease. Of course, transmission diseases such as HIV, sexually transmitted infections, and other infections that might be transmitted via sperm donation have to be screened before selecting the donors.

Medical examinations for the sperm donor

Sperm donors should be given a complete examination, including assessment for urethral discharge and penile warts and ulcers, plus routine laboratory screening, including blood type and Rhesus factor, before being enrolled as donors. Sperm donors should have follow-up examinations every 6 months for urethral discharge and penile warts and ulcers if they remain sperm donors. There is no 100% guarantee that infectious agents will not be transmitted by AID, but exclusion of potential donors at high risk for HIV and other sexually transmitted infections is important. The Chinese Ministry of Health requires the following tests: HIV-1 and HIV-2, hepatitis C antibody, hepatitis B surface antigen, hepatitis B core antibody, and cytomegalovirus. Semen or urethral tests are evaluated for *Neisseria gonorrhoeae* and *Chlamydia trachomatis*. Semen screening documentation confirming that there is no alteration in the donor's medical history should be recorded at 6 month intervals. If screening is negative, semen samples may be collected and prepared for cryopreservation. After donation, sperm samples must be cryopreserved for a minimum of 180 days before use. The donor must be re-screened for HIV antibody and samples may be used only if the results of repeat testing are negative. Fresh donor sperm is not allowed for AID or IVF in China.

Follow up for the results from sperm donation

Sperm banks are required to follow up AID or IVF results and to keep their records in order to allow a limited number of pregnancies with the same donor. A computer management system is required in the sperm bank to save the data. In China, only five women can be allowed to be pregnant with AID or IVF from a sperm donor. It has been recommended in the USA that, in a population of 800 000, limiting a single donor to no more than 25 births would avoid any significant increased risk of inadvertent consanguineous conception [6]. Since 1992, a limit of 25 offspring for every donor has been imposed in the Netherlands in order to avoid children from donors having a greater risk of consanguineous relationships [8]. These regulations may require modification if the population using AID or IVF represents an isolated subgroup or if the specimens are released over a wide geographic area.

Methods for sperm cryopreservation

Clarke *et al.* [9] evaluated six donor semen samples after 28 years of cryopreservation in liquid nitrogen. Their results showed that the samples retained good post-thaw motility and normal levels of binding to the human zona pellucida and that four of the five samples tested also gave normal levels of zona-induced acrosome reaction.

Conventional semen cryopreservation

As the temperature of a sperm sample is lowered in liquid nitrogen, extracellular ice crystals form, which leads to an increased concentration of solutes in the extracellular fluid. The resulting osmotic gradient results in dehydration as water moves out of the spermatozoa. Damage can occur to the cell if the osmotic gradient is too steep, resulting in water flow that is too rapid. Additionally, excessive dehydration causes increased intracellular solute concentration, which can be toxic to sperm cells, especially affecting sperm motility after thawing. Some experiments have shown that sperm DNA integrity also could be damaged and that sperm DNA fragmentation increases during the freezing–thawing cycle [10]. Sperm freezing has deleterious effects on spermatozoa, especially on plasmalemma, acrosome, and tail. Electron microscopy is the ultimate modality to investigate spermatogenic cells following freeze–thawing [11].

The conventional approach to sperm cryopreservation is to simply dilute semen with cryoprotectant and cryopreserve in liquid nitrogen until the sperm samples are thawed for use. A slow-freezing method consists of gradually cooling the sperm over a period of 1 to 2 hours in two or three steps, either manually or using a programmed freezer. Initial cooling rates of the sperm specimen from room temperature to 5°C have been shown to be optimal at 0.5–1°C/min. The sample is then frozen at a rate of 1 to 10°C/min from 5°C to −30°C, after which the specimen is plunged into liquid nitrogen. Additional information has suggested that holding the specimen at −5°C for 10 minutes and seeding the specimen may improve cryosurvival sperm rate after the frozen–thawing cycle [12].

Vitrification of sperm

Although the conventional slow-freezing approach has given acceptable results, others have shown that vitrification may be a better method for sperm cryopreservation [13]. With the advance of ICSI, theoretically only one sperm is required per oocyte. Therefore, the vitrification method may provide infertile men with severe oligozoospermia a good chance to cryopreserve the limited number of sperm needed [14]. There is a report of vitrifying sperm with the Cryoloop, which could offer an alternative approach for sperm freezing [15]. The ability to cryopreserve oligozoospermic samples has many potential areas for application, including for patients with severe oligozoospermia or asthenozoospermia.

Electroejaculation and sperm cryopreservation

Mammalian spermatozoa were among the very first cells to be successfully cryopreserved. The use of frozen–thawed semen for artificial insemination has come to play an important role in reproductive medicine. Electroejaculation is a valuable approach used to obtain semen samples from sexually mature male mammals and has been used for breeding programs and research purposes in various species, as well as in the treatment of anejaculation and ejaculatory dysfunction in infertile men who have failed other treatments [16].

Anejaculation is caused mainly by psychogenic anejaculation, spinal cord injury, diabetes mellitus, retroperitoneal lymph node dissection, transverse myelitis, and multiple sclerosis. Men who suffer from psychogenic anejaculation are healthy males who cannot intentionally ejaculate even by masturbation. However, they may have normal penile erections and nocturnal emissions. Previous data have shown that electroejaculated sperm have severe asthenozoospermia, sperm motility apparently decreasing in those with spinal cord injury or psychogenic anejaculation [17]. The asthenozoospermia in those with spinal cord injury may be connected with increased scrotal temperature, urinary infection, stasis of seminal fluid, neural effects, and so on. The semen quality of patients with psychogenic anejaculation is similar to that of patients with spinal cord injury, despite the fact that the latter do not have a neurological disorder and its complications [18].

A complete urological check is necessary prior to electroejaculation in order to exclude and treat any urinary tract inflammation. Patients with spinal cord injuries often have a problem with poor sperm production as well as ejaculation after the damage. A diagnostic trial of electroejaculation aims to obtain semen samples and to examine their quality. Good-quality semen samples are cryopresereved for future use. A fresh specimen can be used at a suitable time in a female partner's ovulation induction cycle for IVF or ICSI. Patients are prescribed sodium bicarbonate tablets prior to electroejaculation to alkalinize the urine and make it more suitable for sperm survival, because a retrograde sample may need to be retrieved from the bladder through a catheter.

Electroejaculation is usually performed under a general anesthesia while the patient is placed in lateral decubitus. An electric probe is put into the rectum close to the prostate. The probe transfers a slight electric current that stimulates adjacent nerves, resulting in contraction of the pelvic muscles and ejaculation. Prior to electroejaculation, the bladder is filled with Ham's F-10 medium as a buffer and 20 ml of medium is instilled for gathering of the retrograde-emitted semen sample. Multiple electrical stimulations ranging from 5 to 20 V and lasting for 2 seconds are administered. The urethra is manually milked into a sterile container both during and upon completion of electroejaculation to obtain the maximum volume of antegrade semen. After electroejaculation, a bladder catheterization is routinely performed for collection of retrograde specimens. The sperm obtained in the antegrade and retrograde ejaculates are processed by the discontinuous Percoll gradient, as described elsewhere. The concentration and motility of the antegrade and retrograde portions of electroejaculation are assessed using a Makler counting chamber according to published guidelines [7].

During emission and ejaculation in normal men, the internal urinary sphincter closes under the influence of sympathetic innervation from the T10–L2 spinal cord segments, causing semen to be expelled from the penis. In men with a spinal cord injury, whose innervation may be disrupted, the retrograde ejaculation after electroejaculation could be related to their neuropathology. Retrograde ejaculation does not occur in patients who are neurologically intact. However, most of these patients will have retrograde ejaculation with electroejaculation. These findings suggest that the appearance of a retrograde fraction with electroejaculation in men with a spinal cord injury may reflect methodological issues rather than neuropathology.

After electroejaculation, semen can be used for IVF or cryopreserved for future use and is an effective treatment for anejaculatory infertility. Intrauterine insemination with sperm (either fresh or frozen) obtained by electroejaculation is the first choice for men infertile with anejaculation [19]. The high percentage of pregnancies achieved with systemic assisted reproductive technology (ART) using sperm cryopreservation after electroejaculation means that this is a valuable and safe method for treating infertility with anejaculation [20].

Conclusions

Sperm cryopreservation plays an important role in the field of male infertility and reproductive medicine. A donor sperm cryopreservation program has been developed and improved in mainland China. Standards, guidelines, and a protocol for sperm donor screening and cryopreservation have been practiced since 2001. So far 10 human sperm banks have been set up and licensed by the Chinese Ministry of Health. With the advance of new approaches for sperm vitrification, treatment of male infertility will become more effective without using sperm donors. Using vitrification for cryopreservation of sperm obtained from testicular biopsy, epididymal fluid, or a semen sample after electroejaculation could create new hope for infertile men.

References

1. Sherman JK, Bunge RG. Effect of glycerol and freezing on some staining reactions of human spermatozoa. *Proc Soc Exp Biol Med* 1953; **84**: 179–800.
2. Critser JK. Current status for semen banking in the USA. *Hum Reprod* 1998; **13**: 55–67.
3. Botchan A, Hauser R, Gamzu R, *et al.* Results of 6139 artificial insemination cycles with donor spermatozoa. *Hum Reprod* 2001; **16**: 2298–2304.

4. Crha I, Ventruba P, Zakova J, *et al.* Survival and infertility treatment in male cancer patients after sperm banking. *Fertil Steril* 2009; **91**: 2344–2348.
5. Frith L, Blyth E, Farrand A. UK gamete donors' reflections on the removal of anonymity: implications for recruitment. *Hum Reprod* 2007; **22**: 1675–1680.
6. Practice Committee of the American Society for Reproductive Medicine. 2006 Guidelines for Gamete and Embryo Donation. *Fertil Steril* 2006; **86** (Suppl 5): S38–S50.
7. World Health Organization. *Laboratory Manual for the Examination of Human Semen and Sperm–Cervical Mucus Interaction,* 4th edn. New York: Cambridge University Press, 1999.
8. Janssens PM. No reason for a reduction in the number of offspring per sperm donor because of possible transmission of autosomal dominant diseases. *Hum Reprod* 2003; **18**: 669–671.
9. Clarke GN, Liu de Y, Baker HW. Recovery of human sperm motility and ability to interact with the human zona pellucida after more than 28 years of storage in liquid nitrogen. *Fertil Steril* 2006; **86**: 721–722.
10. Hu JH, Li QW, Jiang ZL, *et al.* Effects of different extenders on DNA integrity of boar spermatozoa following freezing–thawing. *Cryobiology* 2008; **57**: 257–262.
11. Ozkavukcu S, Erdemli E, Isik A, *et al.* Effects of cryopreservation on sperm parameters and ultrastructural morphology of human spermatozoa. *J Assist Reprod Genet* 2008; **25**: 403–411.
12. Jin B, Yamasaki C, Yamada N, *et al.* The mechanism by which mouse spermatozoa are injured during freezing. *J Reprod Dev* 2008; **54**: 265–269.
13. Isachenko V, Isachenko E, Katkov II, *et al.* Cryoprotectant-free cryopreservation of human spermatozoa by vitrification and freezing in vapor: effect on motility, DNA integrity, and fertilization ability. *Biol Reprod* 2004; **71**: 1167–1173.
14. Desai NN, Blackmon H, Goldfarb J. Single sperm cryopreservation on cryoloops: an alternative to hamster zona for freezing individual spermatozoa. *Reprod Biomed Online* 2004; **9**: 47–53.
15. Isachenko E, Isachenko V, Katkov II, *et al.* DNA integrity and motility of human spermatozoa after standard slow freezing versus cryoprotectant-free vitrification. *Hum Reprod* 2004; **19**: 932–939.
16. Curry MR. Cryopreservation of mammalian semen. *Methods Mol Biol* 2007; **368**: 303–311.
17. Hovavl Y, Sibirsky O, Pollack RN. Comparison between the first and the second electroejaculate qualities obtained from neurologically intact men suffering from anejaculation. *Hum Reprod* 2005; **20**: 2620–2622.
18. DeForge D, Blackmer J, Garritty C, *et al.* Fertility following spinal cord injury: a systematic review. *Spinal Cord* 2005; **43**: 693–703.
19. Kafetsoulis A, Brackett NL, Ibrahim E, *et al.* Current trends in the treatment of infertility in men with spinal cord injury. *Fertil Steril* 2006; **86**: 781–789.
20. Shieh JY, Chen SU, Wang YH, *et al.* A protocol of electroejaculation and systematic assisted reproductive technology achieved high efficiency and efficacy for pregnancy for anejaculatory men with spinal cord injury. *Arch Phys Med Rehabil* 2003; **84**: 535–540.

Chapter 7

Cryopreservation of surgically retrieved sperm

Peter T. K. Chan

Introduction

With increased understanding of reproductive biology in advanced assisted reproductive technologies (ART) such as intracytoplasmic sperm injection (ICSI), complemented with the improved safety and availability of these procedures worldwide, the management of severe male-factor infertility has undergone tremendous changes over the past few years. Indeed, even for men with the most challenging presentation of non-obstructive azoospermia, a small amount of sperm can be surgically retrieved for ICSI to allow many of these men, who were once considered sterile, to father their genetic children. Various issues in the cryopreservation of surgically retrieved sperm will be the focus of this chapter.

Indications for cryopreservation of surgically retrieved sperm

When the male partner is unable to produce an adequate amount of ejaculated sperm with good quality for ICSI, surgical sperm retrieval is indicated. This includes the following scenarios:

- azoospermia caused by obstruction of the male excurrent ductal system or testicular dysfunction
- poor quality and quantity of sperm in the ejaculate, particularly in association with a previous history of recurrent failure to achieve pregnancy with ICSI
- difficulty in ejaculating because of neurological or psychological problems.

For most couples going through in vitro fertilization (IVF)/ICSI cycles, one major advantage of cryopreserving sperm is that the timing of sperm and egg collection does not have be planned for specific dates, making the scheduling of treatment easier and reducing unnecessary stress for the couples. In addition, where it is not certain whether sperm can be found, obtaining sperm and cryopreserving them ahead of time can allow the couples to make a better informed decision about whether they should proceed with the treatment with advanced reproductive technologies, which can be costly financially and emotionally, or whether they should opt for alternative management such as the use of donor sperm or adoption. Other situations where cryopreservation of surgically retrieved sperm is indicated for men who cannot produce ejaculated sperm include:

- men who plan to have multiple cycles of ICSI and are not willing to undergo multiple sessions of sperm retrieval for each subsequent cycle
- men who anticipate a decline in their reproductive status (e.g. undergoing cytotoxic therapy for malignancies)
- men who are not ready for immediate assisted reproduction (e.g. of young age) or who do not have a female partner for reproduction yet
- men who are undergoing complex reconstructive surgeries for the excurrent ductal system (e.g. microsurgical vasoepididymostomy for epididymal obstruction or trans-urethral resection of the ejaculatory duct to relieve obstruction).

Posthumous sperm retrieval represents a special scenario where cryopreservation of surgically retrieved sperm is required. The techniques for posthumous sperm retrieval are identical to those used in living subjects. The psychological, ethical, and legal implications associated with the procedure, which are beyond the scope of this chapter, must be taken into consideration.

Techniques of sperm retrieval

Various techniques have been described and modified for sperm retrieval since the introduction of ICSI

Fertility Cryopreservation, ed. Ri-Cheng Chian and Patrick Quinn. Published by Cambridge University Press.

in 1992. Descriptions of the various commonly used procedures for sperm retrieval will be provided here to illustrate the principles of each technique and the potential drawbacks for subsequent cryopreservation. The three principal sources of sperm are epididymides, testes, and ejaculation. Although techniques for sperm retrieval from the seminal vesicles and vasa deferens have been described, they are less commonly used because of their more invasive nature and variable sperm yields compared with the techniques described below.

Percutaneous epididymal sperm aspiration

Sperm acquire motility during their epididymal transit. Hence the level of motility can be used as a criterion in conjunction with morphology to identify a "good" and viable spermatozoon for ICSI. In men who have obstructive azoospermia, such as post-vasectomy and congenital bilateral absence of vas deferens, epididymal aspiration to retrieve sperm is a preferred technique by many reproductive surgeons and embryologists. The process is generally performed under local anesthesia. An aspiration needle (gauge 21 to 27) is inserted percutaneously to the caput epididymis to aspirate a small amount of epididymal fluid containing sperm [1]. Although no incision is required for this procedure, multiple blind passages of the needle may be required to obtain an adequate amount of sperm, particularly if cryopreservation of sperm is planned. The potential drawbacks of percutaneous epididymal sperm aspiration (PESA), in addition to low yield of sperm, are (1) potentially scarring of the epididymis, making future sperm retrieval more difficult at the same site; (2) risks of causing hematoma and related complications postoperatively; and (3) presence of blood in the retrieved sperm samples, which may complicate the processing of the sample and subsequent selection of sperm for ICSI.

Microsurgical epididymal sperm aspiration

In microsurgical epididymal sperm aspiration (MESA), the epididymis is exposed and explored microsurgically at 25× or higher magnification to identify a single epididymal tubule for sperm aspiration. To obtain the epididymal fluid, the dissected tubule can be punctured with a fine glass pipette to aspirate the fluid within. Alternatively, the tubule can be microsurgically incised with a micro-ophthalmic knife to allow the fluid to be aspirated with micropipettes [1] or angiocatheters. Compared with PESA, MESA provides a higher sperm yield, as a larger quantity of bloodless epididymal fluid can generally be obtained and this allows sperm to be cryopreserved to avoid future sperm retrieval procedures. Hence, for men with obstructive azoospermia, MESA is the preferred choice of sperm-retrieval techniques by many experts in reproductive urology. Potential drawbacks of MESA include (1) the requirement of a scrotal incision, which can be perceived as more invasive, and (2) the requirement of microsurgical skills and instruments on the surgeon's part.

Testicular sperm aspiration

For men with non-obstructive azoospermia, MESA and PESA are inappropriate as there should be no sperm retrievable in the epididymis. Instead, retrieval of testicular sperm for ICSI should be performed. In testicular sperm aspiration (TESA), an aspiration needle is inserted percutaneously to the testis parenchyma to aspirate fluid or small pieces of seminiferous tubules to obtain sperm. This is generally performed under local anesthesia and is the procedure that is technically the easiest to acquire. In fact, in some parts of the world, this procedure is sometimes performed by healthcare professionals with limited urological training to obtain sperm for ICSI. The drawbacks of this technique are (1) low yield of sperm in those with non-obstructive azoospermia, hence requiring multiple passages of the needle to the testes, and (2) risks of hematoma and related complications postoperatively. Hence, TESA is best reserved for men who have obstructive azoospermia but failed to have sperm retrieved from the epididymis.

Testicular sperm extraction

For men with non-obstructive azoospermia, where the rare foci where there are spermatozoa may be difficult to identify with TESA, an open testicular sperm extraction (TESE), in which the testicle is exposed through a scrotal incision to obtain a large piece of seminiferous tubules, may yield a higher success rate for obtaining sperm. In TESE, the scrotum is incised to expose the testicular tunica albuginea, which is, in turn, incised to expose the seminiferous tubules for sperm retrieval. The obtained tubules should be processed intraoperatively by a qualified embryologist to look for sperm, as it is often necessary to obtain multiple samples from different sites of the testis in order to obtain an adequate amount of sperm for most men with non-obstructive azoospermia. Although an incision is required for TESE, making it perceived as an invasive procedure, it can generally be performed as an outpatient procedure under local anesthesia. Since the incision and the exposure of the seminiferous tubules are performed under direct vision, the risks of complications such as wound infection and hematoma are actually well below 1% when TESE is performed properly. The major drawback of TESE is that a large volume of testicular parenchyma is removed non-selectively to obtain enough sampling of the seminiferous tubules for sperm retrieval, and thorough dissection of these tubules is labor intensive and time consuming for the embryologists/andrologists. In addition, the irrecoverable loss of the Leydig cells mass in the interstitium of the testicular parenchyma may increase the risk of the subsequent development of hypogonadism in men who already have testicular dysfunction.

Micro-dissection for testicular sperm extraction

Most expert reproductive urologists prefer to use micro-TESE to obtain sperm from men with non-obstructive azoospermia. Under 25–40× magnification, the entire volume of seminiferous tubules is examined thoroughly through a large incision on the tunica albuginea [1]. Tubules that are more likely to have active spermatogenesis generally appear larger than the fibrotic tubules. The selected tubules are removed microsurgically with minimal disturbance of the interstitium and adjacent tubules. The advantage of micro-TESE is that a much smaller quantity of seminiferous tubules is removed than in conventional TESE. As a result, more time can be focused on the processing of the retrieved seminiferous tubules to obtain sperm. The need to make a large incision in the testicular tunica albuginea producs the perception that micro-TESE is more invasive than conventional TESE. In fact, when properly performed with a microsurgical technique that allows sparing of major tunical vessels, micro-TESE carries a low complication rate [2]. The major drawback of micro-TESE is that it is time consuming. Proper exploration of one testicle of normal size (> 20 ml) generally require approximately 2 hours. In addition, special microsurgical training is required not only for the opening of the incision and the use of microsutures for the closure of incision but also, and most importantly, for the exploration of the seminiferous tubule to allow proper identification of tubules that are most likely to contain sperm.

Vibratory stimulation

Men with normal spermatogenesis but failure to ejaculate from neurological or psychological reasons may benefit from vibratory stimulation. A vibrator, preferably of adjustable frequency and amplitude of vibration, can be applied to the glans penis or the frenulum of the ventral side of the head of the penis to induce orgasm for ejaculation [3]. Vibratory stimulation is relatively non-invasive. In men with spinal cord injury, particularly those with injury above the level of T10, vibratory stimulation can be effective to obtain sperm. Blood pressure monitoring of these patients during the procedure is required to avoid hypertension from autonomic dysreflexia.

Electroejaculation

In electroejaculation, an electric current is applied trans-rectally through an electric probe to the nerves and ejaculatory organs to trigger an ejaculation [3]. This procedure is painful and generally requires anesthesia, except for men with complete spinal cord injury who have no sensation in the lower body. Ejaculation triggered in this way is not always antegrade. Consequently, catheterization of the bladder after orgasm may be required to obtain sperm. The major drawback is that the quality of sperm obtained is variable, since these patients generally are not able to ejaculate often to allow the aged sperm to be emitted. Cryopreservation of sperm obtained by electroejaculation may further comprise the overall quality of the sperm for future use.

Cryopreservation of surgically retrieved sperm

The quantity of sperm retrievable surgically from the epididymides and testes is generally small compared with the amount of ejaculated sperm. Hence, efforts have been made by various investigators to evaluate a wide range of protocols to determine the best procedure to preserve surgically retrieved sperm [4,5]. The optimal carrier should allow cryopreservation of multiple portions of these sperm in small numbers (e.g. ~10 sperm per carrier, depending on the source and quality) for each cycle of ICSI. Repeated freezing–thawing in the specimen (such as when storing a much larger quantity of sperm in one sample) should be avoided.

Various biological and non-biological carriers have been described in the current literature for this purpose. Examples of biological carriers include algae

(*Volvox globator*) [6] and empty zonae from different species including hamster [7], mouse, or human [5,8]. Non-biological carriers include the conventional and modified straws and micropipettes, calcium alginate capsules [9], microdroplets of various media [10,11], agarose gel microspheres, and Cryoloops [12]. Each protocol has its limitations and drawbacks. Interpretation of data from studies attempting to evaluate cryodamage of surgically retrieved sperm is difficult, as there are no universally accepted markers of sperm function. In addition, many studies reported results from a mixed population of men with obstructive (with normal spermatogenesis) or non-obstructive azoospermia (with abnormal spermatogenesis). Various measurements, from sperm motility, morphology, ultramorphology as evaluated by electron microscopy, nuclear chromatin, and DNA integrity, have been used. An increased rate of damage to the junction of the sperm head and midpiece, as observed by light microscopy, has been reported after thawing of testicular sperm and can lead to dysfunction of the parternal centrosome [13]. Using transmission electron microscopy, Nogueira *et al.* [14] observed swelling and rupture of the inner and outer acrosomal and plasma membranes after freezing and thawing of testicular samples from men with obstructive azoospermia. Using the Comet assay, Steele *et al.* [15] were not able to detect any difference between fresh and frozen–thawed testicular spermatozoa from men with obstructive azoospermia with regard to the percentage of damaged DNA.

The use of cryopreserved sperm retrieved by surgery

With epididymal sperm, which are generally retrieved from men with obstructive azoospermia, there are reductions in the concentration of viable spermatozoa as well as a significant decrease (by 50%) in the percentage of motile spermatozoa [16], but there is little evidence to suggest that there is a difference in fertilization, cleavage, and implantation or pregnancy outcomes between cryopreserved or fresh samples [16–25].

The fertilization rates of frozen–thawed testicular sperm with ICSI ranged from 47 to 79%, which were similar to the use of fresh testicular sperm as reported by most investigators [26,27]. Other investigators, however, noted a significantly decreased fertilization rate or embryo cleavage rate with cryopreserved testicular sperm [28–31]. The reported pregnancy rate with frozen–thawed testicular sperm ranged from 26 to 50%, compared with 26–40% with fresh testicular sperm. As in the case of fertilization rates, most investigators reported similar results whether fresh or frozen–thawed testicular sperm were used. It should be noted that most studies did not perform a separate analysis with frozen–thawed testicular sperm from men with obstructive (with normal spermatogenesis) versus non-obstructive azoospermia (with abnormal spermatogenesis). However, studies that analyzed ICSI outcomes with fresh or frozen–thawed testicular sperm from men with non-obstructive azoospermia demonstrated no difference in most parameters, including fertilization, embryo cleavage, implantation, and clinical pregnancy rates [27,32–34].

Conclusions

For men with azoospermia, cryopreservation of sperm retrieved surgically in advance of the fertilization stage can allow better planning for the ICSI cycle and minimize unnecessary ovarian stimulation. Despite some notable controversies, current data suggest that cryopreservation of surgically retrieved sperm from the epididymides or testes, from men with non-obstructive or obstructive azoospermia, provide acceptable results in many reproductive centers. Clinicians must discuss and choose the most appropriate techniques of sperm retrieval with the patients, taking into account the indications and the advantages and disadvantages of each approach. At the same time, clinicians and embryologists must choose the most effective protocol to cryopreserve the small quantity of sperm retrieved for, hopefully, multiple cycles of ICSI, taking into account the limitations of each technique. The various current cryopreservation techniques for surgically retrieved sperm will no doubt continue to be modified and refined. Further clinical trials and research are required to evaluate the efficiency and cost-effectiveness of these techniques to allow clinicians to provide better counseling for couples who need to undergo these procedures.

References

1. Chan PTK, Schlegel PN. Surgical sperm retrieval. In Chan PTK, Goldstein M, Rosenwaks Z, eds. *Reproductive Medicine Secrets*. Philadelphia, PA: Hanley & Belfus, 2004, pp. 249–258.
2. Schlegel PN. Nonobstructive azoospermia: a revolutionary surgical approach and results. *Semin Reprod Med*. 2009; **27**: 165–170.

3. Ohl DA, Quallich SA, Sonksen J. Management of ejaculatory disorders. In Chan PTK, Goldstein M, Rosenwaks Z, eds. *Reproductive Medicine Secrets*. Philadelphia, PA: Hanley & Belfus, 2004, pp. 140–148.
4. Küpker W, Al-Hasani S, Johannisson R, *et al.* The use of cryopreserved mature and immature testicular spermatozoa for intracytoplasmic sperm injection: risks and limitations. *Semin Reprod Med* 2002; **20**: 25–35.
5. Abdel Hafez F, Bedaiwy M, El-Nashar SA, Sabanegh E, Desai N. Techniques for cryopreservation of individual or small numbers of human spermatozoa: a systematic review. *Hum Reprod Update* 2009; **15**: 153–164.
6. Just A, Gruber I, Wöber M, *et al.* Novel method for the cryopreservation of testicular sperm and ejaculated spermatozoa from patients with severe oligospermia: a pilot study. *Fertil Steril* 2004; **82**: 445–447.
7. Walmsley R, Cohen J, Ferrara-Congedo T, Reing A, Garrisi J. The first births and ongoing pregnancies associated with sperm cryopreservation within evacuated egg zonae. *Hum Reprod* 1998; **13**(Suppl 4): 61–70.
8. Borini A, Sereni E, Bonu MA, Flamigni C . Freezing a few testicular spermatozoa retrieved by TESE. *Mol Cell Endocrinol* 2000; **169**: 27–32.
9. Herrler A, Eisner S, Bach V, Weissenborn U, Beier HM. Cryopreservation of spermatozoa in alginic acid capsules. *Fertil Steril* 2006; **85**: 208–213.
10. Gil-Salom M, Romero J, Rubio C, *et al.* Intracytoplasmic sperm injection with cryopreserved testicular spermatozoa. *Mol Cell Endocrinol* 2000; **169**: 15–19.
11. Sereni E, Bonu MA, Fava L, *et al.* Freezing spermatozoa obtained by testicular fine needle aspiration: a new technique. *Reprod Biomed Online* 2008; **16**: 89–95.
12. Desai NN, Blackmon H, Goldfarb J. Single sperm cryopreservation on cryoloops: an alternative to hamster zona for freezing individual spermatozoa. *Reprod Biomed Online* 2004; **9**: 47–53.
13. Verheyen G, Nagy Z, Joris H, *et al.* Quality of frozen–thawed testicular sperm and its preclinical use for intracytoplasmic sperm injection into in vitro-matured germinal-vesicle stage oocytes. *Fertil Steril* 1997; **67**: 74–80.
14. Nogueira D, Bourgain C, Verheyen G, Van Steirteghem AC. Light and electron microscopic analysis of human testicular spermatozoa and spermatids from frozen and thawed testicular biopsies. *Hum Reprod* 1999; **14**: 2041–2049.
15. Steele EK, McClure N, Lewis SE. Comparison of the effects of two methods of cryopreservation on testicular sperm DNA. *Fertil Steril*. 2000; **74**: 450–453.
16. Cayan S, Lee D, Conaghan J, *et al.* A comparison of ICSI outcomes with fresh and cryopreserved epididymal spermatozoa from the same couples. *Hum Reprod* 2001; **16**: 495–499.
17. Oates RD, Lobel SM, Harris DH, *et al.* Efficacy of intracytoplasmic sperm injection using intentionally cryopreserved epididymal spermatozoa. *Hum Reprod* 1996; **11**: 133–138.
18. Devroey P, Silber S, Nagy Z, *et al.* Ongoing pregnancies and birth after intracytoplasmic sperm injection with frozen–thawed epididymal spermatozoa. *Hum Reprod* 1995; **10**: 903–906.
19. Nagy Z, Liu J, Cecile J, *et al.* Using ejaculated, fresh, and frozen–thawed epididymal and testicular spermatozoa gives rise to comparable results after intracytoplasmic sperm injection. *Fertil Steril* 1995; **63**: 808–815.
20. Cha KY, Oum KB, Kim HJ. Approaches for obtaining sperm in patients with male factor infertility. *Fertil Steril* 1997; **67**: 985–995.
21. Friedler S, Raziel A, Soffer Y, *et al.* The outcome of intracytoplasmic injection of fresh and cryopreserved epididymal spermatozoa from patients with obstructive azoospermia: a comparative study. *Hum Reprod* 1998; **13**: 1872–1877.
22. Hutchon S, Thornton S, Hall J, Bishop M. Frozen–thawed epididymal sperm is effective for intracytoplasmic sperm injection: implications for the urologist. *Br J Urol* 1998; **81**: 607–611.
23. Tournaye H, Merdad T, Silber S, *et al.* No differences in outcome after intracytoplasmic sperm injection with fresh or with frozen–thawed epididymal spermatozoa. *Hum Reprod* 1999; **14**: 90–95.
24. Janzen N, Goldstein M, Schlegel PN, *et al.* Use of electively cryopreserved microsurgically aspirated epididymal sperm with IVF and intracytoplasmic sperm injection for obstructive azoospermia. *Fertil Steril* 2000; **74**: 696–701.
25. Patrizio P. Cryopreservation of epididymal sperm. *Mol Cell Endocrinol* 2000; **169**: 11–14.
26. Wald M, Ross LS, Prins GS, *et al.* Analysis of outcomes of cryopreserved surgically retrieved sperm for IVF/ICSI. *J Androl* 2006; **27**: 60–65.
27. Friedler S, Raziel A, Soffer Y, *et al.* Intracytoplasmic injection of fresh and cryopreserved testicular spermatozoa in patients with nonobstructive azoospermia: a comparative study. *Fertil Steril* 1997; **68**: 892–897.
28. Gil-Salom M, Romero J, Minguez Y, *et al.* Pregnancies after intracytoplasmic sperm injection with cryopreserved testicular spermatozoa. *Hum Reprod* 1996; **11**: 1309–1313.
29. de Croo I, Van Der Elst J, Everaert K, de Sutter P, Dhont M. Fertilization, pregnancy and embryo implantation rates after ICSI with fresh or frozen–thawed testicular spermatozoa. *Hum Reprod* 1998; **13**: 1893–1897.
30. Wood S, Thomas K, Schnauffer K, *et al.* Reproductive potential of fresh and cryopreserved epididymal and testicular spermatozoa in consecutive intracytoplasmic

sperm injection cycles in the same patients. *Fertil Steril* 2002; **77**: 1162–1166.

31. Dirnfeld L, Paz M, Yshai D, *et al.* The impact of early testicular sperm extraction or cryopreservation on the outcome of intracytoplasmic sperm injection: a randomized controlled study. *J Assist Reprod Genet* 2003; **20**: 205–209.
32. Küpker W, Schlegel PN, Al-Hasani S, *et al.* Use of frozen–thawed testicular sperm for intracytoplasmic sperm injection. *Fertil Steril* 2000; **73**: 453–458.
33. Prins GS, Dolgina R, Studney P, *et al.* Quality of cryopreserved testicular sperm in patients with obstructive and nonobstructive azoospermia. *J Urol* 1999; **161**: 1504–1508.
34. Verheyen G, Vernaeve V, van Landuyt L, *et al.* Should diagnostic testicular sperm retrieval followed by cryopreservation for later ICSI be the procedure of choice for all patients with non-obstructive azoospermia? *Hum Reprod* 2004; **19**: 2822–2830.

Chapter 8

Testicular tissue cryopreservation

Ariel Revel and Javier Mejia

Introduction

Cancer among children creates substantial public concern. In France, 2000 new cases of cancer in males below age 15 years are reported every year [1]. In the USA, approximately 150 out of every million males under 20 years of age are diagnosed with cancer each year [2]. Consequently, approximately 12 400 children and adolescents in these countries alone are stricken with cancer. Approximately 2300 children and adolescents die of cancer each year in the USA, which makes cancer the most common cause of disease-related mortality in those aged 1–19 years. A male newborn in the USA has 0.32% probability of developing cancer by age 20 (i.e. a 1 in 300 chance).

Children and adolescents show typical cancer types, usually the more aggressive varieties. Among those younger than 20 years of age, 57% of cancers are leukemia, malignant tumors of the central nervous system, or lymphoma. The relative percentage, however, varied by age group. Leukemia is the most common diagnosis in the USA for those under 14 years of age, but the relative proportion decreased with age through the age groups under 5, 5–9 years, and 10–14 years of age: being 36% for those under 5 years and only 12% for adolescents 15–19 years of age. For those aged 15–19 years, lymphomas have been the most common diagnosis, making up 25% of the cases. The second most common type of cancer in the USA was malignant tumors of the central nervous system for those under 9 years of age, lymphoma for those aged 10–14 years, and leukemia for those aged 15–19 years [2]. Interestingly, cancer incidence is generally higher for males than females [2].

While the incidence rates for some forms of childhood cancer have increased since the mid-1970s, death rates have declined dramatically for most childhood cancers, and survival rates have improved markedly. Therapeutic advances in the management of childhood malignancies mean that the majority of children can realistically hope for long-term survival. With survival rates in excess of 70%, it is estimated that 1 in 250 of the young adult population by the year 2010 will be a long-term survivor of childhood cancer [3,4]. The principal reason for the increasing survival in total childhood cancer is the improvement in survival from leukemia, especially acute lymphocytic leukemia, which makes up approximately a third of the pediatric cases. This improvement is primarily a consequence of more efficacious cancer therapy, which includes surgery, chemotherapy, and irradiation; these modalities may be given alone or in combination, depending on the diagnosis, the location of the neoplasm, and the age of the patient [5].

This improvement in survival rates is, however, not without its costs. The most significant long-term adverse effect of anti-cancer therapies appears to be related to gonadal function. It is, therefore, critical to minimize the gonadotoxic effects of cancer treatment and to offer modalities that help to preserve human fertility [6]. It is well established that cytotoxic chemotherapy agents may produce long-lasting or permanent damage to the germinal epithelium, resulting in oligoospermia or azoospermia. The extent of gonadal damage is dependent upon several factors including the agent and its dosage, the type of cancer, and pre-treatment sperm concentrations [7–18]. Since multi-agent regimens with synergistic toxicity are usually utilized, it can be difficult to determine the specific contribution of each individual agent. Nevertheless, it has been established that alkylating agents are the most common agents implicated in gonadotoxicity [19,20]. Indeed, cyclophosphamide, resulting in 90% azoospermia in men treated for sarcoma, appears to be gonadotoxic above a threshold of 7.5 g/m^2 [21]. Non-alkylating agents implicated in gonadal damage include procarbazine, cisplatin, and vinblastine [8,9,11–17].

Fertility Cryopreservation, ed. Ri-Cheng Chian and Patrick Quinn. Published by Cambridge University Press. Copyright © Cambridge University Press 2010.

Whenever possible, less-gonadotoxic agents should be selected. For example, when the ABVD combination (adriamycin, bleomycin, vinblastine, and decarbazine) is used, which contains neither an alkylating agent nor procarbazine, temporary azoospermia is observed in only 33% of patients and oligozoospermia in only 21%. Moreover, full recovery can be expected after 18 months in most, if not all, patients [16,22].

The major challenge faced by pediatric oncologists today is to maintain the excellent survival rates while striving to achieve optimal quality of life. Since infertility is the most frequently encountered and psychologically distressing late complication of radiotherapy and chemotherapy for childhood cancer, developing techniques to preserve fertility have become a focus of attention for this patient group. It is commonly thought that the prepubertal stage is a protective factor for the gonad from the effects of chemotherapeutic treatment. It has been proved, however, that being prepubertal at exposure is not protective, and the risk of infertility appears to increase with higher doses of therapy [23–26] even though survivors of childhood cancer can expect to achieve normal pubertal development and physiological testosterone production. Though Leydig cell insufficiency has been suggested as an explanation [20], the clinical significance of this abnormality beginning at a young age is unknown. Since spermatogenesis is affected by chemotherapy at any age, fertility preservation should be addressed by physicians when discussing the long-term effects of cancer treatment with young male patients and their parents.

Preservation of fertility potential in boys: cryopreservation of sperm when possible

Advances in assisted reproductive technology (ART) have created opportunities for preservation of the reproductive potential of young males with cancer. Semen cryopreservation is possible in most adolescents with cancer regardless of age or diagnosis [27]. Even semen obtained from prepubertal boys has been shown to be useful for assisted reproduction techniques. There was no cancer group analyzed from which sperm could not be stored [28]. In order to obtain sperm from younger patients, provision of high-quality information and more open discussion of the technique are needed [29].

Nevertheless, the presence of an accompanying person had a three-fold negative effect on the ability of adolescents to produce a sperm sample [30]. Penile vibration or electroejaculation under general anesthesia [31] should be offered only when the adolescent cannot produce a sperm sample by masturbation [32]. Anecdotal evidence suggests that for boys who are unable to ejaculate, taking a urine sample after masturbation may help to isolate some sperm [28]. With modern in vitro fertilization (IVF) techniques, in particular intracytoplasmic sperm injection (ICSI), which involves the injection of a single sperm directly into an oocyte, the problems of low numbers of sperm and poor sperm motility may be circumvented [33–35]. Pregnancies have also been achieved with ICSI using immature spermatids and secondary spermatocytes extracted from testicular tissue in men with spermatogenic arrest [36–41].

Increased awareness of advances in reproductive techniques among hemato-oncologists and other physicians treating males with cancer is of high priority. The UK and the American Society of Clinical Oncology guidelines recommend that the implications of oncological treatment for fertility are discussed with all patients [42]. Although all hemato-oncologists recognize that semen cryopreservation helps the patient psychologically, the vast majority will not refer young men and adolescents and many believe that semen freezing delays cancer treatment. In an Irish study, 54% of consultant oncologists, haematologists, and urologists had heard of ICSI, but 88% were unaware of its benefits for patients with low sperm counts [43]. Older studies described only 20–30% of young patients with cancer considering sperm banking, and only 10–20% reportedly banked their sperm [44–47]. Sperm banking prior to chemotherapy has become significantly more available in recent years. Even so, awareness should be encouraged especially in adolescents and the young adult population. It appears that there is a discrepancy between medical possibilities and how they are perceived and conveyed to young male patients and their parents. In consequence, the possibility of childhood cancer survivors achieving genetic fatherhood is sometimes overlooked. Sperm cryopreservation before cancer chemotherapy should always be made available for young patients with cancer.

Fertility preservation also offers hope to young patients as they observe that planning for their future is a part of treatment. For many patients, the knowledge that their fertility potential has been secured helps in their emotional battle against cancer. In one study on the psychological impact of sperm conservation, 80%

declared that sperm cryopreservation helped them in their battle against cancer, but 60% were still worried about infertility in spite of having their sperm cryopreserved [48]. Although this study was performed in adults, we believe that the results can be extrapolated to the pediatric population. Adolescents can be part of a discussion about future fertility together with their parents. Prepubertal boys, however, are probably too young to discuss such issues. Nevertheless, an effort should be made to offer information and potential cryopreservation modalities to the parents and to advise that when cancer survivors reach adulthood a meeting with a fertility specialist is very important, especially when azoospermia or severe oligospermia is detected.

Preservation of fertility potential in boys when freezing sperm is impossible

Awareness by physicians is even more essential when dealing with younger populations. Physicians will probably never discuss the negative impact of chemotherapy on future spermatogenesis with young boys or with their parents. This is quite understandable as before adolescence boys cannot cryopreserve sperm because there are no haploid spermatozoa and spermatids in their testes.

Theoretically, testicular tissue from prepubertal boys facing gonadotoxic treatment could be banked for many years for spermatogonial stem cell transplantation. Stem cells, which are defined by their biological function, have the ability to both self-renew and to produce daughter cells that undergo differentiation. Human testicular cells might be harvested, cryopreserved before the start of chemotherapy, and re-introduced into the testis upon its completion.

In contrast to the situation in the ovary, it is well established that spermatogonial stem cells (SSC) exist in the testis and are responsible for maintaining spermatogenesis from puberty for the lifetime of the male. These testicular stem cells originate from the primordial germ cells that travel to the gonadal ridges during embryonic development [49]. Male germline stem cells are the only cells in postnatal mammals that undergo self-renewal and transmit genes to subsequent generations, since all female germline stem cells cease their proliferation before birth. The SSCs produce large numbers of differentiating germ cells, which develop into spermatozoa throughout postnatal life. Although many adult tissues are maintained by tissue-specific stem cells, only spermatogonial and a few other types of stem cell (hematopoietic, epidermal) have been unequivocally identified by a functional assay in mice [50,51]. Monoclonal antibodies can be used to detect spermatogonia in the non-human primate (macaque) testis but could not be achieved in humans [52].

The feasibility of germ cell isolation from testicular biopsies for low temperature banking was shown in biopsies obtained from men undergoing routine urological surgery [53]. Slow programmed freezing with dimethyl sulfoxide (DMSO) as a cryoprotectant was recently shown to be efficient in maintaining spermatogonia, Sertoli cells, and stromal compartment during freezing, thawing, and tissue culture [54]. A previous study by the same group has shown that DMSO as a cryoprotectant (at a 0.7 mol/l concentration) maintained the structure of testicular tissue, especially spermatogonia, after cryopreservation. In comparison, the structure of the basal compartment of the tubules was severely damaged when glycerol was used [55]. Long-term cryopreservation appears to have no adverse effect on meiotic re-combination when compared with fresh samples [56,57]. Testicular tissue and male germline stem cells seem to tolerate cryopreservation quite well. This step in the procedure appears to be less critical than is the case when preparing ovarian tissue for grafting.

In the hope that future technologies can utilize their immature gametes, there may be benefits in considering gonadal tissue preservation for children prior to chemotherapy or radiotherapy [58]. When this cancer survivor boy grows and is cured, his testicular precursor cells, which were retrieved prior to treatment and stored in liquid nitrogen, might then be considered for restoration of fertility. Possibilities include transplantation back into the inactive testes (ipsigeneic germ cell transplantation), maturation in vivo in another host (xenogeneic germ cell transplantation), or in vitro spermatogenesis. Mature sperm could then be used for fertilization by ICSI.

Transplantation of spermatogonial stem cells

Though still experimental, transplantation of SSCs is currently considered the most promising direction for fertility restoration in young cancer patients. Transplantation of SSCs into tubules of infertile men has the potential to restore spermatogenesis. Using the transplantation technique as a functional assay, SSCs can be detected unequivocally in any donor-cell population [49]. The method of testis cell transplantation, therefore, has paved the way to identify and study SSCs on the basis of their biological activity.

It should be possible to successfully cryopreserve SSCs from prepubertal testicular tissue and to transplant them back into the seminiferous tubules at a later date where they can differentiate into mature spermatozoa. Establishing a successful method for testicular stem cell transplantation of frozen–thawed testicular cells is essential for fertility restoration. Feasibility was demonstrated in the mouse testis. Stem cell suspension, isolated from the testes of donor male mice, repopulated sterile testes when injected into seminiferous tubules [51]. Heterologous transplantation from rat to mouse was also shown to be successful [59]. However, a study on four macaque monkeys injected with germ cells into their testes following irradiation did not generate a recovery in the sperm count, demonstrating the complexity of this procedure [60].

Sperm obtained after stem cell transplantation were shown to be able to fertilize mouse oocytes. Fertile offspring were obtained through ART following the establishment of complete spermatogenesis by grafting testis tissue from newborn mice, pigs, or goats into mouse hosts [61,62]. It appears that this was possible only when the graft was obtained from neonatal tissue. The use of adult testicular tissue was unsuccessful [60,63]. The species used for grafting in the xenotransplantation model seem to be important [64]. Whereas spermatogenesis could be obtained in the immunodeficient mouse when grafting tissue from macaque monkeys [65], poor results were obtained grafting marmoset testicular tissue [60,66].

The SSCs are Asingle (As) spermatogonia that either renew themselves or produce Apaired spermatogonia (Apr), which are predestined to differentiate [67]. Thus, SSCs can self-renew to maintain the stem cell population and they can produce large numbers of differentiating cells of the spermatogenic line, eventually leading to mature spermatozoa to transmit the genome to the next generation.

The homeostatic maintenance of fertile testes involves a well-orchestrated balance between the spermatogenic and endocrine compartments. The majority of mitotically active germ cells are depleted from seminiferous epithelium following exposure to high-dose ablative therapy. Therefore, spermatogenetic recovery in cancer survivors will depend on the ability of mitotically quiescent stem spermatogonia to transform into actively dividing stem and progenitor spermatogonia.

In the testis, SSCs reside on the basement membrane of the seminiferous tubule and are almost completely surrounded by somatic Sertoli cells, which form a microenvironment known as a niche. Within the niche, growth factors and extracellular signals regulate the decisions of SSCs either to self-renew or to form daughter cells that will begin the complex differentiation process of spermatogenesis, resulting in mature spermatozoa after approximately 35 days in the mouse and 64 days in the human [68]. The timing of sequential steps in spermatogenesis is tightly regulated by genes of the germ cell, and Sertoli cells support the differentiation process. Spermatogenesis thus depends on proper SSC function. The genes and the signaling pathways that regulate SSC function are, nonetheless, not yet well defined. Genes known to be important in mice include glial cell-derived neurotropic factor (GDNF) [69] and the lipid kinase phosphoinositide 3-kinase [70], which seem to be required for spermatogonial self-renewal in mice. No such factors have been reported in humans.

Three different methods of introducing donor cells into the recipient tubules have been developed using mice and rats [71]. As detailed in Figure 8.1a, cells can be injected directly into the seminiferous tubules using a micropipette, and the cells flow to other tubules through the rete testis, to which all tubules are connected. A second method is to insert a micropipette directly into the rete testis (Figure 8.1b). The third method is to inject donor cells into a large efferent duct, which leads to the rete testis (Figure 8.1c). Because all tubules access the rete testis, a cell suspension entering the rete testis can potentially fill a whole system of seminiferous tubules. Whereas all three methods have been used for mice and rats [51,71], only injection of donor cells directly into the rete testis has been used for cynomolgus monkeys [60] and humans [72].

Following microinjection by any of the three methods, only a small percentage of the donor SSCs colonize the basement membrane of the seminiferous tubules and begin proliferating. In humans, the average total number of SSCs in boys varies from 13×10^6 to 83×10^6 during childhood (0–10 years) [73]. This percentage of donor SSCs colonizing the basement membrane probably varies among species and for the mouse is estimated to be 5–12% [74,75]. Restoration of spermatogenesis and fertility was recently shown in mouse recipients who had undergone high-dose ablative treatment before freeze–thawed SSC allotransplantation [76].

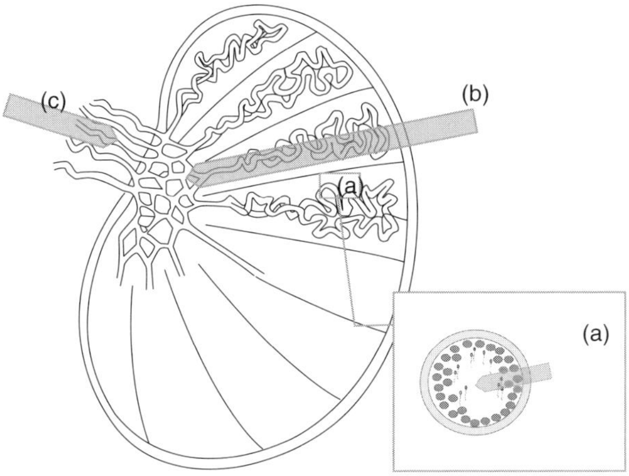

Figure 8.1. Methods of introducing donor cells into recipient tubules using a micropipette. Donor cells can be injected directly into the seminiferous tubules (a), directly into the rete testis (b), or into a large efferent duct leading to the rete testis (c).

In the mouse model, a majority of proliferating donor-derived cells are still located on the basement membrane during the first month after transplantation. By 2 months after transplantation, however, differentiated germ cells begin to fill the tubule from the basement membrane toward the lumen, and spermatozoa appear in the lumen of the donor-cell-derived colonies. The reconstituted spermatogenic colonies continuously produce spermatozoa throughout the remaining life of the recipient males. It has been demonstrated that each donor-derived spermatogenic colony generally arises from a single SSC [77–79].

No human pregnancy using this technique has been reported. Research is in progress to investigate whether testicular cells harvested and cryopreserved before the start of chemotherapy can be reintroduced to the testes after treatment and resume normal spermatogenesis [80]. Grafting adult human testicular tissue into immunodefficient mice has resulted in the ability to maintain spermatogonia for 195 days. In this experiment 13 pieces of human adult testicular tissue were grafted to immunodefficient mice. Most grafts presented with severe sclerosis. Moreover, in no sample was any spermatogenesis observed [63].

Xenotransplantation of cryptorchid testis from young boys into the scrotum of immunodefficinent mice for 3 weeks showed survival, albeit with no spermatogenesis. As identified by the MAGE A4 antibody, 14.5% of the initial spermatogonial population remained. Moreover, 32% of these cells showed proliferative activity as evidenced by production of the proliferation linked protein Ki67 [81]. A recent study has shown survival for 9 months for human prepubertal spermatogonia and Sertoli cells grafted on to the backs of six Swiss nude mice. The grafts were taken from testes of two patients who had severe sickle-cell anemia and who needed to undergo chemotherapy and bone marrow transplantation [82].

In vitro culture and expansion of spermatogonial stem cells

Culturing SSCs in vitro could increase the efficiency of the transplantation technique dramatically, since a high number of pure stem cells can be injected. Moreover, using a SSC-specific culture protocol might provide an efficient method of extracting malignant cells from germ cells. Nagano *et al.* [83] were the first group to report long-term survival of mouse spermatogonial stem cells in vitro. Moreover, they suggested that the in vitro maintenance of the stem cells could be improved by blocking spermatogonial differentiation [84].

While the signaling pathways involved are not understood, glial cell-derived neurotropic factor GDNF, a member of the transforming growth factor β superfamily produced by Sertoli cells, has been identified as an important growth factor in regulating SSC self-renewal and maintenance in culture. Indeed, not only long-term survival but also proliferation of spermatogonial stem cells was accomplished [85]. In the presence of GDNF, epidermal growth factor, basic fibroblast growth factor, and leukemia inhibitory factor, gonocytes isolated from neonatal mouse testis proliferated up to 1014-fold over a 5 month period. The cells maintained their functional capacity, as proven by the restoration of fertility after transplantation of the cultured cells to infertile recipient mice.

Expansion and meiotic entry of SSC appear to be blocked in cultures of testicular cell suspensions, and it is, therefore, impossible to apply the existing in vitro approaches to generate sperm for tumor survivors whose only remaining germ cells are diploid spermatogonia. In vitro growth factor requirements for mouse spermatogonial stem cells have been identified using defined culture conditions [49]. Co-culture in a novel three-dimensional soft agar culture system allowed germ cells to enter meiosis.

Problems with spermatogonial stem cells for restoration of spermatogenesis

The main problems in the application of cryopreservation of testicular tissue for restoring fertility appear to be the small number of SSCs present in the testicular biopsy and the potential for contamination by malignant cells. In mice, it is estimated that only two stem cells are present in 10 000 germ cells [86]. Although this ratio may be higher in humans, the low number of SSCs makes this procedure very inefficient for fertility preservation in prepubertal boys [87]. The low number of SSCs in the testis necessitates an effective purification and isolation technique. Effective purification will most likely require specific antibody probes to distinguish SSCs from other cells [88].

A second serious problem is the risk of contamination by malignant cells. In animal models even as few as 20 leukemic cells can cause a malignant recurrence in the recipient [89,90]. In humans, the threshold for malignant contamination is not known. As the majority of pediatric malignancies are capable of metastasizing through blood, a significant risk of contamination of the collected testicular tissue must be considered [91]. No technique currently exists for the separation of testicular cells from malignant cells. Neither magnetic activated cell sorting nor fluorescence activated cell sorting appears to be adequate for complete depletion of malignant cells from testicular tissue.

Molecular techniques can currently detect one single cancer cell among 10 million normal human cells [92,93]. Although more research on alternative decontamination techniques is obviously necessary, developing a reliable method to screen a priori testicular tissue for malignant cells could be equally important [90]. Therefore, transplantation of cells into the testis in malignancies that metastasize through blood should not yet be performed. Patients treated by chemotherapy for non-malignant hematological disease are obviously the first candidates for transplantation of frozen–thawed testicular tissue. In a mouse lymphoma model, cancer cells were eliminated from the testis-cell suspension by fluorescence activated cell sorting before transplantation [94].

The ethical aspect of this technique is quite intricate. Offering clinical treatment to a child requires consent from his parents and when the benefit to the child is clear, it is justifiable. When, however, a surgical procedure is offered for an experimental approach, this becomes much more controversial. The advantages and disadvantages of ovarian cryopreservation for young girls with cancer prior to chemotherapy have been investigated and documented [95]. The issue of informed consent is quite difficult in young children. Guidelines are required to ensure that this procedure is applied correctly. The rights of parents to consent to, or even request, a procedure that is still at the experimental stage need to be addressed. A multidisciplinary team familiar with these issues should be involved and decisions need to be made on an individual basis.

Future possibilities for restoring fertility

Future possible methods of restoring fertility might include the derivation of mature sperm cells from human embryonic stem cells [96]. Embryoid bodies were shown to support maturation of the primordial germ cells into haploid male gametes, which when injected into oocytes round off the somatic diploid chromosome complement and develop into blastocysts [97]. Moreover, the pluripotent properties of SSCs have recently enabled the establishment of human adult germline stem cells derived from spermatogonial cells of adult human testis. The cellular and molecular characterization of these cells revealed many similarities to human embryonic stem cells [98].

Conclusions

Spermatogonial stem cells are the viable stem cells that can transmit genetic information to the offspring, and their enormous proliferation contributes to fertilization throughout the male lifespan. Although the process of spermatogenesis is relatively efficient and resistant to damage, male infertility can result from exposure to toxic agents such as chemotherapeutic regimens, radiation, or occupational chemicals. Cancer and its treatment commonly cause male infertility and thus impair the chances of post-treatment paternity. The effect of the treatment on future fertility should be discussed with the patient prior to choosing and initiating treatment for cancer. The various options are detailed in Figure 8.2. Moreover, preventive measures should be considered in a multidisciplinary cooperation with oncologists, urologists, andrologists, and fertility specialists.

The first option for fertility preservation is pretreatment sperm cell cryopreservation. With developing technology in mind, today's experimental techniques of harvesting gonadal tissue can be considered in young males; however, it is important to avoid giving these patients and their parents unrealistic expectations of future fertility. Testicular tissue or spermatogonial cryopreservation and transplantation or testis xenografting are in the early phase of experimentation

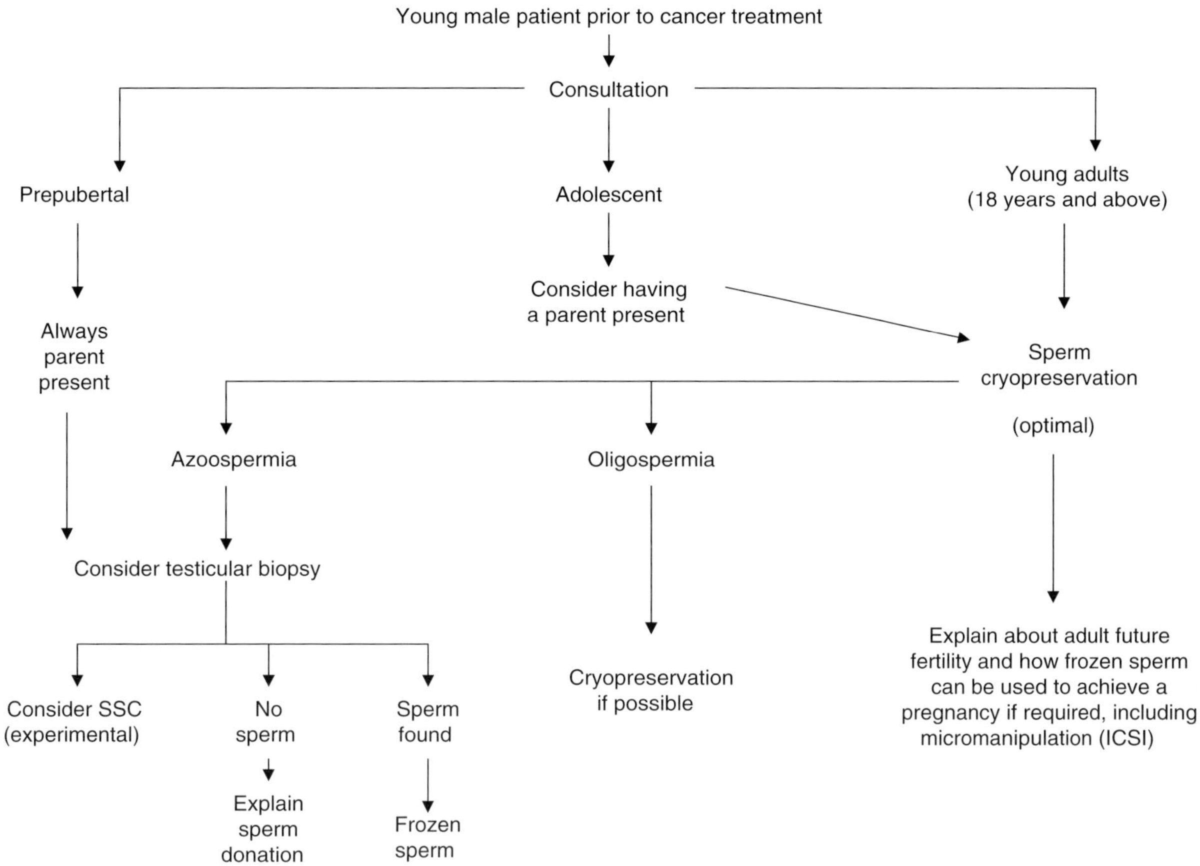

Figure 8.2. Algorithm for counseling patients and parents on potential methods to preserve fertility prior to initiating treatment for cancer.

and have not yet been successfully tested in humans. Recent studies in animal models have demonstrated that isolated testicular germ cells collected from testes may be transplanted into sterile recipient mice to regenerate spermatogenesis. This technology will have widespread applications in efforts to manipulate the genome and produce transgenic offspring, to improve agricultural species, to enhance sperm production in endangered species, to improve our understanding of the control mechanisms regulating spermatogenesis, and to treat male infertility. Nevertheless, it must be remembered that the association of cancer and fertility preservation in young patients raises ethical, legal, and policy issues for oncologists and cancer survivors.

References

1. Guerin JF. [Testicular tissue cryoconservation for prepubertal boys: indications and feasibility.] *Gynecol Obstet Fertil* 2005; **33**: 804–808.
2. Linet MS, Ries LA, Smith MA, Tarone RE, Devesa SS. Cancer surveillance series: recent trends in childhood cancer incidence and mortality in the United States. *J Natl Cancer Inst* 1999; **91**: 1051–1058.
3. Wallace W. Growth and endocrine function following the treatment of childhood malignant disease. In Pinkerton CR, Plowman PN, eds. *Paediatric Oncology: Clinical Practice and Controversies,* 2nd edn. London: Chapman & Hall, 1997, pp. 706–731.
4. Bleyer WA. The impact of childhood cancer on the United States and the world. *CA Cancer J Clin* 1990; **40**: 355–367.
5. Muller J. Impact of cancer therapy on the reproductive axis. *Horm Res* 2003; **59**(Suppl 1): 12–20.
6. Mitwally MF. Fertility preservation and minimizing reproductive damage in cancer survivors. *Expert Rev Anticancer Ther* 2007; **7**: 989–1001.
7. Waring AB, Wallace WH. Subfertility following treatment for childhood cancer. *Hosp Med* 2000; **61**: 550–557.
8. Mackie EJ, Radford M, Shalet SM. Gonadal function following chemotherapy for childhood Hodgkin's disease. *Med Pediatr Oncol* 1996; **27**: 74–78.
9. Papadakis V, Vlachopapadopoulou E, van Syckle K, *et al.* Gonadal function in young patients successfully treated

for Hodgkin disease. *Med Pediatr Oncol* 1999; **32**: 366–372.

10. Whitehead E, Shalet SM, Jones PH, Beardwell CG, Deakin DP. Gonadal function after combination chemotherapy for Hodgkin's disease in childhood. *Arch Dis Child* 1982; **57**: 287–291.
11. Shalet SM, Hann IM, Lendon M, *et al.* Testicular function after combination chemotherapy in childhood for acute lymphoblastic leukaemia. *Arch Dis Child* 1981; **56**: 275–278.
12. Wallace WH, Shalet SM, Lendon M, Morris-Jones PH. Male fertility in long-term survivors of childhood acute lymphoblastic leukaemia. *Int J Androl* 1991; **14**: 312–319.
13. Wallace WH, Shalet SM, Crowne EC, *et al.* Gonadal dysfunction due to cis-platinum. *Med Pediatr Oncol* 1989; **17**: 409–413.
14. Watson AR, Rance CP, Bain J. Long term effects of cyclophosphamide on testicular function. *Br Med J* 1985; **291**: 1457–1460.
15. Heikens J, Behrendt H, Adriaanse R, Berghout A. Irreversible gonadal damage in male survivors of pediatric Hodgkin's disease. *Cancer* 1996; **78**: 2020–2024.
16. Viviani S, Santoro A, Ragni G, *et al.* Gonadal toxicity after combination chemotherapy for Hodgkin's disease. Comparative results of MOPP vs ABVD. *Eur J Cancer Clin Oncol* 1985; **21**: 601–605.
17. da Cunha MF, Meistrich ML, Fuller LM, *et al.* Recovery of spermatogenesis after treatment for Hodgkin's disease: limiting dose of MOPP chemotherapy. *J Clin Oncol* 1984; **2**: 571–577.
18. Trottmann M, Becker AJ, Stadler T, *et al.* Semen quality in men with malignant diseases before and after therapy and the role of cryopreservation. *Eur Urol* 2007; **52**: 355–367.
19. Howell SJ, Shalet SM. Spermatogenesis after cancer treatment: damage and recovery. *J Natl Cancer Inst* 2005; **34**: 12–17.
20. Kenney LB, Laufer MR, Grant FD, Grier H, Diller L. High risk of infertility and long term gonadal damage in males treated with high dose cyclophosphamide for sarcoma during childhood. *Cancer* 2001; **91**: 613–621.
21. Meistrich ML, Wilson G, Brown BW, da Cunha MF, Lipshultz LI. Impact of cyclophosphamide on long-term reduction in sperm count in men treated with combination chemotherapy for Ewing and soft tissue sarcomas. *Cancer* 1992; **70**: 2703–2712.
22. Viviani S, Ragni G, Santoro A, *et al.* Testicular dysfunction in Hodgkin's disease before and after treatment. *Eur J Cancer* 1991; **27**: 1389–1392.
23. Ben Arush MW, Solt I, Lightman A, Linn S, Kuten A. Male gonadal function in survivors of childhood Hodgkin and non-Hodgkin lymphoma. *Pediatr Hematol Oncol* 2000; **17**: 239–245.
24. Rafsanjani KA, Faranoush M, Hedayatiasl AA, Vossough P. Gonadal function and fertility in male survivors treated for Hodgkin's disease in Iran. *Saudi Med J* 2007; **28**: 1690–1693.
25. Brougham MF, Kelnar CJ, Sharpe RM, Wallace WH. Male fertility following childhood cancer: current concepts and future therapies. *Asian J Androl* 2003; **5**: 325–337.
26. Brougham MF, Wallace WH. Subfertility in children and young people treated for solid and haematological malignancies. *Br J Haematol* 2005; **131**: 143–155.
27. Kliesch S, Behre HM, Jurgens H, Nieschlag E. Cryopreservation of semen from adolescent patients with malignancies. *Med Pediatr Oncol* 1996; **26**: 20–27.
28. Bahadur G, Ling KL, Hart R, *et al.* Semen quality and cryopreservation in adolescent cancer patients. *Hum Reprod* 2002; **17**: 3157–3161.
29. Edge B, Holmes D, Makin G. Sperm banking in adolescent cancer patients. *Arch Dis Child* 2006; **91**: 149–152.
30. Bahadur G, Ling KL, Hart R, *et al.* Semen production in adolescent cancer patients. *Hum Reprod* 2002; **17**: 2654–2656.
31. Schmiegelow ML, Sommer P, Carlsen E, *et al.* Penile vibratory stimulation and electroejaculation before anticancer therapy in two pubertal boys. *J Pediatr Hematol Oncol* 1998; **20**: 429–430.
32. Muller J, Sonksen J, Sommer P, *et al.* Cryopreservation of semen from pubertal boys with cancer. *Med Pediatr Oncol* 2000; **34**: 191–194.
33. Rosenlund B, Sjoblom P, Tornblom M, Hultling C, Hillensjo T. In-vitro fertilization and intracytoplasmic sperm injection in the treatment of infertility after testicular cancer. *Hum Reprod* 1998; **13**: 414–418.
34. Aboulghar MA, Mansour RT, Serour GI, *et al.* Fertilization and pregnancy rates after intracytoplasmic sperm injection using ejaculate semen and surgically retrieved sperm. *Fertil Steril* 1997; **68**: 108–111.
35. Chen SU, Ho HN, Chen HF, *et al.* Pregnancy achieved by intracytoplasmic sperm injection using cryopreserved semen from a man with testicular cancer. *Hum Reprod* 1996; **11**: 2645–2647.
36. Tesarik J, Mendoza C. Spermatid injection into human oocytes. I. Laboratory techniques and special features of zygote development. *Hum Reprod* 1996; **11**: 772–779.
37. Tesarik J, Mendoza C, Testart J. Viable embryos from injection of round spermatids into oocytes. *N Engl J Med* 1995; **333**: 525.
38. Fishel S, Green S, Hunter A, *et al.* Human fertilization with round and elongated spermatids. *Hum Reprod* 1997; **12**: 336–340.
39. Sofikitis N, Mantzavinos T, Loutradis D, *et al.* Ooplasmic injections of secondary spermatocytes for non-obstructive azoospermia. *Lancet* 1998; **351**: 1177–1178.

40. Vanderzwalmen P, Zech H, Birkenfeld A, *et al.* Intracytoplasmic injection of spermatids retrieved from testicular tissue: influence of testicular pathology, type of selected spermatids and oocyte activation. *Hum Reprod* 1997; **12**: 1203–1213.
41. Bernabeu R, Cremades N, Takahashi K, Sousa M. Successful pregnancy after spermatid injection. *Hum Reprod (Oxford)* 1998; **13**: 1898–1900.
42. Lee SJ, Schover LR, Partridge AH, *et al.* American Society of Clinical Oncology recommendations on fertility preservation in cancer patients. *J Clin Oncol* 2006; **24**: 2917–2931.
43. Allen C, Keane D, Harrison RF. A survey of Irish consultants regarding awareness of sperm freezing and assisted reproduction. *Irish Med J* 2003; **96**: 23–25.
44. Schover LR, Rybicki LA, Martin BA, Bringelsen KA. Having children after cancer. A pilot survey of survivors' attitudes and experiences. *Cancer* 1999; **86**: 697–709.
45. Hartmann JT, Albrecht C, Schmoll HJ, *et al.* Long-term effects on sexual function and fertility after treatment of testicular cancer. *Br J Cancer* 1999; **80**: 801–807.
46. Rieker PP, Fitzgerald EM, Kalish LA, *et al.* Psychosocial factors, curative therapies, and behavioral outcomes. A comparison of testis cancer survivors and a control group of healthy men. *Cancer* 1989; **64**: 2399–2407.
47. Rieker PP, Fitzgerald EM, Kalish LA. Adaptive behavioral responses to potential infertility among survivors of testis cancer. *J Clin Oncol* 1990; **8**: 347–355.
48. Saito K, Suzuki K, Iwasaki A, Yumura Y, Kubota Y. Sperm cryopreservation before cancer chemotherapy helps in the emotional battle against cancer. *Cancer* 2005; **104**: 521–524.
49. Kubota H, Brinster RL. Technology insight: in vitro culture of spermatogonial stem cells and their potential therapeutic uses. *Natl Clin Pract Endocrinol Metab* 2006; **2**: 99–108.
50. Brinster RL, Avarbock MR. Germline transmission of donor haplotype following spermatogonial transplantation. *Proc Natl Acad Sci USA* 1994; **91**: 11303–11307.
51. Brinster RL, Zimmermann JW. Spermatogenesis following male germ-cell transplantation. *Proc Natl Acad Sci USA* 1994; **91**: 11298–11302.
52. Muller T, Eildermann K, Dhir R, Schlatt S, Behr R. Glycan stem-cell markers are specifically expressed by spermatogonia in the adult non-human primate testis. *Hum Reprod* 2008; **23**: 2292–2298.
53. Brook PF, Radford JA, Shalet SM, Joyce AD, Gosden RG. Isolation of germ cells from human testicular tissue for low temperature storage and autotransplantation. *Fertil Steril* 2001; **75**: 269–274.
54. Keros V, Hultenby K, Borgstrom B, *et al.* Methods of cryopreservation of testicular tissue with viable spermatogonia in pre-pubertal boys undergoing gonadotoxic cancer treatment. *Hum Reprod* 2007; **22**: 1384–1395.
55. Keros V, Rosenlund B, Hultenby K, *et al.* Optimizing cryopreservation of human testicular tissue: comparison of protocols with glycerol, propanediol and dimethylsulphoxide as cryoprotectants. *Hum Reprod* 2005; **20**: 1676–1687.
56. Lyrakou S, Mantas D, Msaouel P, *et al.* Crossover analysis using immunofluorescent detection of MLH1 foci in frozen–thawed testicular tissue. *Reprod Biomed Online* 2007; **15**: 99–105.
57. Li J, Leng M, Ma T, Yu D, Shi H, Shi Q. Cryopreservation has no effect on meiotic recombination and synapsis in testicular tissues. *Fertil Steril* 2009; **91**: 2734–2763.
58. Bahadur G, Ralph D. Gonadal tissue cryopreservation in boys with paediatric cancers. *Hum Reprod* 1999; **14**: 11–17.
59. Clouthier DE, Avarbock MR, Maika SD, Hammer RE, Brinster RL. Rat spermatogenesis in mouse testis. *Nature* 1996; **381**: 418–421.
60. Schlatt S, Foppiani L, Rolf C, Weinbauer GF, Nieschlag E. Germ cell transplantation into X-irradiated monkey testes. *Hum Reprod* 2002; **17**: 55–62.
61. Honaramooz A, Snedaker A, Boiani M, *et al.* Sperm from neonatal mammalian testes grafted in mice. *Nature* 2002; **418**: 778–781.
62. Schlatt S, Honaramooz A, Boiani M, Scholer HR, Dobrinski I. Progeny from sperm obtained after ectopic grafting of neonatal mouse testes. *Biol Reprod* 2003; **68**: 2331–2335.
63. Geens M, de Block G, Goossens E, *et al.* Spermatogonial survival after grafting human testicular tissue to immunodeficient mice. *Hum Reprod* 2006; **21**: 390–396.
64. Schlatt S, Kim SS, Gosden R. Spermatogenesis and steroidogenesis in mouse, hamster and monkey testicular tissue after cryopreservation and heterotopic grafting to castrated hosts. *Reproduction* 2002; **124**: 339–346.
65. Honaramooz A, Li MW, Penedo MC, Meyers S, Dobrinski I. Accelerated maturation of primate testis by xenografting into mice. *Biol Reprod* 2004; **70**: 1500–1503.
66. Wistuba J, Mundry M, Luetjens CM, Schlatt S. Cografting of hamster (*Phodopus sungorus*) and marmoset (*Callithrix jacchus*) testicular tissues into nude mice does not overcome blockade of early spermatogenic differentiation in primate grafts. *Biol Reprod* 2004; **71**: 2087–2091.
67. de Rooij DG. Proliferation and differentiation of spermatogonial stem cells. *Reproduction* 2001; **121**: 347–354.
68. Brinster RL. Germline stem cell transplantation and transgenesis. *Science* 2002; **296**: 2174–2176.
69. Naughton CK, Jain S, Strickland AM, Gupta A, Milbrandt J. Glial cell-line derived neurotrophic

factor-mediated RET signaling regulates spermatogonial stem cell fate. *Biol Reprod* 2006; **74**: 314–321.

70. Lee J, Kanatsu-Shinohara M, Inoue K, *et al.* Akt mediates self-renewal division of mouse spermatogonial stem cells. *Development* 2007; **134**: 1853–1859.
71. Ogawa T, Arechaga JM, Avarbock MR, Brinster RL. Transplantation of testis germinal cells into mouse seminiferous tubules. *Int J Dev Biol* 1997; **41**: 111–122.
72. Radford J, Shalet S, Lieberman B. Fertility after treatment for cancer: questions remain over ways of preserving ovarian and testicular tissue. *Br Med J* 1999; **319**: 935–936.
73. Muller J, Skakkebaek NE. Quantification of germ cells and seminiferous tubules by stereological examination of testicles from 50 boys who suffered from sudden death. *Int J Androl* 1983; **6**: 143–156.
74. Nagano MC. Homing efficiency and proliferation kinetics of male germ line stem cells following transplantation in mice. *Biol Reprod* 2003; **69**: 701–707.
75. Ogawa T, Ohmura M, Yumura Y, Sawada H, Kubota Y. Expansion of murine spermatogonial stem cells through serial transplantation. *Biol Reprod* 2003; **68**: 316–322.
76. Wang X, Ding Q, Zhang Y, *et al.* Two allogeneic descendents derived from the high-dose busulfan-treated infertile mouse model after freeze–thawed spermatogonial stem cell transplantation. *Fertil Steril* 2008; **90**: 1538–1549.
77. Dobrinski I, Ogawa T, Avarbock MR, Brinster RL. Computer assisted image analysis to assess colonization of recipient seminiferous tubules by spermatogonial stem cells from transgenic donor mice. *Mol Reprod Dev* 1999; **53**: 142–148.
78. Nagano M, Avarbock MR, Brinster RL. Pattern and kinetics of mouse donor spermatogonial stem cell colonization in recipient testes. *Biol Reprod* 1999; **60**: 1429–1436.
79. Zhang X, Ebata KT, Nagano MC. Genetic analysis of the clonal origin of regenerating mouse spermatogenesis following transplantation. *Biol Reprod* 2003; **69**: 1872–1878.
80. Radford J. Restoration of fertility after treatment for cancer. *Hormone Res* 2003; **59**(Suppl 1): 21–23.
81. Wyns C, Curaba M, Martinez-Madrid B, *et al.* Spermatogonial survival after cryopreservation and short-term orthotopic immature human cryptorchid testicular tissue grafting to immunodeficient mice. *Hum Reprod* 2007; **22**: 1603–1611.
82. Goossens E, Geens M, de Block G, Tournaye H. Spermatogonial survival in long-term human prepubertal xenografts. *Fertil Steril* 2008; **24**: 2019–2022.
83. Nagano M, Avarbock MR, Leonida EB, Brinster CJ, Brinster RL. Culture of mouse spermatogonial stem cells. *Tissue Cell* 1998; **30**: 389–397.
84. Nagano M, Ryu BY, Brinster CJ, Avarbock MR, Brinster RL. Maintenance of mouse male germ line stem cells in vitro. *Biol Reprod* 2003; **68**: 2207–2214.
85. Kanatsu-Shinohara M, Ogonuki N, Inoue K, *et al.* Restoration of fertility in infertile mice by transplantation of cryopreserved male germline stem cells. *Hum Reprod* 2003; **18**: 2660–2667.
86. Tegelenbosch RA, de Rooij DG. A quantitative study of spermatogonial multiplication and stem cell renewal in the C3H/101 F1 hybrid mouse. *Mut Res* 1993; **290**: 193–200.
87. Aslam I, Fishel S, Moore H, Dowell K, Thornton S. Fertility preservation of boys undergoing anti-cancer therapy: a review of the existing situation and prospects for the future. *Hum Reprod* 2000; **15**: 2154–2159.
88. Aslam I, Robins A, Dowell K, Fishel S. Isolation, purification and assessment of viability of spermatogenic cells from testicular biopsies of azoospermic men. *Hum Reprod* 1999; **13**: 639–645.
89. Jahnukainen K, Hou M, Petersen C, Setchell B, Soder O. Intratesticular transplantation of testicular cells from leukemic rats causes transmission of leukemia. *Cancer Res* 2001; **61**: 706–710.
90. Geens M, van de Velde H, de Block G, *et al.* The efficiency of magnetic-activated cell sorting and fluorescence-activated cell sorting in the decontamination of testicular cell suspensions in cancer patients. *Hum Reprod* 2007; **22**: 733–742.
91. Jahnukainen K, Ehmcke J, Soder O, Schlatt S. Clinical potential and putative risks of fertility preservation in children utilizing gonadal tissue or germline stem cells. *Pediatric Res* 2006; **59**: 40R–47R.
92. Willemse MJ, Seriu T, Hettinger K, *et al.* Detection of minimal residual disease identifies differences in treatment response between T-ALL and precursor B-ALL. *Blood* 2002; **99**: 4386–4393.
93. Jolkowska J, Derwich K, Dawidowska M. Methods of minimal residual disease (MRD) detection in childhood haematological malignancies. *J Appl Genet* 2007; **48**: 77–83.
94. Fujita K, Ohta H, Tsujimura A, *et al.* Transplantation of spermatogonial stem cells isolated from leukemic mice restores fertility without inducing leukemia. *J Clin Invest* 2005; **115**: 1855–1861.
95. Weintraub M, Gross E, Kadari A, *et al.* Should ovarian cryopreservation be offered to girls with cancer. *Pediatr Blood Cancer* 2007; **48**: 4–9.
96. Ko K, Scholer HR. Embryonic stem cells as a potential source of gametes. *Sem Reprod Med* 2006; **24**: 322–329.
97. Geijsen N, Horoschak M, Kim K, *et al.* Derivation of embryonic germ cells and male gametes from embryonic stem cells. *Nature* 2004; **427**: 148–154.
98. Conrad S, Renninger M, Hennenlotter J, *et al.* Generation of pluripotent stem cells from adult human testis. *Nature* 2008; **456**: 344–349[errata in *Nature* 2009; **460**: 1044].

Section 3 Chapter 9

Cryopreservation of embryos

Cryopreservation of embryos: an overview

David H. Edgar and Debra A. Gook

The role of embryo cryopreservation in fertility management

Evolution of clinical-assisted reproduction

The first reported observations of the genesis and early development of the human embryo ex vivo [1] initiated a chain of events that revolutionized the management of human subfertility and laid the foundations of modern reproductive medicine. Although the first clinical pregnancies from in vitro fertilization and embryo transfer (IVF/ET) were obtained using oocytes retrieved in the natural menstrual cycle [2], subsequent successes in controlled ovulatory cycles [3] led to the widespread adoption of ovarian stimulation as a routine component of assisted reproductive technology (ART). The availability of multiple mature oocytes obtained from a single cycle of ovarian stimulation inevitably increased the probability of establishing a clinical pregnancy. It not only allowed selection of oocytes that could undergo normal fertilization and development, it also allowed in many cases the transfer of multiple cleaving embryos in attempts to overcome the frequently disappointing implantation rates observed in the early days of IVF/ET.

The advantages associated with the availability and transfer of multiple embryos were, however, offset by the incidence of multigestation pregnancies. Multigestation pregnancy, while considered a potential bonus by many patients who had experienced long periods of infertility, is widely recognized as a major clinical complication of ART [4], with associated healthcare cost implications [5]. As success rates from IVF/ET increased, much attention was turned to developing treatment strategies designed to minimize the frequency of multiple gestation. By the end of the 1990s, many groups had reduced the number of fresh embryos being transferred and it had been demonstrated that restricting the number of embryos transferred after IVF to two could reduce the risk of multiple births without significantly affecting the pregnancy rate [6]. The practice of transferring only two fresh embryos was, however, already under scrutiny as the risks associated with twin pregnancies were emphasized, and the use of single embryo transfer was soon advocated [7] and subsequently justified on the basis of both health and economic considerations [8]. In our unit in Melbourne, for the period between 2004 and 2007, transfer of two embryos (on day 2 of development) to a woman under 36 resulted in a clinical pregnancy (at least one fetal heartbeat) rate of 37% and a multigestation pregnancy rate of 36%. Over the same period, and in the same age group, the transfer of a single day 2 embryo resulted in a clinical pregnancy rate of 31% but a multigestation pregnancy rate of only 1.3%. Currently in our unit, 76% of patients in this age group undergo single embryo transfer. Maximizing the efficiency of ART, however, requires that the pregnancy potential of the embryos that are not transferred is retained.

Avoiding multigestation pregnancy while maintaining the efficiency of assisted reproduction

It was recognized from the early days of IVF/ET that many of the potential problems associated with the simultaneous transfer of multiple embryos could be circumvented if the non-transferred embryos could be stored for future use. Pregnancies and live births from human cryopreserved IVF embryos [9,10] provided proof of principle and led to the adoption of embryo cryopreservation as a routine adjunct to IVF/ET. When surplus embryos are cryopreserved in conjunction with the transfer of fresh embryos, the practicalities of evaluating success rates from oocyte retrieval cycles

Fertility Cryopreservation, ed. Ri-Cheng Chian and Patrick Quinn. Published by Cambridge University Press.

must be considered and account taken of pregnancies that result from subsequent transfer of thawed embryos [11]. This is true when assessing the impact of cryopreservation on pregnancy and multigestation rates in circumstances where more than one fresh embryo is transferred [12], but the value of cryopreservation is most evident when assessed in the context of single embryo transfer [13]. The importance of assessing the cumulative pregnancy rate from the use of fresh and cryopreserved embryos is emphasized when comparing outcomes from single or double embryo transfer in fresh cycles [14,15]. It is now clear that a successful embryo cryopreservation program allows the confident introduction of single embryo transfer into clinical practice in the knowledge that the incidence of multigestation pregnancy will be reduced while the cumulative chance of a pregnancy will remain essentially unaffected.

Although not all cryopreserved embryos will survive freezing and thawing (see below), the pregnancy potential of any individual embryo that is already cryopreserved will not be affected by extending the period of storage. Rationally, this should then lead to a further reduction in the risk of multigestation by the adoption of single embryo transfer in cycles involving transfer of cryopreserved embryos [16,17]. The role of embryo cryopreservation in maximizing the safety and efficiency of ART is highlighted in our unit by the fact that 52% of all embryo transfer procedures involve stored embryos and 42% of all the implantations arising from embryo transfer can be attributed to cryopreserved embryos. The important role that embryo cryopreservation plays in ART is further emphasized when we consider the fact that many patients will return for the transfer of cryopreserved embryos after the birth of one or more children from the same oocyte collection. In our unit, 78% of all women who give birth as a result of a fresh embryo transfer have the prospect of returning for the transfer of stored embryos. In many cases, therefore, families may be completed without the need for further surgical procedures.

Other roles for embryo cryopreservation

Embryo cryopreservation is also an essential tool when embryo transfer is not possible in the cycle of oocyte collection. While this situation may occur for a variety of reasons, the most common consideration is the risk of ovarian hyperstimulation syndrome. In such cases, where pregnancy would be expected to exacerbate the symptoms, routine management often involves the cryopreservation of all the embryos generated in the cycle and replacement in subsequent cycles when ovarian hyperstimulation syndrome is no longer an issue [18,19].

Of increasing interest is the possibility that reproductive potential can be stored for young women at risk of loss of ovarian function as a consequence of cytotoxic therapies used to eliminate malignant disease. In situations where there is no male partner, the emerging technology of oocyte and ovarian tissue cryopreservation offers some hope of future fertility for the increasing numbers of cancer survivors. Where there is a male partner, however, and where there is adequate time available to undergo ovarian stimulation and oocyte collection prior to commencing therapy, the established and predictable outcomes from embryo cryopreservation may, at present, offer the most realistic prospect of post-cure pregnancy.

Limitations

The value of embryo cryopreservation in all the above circumstances is, of course, predicated on the ability of a sufficient number of embryos to survive the cryopreservation process without significant impairment of their ability to establish a normal pregnancy. This is the challenge that has been faced by the cryobiologists and embryologists.

Methodology for embryo cryopreservation

Although it has been possible to cryopreserve animal and human sperm successfully since the 1950s, it was not until the 1970s that similar success was obtained with mammalian embryos. It had been demonstrated that water-miscible substances known as cryoprotectants, which removed much of the intracellular water, were required to overcome some of the problems associated with ice formation when freezing living cells. Glycerol had been used successfully in this context when cryopreserving semen but it was the introduction of the more rapidly permeating cryoprotectant dimethyl sulfoxide (DMSO) that enabled successful cryopreservation of mouse embryos [20]. Translation of this method to early cleavage stage human embryos resulted in the first reports of successful pregnancy and birth from human cryopreserved embryos [9,10]. Use of DMSO was soon replaced by 1,2 propanediol (PROH) as the permeating cryoprotectant of choice when cryopreserving at pronucleate or early cleavage stages using protocols that also included sucrose to increase intracellular dehydration prior to freezing [21,22]. Although this was initially achieved by sequential exposure to PROH and sucrose, we have found subsequently that single-step dehydration is at least as effective for embryos on day 2 of development. Despite the still predominant use of PROH, encouraging results have also been reported using ethylene glycol as a permeating cryoprotectant during slow cooling of human cleavage stage embryos [23].

The freezing protocols used for cryopreservation of early preimplantation development stages usually involve cooling of dehydrated embryos in sealed plastic straws at approximately −2°C/min, manual nucleation of ice formation (seeding) at around −7°C, and further slow cooling at approximately −0.3°C/min to −30°C before storage in liquid nitrogen. Following rapid thawing, the use of higher extracellular concentrations of sucrose during the early stages of post-thaw rehydration can act as a regulator of the rate at which water enters the cells in response to decreasing extracellular PROH concentrations. In our experience, gradual removal of PROH by serial dilution does not seem to be necessary if a sufficiently high concentration of sucrose (0.5 mol/l) is used during the initial stage of thawing.

Although PROH has continued to be the most widely used permeating cryoprotectant for embryos at early stages of preimplantation development, the methodology used for the slow cooling of blastocyst stages of development has predominantly been based on the use of the less-permeable glycerol. Early reports of pregnancies following the frozen storage of expanding human blastocysts involved the stepwise addition of glycerol alone prior to freezing [24], and this method was subsequently modified to include the addition of sucrose [25]. Rapid thawing and rehydration is usually performed according to the principles outlined above for early cleavage stage embryos. Again, there is a paucity of controlled evidence to support the choice of cryoprotectant used, and successful cryopreservation of blastocyst stage embryos that had been biopsied for preimplantation genetic diagnosis at earlier cleavage stages has been reported using PROH [26]. The start temperature and cooling rate may also play a role in the outcome from slow freezing of blastocysts [27].

More recently, successful cryopreservation of embryos has been reported using the technique of vitrification. This approach involves exposure to very high concentrations of cryoprotectants in very small volumes for very short periods of time, together with extremely rapid cooling. Vitrification results in transition of water to a glass-like state without significant formation of intracellular or extracellular ice crystals. Ultrarapid warming in the presence of elevated concentrations of non-permeating cryoprotectant (usually sucrose) results in rapid removal of the very high levels of intracellular permeating cryoprotectant before rehydration is completed by exposure to reducing concentrations of non-permeating cryoprotectant. Although vitrification of mammalian embryos was described more than 20 years ago [28], translation to human clinical application has only been evident more recently and has predominantly been associated with attempts to improve the outcome from cryopreservation of blastocyst stage embryos [29].

Factors affecting the clinical efficiency of embryo cryopreservation

Selection of embryos for cryopreservation

The inclusion criteria for selection of embryos for cryopreservation may differ widely between units. As a result, the proportion of cycles in which cryopreservation occurs may vary from as low as 10% [30] to as high as 59%, and 73% in women under 36 years of age, in our unit. As discussed above, human embryos can be cryopreserved at all stages of preimplantation development from the unicellular pronucleate stage to the peri-implantation blastocyst stage, but the probability of implantation following transfer of cryopreserved embryos at any stage will also be dependent to a major extent on the quality of the embryo(s) transferred in addition to clinical factors such as female age at the time of oocyte collection and uterine receptivity at the time of embryo transfer.

A number of considerations will determine the stage at which cryopreservation occurs. In young women without partners who wish to preserve their fertility, unfertilized oocytes can be stored but the potential of individual oocytes to fertilize, develop, and implant will be relatively unknown. This approach is also the only option in all circumstances when legislation precludes embryo cryopreservation, which was, but is no longer, the situation in Italy. When embryo cryopreservation is permitted, there is an inverse relationship between the number of embryos stored and the extent to which selection criteria have been applied. Cryopreservation at the pronucleate stage guarantees that all stored oocytes have undergone fertilization and this has been used in many cases where embryo transfer does not take place in the cycle of oocyte collection to avoid the risk of ovarian hyperstimulation syndrome [31]. This approach does not allow significant prestorage selection since the relationship between nuclear morphology and implantation potential remains controversial [32,33]. When applied in conjunction with fresh embryo transfer, pronucleate stage cryopreservation will also restrict the ability to select the highest quality embryo(s) for fresh transfer. It does, however, guarantee that all fertilized oocytes will be stored and is still a commonly used approach in countries where legislation does not allow cryopreservation of later stages. Although slow cooling with PROH and sucrose was used for many years when freezing pronucleate stages, it has now been suggested that vitrification may be a more appropriate technique [34].

The most common approach adopted for cryopreservation of human embryos, to date, has been the slow cooling of cleavage stage embryos, although these stages have also been cryopreserved using vitrification [35]. Cryopreservation on either day 2 or day 3 of development is feasible, although there has been some suggestion that embryos may survive slow cooling better if frozen on day 2 [36]. In routine IVF/ET, this allows selection of embryos for fresh transfer on the basis of developmental rate and other morphological characteristics and also the establishment of minimum criteria for cryopreservation. Stricter criteria for storage may improve implantation rates from thawed embryos but it is important to balance this consideration with the need to preserve the full potential of any cycle of ovarian stimulation [37]. This may be particularly important in cases of cryopreservation for fertility issues prior to cytotoxic therapy. For example, many clinics will only cryopreserve an embryo on day 2 if it has reached the 4-cell stage of development. While it is clear that the implantation rate of 4-cell embryos frozen on day 2 is significantly higher than those with fewer than 4 cells, a decision to exclude embryos with fewer than 4 cells will inevitably result in the discarding of some reproductive potential [17,38].

Embryo selection at cleavage stages can also potentially be enhanced by screening for genetic abnormalities after embryo biopsy. Interestingly, although these embryos are more highly selected, their ability to survive standard cryopreservation techniques is significantly compromised [39,40]. However, modified techniques involving an elevated sucrose concentration [41] or a choline-based, sodium-free medium [42] have been successful in improving the cryosurvival of biopsied embryos.

Whether slow cooled or vitrified, the morphological features of a blastocyst stage embryo will also relate to the probability of implantation [43], and the choice of minimum criteria for blastocyst cryopreservation will impact on the outcome. There are a number of reports, some of them conflicting, on the importance for cryopreservation of degree of expansion, rate of development to the blastocyst stage, and reduction of the blastocelic cavity prior to cryopreservation; these have been reviewed by Youssry *et al.* [29]. Again stricter criteria for cryopreservation may improve apparent success rates at the expense of lost potential.

Cryodamage

Having selected the embryos considered suitable for cryopreservation, the most important consideration becomes the possible detrimental effects of freezing and thawing on the embryo. The nature of cryodamage and its implications will vary between developmental stages. Early evidence of improved outcomes associated with cryopreservation at the pronucleate/zygote stage [44] led to adoption of the approach by many clinics, although the disadvantage of limiting selection of fresh embryos resulted in a move towards cryopreservation of early cleavage stages as results improved. However, there are still some countries in which embryos cannot be cryopreserved after nuclear envelope breakdown, leaving zygote cryopreservation as the main available option. When cryopreservation is performed at the pronucleate stage, cryodamage can be assessed in terms of both survival and subsequent cleavage. Rates of survival of approximately 75% after slow cooling of human zygotes have been reported [18,31] in association with cleavage rates similar to those of fresh embryos. An earlier comparative study of vitrification and slow cooling of zygotes [45] demonstrated a significantly higher survival rate after vitrification. However, post-recovery cleavage rates were compromised in both groups and were lower in vitrified zygotes. More recently, a high (89%) survival rate has been reported after vitrification of human zygotes [34]. In this case, post-recovery embryo development was reported to be normal, with the majority of embryos having reached the 4-cell stage with good morphology after 24 hours of culture. Damage to the integrity of pronuclei has also been reported after cryopreservation of pronuclear zygotes [46] and appears to be associated with reduced developmental potential.

The parameters associated with assessment of success in cryopreservation of cleavage stage embryos are also predominantly survival and subsequent development. Consequences of cryopreservation such as zona pellucida damage [47] and perturbation of metabolism [35] have also been reported. Assessment of survival of cleavage stage embryos is different from that of precleavage stages, where cell survival is all or nothing. The phenomenon of partial survival, whereby some, but not all, blastomeres survive, is interesting in itself. The implication may be that there are differences in individual, and ostensibly equivalent, blastomeres within the same embryo that impact on their ability to withstand freezing and thawing. It is tempting to speculate that these differences may relate to differences in membrane water permeability, such as those shown for mouse and human oocytes [48].

The widely accepted criterion for embryo survival and eligibility for transfer in a clinical situation is that a minimum of 50% of the original blastomeres survive. However, partially intact thawed embryos have a reduced ability to develop to the blastocyst stage in vitro and result in blastocysts with reduced total cell numbers [49]. Loss of blastomeres has been shown clearly to result in reduced implantation rates by a number of groups [30,38,50,51] although the loss of a single blastomere at the 4-cell stage has no impact on implantation potential [17]. It has been claimed that the detrimental effect of blastomere loss may result from a negative influence of the necrotic blastomeres and that this may be reversed by removal of the necrotic material [52]. The proportion of cleavage stage embryos that survives fully intact after cryopreservation is not routinely reported but should be in excess of 50% of all embryos [38].

This survival rate may be increased by the use of vitrification [35], and we have recently shown that a slow-cooling technique based on our previous work with biopsied embryos can result in 80% of non-biopsied cleavage stage embryos surviving fully intact [53]. Post-thaw resumption of mitosis is often used as an indicator of appropriate cryosurvival and has been shown to correlate with implantation potential [30,54,55], as has the number of blastomeres dividing during post-thaw culture [17]. Whether this parameter relates to cryodamage or is a reflection of intrinsic growth potential is not clear, but we have observed an increased frequency of post-thaw resumption of mitosis in embryos that underwent an early first cleavage during the pre-freeze culture period.

Assessment of cryodamage in blastocysts is more complex. Cell survival in the trophectoderm compartment may be easier to assess than in the inner cell mass, where the individual cells are much smaller and often highly compacted, although the collapse of the the blastocelic cavity may preclude assessment of both compartments unless re-expansion occurs before transfer. In fact, the ability of a cryopreserved blastocyst to undergo re-expansion may, in itself, indicate functional survival. Assessment of resumption of development in cryopreserved blastocysts is, again, more limited since any increase in the number of cells is difficult to determine because of the small size of the cells and the morphology of the blastocyst, whether collapsed or re-expanded. The occurrence of hatching after blastocyst cryopreservation may be used as an indicator of functional survival, and it has been suggested that assisting this process may increase the implantation rate [56].

Post-cryopreservation selection of embryos for transfer and implantation

The strictness of the inclusion criteria for embryo cryopreservation and the extent of the cryodamage incurred will be important determinants of the probability of implantation following transfer, but equally important will be the strategy for selection of embryos after cryopreservation. For example, when using cryopreserved zygotes, the options would be to thaw/warm until only the surviving zygote(s) required for transfer is/are obtained and transfer all resulting embryos irrespective of development and quality. This approach, which removes the option for selection, is required by law in countries that do not allow embryo freezing after the breakdown of the pronuclear membrane, and this can reduce the apparent efficiency of the treatment by reducing the implantation rate. Alternatively, multiple zygotes may be recovered and cultured for various periods prior to selection of the highest quality embryos for transfer. In this case, the implantation rate could clearly be improved but surplus embryos would either be discarded or cryopreserved for a second time. Serial cryopreservation is possible, including a reported live birth from transfer of a cryopreserved embryo that resulted from the fertilization of a cryopreserved unfertilized oocyte by a cryopreserved sperm [57].

Criteria for selection of thawed cleavage stage embryos for transfer will also influence the clinical efficiency of embryo transfer. Selection of only intact embryos would reduce the number of embryos transferred but increase the implantation rate [30,50,51,58]. Similarly, selection for transfer on the basis of resumption of mitosis during post-thaw culture would be expected to result in an increased implantation rate [17,30,54,55]. However, although implantation was not evident in one study after transfer of partially intact embryos that failed to resume mitosis in vitro after thawing [30], a number of implantations were reported under the same circumstances in a study of single cryopreserved embryo transfers [17].

Post-thaw/warming characteristics of blastocyst stage embryos may also predict which embryos are most likely to implant. Although the extent of cell survival and the ability of cryopreserved blastocysts to re-form a blastocelic cavity and undergo hatching may be associated with increased implantation rates, there is, again, no evidence that implantation will not occur in the absence of these indicators. The balance between the increased efficiency and implantation rates associated with post-thaw embryo selection and the possibility of "throwing the baby out with the bathwater" has been discussed [37] and will be a matter for consideration in a clinical embryo cryopreservation program.

Safety and ethicolegal considerations

Birth outcomes

As with all forms of ART, there has been extensive follow-up of the outcomes from pregnancies resulting from the transfer of cryopreserved embryos. The available evidence suggests that embryo cryopreservation is not associated with any significant increase in the frequency of adverse perinatal outcomes, and that the health of infants born from cryopreserved embryos is not compromised [59–61]. Interestingly, it has been reported that the increased incidence of low birthweight associated with transfer of IVF embryos is not evident when cryopreserved embryos are transferred [62,63]. Since most of the births to date have resulted from the transfer of embryos cryopreserved using slow-cooling methods, it will be important that similar follow-up is carried out on pregnancies resulting from vitrified embryos.

Storage considerations

The transmission of infectious agents as a consequence of storage in liquid nitrogen has been demonstrated in association with the storage of bone marrow and peripheral blood stem cells [64]. While no documented case of disease transmission mediated by liquid nitrogen related to cryostorage of embryos has been reported yet, systems designed to minimize the theoretical possibility from slow cooling or vitrification are an important feature of the technology [65].

There is no theoretical reason to suspect that the length of time in storage will adversely affect cryopreserved embryos, and there have been many reports of pregnancies and births from embryos that have been stored for more than a decade. However, long-term storage of human embryos will increase the likelihood of a number of possibilities, including death of one or both of the gamete providers or separation of a couple who still have embryos in storage. Valid consent processes that cover such possibilities must, therefore, be a routine part of pretreatment counseling when embryo cryopreservation is envisaged. Concerns over the possible implications of long-term storage of human embryos have led to the introduction of specific legislation in some circumstances. For example, in the UK and in our own state of Victoria, Australia, statutory limits apply to the time an embryo can be kept in storage. An important feature of such legislation is the power of a statutory body to grant an extension of the period in appropriate circumstances. This option is particularly important in cases where the embryos are derived from the gametes of young people who are storing their reproductive potential prior to cytotoxic therapy that may destroy their fertility.

Conclusions

Human embryos can be successfully cryopreserved using a range of techniques at all stages of development and can result in the birth of normal, healthy children when transferred back to the uterus. Application of this technology in the context of infertility treatment has had a major impact on the development of more conservative approaches to the number of embryos transferred and the overall cumulative efficiency of treatment. The success rate will be dependent on a number of factors, including the patient characteristics, the extent of cryodamage, and the criteria for embryo selection both prior to and after storage. In the context of fertility preservation, embryo cryopreservation, when appropriate, can offer a realistic and predictable prospect of future pregnancy. This overview has attempted to set the scene for the following chapters, which will cover in depth the current state of the technology associated with embryo cryopreservation.

References

1. Edwards RG, Steptoe PC, Purdy JM. Fertilization and cleavage in vitro of preovulator human oocytes. *Nature* 1970; **227**: 1307–1309.
2. Edwards RG, Steptoe PC, Purdy JM. Establishing full-term human pregnancies using cleaving embryos grown in vitro. *Br J Obstet Gynaecol* 1980; **87**: 737–756.
3. Trounson AO, Leeton JF, Wood C, Webb J, Wood J. Pregnancies in humans by fertilization in vitro and embryo transfer in the controlled ovulatory cycle. *Science* 1981; **212**: 681–682.
4. Multiple gestation pregnancy. The ESHRE Capri Workshop Group. *Hum Reprod* 2000; **15**: 1856–1864.
5. Collins J. Cost efficiency of reducing multiple births. *Reprod Biomed Online* 2007; **15**(Suppl 3): 35–39.
6. Templeton A, Morris JK. Reducing the risk of multiple births by transfer of two embryos after in vitro fertilization. *N Engl J Med* 1998; **339**: 573–577.
7. Gerris J, de Neubourg D, Mangelschots K, *et al.* Prevention of twin pregnancy after in-vitro fertilization or intracytoplasmic sperm injection based on strict embryo criteria: a prospective randomized clinical trial. *Hum Reprod* 1999; **14**: 2581–2587.
8. Gerris J, de Sutter P, de Neubourg D, *et al.* A real-life prospective health economic study of elective single embryo transfer versus two-embryo transfer in first IVF/ICSI cycles. *Hum Reprod* 2004; **19**: 917–923.
9. Trounson A, Mohr L. Human pregnancy following cryopreservation, thawing and transfer of an eight-cell embryo. *Nature* 1983; **305**: 707–709.
10. Zeilmaker GH, Alberda AT, van Gent I, Rijkmans CM, Drogendijk AC. Two pregnancies following transfer of intact frozen–thawed embryos. *Fertil Steril* 1984; **42**: 293–296.
11. Jones HW, Jr., Out HJ, Hoomans EH, Driessen SG, Coelingh Bennink HJ. Cryopreservation: the practicalities of evaluation. *Hum Reprod* 1997; **12**: 1522–1524.
12. Schnorr JA, Doviak MJ, Muasher SJ, Jones HW, Jr. Impact of a cryopreservation program on the multiple pregnancy rate associated with assisted reproductive technologies. *Fertil Steril* 2001; **75**: 147–151.
13. Tiitinen A, Halttunen M, Harkki P, Vuoristo P, Hyden-Granskog C. Elective single embryo transfer: the value of cryopreservation. *Hum Reprod* 2001; **16**: 1140–1144.
14. Thurin A, Hausken J, Hillensjo T, *et al.* Elective single-embryo transfer versus double-embryo transfer in in vitro fertilization. *N Engl J Med* 2004; **351**: 2392–2402.
15. Lundin K, Bergh C. Cumulative impact of adding frozen–thawed cycles to single versus double fresh embryo transfers. *Reprod Biomed Online* 2007; **15**: 76–82.
16. Hyden-Granskog C, Unkila-Kallio L, Halttunen M, Tiitinen A. Single embryo transfer is an option in frozen embryo transfer. *Hum Reprod* 2005; **20**: 2935–2938.
17. Edgar DH, Archer J, McBain J, Bourne H. Embryonic factors affecting outcome from single cryopreserved embryo transfer. *Reprod Biomed Online* 2007; **14**: 718–723.
18. Queenan JT, Jr., Veeck LL, Toner JP, Oehninger S, Muasher SJ. Cryopreservation of all prezygotes in patients at risk of severe hyperstimulation does not eliminate the syndrome, but the chances of pregnancy are excellent with subsequent frozen–thaw transfers. *Hum Reprod* 1997; **12**: 1573–1576.
19. Tiitinen A, Husa LM, Tulppala M, Simberg N, Seppala M. The effect of cryopreservation in prevention of ovarian hyperstimulation syndrome. *Br J Obstet Gynaecol* 1995; **102**: 326–329.
20. Whittingham DG, Leibo SP, Mazur P. Survival of mouse embryos frozen to −196 degrees and −269 degrees C. *Science* 1972; **178**: 411–414.
21. Lassalle B, Testart J, Renard JP. Human embryo features that influence the success of cryopreservation with the use of 1,2 propanediol. *Fertil Steril* 1985; **44**: 645–651.
22. Testart J, Lassalle B, Belaisch-Allart J, *et al.* High pregnancy rate after early human embryo freezing. *Fertil Steril* 1986; **46**: 268–272.
23. Chi HJ, Koo JJ, Kim MY, *et al.* Cryopreservation of human embryos using ethylene glycol in controlled slow freezing. *Hum Reprod* 2002; **17**: 2146–2151.
24. Cohen J, Simons RF, Edwards RG, Fehilly CB, Fishel SB. Pregnancies following the frozen storage of expanding human blastocysts. *J In Vitro Fert Embryo Transf* 1985; **2**: 59–64.
25. Menezo Y, Nicollet B, Herbaut N, Andre D. Freezing cocultured human blastocysts. *Fertil Steril* 1992; **58**: 977–980.
26. Magli MC, Gianaroli L, Grieco N, *et al.* Cryopreservation of biopsied embryos at the blastocyst stage. *Hum Reprod* 2006; **21**: 2656–2660.
27. Gardner DK, Lane M, Stevens J, Schoolcraft WB. Changing the start temperature and cooling rate in a slow-freezing protocol increases human blastocyst viability. *Fertil Steril* 2003; **79**: 407–410.
28. Rall WF, Fahy GM. Ice-free cryopreservation of mouse embryos at −196 degrees C by vitrification. *Nature* 1985; **313**: 573–575.
29. Youssry M, Ozmen B, Zohni K, Diedrich K, Al-Hasani S. Current aspects of blastocyst cryopreservation. *Reprod Biomed Online* 2008; **16**: 311–320.
30. Guerif F, Bidault R, Cadoret V, *et al.* Parameters guiding selection of best embryos for transfer after cryopreservation: a reappraisal. *Hum Reprod* 2002; **17**: 1321–1326.
31. Ferraretti AP, Gianaroli L, Magli C, *et al.* Elective cryopreservation of all pronucleate embryos in women at risk of ovarian hyperstimulation syndrome: efficiency and safety. *Hum Reprod* 1999; **14**: 1457–1460.

32. Scott L, Alvero R, Leondires M, Miller B. The morphology of human pronuclear embryos is positively related to blastocyst development and implantation. *Hum Reprod* 2000; **15**: 2394–2403.
33. James AN, Hennessy S, Reggio B, *et al.* The limited importance of pronuclear scoring of human zygotes. *Hum Reprod* 2006; **21**: 1599–1604.
34. Al-Hasani S, Ozmen B, Koutlaki N, *et al.* Three years of routine vitrification of human zygotes: is it still fair to advocate slow-rate freezing? *Reprod Biomed Online* 2007; **14**: 288–293.
35. Balaban B, Urman B, Ata B, *et al.* A randomized controlled study of human day 3 embryo cryopreservation by slow freezing or vitrification: vitrification is associated with higher survival, metabolism and blastocyst formation. *Hum Reprod* 2008; **23**: 1976–1982.
36. Salumets A, Tuuri T, Makinen S, *et al.* Effect of developmental stage of embryo at freezing on pregnancy outcome of frozen–thawed embryo transfer. *Hum Reprod* 2003; **18**: 1890–1895.
37. Edgar DH, Archer J, Bourne H. The application and impact of cryopreservation of early cleavage stage embryos in assisted reproduction. *Hum Fertil* (Camb) 2005; **8**: 225–230.
38. Edgar DH, Bourne H, Speirs AL, McBain JC. A quantitative analysis of the impact of cryopreservation on the implantation potential of human early cleavage stage embryos. *Hum Reprod* 2000; **15**: 175–179.
39. Joris H, Van Den Abbeel E, Vos AD, Van Steirteghem A. Reduced survival after human embryo biopsy and subsequent cryopreservation. *Hum Reprod* 1999; **14**: 2833–2837.
40. Magli MC, Gianaroli L, Fortini D, Ferraretti AP, Munne S. Impact of blastomere biopsy and cryopreservation techniques on human embryo viability. *Hum Reprod* 1999; **14**: 770–773.
41. Jericho H, Wilton L, Gook DA, Edgar DH. A modified cryopreservation method increases the survival of human biopsied cleavage stage embryos. *Hum Reprod* 2003; **18**: 568–571.
42. Stachecki JJ, Cohen J, Munne S. Cryopreservation of biopsied cleavage stage human embryos. *Reprod Biomed Online* 2005; **11**: 711–715.
43. Gardner DK, Lane M, Stevens J, Schlenker T, Schoolcraft WB. Blastocyst score affects implantation and pregnancy outcome: towards a single blastocyst transfer. *Fertil Steril* 2000; **73**: 1155–1158.
44. Demoulin A, Jouan C, Gerday C, Dubois M. Pregnancy rates after transfer of embryos obtained from different stimulation protocols and frozen at either pronucleate or multicellular stages. *Hum Reprod* 1991; **6**: 799–804.
45. Van Den Abbeel E, Camus M, van Waesberghe L, Devroey P, Van Steirteghem AC. A randomized comparison of the cryopreservation of one-cell human embryos with a slow controlled-rate cooling procedure or a rapid cooling procedure by direct plunging into liquid nitrogen. *Hum Reprod* 1997; **12**: 1554–1560.
46. Isachenko V, Todorov P, Dimitrov Y, Isachenko E. Integrity rate of pronuclei after cryopreservation of pronuclear-zygotes as a criterion for subsequent embryo development and pregnancy. *Hum Reprod* 2008; **23**: 819–826.
47. Van Den Abbeel E, Van Steirteghem A. Zona pellucida damage to human embryos after cryopreservation and the consequences for their blastomere survival and in-vitro viability. *Hum Reprod* 2000; **15**: 373–378.
48. Hunter JE, Bernard A, Fuller BJ, McGrath JJ, Shaw RW. Measurements of the membrane water permeability (Lp) and its temperature dependence (activation energy) in human fresh and failed-to-fertilize oocytes and mouse oocyte. *Cryobiology* 1992; **29**: 240–249.
49. Archer J, Gook DA, Edgar DH. Blastocyst formation and cell numbers in human frozen–thawed embryos following extended culture. *Hum Reprod* 2003; **18**: 1669–1673.
50. Burns WN, Gaudet TW, Martin MB, *et al.* Survival of cryopreservation and thawing with all blastomeres intact identifies multicell embryos with superior frozen embryo transfer outcome. *Fertil Steril* 1999; **72**: 527–532.
51. Van Den Abbeel E, Camus M, van Waesberghe L, Devroey P, Van Steirteghem AC. Viability of partially damaged human embryos after cryopreservation. *Hum Reprod* 1997; **12**: 2006–2010.
52. Rienzi L, Nagy ZP, Ubaldi F, *et al.* Laser-assisted removal of necrotic blastomeres from cryopreserved embryos that were partially damaged. *Fertil Steril* 2002; **77**: 1196–1201.
53. Edgar DH, Karani J, Gook DA. Increasing dehydration of human cleavage-stage embryos prior to slow cooling significantly increases cryosurvival. *Reprod Biomed Online* 2009; **19:** 521–525.
54. Van Der Elst J, Van Den Abbeel E, Vitrier S, Camus M, Devroey P, Van Steirteghem AC. Selective transfer of cryopreserved human embryos with further cleavage after thawing increases delivery and implantation rates. *Hum Reprod* 1997; **12**: 1513–21.
55. Ziebe S, Bech B, Petersen K, *et al.* Resumption of mitosis during post-thaw culture: a key parameter in selecting the right embryos for transfer. *Hum Reprod* 1998; **13**: 178–181.
56. Vanderzwalmen P, Bertin G, Debauche C, *et al.* Vitrification of human blastocysts with the Hemi-Straw carrier: application of assisted hatching after thawing. *Hum Reprod* 2003; **18**: 1504–1511.
57. Gook DA, Hale L, Edgar DH. Live birth following transfer of a cryopreserved embryo generated from a cryopreserved oocyte and a cryopreserved sperm: case report. *J Assist Reprod Genet* 2007; **24**: 43–45.

58. Edgar DH, Bourne H, Jericho H, McBain JC. The developmental potential of cryopreserved human embryos. *Mol Cell Endocrinol* 2000; **169**: 69–72.
59. Wada I, Macnamee MC, Wick K, Bradfield JM, Brinsden PR. Birth characteristics and perinatal outcome of babies conceived from cryopreserved embryos. *Hum Reprod* 1994; **9**: 543–546.
60. Wennerholm UB, Albertsson-Wikland K, Bergh C, *et al.* Postnatal growth and health in children born after cryopreservation as embryos. *Lancet* 1998; **351**: 1085–1090.
61. Sutcliffe AG, D ' Souza SW, Cadman J, *et al.* Minor congenital anomalies, major congenital malformations and development in children conceived from cryopreserved embryos. *Hum Reprod* 1995; **10**: 3332–3337.
62. Aytoz A, Van Den Abbeel E, Bonduelle M, *et al.* Obstetric outcome of pregnancies after the transfer of cryopreserved and fresh embryos obtained by conventional in-vitro fertilization and intracytoplasmic sperm injection. *Hum Reprod* 1999; **14**: 2619–2624.
63. Shih W, Rushford DD, Bourne H, *et al.* Factors affecting low birthweight after assisted reproduction technology: difference between transfer of fresh and cryopreserved embryos suggests an adverse effect of oocyte collection. *Hum Reprod* 2008; **23**: 1644–1653.
64. Tedder RS, Zuckerman MA, Goldstone AH, *et al.* Hepatitis B transmission from contaminated cryopreservation tank. *Lancet* 1995; **346**: 137–140.
65. Vajta G, Nagy ZP. Are programmable freezers still needed in the embryo laboratory? Review on vitrification. *Reprod Biomed Online* 2006; **12**: 779–796.

Chapter 10

Cryopreservation of pronuclear stage human embryos

Barry Behr and Yimin Shu

Introduction

In vitro fertilization (IVF), embryo transfer in its current form, leads to the generation of multiple oocytes and often supernumerary embryos. The high incidence of multiple births associated with assisted reproductive technology (ART) has become a major concern. A remarkable 29.3% of all births following IVF in 2002 in the USA were twins and another 7.4% births were of three or more infants [1]. The most effective strategy to reduce the risk of multiple births in IVF is to limit the number of embryos replaced per transfer cycle. Many countries (e.g. Brazil, Denmark, Germany, Hungary, Saudi Arabia, Singapore, Sweden, Switzerland, and the UK) have enacted strict laws limiting the number of embryos that can be transferred per cycle [2]. In the USA, there has been a consistent trend toward the transfer of fewer embryos per cycle since the late 1990s [3]. It is, therefore, necessary to have a reliable method to cryopreserve embryos that are surplus to immediate embryo transfer requirements and to store them for future use. Supernumerary embryos may be cryopreserved as early as day 1 (pronuclear stage) and up to day 6 or day 7 (blastocyst stage). This chapter will focus on the crypreservation of pronuclear stage embryos on day 1.

Basic technique

The earliest human embryo cryopreservation protocols were largely borrowed from the existing mammalian animal models of embryo cryopreservation. Live births following frozen–thawed embryo transfer were first reported in mice in 1972 [4]. Later, Wilmut and Rowson [5] reported the first live calf following a frozen embryo transfer with embryos that were produced in vivo. Cryopreservation of oocytes and embryos routinely involves the use of cryoprotectants. The cryoprotectants act as "antifreeze" in several different ways. Freezing point depression through to the colligative properties of permeating cryoprotectants prevents the formation of destructive intracellular ice crystals. The mixture of permeating and non-permeating cryoprotectants aids in cellular dehydration during the cryopreservation process. In addition, the use of non-permeating macromolecules produces an osmotic counterforce to restrict water movement across the membranes and prevent excessive swelling of the cells during the removal of cryoprotectant [6,7]. While glycerol and dimethyl sulfoxide contributed to the first pregnancy following transfer of a frozen–thawed 8-cell stage human embryo [8], slow-freezing/rapid thawing protocols using 1,2-propanediol and sucrose as cryoprotectants have been the standard protocols of pronuclear and early cleavage stage embryos for years [9–12].

Currently there are two main methods used for the cryopreservation of human oocytes and embryos: slow freezing and vitrification. The principle behind conventional slow-freezing procedures is to induce ice formation extracellularly, thereby raising the solute concentration. The cryopreservation procedure can be divided into the following phases: pre-freeze, freezing, storage, thawing, and post-thaw [13]. The pre-freeze phase gives the cells a brief equilibration period to take up the cryoprotectants. When the cells are transferred from isotonic solution to hyperosmotic solutions with permeating cryoprotectants, they shrink immediately as water leaves in response to the difference in osmotic pressure between intracellular and extracellular solutions. As the cryoprotectant permeates, water enters the cells to maintain intracellular osmotic equilibrium. Shrinkage stops when equilibrium is reached between the efflux of water and the influx of cryoprotectants. After that, the cryoprotectant enters the cells at a rate dependent on its permeability characteristics at the given temperature. Equilibration is complete when no

Fertility Cryopreservation, ed. Ri-Cheng Chian and Patrick Quinn. Published by Cambridge University Press.

further osmotic and chemical gradients with regard to the cryoprotectants as well as water exist. Optimal equilibration prior to slow cooling should be long enough for permeating cryoprotectants to enter the cells while minimizing the exposure to the toxic effects of the cryoprotectants.

The optimal cooling rate is determined by a number of biophysical factors and is specific to the cell type. A cooling rate of 1–3°C/min is satisfactory for most animal cell types. Oocytes and embryos have lower surface-to-volume ratio and larger size than somatic cells. Accordingly, a slower cooling rate is required to allow enough time for cell dehydration. After being loaded into plastic straws or vials, oocytes or embryos are cooled at a rate of 1–2°C/min from room temperature to a temperature slightly below the melting point of the solution, which is approximately −5° to −7°C. At this temperature, manual seeding is performed by touching the straw or vial with forceps or spatulas pre-chilled with liquid nitrogen to initiate extracellular ice formation in a controlled manner and avoid super-cooling. The oocytes and embryos are again allowed to equilibrate for 5–10 minutes and the temperature is lowered at a rate of 0.3–0.5°C/min until below −30°C. Osmotic imbalance caused by the increasing extracellular solute concentrations following extracellular ice formation drives the remaining water out of the cells. As ice crystals grow, the extracellular solution becomes more concentrated and the cells are exposed to an increasingly hypertonic environment. The cooling process continues until the intracellular cryoprotectant concentration is high enough to allow vitrification, preventing intracellular ice formation when the cell is plunged into liquid nitrogen. The frozen oocytes and embryos are then stored in a liquid nitrogen tank for future use. As shown in a sample human freezing protocol (Table 10.1), embryos are slow cooled to −35°C before rapid cooling by direct immersion in liquid nitrogen (−196°C).

The stage of embryo cryopreservation and the freezing–thawing protocols vary significantly between clinics and are usually dependent upon the preferences and workload of the individual laboratories. Because of the lack of suitable culture medium to support embryonic development for several days in vitro, embryo transfer was usually performed on day 1 or day 2 in the early days of human IVF. Therefore, most embryos are frozen at pronuclear or 2- to 4-cell stages. The pronuclear stage appeared to be the optimal stage for cryopreservation [14,15]. The unicellular form and lack of spindle apparatus may account for its high post-thaw survival and implantation potential. Because it is difficult to evaluate embryo quality at the pronuclear stage, it is a common practice to cryopreserve all supernumerary pronuclear stage embryos irrespective of future embryonic developmental potential. While different pronuclear scoring systems have been proposed as a predictor of embryo quality, selection based on the morphology of pronuclei and nucleoli is still highly controversial in the literature [16–20]. The freezing strategy utilizing embryos at the cleavage or blastocyst stages differs from the pronuclear stage in that only good-quality embryos are selected for cryopreservation. Fewer embryos are, therefore, cryopreserved per retrieval cycle if the freezing is performed at cleavage or blastocyst stages than if it occurs at the pronuclear stage. Culturing embryos to multicellular or blastocyst stages allows for better selection of high-quality embryos for transfer and freezing of only robust embryos.

Because of the dynamic nature of pronuclear development, timing is a critical issue in the cryopreservation of pronuclear stage embryos. Several authors have investigated the timing of pronuclear formation, pronuclear migration, DNA synthesis, and cleavage in the human 1-cell embryo [21–23]. According to a time-lapse video cinematography study [23], male and female pronuclei were visible as early as 2 hours 51 minutes after sperm injection. By 5 hours after sperm injection, 51% of the oocytes had formed pronuclei. At 8 hours, 80% of the normally fertilized oocytes revealed two pronuclei. The peak or the end of the peak of the two-pronuclei appearance curve was at 16 hours, when all but one oocyte revealed both pronuclei, and at 20 hours this fell to 68%. Pronuclei migrate to the center of the oocyte and remain there from approximately 6 to 8 hours after fertilization, until just before syngamy is reached. Based on the above data, the freezing process must be initiated before the zygote proceeds to syngamy (20–22 hours after insemination/injection for IVF).

Thawing is the reverse of the freezing process and is as equally important. Thawing involves the removal of the frozen straws or vials from liquid nitrogen, removal of cryoprotectant from the frozen cells by stepwise dilution, and warming the thawed cells to 37°C. The optimal thawing protocol depends on the specific freezing protocol and cryoprotectants used. If the cooling is terminated at a high subzero temperature of −30 to −40°C, a moderately rapid warming (200–350°C/min) is required to maximize the survival rate. Embryos

Table 10.1. Freezing and thawing protocols for pronuclear stage human embryos

Protocol steps	Instructions
Freeezing	
1.	Prepare 1.5 M PROH, 1.5 M PROH + 0.1 M sucrose freezing media in a HEPES-buffered mHTF (CooperSurgical, Trumbull, CT, USA) supplemented with 20% SPS
2.	Equilibration with the freezing media is carried out at room temperature. Embryos are first exposed to the 1.5 M PROH for 10 min then to 1.5 M PROH + 0.1 M sucrose solution for another 10 min
3.	Embryos are then loaded into cryostraws (Cryo Bio System, IMV Technologies, Paris, France) and placed in a programmable freezer (CL-8000, Cryologic, Mulgrave, Victoria, Australia)
4.	It is important to make sure that the embryos are well mixed with the freezing solutions by pipetting the embryos up and down in the solution several times after adding them to the freezing solution
5.	The cryostraws are cooled from 20°C down to −6.5°C at a rate of 2.0°C/min, at which point a 2 min pre seeding hold is maintained before manual seeding is performed using pre-cooled forceps or a cotton swab. An additional 8 min hold at −6.5°C is provided for further equilibration. Cooling resumes at a rate of 0.3°C/min to −35°C before the cryostraws are plunged and stored in liquid nitrogen
Thawing	
1.	Prepare 0.5 M sucrose and 0.2 M sucrose thawing media in mHTF with 20% SPS
2.	The thawing procedure is performed at room temperature
3.	Cryostraws are removed from liquid nitrogen and exposed in air for 30 s and then warmed in a water bath at 31°C until the ice has fully melted. The slow cooling is terminated at −35°C in this protocol and a moderately rapid warming (200–350°C/min) is required to maximize the survival rate
4.	The frozen embryos are expelled out of the straw using the stylet and quickly located. The frozen embryos are picked up in a minimal amount of solution and transferred to a 0.5 M sucrose solution and left for 10 min before 0.2 M sucrose solution is added for another 10 min
5.	The thawed embryos are then washed in mHTF with 20% SPS without sucrose and then transferred to Quinn's Advantage Cleavage Medium with 20% SPS and further cultured at 37°C with 5% CO_2, 5% O_2, and 90% N_2 until transfer

PROH, 1,2-propanediol; mHTF, human tubal fluid medium; SPS, Serum Protein Substitute.

cooled slowly to temperatures below −60°C prior to being plunged into liquid nitrogen require a rather slow warming rate of approximately 25°C/min or less. As oocytes and embryos are more permeable to water than to cryoprotectants, the frozen cells will swell or burst if they are placed directly in a medium without cryoprotectants after thawing. For this reason, a high concentration of non-permeating cryoprotectants (such as sucrose) is usually used as an osmotic buffer to counteract the high concentration of cryoprotectants in the cell.

Indications

While embryo cryopreservation has been successfully performed at various developmental stages, cryopreservation of human embryos at the pronuclear stage is more acceptable to some patients for ethical, moral, and religious reasons. Pronuclear-stage cryopreservation has been applied extensively in some European countries with legal restrictions to embryo selection and embryo cryopreservation, such as Germany, Switzerland, and Italy. The German Embryo Protection Law defines the embryo as "the fertilized human egg cell capable of development, from the moment of fusion of the pronuclei" [24]. According to this law, no more than three oocytes can be cultured further than the two-pronuclear (2PN) stage and no embryos can be frozen. After fusion of the pronuclei, the embryos must be transferred and cannot be discarded or used for other purposes, thus limiting the choice to freezing either unfertilized oocytes or fertilized oocytes with two pronuclei [25]. Despite the recent advances on oocyte cryopreservation obtained with the use of vitrification, this procedure is still considered to be experimental and advised to be performed under institutional review board research protocol by the American Society for Reproductive Medicine. Cryopreservation of fertilized oocytes with two pronuclei, therefore, remains the main focus of female fertility preservation in these countries.

Ovarian hyperstimulation syndrome (OHSS) is the most severe complication of controlled ovarian stimulation and complicates 3–8% of IVF cycles; severe OHSS is rare and complicates 1% of cycles. This syndrome may occur either with an early (early onset)

Table 10.2. Outcomes of elective cryopreservation of all pronuclear stage embryos in patients with high risk of ovarian hyperstimulation syndrome

Study	Number of patients	Pregnancy/transfer cycle (%)	Cumulative pregnancy/ patient (%)
Wada *et al.* (1993) [30]	78	26	NA
Pattinson *et al.* (1994) [31]	69	25.2	40.6
Tiitinen *et al.* (1995) [32]	23	32.6	68.2
Frederick *et al.* (1995) [33]	36	31.8	58.3
Shaker *et al.* (1996) [34]	13	38.6	NA
Awonuga *et al.* (1996) [35]	62	12.5–26.7	NA
Queenan *et al.* (1997) [36]	15	58	67
Ferraretti *et al.* (1999) [37]	58	35.4	48.3
Endo *et al.* (2002) [38]	68	32.4	NA
Vyjayanthi *et al.* (2006) [29]	260	31.5	46
Griesinger *et al.* (2007) [39]	20	31.6	36.8

NA, not available.

or a late pattern (late onset) in IVF cycles [26]. As a management strategy for OHSS, elective cryopreservation of all produced embryos has been shown to be effective in the prevention of the late-onset OHSS. A systematic review of the literature for patients at high risk of OHSS shows that elective embryo cryopreservation was performed at the pronuclear stage in almost all the published reports. This is probably because pronuclear zygotes survive the freezing and thawing procedures better than cleavage stage embryos [14,27,28]. Table 10.2 summarizes the clinical outcome of elective cryopreservation of all pronuclear stage embryos in patients with high risk of OHSS. As demonstrated by Vyjayanthi *et al.* [29], elective embryo cryopreservation and subsequent frozen embryo transfer in patients at risk of OHSS does not compromise the cumulative pregnancy rate per patient.

The success rate following pre-implantation genetic diagnosis is directly proportional to the number of embryos suitable for biopsy. For patients with a limited number of embryos, cleavage stage embryos from several retrieval cycles are usually cryopreserved for a future embryo biopsy. However, blastomeres of cryopreserved embryos seem to have a more fragile and brittle cell membrane, which makes embryo biopsy and fixation more difficult. Cryopreservation of pronuclear stage embryos can potentially alleviate this problem by allowing the pronuclear stage embryos to cleave in culture for 2 days prior to biopsy on day 3. This culture interval tends to allow the embryos to recover from the cryopreservation and provides embryos with a more "fresh-like" cell membrane.

There are various forms of stress (i.e. cold, shock, osmotic stress) associated with cell and tissue cryopreservation. Human oocytes and early embryos are very sensitive to chilling and cryopreservation and may suffer considerable morphological and functional damage during cryopreservation. It is, therefore, expected that some frozen embryos will not survive the freezing and thawing process. Pronuclear stage embryos are considered to have survived the freezing–thawing procedure if they regain their original volume without obvious damage to the zona pellucida, oolemma, or cytoplasm after the removal of the cryoprotectants. In general, 60–80% of frozen pronuclear stage embryos survive the thawing [40–42]. In a small percentage of patients, none of the cryopreserved pronuclear stage embryos survives, and no embryo transfer takes place [43].

To verify further embryo development, frozen–thawed pronuclear stage embryos are usually cultured for 1 to 2 more days prior to embryo transfer. Overnight culture and examination for mitotic resumption of frozen–thawed pronuclear stage embryos is considered essential to the selection of viable embryos after thawing [40]. In a recent study performed by Isachenko *et al.* [44], higher rates of blastocyst formation have been reported for cryopreserved pronuclear stage embryos with high integrity rates for pronuclei. Moreover, transfer of the 5-day blastocysts derived from pronuclear stage embryos with high integrity rate for pronuclei resulted in a significantly higher rate of pregnancy compared with those blastocysts from pronuclear stage embryos with low integrity rates (43% and 10%, respectively). The authors concluded that the integrity rate for pronuclei after cryopreservation of pronuclear stage embryos was a predictor of future embryo development and implantation. Because of the negative effect of cryopreservation on embryo viability, relatively more embryos are potentially transferred in a frozen cycle compared with a fresh cycle. Sometimes more pronuclear stage embryos are required to be thawed if the first set fails to undergo further development.

Factors affecting the success of embryo transfer

The clinical outcome of transfer of frozen pronuclear stage embryos varies substantially between studies. Several factors might contribute to the between-study variants, including patient's age, embryo quality before freezing, the number of embryos transferred, freezing and thawing protocol, and endometrial preparation. Maternal age is one of the most important factors affecting the success of fresh embryo transfer. By analysing 103 transfer cycles of cryopreserved embryos at the pronuclear stage, Damario *et al.* [45] observed an apparent trend toward a decline in delivery rate per frozen embryo transfer associated with increasing female age. In both fresh and frozen embryo transfers of a single oocyte retrieval, the chances of at least one live birth for women aged < 35, 35–39, and > 39 years were 61.2%, 59.7%, and 18.5%, respectively. A similar trend has also been noted following the transfer of embryos cryopreserved at cleavage stage [46,47].

The success of a frozen–thawed embryo transfer has been shown to be associated with the outcome of the fresh cycle from which the embryos were derived. Lin *et al.* [48] compared the outcome of two groups of patients who underwent frozen–thawed embryo transfer with a clinical pregnancy or without a pregnancy during the fresh cycle from which the frozen embryos were derived. They reported a significantly higher pregnancy rate (24.1%) in the frozen transfer cycles where a clinical pregnancy was achieved during the fresh cycle than in the frozen transfer cycle following a failed fresh cycle (8.5%). Similar results were also reported by Gabrielsen [49], who found the chance of embryo implantation following a frozen cycle is significantly higher if a pregnancy was established in the prior fresh cycle. A successful fresh cycle, therefore, reflects better embryo quality and can be used to predict the chances of pregnancy of the following frozen–thawed embryo transfer cycle. The number of embryos transferred is another factor affecting the success rate of frozen–thawed embryo transfer. As reported by Testart *et al.* [50], transfer of two frozen–thawed pronuclear stage embryos yields a two-fold increase in pregnancy rate compared with a single pronuclear stage embryo transfer. Similarly, significantly higher rates of pregnancy were obtained after the transfer of three or four frozen–thawed pronuclear stage embryos than with the transfer of one or two [51].

After fertilization, the zona pellucida plays an important role in maintaining the integrity of the embryo. Zona pellucida manipulation, including intracytoplasmic sperm injection (ICSI), assisted hatching, and embryo biopsy, involves an artificial breach of the zona pellucida and there has been concern that manipulation of the zona pellucida could interfere with the diffusion of the cryoprotectants during the dehydration and rehydration process. The impact of the fertilization method on the rates of post-thaw survival and clinical outcome of cryopreserved pronuclear stage embryos has been addressed in several reports. According to Damario *et al.* [15], embryos from both IVF and ICSI survived very well after thawing (IVF 90.4%; ICSI 91.1%). Implantation rate (IVF 19.1%; ICSI 19.9%) and delivery rate (IVF 36.5%; ICSI 39.8%) were also comparable. Similarly, Al-Hasani *et al.* [27] observed comparable rates of post-thaw embryo survival, clinical pregnancy, and spontaneous abortion between cryopreserved pronuclear stage embryos resulting from ICSI ($n = 744$) and conventional IVF ($n = 333$). Opposing results were revealed in the study of Macas *et al.* [52], where a significantly lower implantation rate was seen in the ICSI group (10.9%) compared with the IVF group (25.0%). Moreover, a trend to a higher rate of preclinical and clinical abortions was noted following the transfer of frozen embryos derived from ICSI (8/14 [57.1%]) compared with IVF (2/11 [11.8%]) in the same study. Taking into account the fact that 11.5% of ICSI and only 2.0% of IVF embryos were found in a stage of syngamy at the time of freezing, the overly long post-insemination time of 20 hours seems to be the principal reason for the lower developmental potential of cryopreserved pronuclear stage embryos from ICSI.

In another study, conducted by Simon *et al.* [53], a significantly lower clinical pregnancy rate was achieved from frozen transfer cycles utilizing cleavage stage embryos arising from ICSI than from IVF (20% versus 32.5%). However, there was a higher proportion of good-quality embryos before freezing in conventional IVF cycles compared with ICSI cycles in their study, suggesting that the differences in pregnancy rates found between the groups could not be simply attributed to the use of micromanipulation for ICSI. Based on the current data available, the ICSI procedure does not compromise the ability of pronuclear stage embryos to withstand cryopreservation and their further developmental potential after freezing and thawing. An intact zona pellucida is not necessary for a successful mouse embryo cryopreservation [54]. As reported by Hershlag and Feng [55], a 30 μm diameter defect created in the zona pellucida during assisted hatching before freezing does not hinder post-thaw mouse embryonic development. For humans, a promising clinical pregnancy rate (31.4%) has been obtained following the transfer of cryopreserved blastocysts that underwent laser-assisted hatching on the zona on day 3 [56]. A larger hole is drilled in the zona pellucida for embryo biopsy than used in ICSI and assisted hatching. An adverse effect of embryo biopsy on post-thaw embryo survival has been demonstrated, and vitrification has been shown to be an effective method for improving the survival rate of biopsied embryos at cleavage and pronuclear stages [57–59]. A recent study reported a successful pregnancy following vitrification of pronuclear stage oocytes biopsied for polar body aneuploidy screening [60].

The endometrium plays a crucial role in embryo implantation and pregnancy establishment. Cryopreserved embryos have been successfully replaced in both natural ovulation cycles and hormone replacement cycles. The main advantage of the natural cycle is the lack of medication, whereas the downregulated hormone controlled cycle is more convenient for programming the day of frozen embryo transfer and planning the workload for the IVF practice in advance. In a retrospective study by Al-Shawaf *et al.* [61], natural-cycle frozen embryo transfer was performed for 77 patients with proven ovulation and regular menstrual cycles and hormone replacement cycle was used for patients with anovulation, irregular cycles, or older age. No significant difference in pregnancy rates (26% and 25%, respectively), ongoing/delivery rate (20.8% in both groups), and implantation rate (10.3% and 10.6%, respectively) were found between natural and hormone replacement cycles. In another study, Gelbaya *et al.* [62] compared the outcome of frozen embryo transfers in natural and downregulated hormone replacement cycles in patients with regular menstrual cycles. The rates of embryo implantation, clinical pregnancy, or live birth rates per cycle or per transfer were similar in both groups.

Impact of developmental stage at freezing on clinical outcome

There has been no universal agreement as to which stage of embryonic development at freezing provides a clear advantage for the outcome of a frozen embryo transfer cycle [63]. As shown in Table 10.3, controversial results have been obtained concerning the rates of survival and the developmental competence between embryos frozen at the pronuclear and early cleavage stages.

In a prospective study performed by Horne *et al.* [41], similar rates of embryo survival were found between embryos frozen at the pronuclear (96/129 [74.4%]) and day 2 cleavage (79/102 [77.4%]) stages. Salumets *et al.* [66], in a large series involving a total of 4006 embryos thawed in 1657 cycles, directly compared the survival rates between three cryopreservation strategies utilizing pronuclear, day 2, or day 3 embryo freezing. Their results showed that frozen pronuclear stage embryos survived better (86.5%) than either day 2 (61.7%) or day 3 (43.1%) embryos. On the contrary, Kattera *et al.* [65] reported that supernumerary IVF-generated embryos frozen on day 2 had significantly higher survival rates (73.9%) than those frozen at the pronuclear stage (64.4%). The pregnancy rate following the transfer of embryos frozen at the cleavage stage was also higher than at the pronuclear stage. Others have reported either similar or higher rates of pregnancy and embryo implantation after the transfer of embryos frozen at the pronuclear stage than on day 2 [41,64,66]. As shown by Horne *et al.* [41], while the live birth rate of fresh embryo transfer performed on day 2 was significantly higher than at the pronuclear stage, a trend to higher live birth rate was observed following the transfer of embryos frozen at pronuclear stage (11/44 [25%] versus 4/38 [11%]). Moreover, comparable rates of cumulative viable pregnancy were reached following one fresh and two frozen–thawed embryo replacements in their study (40.2% and 41.4% for pronuclear and cleavage stage, respectively). Demoulin *et al.* [64] have reported higher rates of pregnancy (23.2% vs. 8.2%) and embryo implantation (10.7% vs. 4.7%) following the transfer of embryos frozen at the pronuclear stage than at the multicellular stage. However, most of the embryos frozen at the pronuclear stage were derived from protocols utilizing

Table 10.3. Direct comparison of survival and pregnancy outcomes between transfer of embryos frozen at the pronuclear and early cleavage stages

Study	Developmental stage	Survival rate (%)	Pregnancy per transfer (%)	Implantation rate (%)
Demoulin *et al.* (1991) [64]	Pronuclear	277/494 (56)	26/112 (23.2)	27/252 (10.7)
	Day 2	231/49247 (47)	9/110 (8.2)	4.7 (9/191)
Troup *et al.* (1991) [40]	Pronuclear	44/61 (72)	8/17 (47)	NA
	Day 2	48/80 (60)	3/21 (14)	NA
Horne *et al.* (1997) [41]	Pronuclear	96/129 (74.4)	13/59 (22.0)	14/96 (14.6)
	Day 2	79/102 (77.4)	6/46 (13.0)	6/79 (7.6)
Kattera *et al.* (1999) [65]	Pronuclear	325/504 (64.4)	6/46 (14.8)	NA
	Day 2	165/223 (73.9)	13/56 (22.8)	NA
Salumets *et al.* (2003) [66]	Pronuclear	486/562 (86.5)	47/234 (20.1)	55/393 (14.0)
	Day 2	1935/3136 (61.7)	263/1234 (21.1)	296/2066 (14.3)
	Day 3	134/320 (43.1)	20/109 (18.3)	22/176 (12.5)
Senn *et al.* (2006) [42]	Pronuclear	804/1000 (80.4)	64/329 (19.5)	183/787 (10.5)
	Day 2	438/610 (71.8)	21/192 (10.9)	26/439 (5.9)

gonadotropin-releasing hormone agonist and human menopausal gonadotropin, whereas 69% of the embryos frozen at cleavage stage were from stimulation cycles using clomiphene citrate and human menopausal gonadotropin. It seems more likely that the stimulation protocol was responsible for the difference in pregnancy outcome rather than developmental stage of embryos at freezing.

Very few data are available regarding the pregnancy outcome between embryos frozen at pronuclear and blastocyst stages. A recent study compared the outcome following cryopreservation of all embryos at either the pronuclear or the blastocyst stage [67]. Despite the relatively lower rate of embryo survival for frozen blastocysts (70% versus 85.5%), these led to significantly higher rates of clinical pregnancy (67.7% versus 41.1%) and implantation (40.8% versus 21.5%) in the first frozen transfer cycle. In addition, fewer embryos were replaced in frozen blastocyst transfer cycles (2.5 ± 0.6 versus 3.2 ± 1.1). The extended culture of embryos allows for more optimal embryo selection after the initiation of embryonic genome activation; however, there is risk of failure to achieve blastocyst transfer.

Vitrification of pronuclear stage embryos

Although controlled slow freezing remains the main method of cryopreservation in most IVF programs, the vitrification technique has entered the mainstream of human ART more and more. As the name implies, vitrification is a cryopreservation strategy where cells are converted into a glass-like amorphous solid that is free of any crystalline structure. As a non-equilibrium cryopreservation method, vitrification is achieved by the combination of high concentration of cryoprotectants and an extremely high cooling rate. The rapid-cooling rate used to achieve vitrification allows less time for ice formation. Compared with slow freezing, vitrification is simpler and more convenient and does not require expensive equipment (i.e. a controlled rate freezer). Vitrification involves a very high cooling rate and passages rapidly through the dangerous temperature zone between +15 and −5°C, thus significantly decreasing chilling injury to the oocytes and embryos [68]. Vitrification is also able to eliminate the ice crystal formation in the intra- and extracellular spaces.

Successful pregnancies and live births have been achieved by vitrification of human oocytes and embryos using different carrier systems: open pulled straws [69], Cryotop [70], Cryoleaf [71], and Cryotip [72]. Relatively limited data are available regarding the application of vitrification in the cryopreservation of pronuclear stage human embryos [39,59,72–74]. This might be because acceptable rates of embryo survival and pregnancy have been achieved using the slow-freezing method. Liebermann *et al.* [73], using a single pronucleate and three pronucleate embryos,

Table 10.4. Vitrification protocol for pronuclear stage human embryos

Protocol steps	Instructions
Vitrification	
1.	Embryo vitrification is performed at room temperature with Irvine Vit Kit (Irvine Scientific, Santa Ana, CA, USA). Equilibration, vitrification, thawing, dilution, and washing solutions are equivalents to those in Vit Kit
2.	Embryos are first transferred into equilibration solution consisting of 1.5% (v/v) EG and 7.5% (v/v) DMSO dissolved in TCM 199 supplemented with 20% SSS (Irvine Scientific) at 27°C for 5–15 min
3.	After an initial shrinkage, embryos regain their original volume and are transferred into three 20 μl drops of vitrification solution consisting of 15% (v/v) EG, 15% (v/v) DMSO, and 0.5 M sucrose dissolved in TCM 199 supplemented with 20% SSS
4.	After incubation of each drop for 20 s, embryos are loaded in approximately 1 μl solution into the narrow part of a Cryotip without any air bubbles by aspiration of medium, embryo, and medium, by a connected syringe
5.	The straw with embryos is heat sealed at both ends; the protective sleeve is pulled over the narrow part and the device is plunged into liquid nitrogen. The total time period required for loading, sealing, adjustment of the sleeve, and plunging should be less than 90 s
Warming	
1.	The Cryotip is removed from liquid nitrogen, plunged into a 37°C water bath for 3 s, wiped with ethanol and a paper towel, and the sealed ends cut with a sterile scissor. By using a syringe adjusted to the thick end of the straw, the contents can be expelled on to a sterile Petri dish
2.	Solutions used for further manipulations are kept at room temperature. A portion of TS consisting of 1.0 M sucrose in TCM 199 plus 20% SSS is placed adjacent to the expelled drop and merged subsequently with the other drop containing the embryos
3.	After 1 min, embryos are retrieved and transferred to a second drop of TS for 1 min; then transferred to two sequential 20 μl drops of dilution solution (DS) consisting of 0.5 M sucrose in TCM 199 plus 20% SSS for 2 min in each
4.	After three subsequent washings through three successive 20 μl drops of washing solution (TCM 199 supplemented with 20% SSS) for 3 min each, embryos are transferred into l00 μl droplets of Cleavage Medium (Irvine Scientific) and cultured in a CO_2 incubator until embryo transfer

DMSO, dimethyl sulfoxide; EG, ethylene glycol; SSS, Synthetic Serum Substitute; TS, thawing solution.
Source: Kuwayama *et al.* (2005) [72].

demonstrated that vitrification did not impact the developmental potential of human pronuclear stage embryos. Similar rates of embryo cleavage, cavitation, and blastocyst formation were obtained between vitrified groups and the unvitrified control groups in their study. In another study, similar results were obtained by ultra-rapid freezing using an electron microscope EM grid [75]. As demonstrated by Griesinger *et al.* [39], elective cryopreservation of all pronuclear stage embryos by vitrification yielded an ongoing pregnancy rate of 31.6% per first frozen transfer and a cumulative ongoing pregnancy rate of 36.8%. These results demonstrated the effectiveness of vitrification in the cryopreservation of pronuclear stage embryos. A sample of a vitrification protocol for pronuclear stage embryos is given in Table 10.4.

Existing data support the proposition that vitrification yields improved embryo survival compared with slow freezing [76]. Kuwayama *et al.* compared the efficacy of vitrification and slow freezing with 7825 pronuclear stage human embryos [72]: 100% of vitrified human pronuclear stage embryos survived and 52% developed to blastocysts, compared with 89% survival and 41% blastocyst development after slow cooling. This was confirmed by a recent study performed in a mouse model, where the blastocyst formation rate of pronuclear stage mouse embryos cryopreserved by a conventional method (30.4%) was significantly lower than in those vitrified by a straw method (56.9% to 69.1%) or by open pulled straw method (66.0% to 85.7%) [77]. As reported in a retrospective study by Al-Hasani *et al.* [78], the pregnancy rate obtained with vitrification of pronuclear stage embryos (36.9%) was three times higher than that obtained with the slow-rate freezing method (10.2%) used previously in the same center. Because of the limited sample sizes in these studies, further prospective trials are needed to evaluate the two cryopreservation methods in terms of clinical outcomes.

High concentration of cryoprotectants is a negative factor in vitrification. The total concentration of cryoprotectant ranges from 5 to 8 mol/l in vitrification protocols currently used in the cryopreservation of human oocyte and embryos [72,79]. More severe osmotic stress and toxic effects are potentially imposed upon the cells during the vitrification and warming processes than in the slow-freezing process. It is, therefore, of critical importance to restrict the concentration of cryoprotectants to the minimal level to achieve vitrification. A stepwise addition of cryoprotectants can help to reduce the toxic and osmotic damage induced by cryoprotectants at high concentrations [80]. Increasing the viscosity or the cooling/warming rates [81] or decreasing the volume [82] will each independently increase the probability of vitrification. Based on the fact that the higher the cooling rate is, the lower the required cryoprotectant concentration for vitrification, He *et al.* [83] recently developed a novel ultra-fast vitrification approach using a small quartz microcapillary with an inner diameter less than 0.4 mm. According to their study, only 2 M 1,2-propanediol is required to achieve apparent vitrification using the quartz microcapillary plunged into liquid nitrogen, with the intracellular concentration (2 M) of cryoprotectants being in the range of that used for slow freezing.

Second, attention should be paid to the safety aspects involved in vitrification, storage, and transportation. In order to increase the cooling rate, most vitrification carrier systems require the direct contact between oocyte or embryo and liquid nitrogen, which makes it possible for cross-contamination of samples to occur in liquid nitrogen storage tanks [84]. A number of viruses, including the human immunodeficiency virus and hepatitis B and C viruses, can survive in liquid nitrogen [84]. While there is no direct evidence of cross-contamination of human gametes and embryos stored in the same tank, transmission of viral pathogens to embryos vitrified and stored in open containers by experimentally contaminated liquid nitrogen has been reported in a bovine model [85]. The small sample volume also places the vitrified cell at a risk of inadvertent thawing as temperature increases when being moved from tank to tank or during inventory.

To guarantee complete isolation of embryos and to avoid the potential contamination by pathogens from liquid nitrogen, different methods of closed vitrification systems have emerged. Mouse pronuclear oocytes vitrified using Cryoloop with or without contact with liquid nitrogen had similar rates of embryo survival and blastocyst formation. In addition, contact and non-contact vitrification did not alter the mean total cell number and the mean number of cells composing the inner cell mass and trophectoderm of blastocysts from vitrified mouse embryos [86]. Similarly, no adverse effect on the further embryonic development was observed when human pronuclear oocytes were loaded into open pulled straws located in a 0.5 ml closed straw before being plunged into liquid nitrogen for cooling and storage [59]. Although keeping a carrier containing the specimen inside an outer protecting container provides a strategy to eliminate the potential contamination associated with direct contact with liquid nitrogen [87], it does not allow for rapid warming of a small volume and simultaneous removal of the cryoprotectant during the warming process [88]. It is, therefore, of importance to maintain a delicate balance among all the factors that affect the probability of vitrification in order to prevent crystallization, devitrification, recrystallization, glass fractures, and chilling injury. Another strategy to minimize the potential for transmission is the use of nitrogen vapor instead of liquid nitrogen itself. Vapor storage has been proposed to minimize or eliminate the possibility of cross-contamination [89,90]. A major concern of vapor storage is the risk of loss of cell viability. Human sperm survive satisfactorily with good recovery in the vapor of liquid nitrogen [91]. Similar rates of embryo survival and blastocyst formation were obtained between 1-cell mouse embryos stored in liquid nitrogen and nitrogen vapor [90]. Although no published data are available on human embryos, nitrogen vapor storage does not compromise the viability of vitrified human oocytes [92].

References

1. President's Council on Bioethics. *Reproduction and Responsibility: The Regulation of New Biotechnologies*. Washington, DC: US Government Press, 2004. http://www.bioethics.gov/reports/reproductionandresponsibility/chapter2.html.
2. Jones HW, Schnorr JA. Multiple pregnancies: a call for action. *Fertil Steril* 2001; **75:** 11–13.
3. Jain T, Missmer SA, Hornstein MD. Trends in embryo-transfer practice and in outcomes of the use of assisted reproductive technology in the United States. *N Engl J Med* 2004; **350:**1639–1645.
4. Whittingham DG, Leibo SP, Mazur P. Survival of mouse embryos frozen to –196 degrees and –269 degrees C. *Science* 1972; **178:** 411–414.

5. Wilmut I, Rowson LE. Experiments on the low-temperature preservation of cow embryos. *Vet Rec* 1973; **92:** 686–690.
6. Leibo SP. A one-step method for direct nonsurgical transfer of frozen–thawed bovine embryos. *Theriogenology* 1984; **21**: 767–790.
7. Kasai M, Komi JH, Takakamo A, *et al.* A simple method for mouse embryo cryopreservation in a low toxicity vitrification solution, without appreciable loss of viability. *J Reprod Fertil* 1990; **89**: 91–97.
8. Trounson A, Mohr L . Human pregnancy following cryopreservation, thawing and transfer of an eight-cell embryo. *Nature* 1983; **305**: 707–709.
9. Lassalle B, Testart J, Renard JP. Human embryo features that influence the success of cryopreservation with the use of 1,2 propanediol. *Fertil Steril* 1985; **44**: 645–651.
10. Testart J, Lassalle B, Belaisch-Allart J, *et al.* High pregnancy rate after early human embryo freezing. *Fertil Steril* 1986; **46**: 268–272.
11. Mandelbaum J, Junca AM, Plachot M, *et al.* Cryopreservation of human embryos and oocytes. *Hum Reprod* 1988; **3**: 117–119.
12. Edgar DH, Bourne H, Jericho H, McBain JC. The developmental potential of cryopreserved human embryos. *Mol Cell Endocrinol* 2000; **169**: 69–72.
13. Schneider U. Cryobiological principles of embryo freezing. *J In Vitro Fert Embryo Transf* 1986; **3**: 3–9.
14. Veeck LL, Amundson CH, Brothman LJ, *et al.* Significantly enhanced pregnancy rates per cycle through cryopreservation and thaw of pronuclear stage oocytes. *Fertil Steril* 1993; **59:** 1202–1207.
15. Damario MA, Hammitt DG, Galanits TM, Session DR, Dumesic DA. Pronuclear stage cryopreservation after intracytoplasmic sperm injection and conventional IVF: implications for timing of the freeze. *Fertil Steril* 1999; **72:** 1049–1054.
16. Scott L, Alvero R, Leondires M, Miller B. The morphology of human pronuclear embryos is positively related to blastocyst development and implantation. *Hum Reprod* 2000; **15:** 2394–2403.
17. Balaban B, Urman B, Isiklar A, *et al.* The effect of pronuclear morphology on embryo quality parameters and blastocyst transfer outcome. *Hum Reprod* 2001; **16:** 2357–2361.
18. James AN, Hennessy S, Reggio B, Wiemer K, Larsen F, Cohen J. The limited importance of pronuclear scoring of human zygotes. *Hum Reprod* 2006; **21:** 1599–1604.
19. Nicoli A, Valli B, Di Girolamo R, *et al.* Limited importance of pre-embryo pronuclear morphology (zygote score) in assisted reproduction outcome in the absence of embryo cryopreservation. *Fertil Steril* 2007; **88**(Suppl 4): 1167–1173.
20. Guerif F, Le Gouge A, Giraudeau B, *et al.* Limited value of morphological assessment at days 1 and 2 to predict blastocyst development potential: a prospective study based on 4042 embryos. *Hum Reprod* 2007; **22:** 1973–1981.
21. Capmany G, Taylor A, Braude PR, Bolton VN. The timing of pronuclear formation, DNA synthesis and cleavage in the human 1-cell embryo. *Mol Hum Reprod* 1996; **2:** 299–306.
22. Nagy ZP, Liu J, Joris H, Devroey P, Van Steirteghem A. Time-course of oocyte activation, pronucleus formation and cleavage in human oocytes fertilized by intracytoplasmic sperm injection. *Hum Reprod* 1994; **9:** 1743–1748.
23. Payne D, Flaherty SP, Barry MF, Matthews CD. Preliminary observations on polar body extrusion and pronuclear formation in human oocytes using time-lapse video cinematography. *Hum Reprod* 1997; **12:** 532–541.
24. ESHRE Task Force on Ethics and Law. I. The moral status of the pre-implantation embryo. *Hum Reprod* 2001; **16:** 1046–1048.
25. Orief Y, Nikolettos N, Al Hasani S. Cryopreservation of two pronuclear stage zygotes. *Rev Gynaecol Prac* 2005; **5:** 39–44.
26. Papanikolaou EG, Tournaye H, Verpoest W, *et al.* Early and late ovarian hyperstimulation syndrome: early pregnancy outcome and profile. *Hum Reprod* 2005; **20:** 636–641.
27. Al-Hasani S, Ludwig M, Gagsteiger F, *et al.* Comparison of cryopreservation of supernumerary pronuclear human oocytes obtained after intracytoplasmic sperm injection (ICSI) and after conventional in-vitro fertilization. *Hum Reprod* 1996; **11:** 604–607.
28. Hoover L, Baker A, Check JH, *et al.* Clinical outcome of cryopreserved human pronuclear stage embryos resulting from intracytoplasmic sperm injection. *Fertil Steril* 1997; **67:** 621–624.
29. Vyjayanthi S, Tang T, Fattah A, *et al.* Elective cryopreservation of embryos at the pronucleate stage in women at risk of ovarian hyperstimulation syndrome may affect the overall pregnancy rate. *Fertil Steril* 2006; **86**: 1773–1775.
30. Wada I, Matson PL, Troup SA, *et al.* Does elective cryopreservation of all embryos from women at risk of ovarian hyperstimulation syndrome reduce the incidence of the condition? *Br J Obstet Gynaecol* 1993; **100:** 265–269.
31. Pattinson HA, Hignett M, Dunphy BC, Fleetham JA. Outcome of thaw embryo transfer after cryopreservation of all embryos in patients at risk of ovarian hyperstimulation syndrome. *Fertil Steril* 1994; **62:** 1192–1196.
32. Tiitinen A, Husa LM, Tulppala M, Simberg N, Seppälä M. The effect of cryopreservation in prevention

of ovarian hyperstimulation syndrome. *Br J Obstet Gynaecol* 1995; **102:** 326–329.

33. Frederick JL, Ord T, Kettel LM, *et al.* Successful pregnancy outcome after cryopreservation of all fresh embryos with subsequent transfer into an unstimulated cycle. *Fertil Steril* 1995; **64:** 987–990.
34. Shaker AG, Zosmer A, Dean N, *et al.* Comparison of intravenous albumin and transfer of fresh embryos with cryopreservation of all embryos for subsequent transfer in prevention of ovarian hyperstimulation syndrome. *Fertil Steril* 1996; **65:** 992–996.
35. Awonuga AO, Dean N, Zaidi J, *et al.* Outcome of frozen embryo replacement cycles following elective cryopreservation of all embryos in women at risk of developing ovarian hyperstimulation syndrome. *J Assist Reprod Genet* 1996; **13:** 293–297.
36. Queenan JT, Jr., Veeck LL, Toner JP, Oehninger S, Muasher SJ. Cryopreservation of all prezygotes in patients at risk of severe hyperstimulation does not eliminate the syndrome, but the chances of pregnancy are excellent with subsequent frozen–thaw transfers. *Hum Reprod* 1997; **12:** 1573–1576.
37. Ferraretti AP, Gianaroli L, Magli C, *et al.* Elective cryopreservation of all pronucleate embryos in women at risk of ovarian hyperstimulation syndrome: efficiency and safety. *Hum Reprod* 1999; **14:** 1457–1460.
38. Endo T, Honnma H, Hayashi T, *et al.* Continuation of GnRH agonist administration for 1 week, after hCG injection, prevents ovarian hyperstimulation syndrome following elective cryopreservation of all pronucleate embryos. *Hum Reprod* 2002; **17:** 2548–2451.
39. Griesinger G, von Otte S, Schroer A, *et al.* Elective cryopreservation of all pronuclear oocytes after GnRH agonist triggering of final oocyte maturation in patients at risk of developing OHSS: a prospective, observational proof-of-concept study. *Hum Reprod* 2007; **22:** 1348–1352.
40. Troup SA, Matson PL, Critchlow JD, *et al.* Cryopreservation of human embryos at the pronucleate, early cleavage, or expanded blastocyst stages. *Eur J Obstet Gynecol Reprod Biol* 1991; **38:** 133–139.
41. Horne G, Critchlow JD, Newman MC, *et al.* A prospective evaluation of cryopreservation strategies in a two-embryo transfer programme. *Hum Reprod* 1997; **12:** 542–547.
42. Senn A, Urner F, Chanson A, *et al.* Morphological scoring of human pronuclear zygotes for prediction of pregnancy outcome. *Hum Reprod* 2006; **21:** 234–239.
43. Veeck LL. Does the developmental stage at freeze impact on clinical results post-thaw? *Reprod Biomed Online* 2003; **6:** 367–374.
44. Isachenko V, Todorov P, Dimitrov Y, Isachenko E. Integrity rate of pronuclei after cryopreservation of pronuclear-zygotes as a criterion for subsequent embryo development and pregnancy. *Hum Reprod* 2008; **23:** 819–826.
45. Damario MA, Hammitt DG, Session DR, Dumesic DA. Embryo cryopreservation at the pronuclear stage and efficient embryo use optimizes the chance for a liveborn infant from a single oocyte retrieval. *Fertil Steril* 2000; **73:** 767–773.
46. Wang JX, Yap YY, Matthews CD. Frozen–thawed embryo transfer: influence of clinical factors on implantation rate and risk of multiple conception. *Hum Reprod* 2001; **16:** 2316–2319.
47. Salumets A, Hydén-Granskog C, Suikkari AM, Tiitinen A, Tuuri T. The predictive value of pronuclear morphology of zygotes in the assessment of human embryo quality. *Hum Reprod* 2001; **16:** 2177–2181.
48. Lin YP, Cassidentid L, Chacon RR, *et al.* Successful implantation of frozen sibling embryos is influenced by the outcome of the cycle from which they were derived. *Fertil Steril* 1995; **63:** 262–267.
49. Gabrielsen A. Parameters predicting the implantation rate of thawed IVF/ICSI embryos: a retrospective study. *Reprod Biomed Online* 2006; **12:** 70–76.
50. Testart J, Lassalle B, Belaisch-Allart J, *et al.* Human embryo freezing. *Ann N Y Acad Sci* 1988; **541:** 532–540.
51. Irianni FM, Veeck LL, Toner JP, Muasher SJ. Influence of number of pre-embryos transferred, progesterone level and oestradiol/progesterone relation at thaw on pregnancy results during replacement of cryopreserved pre-embryos in natural cycles. *Hum Reprod* 1992; **7:** 797–800.
52. Macas E, Imthurn B, Borsos M, *et al.* Impairment of the developmental potential of frozen–thawed human zygotes obtained after intracytoplasmic sperm injection. *Fertil Steril* 1998; **69:** 630–635.
53. Simon A, Holzer H, Hurwitz A, *et al.* Comparison of cryopreservation outcome following intracytoplasmic sperm injection and conventional in vitro fertilization. *J Assist Reprod Genet* 1998; **15:** 431–437.
54. Garrisi GJ, Talansky BE, Sapira V, Gordon JW, Navot D. An intact zona pellucida is not necessary for successful mouse embryo cryopreservation. *Fertil Steril* 1992; **57:** 677–681.
55. Hershlag A, Feng HL. Effect of pre-freeze assisted hatching on post-thaw survival of mouse embryos. *Fertil Steril* 2005; **84:** 1752–1754.
56. Kung FT, Lin YC, Tseng YJ, *et al.* Transfer of frozen–thawed blastocysts that underwent quarter laser-assisted hatching at the day 3 cleaving stage before freezing. *Fertil Steril* 2003; **79:** 893–899.
57. Magli MC, Gianaroli L, Fortini D, Ferraretti AP, Munné S. Impact of blastomere biopsy and cryopreservation techniques on human embryo viability. *Hum Reprod* 1999; **14:** 770–773.
58. Jericho H, Wilton L, Gook DA, Edgar DH. A modified cryopreservation method increases the survival of

human biopsied cleavage stage embryos. *Hum Reprod* 2003; **18:** 568–571.

59. Isachenko V, Montag M, Isachenko E, van der Ven H. Vitrification of mouse pronuclear embryos after polar body biopsy without direct contact with liquid nitrogen. *Fertil Steril* 2005; **84:** 1011–1016.
60. Naether OG, Rudolf K, Fischer R, *et al.* Pregnancy after vitrification of pronuclear stage oocytes biopsied for polar body aneuploidy screening. *Reprod Biomed Online* 2008; **16:** 268–270.
61. Al-Shawaf T, Yang D, al-Magid Y, *et al.* Ultrasonic monitoring during replacement of frozen/thawed embryos in natural and hormone replacement cycles. *Hum Reprod* 1993; **8:** 2068–2074.
62. Gelbaya TA, Nardo LG, Hunter HR, *et al.* Cryopreserved-thawed embryo transfer in natural or down-regulated hormonally controlled cycles: a retrospective study. *Fertil Steril* 2006; **85:** 603–609.
63. Kolibianakis EM, Zikopoulos K, Devroey P. Implantation potential and clinical impact of cryopreservation: a review. *Placenta* 2003; **24**(Suppl B): S27–S33.
64. Demoulin A, Jouan C, Gerday C, Dubois M. Pregnancy rates after transfer of embryos obtained from different stimulation protocols and frozen at either pronucleate or multicellular stages. *Hum Reprod* 1991; **6**: 799–804.
65. Kattera S, Shrivastav P, Craft I. Comparison of pregnancy outcome of pronuclear- and multicellular-stage frozen–thawed embryo transfers. *J Assist Reprod Genet* 1999; **16:** 358–362.
66. Salumets A, Tuuri T, Mäkinen S, *et al.* Effect of developmental stage of embryo at freezing on pregnancy outcome of frozen–thawed embryo transfer. *Hum Reprod* 2003; **18:** 1890–1895.
67. Surrey ES, Keller JL, Stevens J, *et al.* 'Freeze-all': higher implantation and pregnancy rates with cryopreservation (cryo) at the blastocyst (blast) versus pronuclear (2pn) stage. *Fertil Steril* 2008; **90**(Suppl 1): S27–S28.
68. Ambrosini G, Andrisani A, Porcu E, *et al.* Cryotop vitrification of human oocytes results in high survival rate and healthy deliveries. *Reprod Biomed Online* 2007; **14:** 72–79.
69. Selman H, Angelini A, Barnocchi N, *et al.* Ongoing pregnancies after vitrification of human oocytes using a combined solution of ethylene glycol and dimethyl sulfoxide. *Fertil Steril* 2006; **86**: 997–1000.
70. Antinori M, Licata E, Dani G, *et al.* Cryotop vitrification of human oocytes results in high survival rate and healthy deliveries. *Reprod Biomed Online* 2007; **14:** 72–79.
71. Chian RC, Son WY, Huang JY, *et al.* High survival rates and pregnancies of human oocytes following vitrification: preliminary report. *Fertil Steril* 2005; **84**(Suppl 1): S36.
72. Kuwayama M, Vajta G, Ieda S, Kato O. Comparison of open and closed methods for vitrification of human embryos and the elimination of potential contamination. *Reprod Biomed Online* 2005; **11:** 608–614.
73. Liebermann J, Tucker MJ, Graham JR, *et al.* Blastocyst development after vitrification of multipronuclear zygotes using the Flexipet denuding pipette. *Reprod Biomed Online* 2002; **4**: 146–150.
74. Isachenko V, Montag M, Isachenko E, *et al.* Developmental rate and ultrastructure of vitrified human pronuclear oocytes after stepwise versus direct rehydration. *Hum Reprod* 2004; **19:** 660–665.
75. Park SP, Kim EY, Oh JH, *et al.* Ultrarapid freezing of human multipronuclear zygotes using electron microscope grids. *Hum Reprod* 2000 **15:** 1787–1790.
76. Loutradi KE, Kolibianakis EM, Venetis CA, *et al.* Cryopreservation of human embryos by vitrification or slow freezing: a systematic review and meta-analysis. *Fertil Steril* 2008; **90:** 186–193.
77. Zhao XM, Quan GB, Zhou GB, Hou YP, Zhu SE. Conventional freezing, straw, and open-pulled straw vitrification of mouse two pronuclear (2-PN) stage embryos. *Anim Biotechnol* 2007; **18:** 203–212.
78. Al-Hasani S, Ozmen B, Koutlaki N, *et al.* Three years of routine vitrification of human zygotes: is it still fair to advocate slow-rate freezing? *Reprod Biomed Online* 2007; **14:** 288–293.
79. El-Danasouri I, Selman H. Successful pregnancies and deliveries after a simple vitrification protocol for day 3 human embryos. *Fertil Steril* 2001; **76:** 400–402.
80. Rall WF. Factors affecting the survival of mouse embryos cryopreserved by vitrification. *Cryobiology* 1987; **24:** 387–402.
81. Vajta G, Kuwayama M. Improving cryopreservation systems. *Theriogenology* 2006; **65:** 236–244.
82. Arav A. Vitrification of oocytes and embryos. In Lauria A, Gandolfi F, eds. *New Trends in Embryo Transfer*. Cambridge, UK: Portland Press, 1992, pp. 255–264.
83. He X, Park EY, Fowler A, Yarmush ML, Toner M. Vitrification by ultra-fast cooling at a low concentration of cryoprotectants in a quartz micro-capillary: a study using murine embryonic stem cells. *Cryobiology* 2008; **56:** 223–232.
84. Practice Committee of the American Society for Reproductive Medicine. Guidelines for reducing the risk of viral transmission during fertility treatment. *Fertil Steril* 2006; **86**(Suppl 5): S11–S17.
85. Bielanski A, Nadin-Davis S, Sapp T, Lutze-Wallace C. Viral contamination of embryos cryopreserved in liquid nitrogen. *Cryobiology* 2000; **40:** 110–116.
86. Lane M, Lyons EA, Bavister BD. Cryopreservation reduces the ability of hamster 2-cell embryos to

regulate intracellular pH. *Hum Reprod* 2000; **15:** 389–394.

87. Kuleshova LL, Shaw JM. A strategy for rapid cooling of mouse embryos within a double straw to eliminate the risk of contamination during storage in liquid nitrogen. *Hum Reprod* 2000; **15:** 2604–2609.
88. Isachenko V, Selman H, Isachenko E, *et al.* Modified vitrification of human pronuclear oocytes: efficacy and effect on ultrastructure. *Reprod Biomed Online* 2003; **7:** 211–216.
89. Clarke GN. Sperm cryopreservation: is there a significant risk of cross-contamination? *Hum Reprod* 1999; **14:** 2941–2943.
90. Tomlinson M, Sakkas D. Is a review of standard procedures for cryopreservation needed? Safe and effective cryopreservation: should sperm banks and fertility centres move toward storage in nitrogen vapour? *Hum Reprod* 2000; **15**: 2460–2463.
91. Saritha KR, Bongso A. Comparative evaluation of fresh and washed human sperm cryopreserved in vapor and liquid phases of liquid nitrogen. *J Androl* 2001; **22**: 857–862.
92. Cobo A, Pérez S, Santos MJ, Pellicer A, Remohí J. Comparison between storage of vitrified oocytes by Cryotop method in liquid nitrogen vs. vapour phase of liquid nitrogen tanks. *Fertil Steril* 2007; **88** (Suppl 1): S91.

Chapter 11

Cryopreservation of day two and day three embryos

Yunxia Cao and Zhiguo Zhang

Introduction

Cryobiology studies commenced in earnest in the late 1940s. Initially, cells with a simple structure, such as erythrocytes, were used as models to explore cryopreservation. As theory and technical aspects evolved, cryopreservation was gradually applied to a variety of cells with complex structures, and even tissues. In 1972, the first offspring was achieved after freezing mouse embryos [1]. This study examined the effects of suspending medium, cooling rate, final temperature, and warming rate on embryos up to blastocyst stage. It was found that the maximal recovery rate was obtained with a cooling rate of 0.3°C/min, using 1.0 M dimethyl sulfoxide (DMSO) as a cryoprotectant, and with a warming rate of 4°C/min. However, survival rates varied for embryos at different developmental stages, for example 70% for 2-cell embryos and 20% for blastocysts. After transferring thawed embryos to foster mothers, approximately 65% of the recipients became pregnant and 40% produced normal full-term offspring. In the same year, there were other reports of successful cryopreservation of embryos from mouse and other species using 2.0 M DMSO as a cryoprotectant with a cooling rate of 0.2°C/min [2,3]. Subsequently, cryopreservation methodology for mammalian embryos was established gradually as a slow-freezing method.

Trounson and Mohr (1983) [4] reported the first pregnancy from frozen–thawed human embryos using DMSO as a cryoprotectant, and several successful live births were subsequently reported [5–7]. The first pregnancy and live births from frozen–thawed human embryos are listed in Table 11.1. Now embryo freezing is a routine clinical procedure in every in vitro fertilization (IVF) clinic.

Why cryopreserve human embryos?

With advancing technology in human IVF during the late 1980s, and the development of ovarian stimulation protocols in which exogenous gonadotropins were widely used for ovulation induction, the production of multiple embryos frequently occurred in clinics. Transfer of more than one embryo increased the pregnancy rate but could result in multigestation pregnancy with a high risk of pre- and postnatal complications. Therefore, it becomes apparent that a method of cryopreservation was needed for excess embryos not transferred initially. Cryopreservation of embryos makes it possible to transfer fewer embryos per cycle and minimizes the incidence of multigestation pregnancy, but it does not alter the effectiveness of IVF treatment. In addition, in some medical emergencies, such as the occurrence of ovary hyperstimulation syndrome during treatment, cryopreservation allows all embryos to be safeguarded for later use. Furthermore, if IVF treatment failed from the fresh embryo transfer, the patients could have a further chance for pregnancy and live birth from the frozen–thawed embryos without repeating the controlled ovarian hyperstimulation. If the fresh IVF treatment is successful, the frozen embryos can be stored for later use when the couple wishes to have more children. The following summarizes the main reasons why human embryos are cryopreserved [8]:

- embryos not used in the initial transfer can be cryopreserved for later use, which gives a couple more chance for pregnancy and live birth
- using cryopreserved embryos from an ovarian hyperstimulation cycle can obviate the need of repeated ovarian stimulation and egg collection
- embryo cryopreservation provides an opportunity to detect infectious diseases and genetic anomalies with ample time for proper screening and analysis
- embryo freezing offers the opportunity for fertility preservation and provides a possible source of embryos for donation to other couples.

Fertility Cryopreservation, ed. Ri-Cheng Chian and Patrick Quinn. Published by Cambridge University Press.

Table 11.1. The first pregnancy and live births from frozen–thawed human embryos reported in 1980s

Authors and year	Method of freezing	Embryo stage and cryoprotectant	Pregnancy and live birth
Trounson and Mohr (1983) [4]	Slow freezing	8-cell/DMSO	Pregnancy
Zeilmaker *et al.* (1984) [5]	Slow freezing	8-cell/DMSO	Live birth
Downing *et al.* (1985) [6]	Slow freezing	8-cell/DMSO	Live birth
Cohen *et al.* (1985) [7]	Slow freezing	Blastocyst/DMSO	Live birth

DMSO, dimethyl sulfoxide.

Factors affecting successful cryopreservation of human embryos

There are many factors affecting the viability and developmental potential of the frozen–thawed embryos. There is no doubt that the quality of the thawed embryos directly impacts the subsequent implantation. However, it must be acknowledged that the quality of embryos before cryopreservation is also an important factor affecting the viability of embryos post-thawing. It is a common belief that high-quality embryos may have less damage during the process of cryopreservation, and poor-quality embryos may not survive after freeze–thawing. Therefore, it is difficult to compare different settings for the outcome of frozen–thawed embryos.

After thawing, the embryos must be viable. How are viable embryos identified following thawing? For day 2 or day 3 embryos, the blastomeres of embryos must be intact after freeze–thawing. As mentioned in the previous chapters, the potential for cryodamage is related not only to the quality of the embryos selected for freezing but also to the cryopreservation method chosen. Of course, having viable embryos does not necessarily mean they will have good developmental potential. Viable embryos can have some ultrastructural damage already that is not easily judged through their morphology under light microscopy. Therefore, various suboptimal freezing–thawing protocols might have different degrees of damage to embryos.

A recent study comparing the damage to embryos from freeze–thawing with plastic ministraws and plastic cryovials showed that there was significantly increased damage to the zona pellucida in the embryos frozen–thawed using cryovials [9]. Also it has been indicated that embryo biopsy has a significant impact on embryo survival after freeze–thawing: 61% of non-biopsied embryos survived compared with 38% of embryos that were biopsied prior to freezing in one study [10]. Similarly, another study indicated that the biopsied embryos or embryos with zona drilling had significantly lower amounts of intact blastomeres compared with non-biopsied embryos [11].

Which embryo stage for cryopreservation?

There are some controversies concerning which embryo stage is the most suitable for cryopreservation. Some laboratories like to freeze embryos at cleavage stage; others prefer to cryopreserve at blastocyst stage. In our practice until recent, we cryopreserved the remaining embryos after fresh transfer at day 3 using the slow-freezing method. We have obtained approximately a 35% clinical pregnancy rate constantly with these frozen–thawed embryos. Again it is difficult to compare the pregnancy and live birth rates in different IVF centers, because the selective criteria and freezing protocols vary in different practice settings.

The survival of embryos is not the endpoint. For day 2 or day 3 embryos, it is better practically to culture the thawed embryos further for a period of time before transfer in order to confirm that these embryos resume development. Significantly higher pregnancy and delivery rates have been reported after transferring frozen–thawed embryos that had undergone cleavage compared with those without further development during culture [12]. Therefore, the selection method for post-thawed embryos for transfer directly affects the clinical outcome in terms of pregnancy and live birth rates.

Cryopreservation technique for human embryos

Nowadays, at least two basic techniques have been employed for the cryopreservation of human embryos: slow freezing and vitrification. Slow freezing was used first and is still the most common method for cryopreservation of human embryos [13]. Vitrification is a relatively new technique and has been introduced to cryopreserve human embryos in recent years. Many studies have reported improved success rates in terms of clinical pregnancy and live birth rates with the vitrification technique [14–18].

Propylene glycol (PROH) is the most commonly used permeating cryoprotectant for cryopreservation of human embryos using the slow-freezing protocol. In this protocol, it is normal to use 1.0–1.5 M PROH as cryoprotectant. However, in the vitrification protocol, the concentration of cryoprotectants is higher. Other permeating cryoprotectants, such DMSO and ethylene glycerol, are also used for cryopreservation of human embryos by either the slow-freezing or vitrification method. Additionally a non-permeating cryoprotectant, such as sucrose, has often been used for both slow freezing and vitrification [19].

Human embryos can be cryopreserved at all stages of preimplantation from pronuclear to blastocyst stage [20,21]. Excluding the clinical factors mentioned above, the quality of the thawed embryos directly affects the clinical outcome after transfer of the frozen–thawed embryos. It is also important to select suitable embryos initially for cryopreservation because the quality of embryos impacts their capability for survival of cryopreservation. For day 2 or day 3 embryos, it is important to select or examine the embryos carefully before cryopreservation. The criteria for evaluation of embryos are based on the number of blastomeres, the degree of fragmentation, and the uniformity of cleaved blastomeres. The embryo can be evaluated by different scores based on its morphology: grade A, less than 10% fragmentation and equal blastomeres; grade B, 10% to less than 30% fragmentation and equal blastomeres; grade C, 30–50% fragmentation and/or unequal blastomeres; and grade D, more than 50% fragmentation. Our strategy is to freeze the supernumerary embryos only if they exhibited a favorable grading with less than 30% fragmentation of the blastomeres: that is grade A or B.

Interestingly it has been reported that cryopreservation of supernumerary embryos on day 2 or day 3 provided similar thawing survival parameters, but better implantation pregnancy and live birth rates were obtained with day 3 embryos than with cryopreservation of day 2 embryos [22]. It is possible that day 3 embryos were selected naturally during culture and had better quality than day 2 embryos because a developmental block occurred in the day 2 embryo. So some embryos on day 2 might not be able to develop to day 3 and so would not be selected for cryopreservation on day 3.

Slow-freezing technique

There appears to be no a universal slow-freezing protocol. Computer-controlled automatic freezing devices are often used for slow freezing. In general, the standard slow-freezing protocol consists of two stages: freezing and thawing.

The freezing protocol has the following steps.

1. Embryos are equilibrated first for 5–15 minutes at room temperature in a solution without cryoprotectant and then transferred to a solution containing a low concentration of cryoprotectant for 10 minutes. Finally, the embryos are transferred to a solution containing a final concentration of cryoprotectant (1.0–1.5 M) together with 0.1 M (0.2 or 0.3 M) sucrose for 5 minutes at room temperature.
2. Embryos are loaded into straws or ampules.
3. The samples are then cooled at 2°C/min from room temperature to −6°C and allowed to equilibrate for 10 minutes before "seeding," which may be initiated automatically or manually.
4. The cooling rate is reduced to 0.3°C/min after seeding and the sample cooled to −30°C.
5. In the final cooling, from −30°C to −180°C, the cooling rate is 40°C/min.
6. The samples are then plunged into liquid nitrogen for storage.

The thawing protocol has the following steps.

1. Straws or vials are held in air for 30 to 40 seconds and then transferred to a water bath (31°C) for 60 seconds.
2. The embryos are flushed out from the straws or vials and transferred to a solution containing 0.5 M sucrose at 37°C for 10 minutes.
3. The embryos are transferred to a solution containing 0.2 M of sucrose at 37°C for 10 minutes.
4. The embryos are placed in washing medium containing no sucrose for a washing procedure for 10 minutes at 37°C. They are then cultured in an incubator before embryo transfer.

Figure 11.1 shows embryos at different stages within the freeze–thaw procedure.

It has been reported that the pregnancy rate with frozen–thawed embryos was the same as with non-frozen embryos [21]. A cryosurvival rate of 70–80% can be reached and a 12% implantation rate can be obtained following embryo transfer. However, pregnancy and implantation rates depend upon the quality

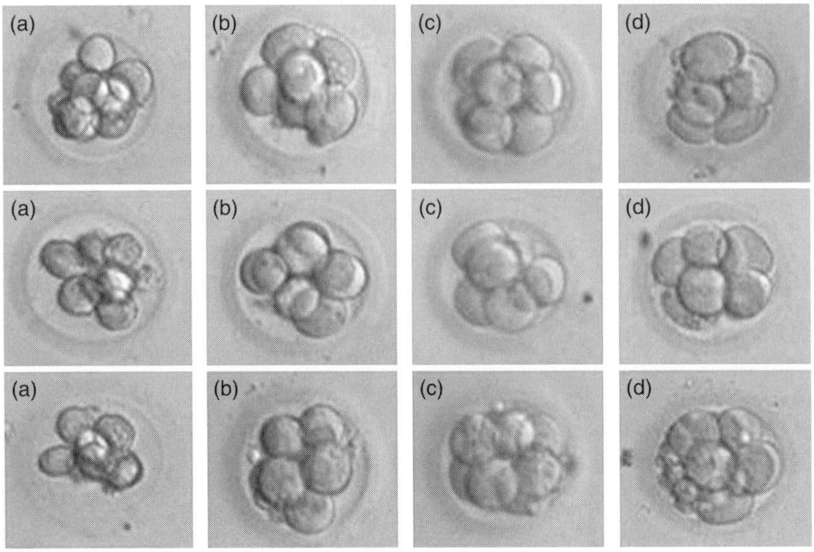

Figure 11.1. Day 3 human embryos during thawing process after slow freezing. There are three sets of thawed human embryos, one set in each row. (a) Embryos in thawing solution 1, containing 0.5 M sucrose; (b) embryos in the thawing solution 2, containing 0.2 M sucrose; (c) embryos in the washing medium; (d) embryos after thawing and before incubation. Magnification 200×.

of embryos after thawing. A higher implantation rate per embryo transfer can be achieved when all the transferred embryos are characterized by fully intact blastomeres compared with that seen with damaged embryos [23].

Vitrification technique

The principal of vitrification is to make samples reach an extremely low temperature in a glassy state and thus avoid the formation of ice crystals. This is achieved by combining the use of a high concentration of cryoprotective solution with an extremely rapid cooling speed. The advantages of vitrification are primarily that it can be carried out rapidly and easily and does not require expensive equipment. However, it can also easily expose freezing samples to osmotic shock and toxicity because of the high concentration of cryoprotectant used, and this may affect the viability of embryos. The common vitrification protocol for embryo cryopreservation also has two stages: cooling and warming.

The cooling protocol has the following steps.

1. The embryos are placed in equilibration solution containing a lower concentration of cryoprotectant (normally 7.5–10.0%) for 5–10 minutes.
2. The embryos are then transferred to a vitrification solution containing a higher concentration of cryoprotectant (normally 15–20%) with sucrose (normally 0.5 M) for 30–60 seconds.
3. The embryos are loaded on to a device for vitrification.
4. The device is plunged directly into liquid nitrogen for storage.

The warming protocol has the following steps.

1. The vitrification device is placed directly into warming solution containing 1.0 M sucrose at 37°C for 1 minute and the embryos are allowed to fall into the solution.
2. The warmed embryos are then transferred to a solution containing 0.5 M sucrose for 3 minutes.
3. The embryos are transferred to a solution containing 0.25 M sucrose for 3 minutes.
4. The embryos are washed twice in a sucrose-free medium for 3 minutes each wash and then transferred to an incubator for culture before transfer.

At present, there are several vitrification devices that have been developed, such as the open pulled straw, Cryotop, Cryoloop, Cryotip, and Cryoleaf. Using these devices, a cooling rate of up to 20 000°C/min can be reached when plunging the devices directly into liquid nitrogen. In addition, various cryoprotectants have been used for vitrifying human embryos, including DMSO, PROH, glycerol, ethylene glycol, and their combinations.

Selection of frozen–thawed embryos for transfer

The importance of selecting high-quality embryos before cryopreservation has been discussed above. But how are frozen–thawed embryos for transfer selected? Practically, it is based on embryo morphology after freeze–thawing. Normally the following criteria are used for selecting embryos: (1) the embryo should have intact blastomeres; (2) the embryo should have a low fragmentation of blastomeres; (3) the embryos should show further development following a period of culture.

It seems the most important factor appears to be to select embryos with continuing development following thawing for transfer, because it has been reported that significantly higher pregnancy and delivery rates have been achieved after transferring these embryos compared with transfer of embryos without further development [23,24]. In our experience, we prefer a culture period of 24 hours after thawing, and then we select the developing embryos for transfer. This procedure confirms that the embryos are viable after freeze–thawing, and this can optimize the success rate following transfer of the embryos.

Conclusions

Cryopreservation of human embryos is an important tool for IVF practice. Human embryos can be cryopreserved efficiently from the pronuclear to blastocyst stage. Human embryo cryopreservation is a proven method for fertility preservation. Successful cryopreservation of human embryos depends predominantly upon the selection of high-quality embryos before freezing, because embryos of differing quality have differing survival rates for freeze–thawing. The method for cryopreservation of embryos can be divided into slow freezing and vitrification, and it seems that vitrification improves embryo survival rate following cryopreservation. However, the clinical outcome needs to be verified by randomized clinical trials. There is controversy concerning cryopreservation of embryos that are on day 2, day 3, or at the blastocyst stage, which directly relates to their condition for the IVF program. Clinical pregnancy and live birth rates are affected by the post-thawing selection of embryos for transfer.

References

1. Whittingham DG, Leibo SP, Mazur P. Survival of mouse embryos frozen to −196 degrees and −269 degrees C. *Science* 1972; **178**: 411–414.
2. Wilmut I. The low temperature preservation of mammalian embryos. *J Reprod Fertil* 1972; **31**: 513–514.
3. Wilmut I. The effect of cooling rate, warming rate, cryoprotective agent and stage of development on survival of mouse embryos during freezing and thawing. *Life Sci* 1972; **11**: 1071–1079.
4. Trounson A, Mohr L. Human pregnancy following cryopreservation, thawing and transfer of an eight-cell embryo. *Nature* 1983; **305**: 707–709.
5. Zeilmaker GH, Alberda AT, van Gent I, Rijkmans CM, Drogendijk AC. Two pregnancies following transfer of intact frozen–thawed embryos. *Fertil Steril* 1984; **42**: 293–296.
6. Downing BG, Mohr LR, Trounson AO, Freemann LE, Wood C. Birth after transfer of cryopreserved embryos. *Med J Aust* 1985; **142**: 409–411.
7. Cohen J, Simons RF, Fehilly CB, *et al.* Birth after replacement of hatching blastocyst cryopreserved at expanded blastocyst stage. *Lancet* 1985; **325**: 647.
8. Wood EC. The future of in vitro fertilization. *Ann N Y Acad Sci* 1988; **541**: 715–721.
9. Van Den Abbeel E, Van Steirteghem A. Zona pellucida damage to human embryos after cryopreservation and the consequences for their blastomere survival and in-vitro viability. *Hum Reprod* 2000; **15**: 373–378.
10. Magli MC, Gianaroli L, Fortini D, Ferraretti AP, Munné S. Impact of blastomere biopsy and cryopreservation techniques on human embryo viability. *Hum Reprod* 1999; **14**: 770–773.
11. Joris H, Van den Abbeel E, Vos AD, Van Steirteghem A. Reduced survival after human embryo biopsy and subsequent cryopreservation. *Hum Reprod* 1999; **14**: 2833–2837.
12. Van der Elst J, Van den Abbeel E, Vitrier S, *et al.* Selective transfer of cryopreserved human embryos with further cleavage after thawing increases delivery and implantation rates. *Hum Reprod* 1997; **12**: 1513–1521.
13. Quinn P, Kerin JF. Experience with the cryopreservation of human embryos using the mouse as a model to establish successful techniques. *J In Vitro Fert Embryo Transf* 1986; **3**: 40–45.
14. Mukaida T, Nakamura S, Tomiyama T, *et al.* Vitrification of human blastocysts using cryoloops: clinical outcome of 223 cycles. *Hum Reprod* 2003; **18**: 384–391.
15. Mukaida T, Takahashi K, Kasai M. Blastocyst cryopreservation: ultrarapid vitrification using cryoloop technique. *Reprod Biomed Online* 2003; **6**: 221–225.
16. Kuwayama M, Vajta G, Ieda S, Kato O. Comparison of open and closed methods for vitrification of human embryos and the elimination of potential contamination. *Reprod Biomed Online* 2005; **11**: 608–614.
17. Rama Raju GA, Haranath GB, Krishna KM, Prakash GJ, Madan K. Vitrification of human 8-cell embryos,

a modified protocol for better pregnancy rates. *Reprod Biomed Online* 2005; **11**: 434–437.

18. Desai N, Blackmon H, Szeptycki J, Goldfarb J. Cryoloop vitrification of human day 3 cleavage-stage embryos: post-vitrification development, pregnancy outcomes and live births. *Reprod Biomed Online* 2007; **14**: 208–213.
19. Jain JK, Paulson RJ. Oocyte cryopreservation. *Fertil Steril* 2006; **86**: 1037–1046.
20. Ménézo Y, Nicollet B, Herbaut N, André D. Freezing cocultured human blastocysts. *Fertil Steril* 1992; **58**: 977–980.
21. Behr B, Gebhardt J, Lyon J, Milki AA. Factors relating to a successful cryopreserved blastocyst transfer program. *Fertil Steril* 2002; **77**: 697–699.
22. Guerif F, Bidault R, Cadoret V, Couet ML, Lansac J, Royere D. Parameters guiding selection of best embryos for transfer after cryopreservation: a reappraisal. *Hum Reprod* 2002; **17**: 1321–1326.
23. American Society for Reproductive Medicine. Day 3 compared with day 2 cryopreservation does not affect embryo survival but improves the outcome of frozen–thawed embryo transfers. *Fertil Steril* 2006; **86**: 1537–1540.
24. Hartshorne GM, Elder K, Crow J, Dyson H, Edwards RG. The influence of in-vitro development upon post-thaw survival and implantation of cryopreserved human blastocysts. *Hum Reprod* 1991; **6**: 136–141.

Chapter 12

Cryopreservation of blastocysts

Yoshiharu Morimoto

Introduction

Cryopreservation is currently limited to sperm or embryos but for extending its use to other fields, such as stem cell research, the technology needs improvement. Recently, cryopreservation of gametes in the form of gonadal tissue, such as testicular and ovarian tissues at various developmental stages, has been achieved [1].

The first successful cryopreservation in the field of reproduction was the freezing of animal spermatozoa, performed in Italy in 1776 [2]. Two centuries later, successful human pregnancies and births from frozen embryos were reported [3]. Nowadays, it is a routine procedure in infertility centers to freeze pronuclear, multicellular embryos, and blastocysts [4]. Successful pregnancies from cryopreserved and thawed human blastocysts were first reported by Cohen *et al.* [5] in 1985. In the early work on the culture of blastocysts, the survival and pregnancy rates after freezing and thawing the blastocysts was low. Ménézo *et al.* [6] applied the technique of co-culture for culturing blastocysts. The blastocysts were cultured on Vero cells before freezing. The embryos showed an increase of pre-embryo cell number and Vero cells enhanced the competence for further development [7]. The benefits of co-culture were thought to derive from the effect of embryotropic factors, including glycoproteins, released from the feeder cell layer and the reduction of the action of toxic compounds such as heavy metals. Another approach was to remove lysed blastomeres from frozen–thawed embryos [8]. The pregnancy rate was much higher in this group than in the unaltered group. This study indicated that necrotic blastomeres may produce some deleterious substances.

Recently, a vitrification method has been developed as another option. Oocytes and ovarian tissues can be cryopreserved using this new technique. Cryopreservation of gametes, embryos, and ovarian tissues is beneficial and safe for infertility treatment in terms of prevention of ovarian hyperstimulation syndrome and thorough improvement of endometrial receptivity. Moreover, cryobiological techniques can be used in association with preimplantation genetic diagnosis (PGD) to prevent hereditary diseases.

Thirty years have passed since the first baby conceived by in vitro fertilization (IVF) was born. Nowadays, minimum stimulations of the ovary have has become one of the topics of interest and single blastocyst transfer is required to prevent multiple pregnancies, which is a risk for both the mothers and the babies. Therefore, cryopreservation techniques for blastocysts are required to preserve surplus blastocysts.

Structural features of the blastocyst

Soon after the morula enters into the uterine cavity, 4 days after fertilization, a blastocele, which is a fluid-filled cavity, appears inside the embryonic mass. Fluid passes through the zona pellucida into the cell from the uterine cavity. Thereafter, cells separate into two parts, the trophectoderm and the inner cell mass. At this stage, the embryo is called a blastocyst. The blastocyst possesses the unique structure of a blastocele and is very different in shape from the other developmental stages of preimplantation embryo. Initially the blastocele is small, but it grows as it accumulates fluid; the embryo enlarges and is known as an expanded blastocyst. Blastocysts expand and contract periodically. Cryopreservation of blastocysts requires careful attention because of their delicate structure. Ice crystal injury may be the main reason for low survival rates after thawing, as blastocysts contain large amounts of water inside the blastocele. In order to address this issue, two methods can be adopted. One is to freeze embryos at the contraction stage and the other is to artificially shrink the blastocele (described in detail below). Consequently, in blastocyst cryopreservation, the structure at each stage should be considered in order to achieve a preferential survival rate after thawing.

Which is the best stage for transfer?

Early cleavage stage embryos such as those at day 2 or day 3 are transferred in routine work. Recently, improvement in culture methods, especially the development of improved media, has made prolonged culture possible, providing another option. Culturing of the blastocyst may be advantageous for the assessment of embryo quality; however, controversy still surrounds the choice of which is the best stage to transfer. Prolonged time in in vitro culture may increase the chances of impairment of embryos through changes in temperature, pH, and osmolality. Meta-analysis of the Cochrane database provides results that have changed over time. In 2002 [9], the study showed little difference in the major outcome for parameters such as birth rates, clinical pregnancies, and implantations per woman between early stage embryo and blastocyst transfer.

In 2005 [10], the database also showed no evidence of difference between the two groups. However, in 2007 [11], blastocyst transfer was proved to be the preferred method, in terms of a better live birth rate than seen with other methods. The study showed that the number of surplus embryos frozen was higher in the early cleaved embryo transfer group and that the transfer cancellation rate was higher in the blastocyst transfer group. This change might reflect improvements in media, culture conditions, and the laboratory techniques used in each laboratory.

Which is the best stage for cryopreservation?

The utilization of blastocysts for transfer has recently been adopted in humans. The development of sequential medium enabled this new technology. Blastocysts that had been cultured in sequential medium were shown to be well preserved by cryopreservation [12].

The effectiveness of blastocyst cryopreservation has been described in many studies. In a 3 year trial of blastocyst cryopreservation, 76% of blastocysts survived and a 59% pregnancy rate was achieved [13].

Many authors have discussed which stage of cell growth is appropriate for cryopreservation. Pantos *et al.* [14] compared the effectiveness of cryopreservation at each stage of embryo development in a retrospective study. In 170 cycles, using day 6 blastocysts, the survival rate was much better in cleaved embryos (89%) than in blastocysts (56%). The review also identified the same tendency in implantation rate. Troup *et al.* [15] compared the survival rates after thawing at the pronuclear, cleaved embryo, and blastocyst stages. A greater survival rate was shown at the pronuclear (72%) and cleavage embryo (60%) stages than at the expanded blastocyst stage (38%). The proportion of patients who required embryo replacement was also much higher in the pronuclear and cleaved embryo stages. Moreover, Liebermann and Tucker [16], in their comparison of day 5 and day 6 blastocysts in 254 vitrified transfer cycles, showed no difference between the two groups in terms of survival rate, implantation rate, and pregnancy rate. The result was the same with slow-freezing cycles. In contrast, cryopreservation at the blastocysts stage has been reported as being more effective in some studies.

Which stage, pronuclear or blastocyst, yields more transferable embryos has not yet been identified. We have compared two stages, where both the pronuclear and blastocyst stage embryos had been cryopreserved for the same patient [17]. There was no difference in the number of transferable blastocysts between two groups. However vitrification at the blastocyst stage is more beneficial for patients and laboratories in terms of cost and space, because the number of vitrified pronuclear and cleaved embryos is approximately five times that of embryos vitrified at the blastocyst stage.

Selection of culture methods and effectiveness of blastocyst cryopreservation

Culture methods

The development of a culture method for blastocysts was a breakthrough in assisted reproductive tech nology (ART) [18]. Sequential media for human blastocyst culture was first described by Gardner and Lane [19] and is now used all over the world as a routine procedure for IVF. Even with more options for ART procedures, there is still controversy over which is the best stage for transfer. Some patients conceive with day 2 or day 3 stage embryo transfer after failure with transfer of an embryo at the blastocyst stage. More studies are needed to clarify whether blastocysts have the highest competence for further embryonic development into a fetus.

Currently there are two kinds of strategy for blastocyst stage culture. One is a sequential culture method and the other is single-phase culture. These have been developed based on embryo developmental biology. Essential ingredients differ according to the developmental stage of the embryos, and sequential media can tailor nutrients, energy, and protein sources for each stage. Sequential media have been used in many centers; however, recently it has been questioned whether sequential media are really essential for blastocyst culture. A new single-phase medium (Blastocyst, LifeGlobal, Nashville, TN, USA) has been designed, based on KSOM (potassium simplex optimized medium), and has been successfully used for the culture of mice blastocyst [20] and humans [21] with the same effectiveness as the sequential media.

Blastocyst stage transfer

We now consider the potential advantage of blastocyst stage transfer. When embryos at early stages, such as 4- to 8-cell embryos, are prematurely transferred into the uterus, they are not fully prepared for implantation. The embryos, therefore, remain on the premature endometrium, incurring metabolic stress [22]. Consequently, these embryos transferred early may be impaired and lose the competence for further development. In these premature embryos, identification of embryos possessing developmental potential is not possible, as transcription of embryonic genomes may be at an initial stage. Assessment of the quality of embryos at the pronuclear and cleavage stages has been attempted; however, these methods have not been successful in identifying embryos that have the potential to develop and be implanted on the endometrium.

Currently, there is a trend for late marriages and for patients to visit infertility centers in their late thirties and early forties. This means that centers are treating older patients who produce more embryos with abnormal chromosomes. Even if some of the abnormal embryos develop into blastocysts, most of them could be excluded naturally during culture to blastocyst stage, and this would be an advantage in blastocyst transfer.

In our centers, all surplus embryos are cultured to the blastocyst stage and only transferable blastocysts are frozen. This may benefit patients by preventing the waste of energy, time, and money in unnecessary transfers. It also benefits the laboratory by saving space and human resources, because embryos with lower potential are excluded by culture to the blastocyst stage. However, as discussed above, there remains the important question of whether the embryos that do not reach the blastocyst stage are not truly competent for further development. During in vitro culture, embryos are exposed to poor conditions, which may cause the errors in genetic and epigenetic modifications. Therefore, the fact that embryos develop to the blastocyst stage does not ensure that they have the competence to develop to fetuses.

Over 30 years, ART has been improved in quality and safety. In the modern program, the minimum numbers of follicles are grown and single embryo transfer is preferred. From this view point, blastocyst culture and cryopreservation will become more frequent.

Methods of cryopreservation

Initially, cryopreservation of the blastocyst was mainly carried out with a slow-freezing technique using programmed freezers. Many such programmable freezers, with features such as easy loading and various temperature settings, have become commercially available. In the slow-freezing method, stress to the cell can be minimized by inactivating cell metabolism as the temperature drops below zero Celsius. Intracellular dehydration may prevent the formation of intracellular ice crystals. However, as a typical container for embryos, a cryostraw, includes both liquid (cryoprotectant) and solids (artificial crystal and bubble), a slow change in temperature is needed to preserve cell structure.

A vitrification technique has been introduced from animal research to the human field. Initially it was tested using straws; however, acceptable results were not achieved, except in a few cases [36]. Later, electron microscope grids were used to load the embryos [23]. The grids are copper meshes, 3 mm in diameter and 25 μm thick, available in different mesh sizes (Figure 12.1). Very low temperatures can be rapidly attained because copper is a good heat conductor. The grids are, therefore, considered to be suitable carriers for embryo vitrification. Cho *et al.* [43] used electron microscope grids for vitrification of human blastocysts with a six-step thawing technique; this substantially

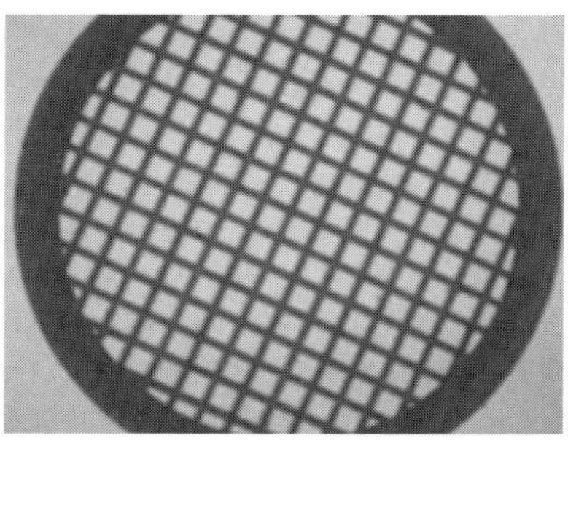

Figure 12.1. The electron microscopy grid for the vitrification.

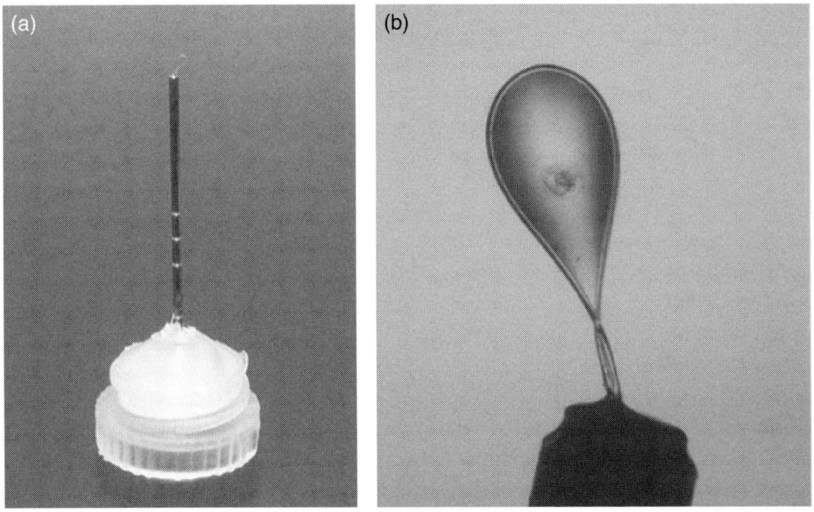

Figure 12.2. Cryoloop. (a) A blastocyst is loaded in the cryovial with the culture medium. (b) The loop is attached to a stainless steel rod.

reduced osmotic shock to the blastocysts and achieved preferable results.

Support devices for vitrification

Use of a Cryoloop is a good alternative as a supporter for the blastocyst in vitrification. The loop can be handled with a magnet attached to a stainless steel rod. Embryos are preserved in a cryovial (Figure 12.2). The Cryoloop consists of a small nylon loop (20 μm thick and 0.5–0.7 mm in diameter) that is mounted on a stainless steel tube inserted into the lid of the cryovial. The cap is attached to a stainless steel handling rod with a small magnet for manipulation of the loop at low temperatures [24].

The Cryotop was developed explicitly for the cryopreservation of human embryos. Embryos are loaded on to a specially constructed fine polypropylene strip attached to a plastic handle (Figure 12.3). The efficacy of this method for cryopreservation of human oocytes [25,26], embryos, and blastocysts [27], and bovine oocytes [28] has been reported. The Cryotop is an open vitrification system, and there was a concern that open systems were at risk of viral contamination from the liquid nitrogen. To address this issue, Kuwayama *et al.* [29] developed a new device, the CryoTip, to close the vitrification system and prevent contamination. The CryoTip consists of a thin plastic straw (250 μm inner diameter, 20 μm wall thickness, and 3 cm length) connected to a thicker part (200 μm inner diameter, 150 μm wall thickness, and 4.5 cm length, and equipped with a movable protective metal sleeve). Their study indicated no difference

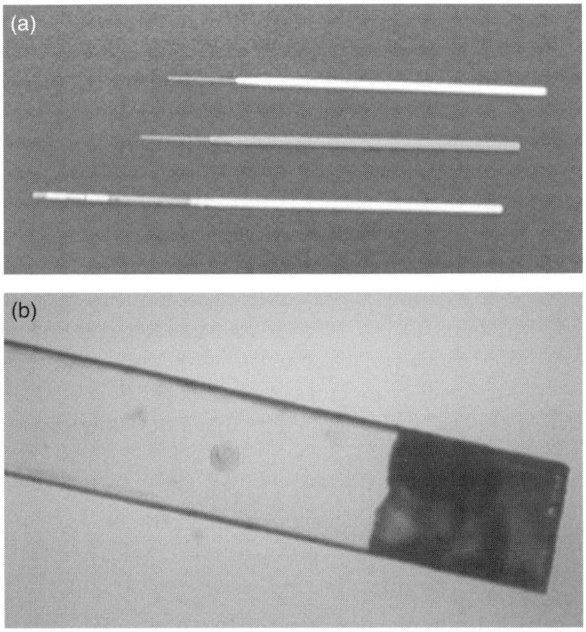

Figure 12.3. Cryotop. (a) A fine polypropylene strip attached to a plastic handle. (b) A blastocyst is loaded on to the strip.

in blastocyst survival and pregnancy rates between the Cryotop and the CryoTip groups.

No studies have provided evidence of contamination by pathogens from liquid nitrogen; however, in order to encourage further application of this method of cryopreservation, the issue of infection should be eliminated. One way to solve the problem is to filter liquid nitrogen through a 0.2 μm pore size filter, and this has been applied in many laboratories. Another way is to use individual tanks to prevent the spread of infectious diseases; however, this method requires a spacious laboratory.

Slow freezing

The slow-freezing technique has long been applied as a routine method for cryopreservation of human embryos. This method utilizes equilibrium power to drive cellular dehydration by stepping down temperatures using a programmed freezer. Artificial seeding is then needed before cryopreservation by slow freezing and with low concentrations of cryoprotectants mixed with sucrose. Dimethyl sulfoxide (DMSO) and 1,2-propanediol are the main cryoprotectants used in blastocyst freezing, but glycerol can be used as an alternative [6]. The slow-cooling method for cryopreservation of blastocysts has not given good results, so far. This may be because of cell damage by ice crystal formation within the unique structure of the blastocyst.

Vitrification

The vitrification method developed for mammals [30–34] has recently been applied to human embryos [35,36]. In vitrification, short periods of application of cryoprotectants at high concentration may reduce or eliminate ice crystal formation in cells. The effectiveness of vitrification for human embryo preservation has been reported in several studies. Stehlik *et al.* [37] performed a retrospective study comparing the slow-freezing method and the vitrification method for day 5 and day 6 blastocysts. This study showed an 83% survival rate with slow freezing and a 100% survival rate with vitrification. A study by Loutradis *et al.* [38] demonstrated a significantly higher survival rate with vitrification than with slow freezing. Libermann and Tucker [16] reported survival and implantation rates, respectively, of 96% and 33% with vitrification and 91% and 30% with slow freezing; that is, there was no difference between the two methods. The vitrification method is safer in terms of avoiding injury by ice crystal formation in the cytoplasm, but high concentrations of cryoprotectants may be harmful to the cell viability.

Recently, Huang *et al.* (2005) [39] reported successful pregnancies following blastocyst cryopreservation by supercooling ultra-rapid vitrification in mice. They preserved mouse blastocysts in supercooled liquid nitrogen at −205°C. The survival and pregnancy rates were 77% and 54%, respectively. This new technology holds promise for the development of blastocyst freezing technology in humans.

Cryoprotectant

The selection of cryoprotectant and its concentration may affect the success of the cryopreservation of blastocysts. In the slow-freezing method, propanediol and DMSO were the main cryoprotectants; however, ethylene glycol has also been used because of its low molecular weight and high permeability into cells. Chi *et al.* [40] showed improved implantation and pregnancy rates with ethylene glycol compared with use of propanediol. In general, DMSO is appropriate for cryopreservation of cleavage stage embryos and propanediol is used for pronuclear stage embryos. For vitrification, ethylene glycol and DMSO are usually used, and optimal concentrations have been studied in pigs [41,42]. Two issues must be considered concerning cryoprotectants. One is permeability into the cell and the other is potential toxicity, which may affect cell viability.

For thawing, a six step method prevented osmotic shock and improved the survival rate of blastocysts [43].

Table 12.1 outlines a vitrification procedure for cryopreservation of blastocysts (Cryotop method). Careful observation is needed to assess the quality of blastocysts after thawing. The blastocyst changes its shape by periodical contraction of the cells themselves (Figure 12.4).

Artificial shrinkage of the blastocele

Damage to blastocysts during cryopreservation is considered to be caused by intracellular ice formation, fracture damage, and osmotic swelling during the removal of cryoprotectant from the embryo. As the structure of blastocysts is unique, they cannot be frozen by the same strategy as other embryos and zygotes. Blastocysts contain a fluid-filled cavity, called the blastocele. In particular, expanded blastocysts contain large amounts of water inside the cells and are, therefore, easily impaired by ice crystal formation. In mice [44] and cattle [45], it has been shown that the survival rate of blastocysts depends on their stage. Miyake *et al.* [32] described a negative relationship between the survival rate and the volume of blastocysts in mice. However, this has not been observed in human blastocysts. Efforts for improving survival rate have been made, such as changing the cryoprotectant concentration [46] and the numbers of equilibration steps [47]. Vanderzwalmen *et al.* [48] suggested that shrinkage of the blastocele volume might improve survival during the cryopreservation of human blastocysts. Their report showed blastocele shrinkage before a fresh transfer resulted in no harmful effects and showed a better rate of survival, re-expansion, and hatching compared with a procedure involving no

Table 12.1. Vitrification procedure for cryopreservation of blastocysts (Cryotop method)

Protocol steps	Instructions[a]
Preparation	Prepare equilibration solution (ES), vitrification solution (VS), thawing solution (TS), diluting solution (DS), and washing solution (WS); at room temperature; two dishes (Falcon 3037); Cryotop; liquid nitrogen; timer, pipette (200 μm); tweezers, cane for cryopreservation
Vitrification	
1.	Take blastocyst from incubator
2.	Load the blastocyst on to the tip of the pipette with minimal volume of medium
3.	Place the blastocyst on the surface of ES; the embryo shrinks and sinks into the bottom
4.	When the blastocyst recovers its volume, proceed to the next step; usually pronuclear stage and cleaved embryos recover their size in 7–8 min but blastocysts take up to 15 min
5.	The next step should be completed in 45–60 s because evaporation of water may cause dryness and damage owing to the high concentration of cryoprotectant. Place the embryo onto the surface of the ES loading a minimum volume of medium. Place the ES in the pipette into the other well and wash the pipette with VS several times. Pipette VS rapidly into the VS dish covering the area until the margin of ES fluid disappears. Place the blastocyst on the tip of the Cryotop with minimum VS. Pull surplus VS onto the Cryotop. It is important to pull surplus medium from the proximal edge with a pipette of smaller diameter than the blastocyst in order not to pull the embryo, especially for expanded blastocysts
6.	Soak the Cryotop into liquid nitrogen
7.	Shake the Cryotop in order to remove small bubbles that may disturb rapid cooling
8.	Cap in liquid nitrogen
Thawing	
1.	Heat TS to 37°C for 1 h before the start of thawing
2.	Keep DS and WS1 at room temperature
3.	Keep WS2 on a warm plate
4.	Take the cane from the liquid nitrogen in the tank and transfer rapidly into a dish filled with liquid nitrogen
5.	Take out the Cryotop and remove the cap from it and soak it in TS fluid. It is essential to keep TS at 37°C, because rapid warming is needed to prevent ice crystal formation in the blastocyst
6.	Once the blastocyst no longer adheres to the sheet, place it on the surface of TS
7.	Transfer the blastocyst into DS for 1 min
8.	Transfer the blastocyst into WS1 solution for 3 min
9.	Transfer the blastocyst into WS2 solution for 5 min
10.	Transfer the blastocyst into the culture medium for 5 min
11.	The blastocyst should be cultured for a few hours and the viability of cell should be confirmed after expansion of the blastocele

[a] Media for the vitrification technique are provided by Kitazato BioPharma (Tokyo, Japan); for vitrification, Kitazato Vitrification Kit Vitrification Media was used; for thawing, Kitazato Vitrification Kit Thawing Media was used.

shrinkage; however, there was no statistical significance. Hiraoka *et al.* [49] reported a very good survival rate of 98% in vitrification of day 5 and day 6 expanded blastocysts using the artificial shrinkage technique. In this report, a handmade glass pipette (< 140 μm in diameter) was used for artificial shrinkage. After confirmation of a slight reduction of the blastocele puncturing with this pipette, a smaller diameter (100–120 μm) pipette was used and the procedure was repeated a few times. Careful attention, a fine technique, and confirmation of no injury to the trophectoderm and inner cell mass are required to carry out this method successfully. Mukaida *et al.* [50] used a laser pulse to make a hole in the trophectoderm and collapse the blastocele, instead of using a pipette. This method had a positive effect, achieving a 98% survival rate and a 49% implantation rate.

Cryopreservation may be sometimes disruptive to the cellular cytoskeleton of embryos and may damage the plasma membrane. Dobrinsky *et al.* [51] proposed the use of a microfilament stabilizer for vitrification of porcine embryos; however, using the same technique for mouse blastocysts did not show any significant improvement in results [52]. It is possible that this technique may induce improved clinical results for human blastocysts.

Day 6 blastocyst transfer

The cryopreservation of surplus blastocysts is beneficial, especially for day 6 blastocysts [53]. In our centers, morula or very early blastocysts at day 5 are cultured for

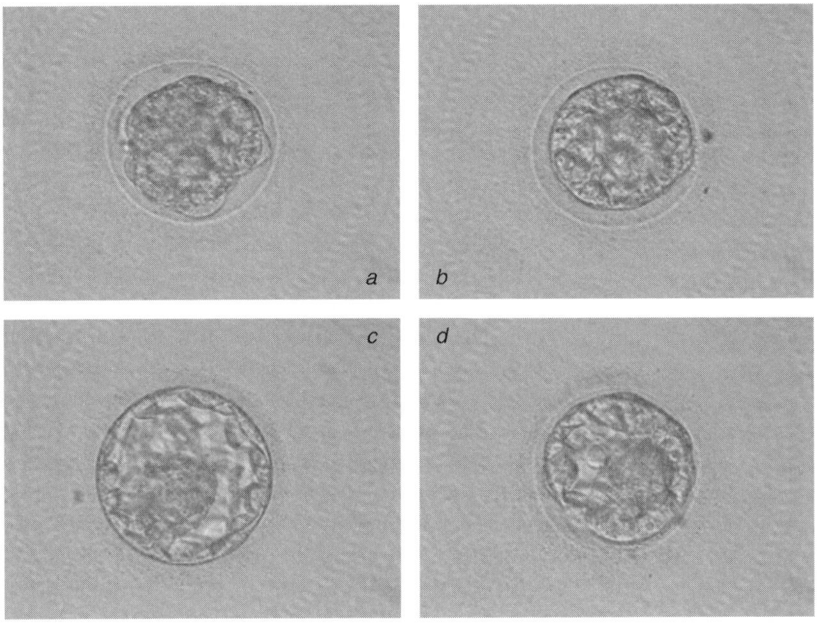

Figure 12.4. The change of a blastocyst after thawing. (a) Just after the thawing, the blastocele is contracted completely. (b) at 1 h after the thawing; (c) at 2 h after thawing, the blastocyst has recovered its shape; (d) before the embryo transfer, when the blastocyst is again a little contracted.

one extra day. However, even if these embryos develop to mature blastocysts and are transferred to the uterus, the implantation rate is low. If these embryos have formed a good-quality blastocyst on day 6, they should be frozen. Day 6 blastocysts contain embryos that possess potential for implantation. We had a much better pregnancy rate with frozen–thawed day 6 blastocysts (27%) compared with the transfer of fresh embryos (6%) [54]. Hence, the low implantation rate in day 6 blastocysts is caused not only by the quality of blastocysts but also by a mismatch of blastocysts with the implantation window.

Endometrial preparation

When cryopreserved and thawed blastocysts are transferred into the uterus, two methods of endometrial preparation for transfer are available. One is transferring to the endometrium in the natural menstrual cycle and the other is to an endometrium prepared by hormone replacement. In the former method, precise confirmation of ovulation is necessary. Ultrasound monitoring is carried out from day 10 if the patient has a regular menstrual cycle of 28 days. Five or six days after ovulation confirmation, the blastocyst can be transferred. Ovulation confirmation is sometimes difficult and it can be confirmed by the disappearance of the dominant follicle or the existence of the corpus luteum. Ovulation induction is sometimes necessary for patients with irregular menstrual cycles; however, clomiphene citrate cannot be recommended because of its antiestrogenic effect. For natural cycle transfer, no medication after transfer is needed; however, low-dose aspirin, drugs to prevent uterine contraction, or vitamins are sometimes administered depending on clinical need.

In our center, frozen and thawed blastocysts are transferred to an endometrium that is prepared by hormone replacement in most cases. During the previous cycle, a progesterone and estrogen combination drug (Norluten D [Shionogi, Osaka, Japan]; 5 mg norethisterone + 0.05 mg mestranol) is started from day 16 for 10 days. From day 21 to the date of transfer, buserelin, a gonadotropin-releasing hormone agonist (Sprecur [Mochida Parmaceutical, Tokyo, Japan] nasal spray, 600 μg/day) is taken. From day 1 of the transfer cycle, estradiol valerate (Progynova [Bayer Shering Pharma, Switzerland]; 2–10 mg, step-up increase) is administered to produce an endometrium of over 8 mm thickness. In our center, blastocyst transfer by hormone replacement is usually preferred by the patient, because it requires only two visits to the clinic. In contrast, the blastocyst transfer by natural cycle needs frequent visits and is inconvenient for patients.

Table 12.2. Survival rates of embryos after thawing from vitrification and slow freezing: clinical results in the IVF Namba Clinic from 2005 to 2008

Stage cryopreserved	No. thawed	No. survived (%)	No. transferable (%)
Vitrification			
Pronuclear	7068	6809 (96.3)[a]	–
Cleaved	1361	1186 (87.1)[b]	1327 (97.5)[d]
Blastocyst	881	785 (89.1)[b]	839 (95.2)[e]
Slow freezing			
Pronuclear	315	231 (73.3)[c]	–

a,b,c $p < 0.01$ for *a* vs. *b,c*; *b* vs. *a,c*; *d* vs. *e*.

Cryopreservation of preimplantation genetically diagnosed blastocyst

For patients who have a chromosomal abnormality, PGD is applied for in order to choose normal embryos. Aneuploidy may be the most common indication PGD and this may enable embryos to be identified without genetic and chromosomal abnormalities. For PGD, cryopreservation of the biopsied blastocyst is essential and both slow freezing [55] and vitrification [56] have been applied in cryopreservation of biopsied blastocysts. Several issues should be considered in the cryopreservation of biopsied blastocysts. Biopsied blastocysts have a breach in the zona pellucida, which may alter the diffusion by cryoprotectant. The manner of dehydration of the fluid and permeation of cryoprotectant may differ from blastocysts with intact zona. Cryoprotectant can easily invade the perivitelline space through the hole in the zona. Therefore, the time for permeation should be changed from that used for cryopreservation with intact zona. Furthermore, space left after the removal of blastomeres may impair the viability of blastocysts. The vitrification method can be also applied for biopsied blastocyst cryopreservation. Escribá *et al.* [56] showed parallel survival rates by vitrification at cavitated, expanded, and hatching blastocysts between PGD assessed and non-PGD groups. Further study is needed to identify the optimal sort of cryoprotectant, its amounts, and the time for permeation in order to ensure surviving blastocyst after PGD and cryopreservation.

Clinical outcome

In our centers, almost all of the embryos are cryopreserved by the Cryotop method (vitrification). The slow-freezing method is rarely applied in cases where many oocytes are retrieved and embryos are cryopreserved at

Table 12.3. Pregnancy and baby take-home rates with embryos transferred at the cleaved stage or the blastocyst stage in fresh transfers and for embryos transferred at the blastocyst stage but cryopreserved at either blastocyst stage or the cleaved embryo stage: clinical results in the IVF Namba Clinic from 2005 to 2008

	Freezing stage	No. transferred	No. pregnancies (%)	Implantation (%)	Take-home babies (%)
Embryo transfers at cleaved stage					
Vitrification	Pronuclear	719	210 (29.2)[a]	19.3	66.5[d]
	Cleaved	165	52 (31.5)[b]	18.2	74.4
Fresh embryo transfer		918	376 (41)[c]	20.8	78.7[e]
Embryo transfers at blastocyst stage					
Vitrification	Pronuclear	111	59 (53.2)	43.1[ah]	76.5
	Cleaved	99	64 (64.6)[f]	50.9[i]	69.4
	Blastocyst	475	249 (52.4)[g]	42.3[j]	78.1
Fresh embryo transfer		144	75 (52.1)	32[c]	84.1

$p < 0.05$ for *b* vs. *c*, *f* vs. *g*, *h* vs. *j*; $p < 0.01$ for *a* vs. *c*, *d* vs. *e*, *i* vs. *j*.

pronuclear stage, because it wastes a lot of time to cryopreserve many embryos with vitrification. The survival rate after thawing was acceptable in both vitrification and slow freezing; however, it was significantly better in vitrification (Table 12.2). With vitrification, the survival rate was the best in the embryos cryopreserved at pronuclear stage. The embryos that were frozen at the blastocyst stage showed higher survival, but fewer were transferrable compared with the embryos frozen at the cleavage stage. This might be because that the surviving blastocysts included embryos with partial degeneration.

Table 12.3 shows pregnancy and baby take-home rates with embryos transferred at the cleaved stage or the blastocyst stage. Cleaved embryos were transferred after thawing in 884 cases and when fresh in 918 cases from 2005 to 2007 in our centers. The fresh transfer group showed better pregnancy and baby take-home rates where transfer occurred at the cleaved stage than when it occurred at the blastocyst stage. In transfers at the blastocyst stage, the pregnancy and implantation rate were lower for embryos cryopreserved at blastocyst stage than at the cleaved embryo stage. These data are easier to understand if it is remembered that premature blastocysts are included in the number of blastocysts.

References

1. Woods EJ, Benson JD, Agca Y, *et al.* Fundamental cryobiology of reproductive cells and tissues. *Cryobiology* 2004; **48:** 146–156.
2. Bredkjaer HE, Grudzinskas JG. Cryobiology in human assisted reproductive technology. Would Hippocrates approve? *Early Pregnancy* 2001; **5:** 211–213.
3. Trounson A, Mohr L. Human pregnancy following cryopreservation, thawing and transfer of an eight-cell embryo. *Nature* 1983; **305:** 707–709.
4. Byrd W. Cryopreservation, thawing, and transfer of human embryos. *Semin Reprod Med* 2002; **20:** 37–43.
5. Cohen J, Simons RF, Edwards RG, *et al.* Pregnancies following the frozen storage of expanding human blastocysts. *J In Vitro Fert Embryo Transf* 1985; **2:** 59–64.
6. Ménézo Y, Nicollet B, Herbaut N, *et al.* Freezing cocultured human blastocysts. *Fertil Steril* 1992; **58:** 977–980.
7. Kaufman RA, Ménézo Y, Hazout A, *et al.* Cocultured blastocyst cryopreservation: experience of more than 500 transfer cycles. *Fertil Steril* 1995; **64:** 1125–1129.
8. Nagy ZP, Taylor T, Elliott T, *et al.* Removal of lysed blastomeres from frozen–thawed embryos improves implantation and pregnancy rates in frozen embryo transfer cycles. *Fertil Steril* 2005; **84:** 1606–1612.
9. Blake D, Proctor M, Johnson N, Olive D. Cleavage stage versus blastocyst stage embryo transfer in assisted conception. *Cochrane Database Syst Rev* 2002; **2:** CD002118.
10. Blake D, Proctor M, Johnson N, *et al.* Cleavage stage versus blastocyst stage embryo transfer in assisted conception. *Cochrane Database Syst Rev* 2005; **4:** CD002118.
11. Blake DA, Farquhar CM, Johnson N, *et al.* Cleavage stage versus blastocyst stage embryo transfer in assisted conception. *Cochrane Database Syst Rev* 2007; **4:** CD002118.
12. Virant-Klun I, Tomaźević T, Baćer-Kermavner L, *et al.* Successful freezing and thawing of blastocysts cultured in sequential media using a modified method. *Fertil Steril* 2003; **79:** 1428–1433.
13. Veeck LL, Bodine R, Clarke RN, *et al.* High pregnancy rates can be achieved after freezing and thawing human blastocysts. *Fertil Steril* 2004; **82:** 1418–1427.
14. Pantos K, Stefanidis K, Pappas K, *et al.* Cryopreservation of embryos, blastocysts, and pregnancy rates of blastocysts derived from frozen–thawed embryos and frozen–thawed blastocysts. *J Assist Reprod Genet* 2001; **18:** 579–582.
15. Troup SA, Matson PL, Critchlow JD, *et al.* Cryopreservation of human embryos at the pronucleate, early cleavage, or expanded blastocyst stages. *Eur J Obstet Gynecol Reprod Biol* 1991; **38:** 133–139.
16. Liebermann J, Tucker MJ. Comparison of vitrification and conventional cryopreservation of day 5 and day 6 blastocysts during clinical application. *Fertil Steril* 2006; **86:** 20–26.
17. Sawada N, Akamatsu Y, Tsuji Y, *et al.* Effects of developmental stage of human embryos on the development to transferable blastocyst following vitirfication and warming. *Reprod Biomed Online* 2008; **16**(Suppl 2): S28–S29.
18. Youssry M, Ozmen B, Zohni K, *et al.* Current aspects of blastocyst cryopreservation. *Reprod Biomed Online* 2008; **16:** 311–320.
19. Gardner DK, Lane M. Culture and selection of viable blastocysts: a feasible proposition for human IVF? *Hum Reprod Update* 1997; **3:** 367–382.
20. Lawitts JA, Biggers JD. Culture of preimplantation embryos. *Method Enzymol* 1993; **225:** 153–164.
21. Biggers JD, Racowsky C. The development of fertilized human ova to the blastocyst stage in KSOM(AA) medium: is a two-step protocol necessary? *Reprod Biomed Online* 2002; **5:** 133–140.
22. Gardner DK, Michelle L. Culture systems for the human embryo. In Gardner DK, Weissman A, Howles CM, *et al.*, eds. *Textbook of Assisted Reproductive Techniques: Laboratory and Clinical Perspectives*, 2nd edn. London: Taylor & Francis, 2004, pp. 211–234.

23. Choi DH, Chung HM, Lim JM, *et al.* Pregnancy and delivery of healthy infants developed from vitrified blastocysts in an IVF-ET program. *Fertil Steril* 2000; **74:** 838–839.
24. Mukaida T, Takahashi K, Kasai M. Blastocyst cryopreservation: ultrarapid vitrification using cryoloop technique. *Reprod Biomed Online* 2003; **6:** 221–225.
25. Cobo A, Bellver J, Domingo J, *et al.* New options in assisted reproduction technology: the Cryotop method of oocyte vitrification. *Reprod Biomed Online* 2008; **17:** 68–72.
26. Kuwayama M, Vajta G, Kato O, *et al.* Highly efficient vitrification method for cryopreservation of human oocytes. *Reprod Biomed Online* 2005; **11:** 300–308.
27. Kuwayama M. Highly efficient vitrification for cryopreservation of human oocytes and embryos: the Cryotop method. *Theriogenology* 2007; **67:** 73–80.
28. Morató R, Izquierdo D, Paramio MT, *et al.* Cryotops versus open-pulled straws (OPS) as carriers for the cryopreservation of bovine oocytes: effects on spindle and chromosome configuration and embryo development. *Cryobiology* 2008; **57:** 137–141.
29. Kuwayama M, Vajta G, Ieda S, *et al.* Comparison of open and closed methods for vitrification of human embryos and the elimination of potential contamination. *Reprod Biomed Online* 2005; **11:** 608–614.
30. Kuwayama M, Hamano S, Nagai T. Vitrification of bovine blastocysts obtained by *in vitro* culture of oocytes matured and fertilized *in vitro. J. Reprod Fertil* 1992; **96:** 187–193.
31. Massip A, Vanderzwalmen P, Scheffen B, *et al.* Pregnancies following transfer of cattle embryos preserved by vitrification. *Cryo Letters* 1986; 7: 270–273.
32. Miyake T, Kasai M, Zhu SE, *et al.* Vitrification of mouse oocytes and embryos at various stages of development in an ethylene glycol-based solution by a simple method. *Theriogenology* 1993; **40:** 121–134.
33. Vanderzwalmen P, Gaurois B, Ectors FJ, *et al.* Some factors affecting successful vitrification of mouse blastocysts. *Theriogenology* 1988; **30:** 1177–1183.
34. Dattena M, Ptak G, Loi P, *et al.* Survival and viability of vitrified in vitro and in vivo produced ovine blastocysts. *Theriogenology* 2000; **53:** 1511–1519.
35. Choi DH, Chung HM, Lim JM, *et al.* Pregnancy and delivery of healthy infants developed from vitrified blastocysts in an IVF-ET program. *Fertil Steril* 2000; **74:** 838–839.
36. Yokota Y, Sato S, Yokota M, *et al.* Birth of a healthy baby following vitrification of human blastocysts. *Fertil Steril* 2001; **75:** 1027–1029.
37. Stehlik E, Stehlik J, Katayama KP, *et al.* Vitrification demonstrates significant improvement versus slow freezing of human blastocysts. *Reprod Biomed Online* 2005; **11:** 53–57.
38. Loutradis KE, Kolibianakis EM, Venetis CA, *et al.* Cryopreservation of human embryos by vitrification or slow freezing: a systematic review and meta-analysis. *Fertil Steril* 2008; **90:** 186–193.
39. Huang CC, Lee TH, Chen SU, *et al.* Successful pregnancy following blastocyst cryopreservation using super-cooling ultra-rapid vitrification. *Hum Reprod* 2005; **20:** 122–128.
40. Chi HJ, Koo JJ, Kim MY, *et al.* Cryopreservation of human embryos using ethylene glycol in controlled slow freezing. *Hum Reprod* 2002; **17:** 2146–2151.
41. Berthelot F, Venturi E, Cognié J, *et al.* Development of OPS vitrified pig blastocysts: effects of size of the collected blastocysts, cryoprotectant concentration used for vitrification and number of blastocysts transferred. *Theriogenology*. 2007; **68:** 178–185.
42. Cuello C, Sanchez-Osorio J, Almiñana C, *et al.* Effect of the cryoprotectant concentration on the in vitro embryo development and cell proliferation of OPS-vitirified porcine blastocysts. *Cryobiology* 2008; **56:** 189–194.
43. Cho HJ, Son WY, Yoon SH, *et al.* An improved protocol for dilution of cryoprotectants from vitrified human blastocysts. *Hum Reprod* 2002; **17:** 2419–2422.
44. Scheffen B, Vanderzwalmen P, Massip A. A simple and efficient procedure for preservation of mouse embryos by vitrification. *Cryo Letters* 1986; **7:** 260–269.
45. Vanderzwalmen P, Touati K, Ectors FJ, *et al.* Vitrification of bovine blastocysts. *Theriogenology* 1989; **31:** 270.
46. Ali J, Shelton JN. Successful vitrification of day-6 sheep embryos. *J Reprod Fertil* 1993; **99:** 65–70.
47. Kuwayama M, Hamano S, Nagai T. Vitrification of bovine blastocysts obtained by *in vitro* culture of oocytes matured and fertilized *in vitro. J Reprod Fertil* 1992; **96:** 187–193.
48. Vanderzwalmen P, Bertin G, Debauche C, *et al.* Births after vitrification at morula and blastocyst stages: effect of artificial reduction of the blastocoelic cavity before vitrification. *Hum Reprod* 2002; **17:** 744–751.
49. Hiraoka K, Hiraoka K, Kiunutani M, *et al.* Blastocoele collapse by micropipetting prior to vitrification gives excellent survival and pregnancy outcomes for human day 5 and 6 expanded blastocysts. *Hum Reprod* 2004; **19:** 2884–2888.
50. Mukaida T, Oka C, Goto T, *et al.* Artificial shrinkage of blastocoeles using either a micro-needle or a laser pulse prior to the cooling steps of vitrification improves survival rate and pregnancy outcome of vitrified human blastocysts. *Hum Reprod* 2006; **21:** 3246–3252.
51. Dobrinsky JR, Pursel VG, Long CR, *et al.* Birth of piglets after transfer of embryos cryopreserved by cytoskeletal stabilization and vitrification. *Biol Reprod* 2000; **62:** 564–570.
52. Chen SU, Lee TH, Lien YR, *et al.* Microsuction of blastocoelic fluid before vitrification increased survival

and pregnancy of mouse expanded blastocysts, but pretreatment with the cytoskeletal stabilizer did not increase blastocyst survival. *Fertil Steril* 2005; **84**(Suppl 2): 1156–1162.

53. Urman B, Balaban B, Yakin K, *et al.* Outcome of blastocyst transfer according to availability of excess blastocysts suitable for cryopreservation. *Reprod Biomed Online* 2003; **7:** 587–592.

54. Murata Y, Oku H, Morimoto Y, *et al.* Freeze–thaw programmes rescue the implantation of day 6 blastocysts. *Reprod Biomed Online* 2005; **11:** 428–433.

55. Magli MC, Gianaroli L, Grieco N, *et al.* Cryopreservation of biopsied embryos at the blastocyst stage. *Hum Reprod* 2006; **21:** 2656–2660.

56. Escribá MJ, Zulategui JF, Galán A, *et al.* Vitrification of preimplantation genetically diagnosed human blastocysts and its contribution to the cumulative ongoing pregnancy rate per cycle by using a closed device. *Fertil Steril* 2008; **89:** 840–846.

Chapter 13

Aseptic vitrification of human blastocysts: protocol development and clinical application

Pierre Vanderzwalmen, Luc Grobet, Yannis Prapas, Patricia Frias, and Nicolas Zech

Introduction

After the initial application of vitrification to cleaving embryos [1] and blastocysts, in closed 0.25 ml insemination straws [2,3], the trend was to increase considerably the cooling and warming rates from <2000°C/min to >20 000°C/min [4]. With higher cooling and/or warming rates, the formation of ice crystals decreases considerably. In order to cool biological samples instantaneously below the glass transition temperature (T_g), thus capturing cells in an amorphous state, embryo carrier devices were designed to allow direct contact of the biological sample with liquid nitrogen (LN_2). Under such fast cooling conditions, it is possible to avoid ice crystal formation, even if cells are exposed for only a short period of time to higher concentrations of cryoprotectant agent (CPA). At present, non-aseptic devices such as the Cryotop, the open pulled straw, the hemi-straw, the Cryoloop or electron microscopy grids are mostly used for ultra-rapid cooling of embryos [5].

One major drawback of the ultra-rapid cooling process is the risk of bacterial as well as viral contamination of the biological sample during the cooling process as well as during long-term storage [6,7]. Even though the concerns of contamination during LN_2 storage are rather debatable [8], an European Parliament directive (EU Tissues and Cells Directive 2004/23/EC) [9], which was actualized in 2006 (COMMISSION Directive 2006/86/EC) [10], defines medical safety requirements for the cryopreservation of human cells. The directive mentions that cooling and storage of embryos has to be performed in a way that guarantees aseptic conditions. It was, therefore, necessary to switch from non-aseptic vitrification protocols to a protocol that entails complete isolation of the samples from LN_2 during every step, while providing good rates of survival.

Hermetically closed containers were already developed to vitrify mice [11,12] and human [13–15] oocytes and embryos. Although such aseptic systems have been developed, their use remained sporadic. Even Kuwayama, who developed the aseptic CryoTip device, recognized the superiority of the open Cryotop system [16]. If the embryos are not sufficiently exposed to the CPA solutions, aseptic cooling that isolates the embryo from the LN_2 may have an adverse effect on survival after warming. Knowing that the probability to bring the intracellular part into a "glass-like state" depends on the speed of cooling/re-warming and the concentrations of CPA [17], it is obvious that the likelihood of ice crystal formation will increase if the cells are not well protected through too short an exposure time to CPA solutions. The conversion of a solution into a glassy state is only achieved if its temperature is very rapidly lowered beneath the glass transition temperature. Before reaching this glass transition temperature, the solution has to cross a temperature zone of high risk for ice crystal formation very quickly. The bandwidth of this dangerous zone can be narrowed by increasing the concentration and viscosity of the solute. Therefore, when developing protocols using a closed system, procedures need to be modified to compensate for the reduced cooling rate resulting from the heat-insulating barrier.

The key to success is to find an optimal balance between the speed of cooling and re-warming with aseptic devices and the necessary quantity of CPA to obtain the vitrified state without being toxic to the cells. In 2003, we published an ultra-rapid vitrification technique for embryos at different stages of development using the hemi-straw as a carrier device [18]. After two short exposures of 2 to 4 minutes in 10% dimethyl sulfoxide (DMSO) and 10% ethylene glycol (EG) and

Fertility Cryopreservation, ed. Ri-Cheng Chian and Patrick Quinn. Published by Cambridge University Press.

30 seconds in 20% DMSO plus 20% EG, embryos are placed on the tip of a small gutter before plunging them directly into contact with LN_2. As published earlier, with such a strategy an overall survival rate of 77% was obtained after ultra-rapid vitrification of blastocysts.

The aims of the study described in this chapter are (1) to determine, with human blastocysts, the best protocol to prepare the embryos before cooling under aseptic conditions; (2) to produce an aseptic embryo carrier device that is easy to handle and that ensures the medical safety of vitrified human embryos; and (3) to present results on the clinical application of aseptic vitrification of blastocysts that originated from a conventional assisted reproductive technology (ART) program, including male and female infertility factors as well as egg donation and in vitro maturation (IVM).

Materials and methods

Embryo carrier devices

Non-aseptic embryo carrier: hemi-straw

The Hemi-straw (Astro-Med-tec, Salzburg, Austria), previously described [18], is an embryo carrier that consists of a large gutter on which a small quantity of CPAs (< 1 μl) containing the embryos is deposited (Figure 13.1). An ultra-rapid cooling rate of > 20 000°C/min was achieved by allowing direct contact of the biological material with LN_2. The Hemi-straw was subsequently inserted into a larger pre-cooled 0.5 ml straw (CBS, Cryo Bio System, Grenoble, France) under LN_2 (Figure 13.2). Prior to the commencement of the warming process the Hemi-straw was pulled out of the larger straw under LN_2. In order to achieve a warming rate of > 20 000°C /min, the tip of the Hemi-straw was instantaneously immersed into a petri dish containing a sucrose solution.

Aseptic embryo carrier: Vitrisafe

Vitrisafe (VitriMed, Austria) is a modification of our previous Hemi-straw vitrification plug [18] that allows a complete insertion inside a high security 0.5 ml straw (Figure 13.3). The Vitrisafe consists of a large gutter that is totally inserted into a larger pre-cooled 0.5 ml straw (CBS, Cryo Bio System, France). Only after welding both ends of the 0.5 ml straw to ensure complete isolation of the biological sample is the complete straw plunged into LN_2. A cooling rate of 1300°C/min is achieved.

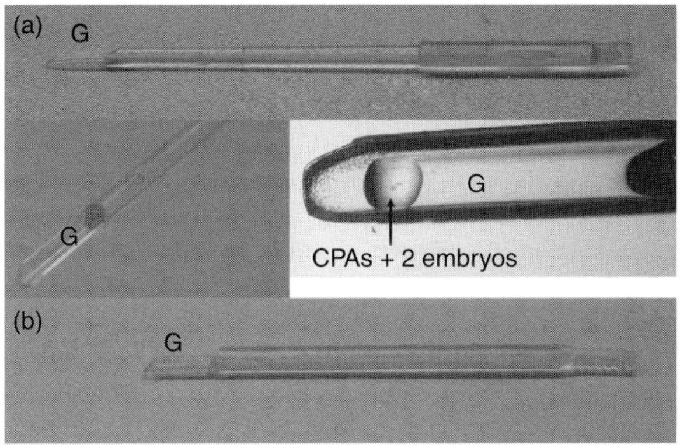

Figure 13.1. Design of the Vitriplug (a) and the Vitrisafe plug (b). G, gutter, where the embryos and cryoprotectants (CPAs) are placed.

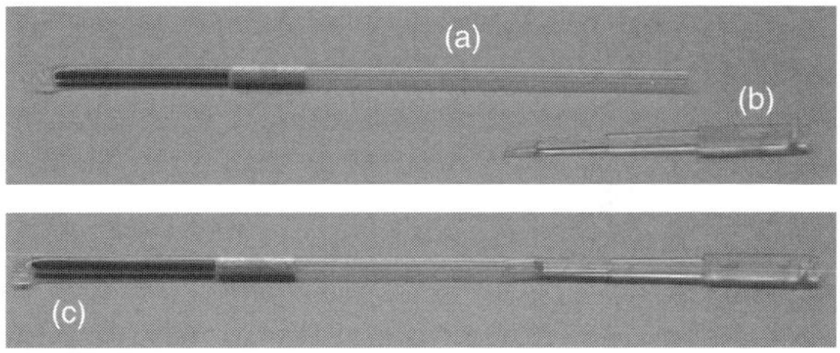

Figure 13.2. Non-aseptic vitrification of embryos using the Vitriplug hemi-straw embryo carrier device. (a) The 0.5 ml high-security straw for the embryo or sperm. (b) The hemi-straw. The embryos are loaded into the gutter and the two parts (a and b) are plunged separately into liquid nitrogen. (c) The hemi-straw is inserted into the high-security straw under the surface of the liquid nitrogen.

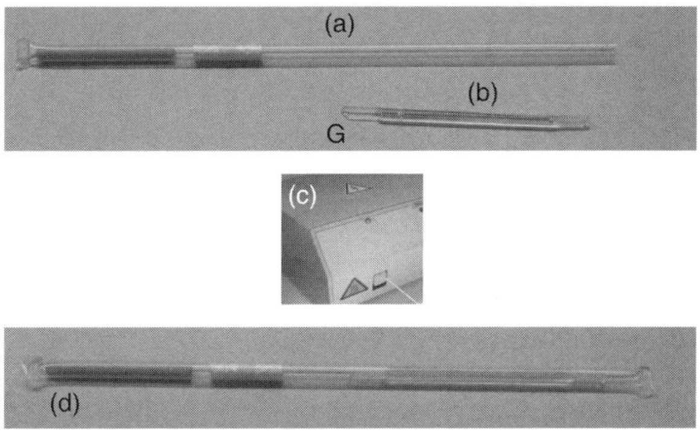

Figure 13.3. Aseptic vitrification of embryos using the Vitrisafe embryo carrier device. (a) The 0.5 ml high-security straw for the embryo or sperm. (b) The Vitrisafe device. The embryos are loaded into the gutter (G) and the Vitrisafe is inserted into the high-security straw. (c) The ends of the straw are welded. (d) The welded unit is plunged into liquid nitrogen.

For warming, the gutter is removed from the outer straw without contact with LN_2 and the tip containing the biological material is directly plunged into the dilution solution in order to achieve ultra-rapid warming.

Vitrification: solutions and protocols

Vitrification solutions

Three non-vitrifying solutions (NVS), NVS 2.5/2.5, NVS 5/5, and NVS 10/10, and one vitrification solution (VS) were prepared. The NVS 10/10 solution contained 10% EG (v/v) and 10% DMSO (v/v) (Fertipro, Bernem, Belgium). The NVS 2.5/2.5 and NVS 5/5 solutions were prepared by diluting NVS 10/10 with Global–HEPES 20% human serum albumin (HSA) (IVFOnline, LifeGlobal, Ontario, Canada) or phosphate-buffered saline (PBS) 20% HSA. The VS (Fertipro) comprised 20% EG (v/v), 20% DMSO (v/v), 25 μM (10 mg/ml) Ficoll (70 000 MW), and 0.75 M sucrose (VS 20/20).

Solutions used for dilution after warming

The solutions for warming contained 1, 0.5, 0.25, and 0.125 M sucrose in Global HEPES 20% HSA or PBS 20% HSA (Fertipro).

Development of an aseptic vitrification protocol

Before application of aseptic vitrification to human blastocysts in a clinical setting, spare human embryos otherwise not eligible for a fresh embryo transfer or for cryopreservation in a subsequent transfer cycle were used after informed consent of the patients.

In vitro survival of vitrified blastocysts was evaluated immediately after warming and after 24 hours of further culture.

The analysis of the effect of a reduction of the cooling rate was done after comparing the "in vitro" survival capacity of human blastocyts that were cooled ultra-rapidly (non-aseptic cooling) or more slowly (aseptic cooling) (Table 13.1).

For the development of the aseptic vitrification protocol, the blastocysts were first exposed to different combinations of the three NVS at room temperature (Table 13.2). After this step, the embryos were exposed for 40 to 60 seconds in VS 20/20. During this period, the blastocysts were placed into VS 20/20 and deposited into the gutter of the Vitrisafe plug, which was then inserted into the outer protective straw and welded before being plunged into LN_2. This part of the procedure may be considered as the critical part. When blastocysts are placed in the VS 20/20 droplet, it must be ensured that they are well encapsulated in the solution. Embryos were transferred in the gutter of the devices when a quite intense collapsing was observed during some in and out movement of the embryos in the VS 20/20 by means of a stripper pipette.

Table 13.1. "In vitro" development of human blastocysts exposed for 2–4 minutes to non-vitrifying solution 10/10 and for 45 seconds to vitrifying solution 20/20 before vitrification in aseptic and non-aseptic conditions

Vitrification conditions	No. blastocysts	Survival at	
		0 h	24 h
Non-aseptic	21	16 (76%)	15 (71%)
Aseptic	20	8 (40%)*	7 (35%)*

Analysis by chi square for non-aseptic versus aseptic at each time point: *$p < 0.02$

Clinical aseptic vitrification protocol

All the procedures occurred at room temperature. The embryos were exposed to NVS 5/5 and NVS 10/10. Drops of 100 μl covered with oil were prepared. Embryos were first exposed for 5 to 10 minutes in NVS 5/5 according to the degree of the blastocelic cavity expansion. In general, early blastocysts were exposed for 5 minutes and more expanded blastocysts for longer times, up to 10 minutes. They were subsequently exposed to NVS 10/10 for 4 minutes. When the embryos were in NVS 10/10, two 50 μl drops of VS 20/20 were placed into a petri dish but without a covering of oil. After this step, the embryos were exposed for 40–60 seconds to VS 20/20. This time was necessary to place and mix the embryos into the VS 20/20, load them into the gutter, insert them into the outer protective straw, and to weld the straw before finally plunging the closed system into LN_2.

The warming procedure was identical for both vitrification devices. A Dewar flask of LN_2 containing the devices was placed close to the microscope. Avoiding contact with LN_2, the plug was pulled out of the larger straw and the tip of the gutter holding the embryos was immediately immersed in 1 ml of 1 M sucrose. After 2 minutes, the blastocysts were transferred to 0.5, 0.25, and 0.125 M sucrose at intervals of 4 minutes. All procedures were performed at room temperature. The blastocysts were then washed several times in Global medium supplemented with 7.5% HSA and cultured for an additional period of 24 hours.

Clinical application of aseptic vitrification of blastocysts

Aseptic vitrification was carried out on blastocysts originating from three groups of patients. Group I included couples entering the in vitro fertilization (IVF) program for different types of female (tubal, endometriosis,

Table 13.2. "In vitro" development of human blastocysts after exposure for different time periods to distinct non-vitrifying solutions before vitrification in aseptic conditions

No. blastocysts	Time in solutions				Survival at	
	NVS 2.5/2.5	NVS 5/5	NVS 10/10	VS 20/20	0 h	24 h
10			2–4 min	40–60 s	4 (40%)	2 (20%)
31			7–8 min	40–60 s	22 (71%)	17 (55%)
31		5 min	3–4 min	40–60 s	29 (94%)	26 (83%)
12		7.5 min	3–4 min	40–60 s	11 (92%)	9 (75%)
23		10 min	3–4 min	40–60 s	22 (96%)	20 (87%)
21	5 min	10 min	3–4 min	40–60 s	20 (95%)	20 (95%)

NVS, non-vitrifying solution; VS, vitrifying solution.
Analysis by chi square was non-significant for comparison of all combinations of varying times of exposure to NVS.

ovarian hyperstimulation syndrome, idiopathic) and/or male infertility (oligoasthenoteratozoospermia with freshly ejaculate sperm only). In a second group (II), the embryos that were vitrified originated from egg donation cycles. The last group (III) consisted of women with polycystic ovary syndrome whose eggs underwent IVM and further culture to the blastocyst stage after intracytoplasmic sperm injection.

Before embryo transfer, hormonal replacement therapy was administered to each group of patients. After confirming steroid downregulation (gonadotropin-releasing hormone agonist), estrogen therapy was started, consisting of increasing doses of oestradiol valerate (Progynova, Schering, Berlin, Germany) until an appropriate thickness of the endometrium (> 8 mm)is achieved. From that day on, intramuscular or intravaginal progesterone was administered.

Ongoing pregnancy was defined by observing one or more gestational sacs with beating hearts using ultrasound scan at 6 weeks after the last menstrual period. The implantation rate represents the percentage of gestational sacs with fetal heartbeat divided by the total number of embryos transferred.

Results

Development of an aseptic vitrification protocol

The in vitro development of blastocysts vitrified in aseptic and non-aseptic conditions after a short exposure (4 minutes maximum) to NVS 10/10 is shown in Table 13.1. There was a significant increase in survival rates when the speed of cooling was > 20 000°C/min (non-aseptic). A decrease in the cooling rate to < 2000°C/min as a result of isolating the sample from the LN_2 dramatically reduced the survival rate to 35%. Table 13.2 shows the results of a pre-incubation of blastocysts in different solution of NVS and for different time periods.

A benefit of increasing the exposure time in the NVS 10/10 to 7–8 minutes instead of 2–4 minutes before applying aseptic vitrification can be seen. In spite of a survival rate of 71% after warming, only 55% continued further their re-expansion. Even though these observations do not reach statistical significance, the trend shows a beneficial effect of increasing the time of incubation, as had been shown previously in the mice model [26].

Compared with the one-step addition to NVS 10/10 (Table 13.2), a survival rate of almost 90% was observed when incubation in NVS 5/5 was performed before addition to NVS 10/10. No significant difference in survival rates was observed regardless of whether the blastocysts were exposed to NVS 5/5 for 5 minutes or 10 minutes. Even though the difference was not statistically significant, a tendency for higher survival rates could be seen when stepwise addition of NVS occurred in four steps starting with NVS 2.5/2.5.

Clinical aseptic vitrification

Table 13.3 summarizes embryo survival, development, pregnancy rate, ongoing pregnancies, and implantation rates for vitrified blastocysts that originated from a population of patients with female and/or male infertility factors (group I), were generated from egg donation cycles (group II), and after 15 IVM cycles (group III).

Discussion

Isolation of embryos inside a closed straw guarantees safety against contamination from LN_2 during

Table 13.3. Survival, ongoing pregnancies, and implantation rates after aseptic vitrification of blastocysts using the Vitrisafe carrier devices for different groups of patients

	Groups		
	I	II	III
No. patients	87	56	15
Women's age (mean years [SD])	34.3 (3.7)	27.6 (2.8)	32.1 (4.8)
No. vitrification–warming cycles	102	56	15
No. vitrified (warmed) blastocysts	263 (263)	238 (141)	40 (40)
Survival after warming	224 (85%)	137 (97%)	32 (80%)
Survival before embryo transfer	191 (73%)	131 (93%)	26 (65%)
Embryo transfers	94 (92%)	56 (100%)	14 (93%)
Blastocyst transfers (mean)	177 (1.9)	120 (2.1)	26 (1.9)
Preganancy rate/ vitrification–warming cycle	62 (60%)	38 (68%)	11 (73%)
Miscarriages	15 (24%)	4 (11.0%)	3 (27%)
Ongoing pregnancy rate/ vitrification–warming cycles	47 (46%)	34 (61%)	8 (53%)
No. with fetal heart beat	56	44	10
Implantation rate	32%	37%	38%

vitrification and during long-term storage in tanks. The results described in this chapter show that satisfactory survival rates of blastocysts and ongoing pregnancies can be achieved after aseptic vitrification in spite of reduced cooling rates. This is possible if the intracellular concentration of CPAs is well adapted to the needs of the cells without inducing a toxic effect.

Before an aseptic vitrification could be implemented into our routine clinical program, two issues had to be solved: to design an embryo carrier device allowing cooling and storage without contact with LN_2, and to determine the optimal protocol for exposing blastocysts to CPAs before the cooling step.

We designed an embryo carrier, the Vitrisafe, which is a modification of the original Hemi-straw device [18]. Blastocysts are deposited on the end of a gutter before complete insertion into a protective straw, which is welded before being plunged into LN_2. This results in a cooling rate of –1300°C/min. The advantages of the Vitrisafe plug are that a large gutter allows easier visualization and deposition of the embryos. Moreover, the drop of CPA containing the biological material is better protected during its insertion in the outer straw because no contact with the inner wall of the protective straw is possible. The fundamental issue to be solved in all vitrification methods is to be able to achieve and maintain conditions within the embryos that guarantee an amorphous state throughout the cooling as well during the warming process.

It is well known that for any given concentration of CPA the critical warming rates are much higher than the critical cooling rates [19,20]. Consequently, for a given volume and with constant speeds of cooling and re-warming, the minimal concentration of CPAs to prevent crystallization during warming must be higher than during cooling. Therefore, if the warming rate is lowered by using devices that separate the drop containing the embryos from the LN_2, higher intracellular concentrations of CPA are needed in order to reduce the likelihood of re-crystallization, which might be detrimental to further development. Consequently, in order to avoid increasing the concentration of CPA too much, the Vitrisafe was conceived to guarantee high warming rates of > 20 000°C/min without neglecting aseptic conditions. Indeed, ultra-fast warming rates can be achieved by instantly plunging the tip of the gutter directly into a solution of sucrose.

The second issue concerns the determination of a protocol for exposing blastocysts to CPAs before vitrification in conditions where cooling rates are reduced because of the heat-insulating barrier of the straw in which the blastocysts are kept. Yavin and Arav [17] reported that the probability of obtaining and maintaining a vitrified and thus amorphous state is directly correlated to the speed of cooling/warming and the intracellular viscosity, whereas it is inversely proportional to the size of the carrier and of the drop containing the embryo. We have shown the advantage of prolonging exposure of supernumerary human embryos to gradually increasing concentrations of CPA before vitrifying blastocysts aseptically in reduced cooling rate conditions. From the various combinations of CPAs evaluated on supernumerary blastocysts, the protocol implemented in our routine clinical program was derived. This consists of a stepwise addition of the CPAs in increasing concentrations. Blastocysts were first exposed for 5 to 10 minutes to NVS 5/5, followed by a shorter exposure of 4 minutes in NVS 10/10, and 40–60 seconds in VS 20/20.

The results shown here indicate that stepwise addition of the CPAs and vitrification in an aseptic embryo carrier device enables vitrification of blastocysts derived from couples presenting male and/or female infertility factors, and also from egg donor cycles and from IVM cycles. In addition to the aseptic safety achieved, this system of vitrification is simple, very flexible, and allows the handling of the embryos without the pressure of time. It is generally acknowledged that the quality of the blastocysts is an important factor affecting the outcome in terms of survival and pregnancies. Therefore, application of aseptic vitrification for blastocysts that originated from the ovum donor program can be considered as the reference standard group to assess the efficiency of this vitrification technique. The corresponding oocytes are retrieved from young women and only good-quality blastocysts were selected for vitrification.

The application of aseptic vitrification methods seems also very promising for blastocysts that developed from IVM oocytes. In fact, the implantation rates for embryos developing from IVM oocytes are said to be lower than after classical IVF techniques [21]. Obviously, good implantation rates for IVM oocytes were not yet achieved after fresh embryo transfer, which appears to be a drawback of this technique. The results shown here indicate an improvement if embryos generated from IVM oocytes were vitrified in aseptic conditions and then replaced in a further estradiol/progesterone-supplemented cycle. This highlights that endometrial quality or an inappropriate hormonal preparation of the selected population, who had polycystic ovary syndrome, may negatively influence implantation.

In view of the efficiency of our aseptic vitrification method with good-quality blastocysts, we may consider adapting our policy to embryo selection before fresh embryo transfer. The receptivity of the endometrium largely contributes to the clinical outcome of IVF/ICSI treatment, especially in stimulation cycles. The high implantation rates observed in an egg donation program are related to the high potential of good blastocysts to survive aseptic vitrification methods and this also reinforces the concept of good endometrial receptivity being achieved in hormone replacement cycles. From these observations, assuming that the receptivity of stimulation cycles is not always optimal and patients may already have a history of repeated implantatory failure, we may consider vitrifying the good-quality blastocysts and transferring those with moderate quality in the fresh cycles. Moreover, according to the current tendency of transferring only one embryo per cycle [22], it is more reasonable to present the results in terms of pregnancy per egg retrieval. As a consequence, in order to present the results in term of cumulative pregnancy rates, a good cryopreservation technique is mandatory when single embryo transfer is applied [23].

Another advantage of our aseptic vitrification protocol is that it does not necessitate the collapse of the blastocelic cavity. As confirmed by other teams working in this area, we have demonstrated previously the beneficial effect of reducing the blastocele volume prior to ultra-rapid vitrification [3]. In ultra-rapid vitrification, the blastocysts are left for a short period in the NVS 10/10. We assume, therefore, that the cavity was not well protected and that a vitrified state was not well established. Conversely, in the approach described here, where there is an initial exposure of the embryos to a lower concentration of CPA (NVS 5/5 for 5 to 10 minutes), sufficient CPA is present inside the cavity to prevent intracellular ice crystal formation at the virtrification point.

More than 20 years ago, in the 1980s, we reported acceptable survival rates followed by births of mice [20] and bovine [24] blastocysts that were vitrified in 0.25 ml French mini-straws. Recently Stachecki *et al.* [25] have reported excellent results after vitrification of human blastocysts loaded in a 0.25 ml straw, guaranteeing also the safety of the vitrification technique. The ultra-rapid way to vitrify blastocysts has to be finally revised, and cooling at lower rate is sufficient if the embryo is well prepared. After vitrification in straws, in open systems, and in aseptic devices, it will not be long before vitrification will occur definitely in straws [25,26].

In spite of reduced cooling rates inherent in the aseptic vitrification conditions, acceptable results are obtainable if the intracellular concentrations of CPAs are well adapted to the needs of the cells. If such results could be confirmed on a large scale, aseptic vitrification may become more routine and advantageous for cryopreservation of human blastocysts and also other embryo developmental stages. In a recent study [27], the authors provided evidence that vitrification of day 3 embryos imparts less trauma to cells than the slow-freezing technique and is associated with higher survival and better metabolism and blastocyst formation.

References

1. Mukaida T, Wada S, Takahashi K, *et al.* Vitrification of human embryos based on the assessment of suitable conditions for 8-cell mouse embryos. *Hum Reprod* 1998; **13:** 2874–2879.
2. Yokota Y, Sato S, Yokota M, *et al.* Birth of a healthy baby following vitrification of human blastocysts. *Fertil Steril* 2001; **75:** 1027–1029.
3. Vanderzwalmen P, Bertin G, Debauche CH, *et al.* Births after vitrification at morula and blastocyst stages: effect of artificial reduction of the blastocoelic cavity before vitrification. *Hum Reprod* 2002; **17:** 744–751.
4. Lane M, Schoolcraft WB, Gardner DK. Vitrification of mouse and human blastocysts using a novel cryoloop container-less technique. *Fertil Steril* 1999; **72:** 1073–1078.
5. Vajta G, Nagy Z. Are programmable freezers still needed in the embryo laboratory? Review on vitrification. *Reprod BioMed Online* 2006; **7:** 623–633.
6. Bielanski A. Non-transmission of bacterial and viral microbes to embryos and semen stored in the vapour phase of liquid nitrogen in dry shippers. *Cryobiology* 2005; **50:** 206–210.
7. Morris G. The origin, ultrastructure, and microbiology of the sediment accumulating in liquid nitrogen storage vessels. *Cryobiology* 2005; **50:** 231–238.
8. Kyuwa S, Nishikawa T, Kaneko T, *et al.* Experimental evaluation of cross-contamination between cryotubes containing mouse 2-cell embryos and murine pathogens in liquid nitrogen tanks. *Exp Anim* 2003; **52:** 67–70.
9. European Parliament. *EU Tissues and Cells Directive 2004/23/EC*. Brussels: EU Publications Office, 2004. http://eur-lex.europa.eu/LexUriServ/LexUriServ.do?uri=OJ:L:2004:102:0048:0058:EN:PDF (accessed October 2, 2009).
10. European Commission. *Directive 2006/17/CE of 8 February 2006*. Brussels: EU Publications Office, 2006. http://eur-lex.europa.eu/LexUriServ/site/en/oj/2006/l_038/l_03820060209en00400052.pdf (accessed October 2, 2009).
11. Walker D. (2004) Vitrification versus programmable rate freezing of late stage murine embryos: a randomised comparison prior to application in clinical IVF. *Reprod BioMed Online* 2004; **8:** 558–568.
12. Larman M, Sheehan C, Gardner D. Vitrification of mouse pronuclear oocytes with no direct liquid nitrogen contact. *Reprod BioMed Online* 2006; **12:** 66–69.
13. Kuleshova L, Shaw J. A strategy for rapid cooling of mouse embryos within a double straw to eliminate the risk of contamination during storage in liquid nitrogen. *Hum Reprod* 2000; **15:** 2604–2609.
14. Kuwayama M, Vajta G, Leda S, *et al.* Comparison of open and closed methods for vitrification of human embryos and the elimination of potential contamination. *Reprod BioMed Online* 2005; **11:** 608–614.
15. Isachenko V, Katkov I, Yakovenko S, *et al.* Vitrification of human laser treated blastocysts within cut standard straws (CSS): novel aseptic packaging and reduced concentrations of cryoprotectants. *Cryobiology* 2007; **54:** 305–309.
16. Kuwayama M. Highly efficient vitrification for cryopreservation of human oocytes and embryos: the Cryotop method. *Theriogenology* 2007; **67:** 73–80.
17. Yavin S, Arav A. Measurement of essential physical properties of vitrification solutions. *Theriogenology* 2007; **67:** 81–89.
18. Vanderzwalmen P, Bertin G, Debauche CH, *et al.* Vitrification of human blastocysts with the Hemi-Straw carrier: application of assisted hatching after thawing. *Hum Reprod* 2003; **18:** 1504–1511.
19. Fahy G. Biological effects of vitrification and devitrification. In Pegg DE, Karow AM, Jr., eds. *The Biophysics of Organ Cryopreservation*. New York: Plenum Press, 1987, pp. 265–293.
20. Scheffen B, Vanderzwalmen P, Massip A. A simple and efficient procedure for preservation of mouse embryos by vitrification. *Cryo Letters* 1986; **7:** 260–269.
21. Torre A, Frydman A, Feyereisen E, *et al.* How do we improve implantation rate following in-vitro maturation of oocytes? In Tan SL, Chian R-C, Buckett W, eds. *In-vitro Maturation of Human Oocytes: Basic Science to Clinical Application*. [*Reproductive Medicine and Assisted Reproductive Techniques Series*] London: Informa Healthcare, 2007, pp. 319–331.
22. Zech N, Lejeune B, Puissant F *et al.* Prospective evaluation of the optimal time for selecting a single embryo for transfer: day 3 versus day 5. *Fertil Steril* 2007; **88:** 244–246.
23. Henman M, Catt J, Wood T, *et al.* Elective transfer of single fresh blastocysts and later transfer of cryostored blastocysts reduces the twin pregnancy rate and can improve the in vitro fertilization live birth rate in younger women. *Fertil Steril* 2005; **84:** 1620–1627.
24. Massip A, Vanderzwalmen P, Scheffen B, *et al.* Pregnancies following transfer of cattle embryos preserved by vitrification. *Cryo Letters* 1986; **7:** 270–273.
25. Stachecki J, Garrisi J, Sabino S, *et al.* A new safe, simple and successful vitrification method for bovine and human blastocysts. *Reprod BioMed Online* 2008; **17:** 360–367.
26. Vanderzwalmen P, Ebner T, Zech N. One decade of experience with vitrification of human embryos in

straws, hemi-straws and high security vitrification straws. In Tucker MJ, Liebermann J, eds. *Vitrification in Assisted Reproduction: A User's Manual and Trouble-shooting Guide.* London: Informa Healthcare, 2007, pp. 195–217.

27. Balaban B, Urman B, Ata B, *et al.* A randomized controlled study of human day 3 embryo cryopreservation by slow freezing or vitrification: vitrification is associated with higher survival, metabolism and blastocyst formation. *Hum Reprod* 2008; **23:** 1976–1982.

Section 4 Chapter 14

Cryopreservation of oocytes

Cryopreservation of human oocytes: an overview

Ri-Cheng Chian

Introduction

The development of an effective oocyte cryopreservation system will have a significant impact on the clinical practice of assisted reproduction. In addition to fertility preservation for young women requiring sterilizing medical and surgical treatments, cryobanking of oocytes will benefit a large population of single women who wish to delay motherhood for personal, professional, and financial reasons.

An effective oocyte cryopreservation program will benefit infertile couples with moral or religious objections about cryopreservation of embryos. In fact, oocyte freezing has become the only option of cryopreservation in many countries where the laws forbid cryopreservation of embryos. In a country like Italy, only unfertilized gametes could be cryopreserved until a recent change in the law that again allowed for the cryopreservation of supernumerary embryos.

Women with premature ovarian failure who wish to conceive must rely on donor oocytes. Oocyte donation can be complicated and time consuming, requiring hormonal synchronization of the donor and recipient menstrual cycle. A successful oocyte cryopreservation protocol would eliminate the need for donor–recipient menstrual cycle synchronization and enable the establishment of egg banks, facilitating the logistics of coordinating egg donors with recipients. Furthermore, egg cryopreservation allows for temporary quarantine of donor eggs to test the donors for transmissible diseases. Therefore, the establishment of an effective oocyte cryopreservation program will likely encourage more women to donate their eggs and improve the current shortage of donor eggs.

Oocyte freezing may open a new option for women who worry that childbirth may interfere with their careers. Recently, it has been indicated that the effect of maternal age on the outcome of pregnancy may be best assessed by examining five specific factors that can negatively affect the desired outcome of a pregnancy, namely a healthy mother and a healthy baby: declining fertility, miscarriage, chromosomal abnormalities, hypertensive complications, and stillbirth [1]. Women's fertility declines with age and the rates of spontaneous abortions increase significantly after their mid 30s. The risks of having a baby with Down's syndrome and any chromosomal abnormalities are also higher in the oocytes produced by older women [2]. Although the decade between 25 and 35 years of age would seem to be ideal for women to have a baby, today in North America many women still want to have a baby after these ideal ages, even substantially older, for various reasons, including their professional arena. It has been emphasized that, for women for whom earlier childbearing is not an option, the decade between 35 and 45 years of age remains safe enough that maternal age alone should not be a contraindication to childbearing [1]. Nevertheless, oocyte freezing as a lifestyle option for women to give a birth in the future should be reconsidered socially.

The first report of successful cryopreservation of mouse oocytes was reported in 1958 by Sherman and Lin [3]. Nearly two decades later, the first live offspring from frozen–thawed mouse oocytes was reported by Parkening *et al.* [4] and Whittingham [5] using a slow-freezing method. After these reports, there has been very limited success in oocyte cryopreservation until more recent years.

The first reported human pregnancy and live birth from cryopreserved oocytes were reported by Chen [6] and van Uem *et al.* [7], respectively. However, most early reports of human oocyte cryopreservation showed dismal survival and pregnancy rates [8–11]. In fact, only three cases of clinical pregnancies were reported in the 1980s. Nearly a decade later, when Tucker *et al.* [10] and Porcu *et al.* [11] demonstrated the use of intracytoplasmic sperm injection (ICSI) to overcome hardening

Fertility Cryopreservation, ed. Ri-Cheng Chian and Patrick Quinn. Published by Cambridge University Press.

of the zona pellucida and to achieve pregnancies and a live birth, there was a renewed interest in oocyte cryopreservation.

Since the late 1990s, the number of reported live births resulting from oocyte cryopreservation has increased rapidly. Recently Noyes *et al.* [12] reviewed 58 reports from 1986 to 2008, indicating a total of 936 live births resulted from cryopreserved oocytes. Compared with congenital anomalies occurring in naturally conceived infants, no difference was noted [12,13]. It seems that so far, there are similar numbers of live births from the slow-freezing and the rapid-cooling (vitrification) methods. Therefore, it is important to review the technical development of these methods for oocyte cryopreservation.

Classic slow-freezing method

To date, pregnancies and live births from cryopreserved oocytes using the classic slow-freezing method have been published as case reports and series involving small numbers of patients. Only two large series of human oocyte cryopreservation using the classic slow-freezing protocols have been published [14,15]. Based on 112 in vitro fertilization (IVF) cycles with cryopreserved mature human eggs, a total of 1769 mature eggs were frozen and 1502 eggs were thawed. The survival rate was only 54.1%. The rates of fertilization following ICSI and cleavage were 57.7% and 91.2%, respectively. Sixteen pregnancies and 11 live births were reported. In 2004, Borini *et al.* [15] reported the clinical outcomes of 59 transfer cycles of embryos derived from cryopreserved oocytes. Out of 737 thawed oocytes, the survival rate was only 37%. In this series, 15 pregnancies and 13 live births were achieved.

When considering all pregnancies and live births obtained from cryopreserved oocytes using the classic slow-freezing method, the survival rates averaged approximately 50% and varied tremendously between the reported cases and series (23% to 89%). In fact, taken together for all the reported live births so far, 56 live births have been reported from cryopreserved human oocytes using the conventional slow-freezing procedure. The percentage of live births per thawed egg ranges from 1 to 10% using the classic slow-freezing protocols [16–19].

Modification of slow-freezing techniques

Recently improved survival and pregnancy rates have been reported using modified slow-freezing procedures, particularly increased sucrose concentration in the suspending solution and the use of sodium-free freezing solutions.

Increased sucrose concentration in suspending solution

Based on the hypothesis that the use of a higher sucrose concentration during slow freezing increases oocyte dehydration, thus reducing the formation of intracellular ice, Yang *et al.* [20] and Fabbri *et al.* [21] demonstrated that a higher sucrose concentration (0.2 M and 0.3 M, respectively) in the suspending solution led to a significant improvement in oocyte survival and pregnancy rates. Using a freezing solution containing 0.2 M sucrose and a slow-freezing/rapid thawing protocol, Yang *et al.* [20] first reported a case of successful ongoing twin pregnancy and, subsequently, in a series of 24 transfer cycles reported a survival rate of 71% and a pregnancy rate of 46% that resulted in 14 live births [22]. Using the same slow-freezing protocol, Winslow *et al.* [23] reported a similar frozen–thawed survival rate of 69% and achieved 16 live births in 42 transfer cycles.

Similarly, by increasing the sucrose concentration to 0.3 M and prolonging the exposure time to the freezing media, Fabbri *et al.* [21] reported a significantly higher post-thawing survival rate. In fact, using the 0.3 M sucrose slow-freezing protocol, Chen *et al.* [24] reported a post-thawing survival rate of 100% and an ongoing twin pregnancy. In a small series of seven patients, Fosas *et al.* [25] reported a survival rate of 90%, a pregnancy rate of 57%, and five live births. More recently, based on 21 freezing–thawing cycles, Chen *et al.* [26] reported a survival rate of 75%, a pregnancy rate of 33%, and five live births. Similarly, Li *et al.* [27] reported a survival rate of 90%, a pregnancy rate of 47%, and six live births in a series of 12 patients. Most recently, clinical outcome of two large series of oocyte cryopreservation using 0.3 M sucrose protocols were published [28,29]. Based on cryopreservation of 927 oocytes in 146 patients, Borini *et al.* [28] reported a survival rate of 74.1%, a pregnancy rate of 9.7%, and four live births. Levi Setti *et al.* [29] reported a similar survival rate (69.9%) based on 120 patients and 1087 oocytes but achieved a higher pregnancy rate (12.4%) and 13 live births. Overall, the use of 0.3 M sucrose in slow-freezing protocols appeared to improve the survival rate to approximately 70% and has resulted in 37 live births to date [26–30].

In the last few years, with these modified slow-freezing methods, the efficiency of oocyte cryopreservation has improved tremendously, resulting in cumulative pregnancy rates approaching 50% [31]. Borini *et al.* [32] reported that in 660 thawing cycles up to December 2006, 2205 oocytes survived out of 3238 thawing oocytes, a 68.1% survival rate. Five hundred and ninety cycles were performed for embryo transfer, giving rise to a clinical pregnancy rate per transfer of 15.0% (88/590).

Choline-based freezing media

Another strategy to improve the efficacy of oocyte cryopreservation is to change the composition of the freezing media. As highlighted by work of Stachecki *et al.* [33], the replacement of sodium with choline in the base solution may prevent salt-induced cryopreservation injury, resulting in improved survival rate and embryonic development in vitro using animal models. Another protective mechanism of choline-based media is believed to relate to an increase in viscosity at low temperature. Stachecki *et al.* [33] demonstrated high survival of choline-exposed oocytes despite plunging the oocytes into liquid nitrogen at a higher temperature (−20°C) than used in other slow-freezing protocols.

A total of 11 live births have been reported in several case reports and small series using the choline-based freezing method, although the survival rates were not significantly higher than the conventional slow-freezing method [34–37]. Therefore, larger clinical trials are needed to determine whether the clinical efficacy of oocyte cryopreservation using low-sodium media is superior to the other freezing protocols.

Rapid-cooling (vitrification) method

The rapid-cooling (vitrification) method is a promising novel technique and may be more effective than a slow-freezing procedure for egg cryopreservation [18]. Vitrification of human oocytes and embryos has resulted in relatively high survival rates [38–48]. In fact, many pregnancies and live births have been reported after cryopreservation of mature human oocytes or embryos using vitrification procedures [41,49–57].

In 1999, Kuleshova *et al.* [41] reported the first human live birth following vitrification of 17 mature oocytes using open pulled straws and high concentration of ethylene glycol and sucrose. Eleven eggs survived (65%) after vitrification–warming and five pronuclear zygotes (46%) were obtained after ICSI. In the series of three patients, one patient became pregnant. Yoon *et al.* [49] cryopreserved 90 mature eggs from seven patients by vitrification using electron microscope grids. Fifty-seven eggs survived (63%) after thawing. The fertilization rate was 75% (43/57) following ICSI. Two healthy live births and one ongoing pregnancy were obtained following transfer of 32 embryos, resulting in an implantation rate of 9% (3/32). The use of a vitrification solution mixture of 15% ethylene glycol, 15% dimethyl sulfoxide, and 0.5 M sucrose appeared to enable a dramatic improvement in the survival rate of vitrified human oocytes. Several groups reported high survival rates (89% to 100%) and successful live births using a vitrification method [50,51,55–57]. In fact, tremendous progress has been achieved recently for human oocyte cryopreservation using vitrification procedures [58,59].

Recently a clinical trial of oocyte vitrification indicated that 383 oocytes survived (82.7%) after thawing from a total of 463 oocytes that were vitrified and 17 out of 38 patients became pregnant, with 45% clinical pregnancy rate per embryo transfer [60]. This provides evidence that vitrification of oocytes results in a satisfactory clinical pregnancy rate, with better results than those achieved by the slow-freezing method. It was also demonstrated that pregnancies achieved with vitrification of oocytes do not appear to be associated with adverse pregnancy outcomes, indicating that vitrification of oocytes represents a novel option and efficient method for female fertility preservation [60].

Cryopreservation of oocytes at immature or mature stages

In earlier work when there was a poor survival rate for cryopreserved oocytes, an alternative strategy was considered using a slow-freezing method: to cryopreserve oocytes at the immature germinal vesicle (GV) stage instead of cryopreserving at mature metaphase II (MII) stage. The immature oocytes are at diplotene state of prophase I. Theoretically, given their microstructure, immature GV stage oocytes should be more resistant to the damage caused by cooling and would circumvent the risk of polyploidy and aneuploidies, since the chromatin is diffused and surrounded by a nuclear membrane [61,62]. However, difficulties are associated with in vitro maturation (IVM) of immature oocytes after freeze–thawing. Several attempts have been made with immature human oocytes. Although the survival rates seemed to be improved by the slow-freezing method, poor IVM and fertilization are major problems associated with immature egg freezing [17,63–66]. It has been known that oocyte cytoplasmic maturation requires cumulus cell and cytoplasmic communication using gap junctions [67]. So during freezing and thawing procedures, these gap junctions may be disconnected in the cryopreservative solution because this solution usually is hypertonic.

To date, only one human live birth has been reported following cryopreservation of GV stage oocytes and IVM [68]. Therefore, in all species, cryopreservation of mature oocytes is still more efficient than cryopreservation of immature oocytes [69]. Recently a study determined the efficacy of the vitrification method by vitrifying human oocytes before and after IVM of human oocytes [70]. The immature human oocytes recovered (total of 472 oocytes) were divided into two groups: 219 immature oocytes that were vitrified at the GV stage and 253 immature GV stage oocytes that were first matured in vitro (178 to the MII stage); 79 of the 178 were vitrified and 99 were not vitrified but were processed as controls. After thawing, the oocyte survival, maturation, and fertilization rates as well as embryonic development were compared. The results showed no significant difference between the survival rates of the oocytes vitrified at GV stage and those vitrified at MII stage (85% versus 86%). However, oocyte maturation rates were significantly reduced when oocytes were vitrified at immature GV stage followed by IVM (51%) in comparison with the oocytes without vitrification (70%). This study suggested that better results can be achieved by vitrifying mature oocytes rather than immature oocytes [69]. In fact, recently, several pregnancies and live births were obtained with the immature oocyte retrieval followed by IVM and vitrification [60,71], providing proof-of-principle evidence that the novel fertility preservation strategy of immature oocyte retrieval, IVM, and vitrification of mature oocytes can lead to successful pregnancies and healthy live births.

Conclusions

The development of an effective oocyte cryopreservation system has had a significant impact on the clinical practice of assisted reproduction. With modified slow-freezing methods, particularly increased sucrose concentration in suspending solution, improved survival and pregnancy rates have been obtained. However, rapid cooling (vitrification) of human oocytes has resulted in relatively higher survival rates. Pregnancies achieved with cryopreservation of oocytes, regardless of whether slow freezing or vitrification was used, do not appear to be associated with adverse pregnancy outcomes, indicating that cryopreservation of oocytes represents a novel option and an efficient method for female fertility preservation. It seems that cryopreservation of mature stage oocytes has better results than freezing immature stage oocytes, because oocyte maturation rate will be significantly reduced when the oocytes are cryopreserved at an immature stage followed by IVM after thawing. Although approximately more than 1000 live births obtained from the cryopreserved oocytes showed no difference in congenital anomalies compared with naturally conceived infants, more live born data and long-term monitoring are required to assure the safest and most expeditious development of oocyte cryopreservation technology.

References

1. Heffner LJ. Advanced maternal age: how old is too old? *N Engl J Med* 2004; **351**: 1927–1929.
2. Hook EB, Cross PK, Schreinemachers DM. Chromosomal abnormality rates at amniocentesis and in live-born infants. *JAMA* 1983; **249**: 2034–2038.
3. Sherman JK, Lin TP. Survival of unfertilized mouse eggs during freezing and thawing. *Proc Soc Exp Biol Med* 1958; **98:** 902–905.
4. Parkening TA, Tsunoda Y, Chang MC. Effects of various low temperatures, cryoprotective agents and cooling rates on the survival, fertilizability and development of frozen–thawed mouse eggs. *J Exp Zool* 1976; **197:** 369–374.
5. Whittingham DG. Fertilization in vitro and development to term of unfertilized mouse oocytes previously stored at −196°C. *J Reprod Fertil* 1977; **49**: 89–94.
6. Chen C. Pregnancy after human oocyte cryopreservation. *Lancet* 1986; **327:** 884–886.
7. van Uem JF, Siebzehnrübl ER, Schuh B, *et al.* Birth after cryopreservation of unfertilized oocytes. *Lancet* 1987; **329:** 752–753.
8. Chen C. Pregnancies after human oocyte cryopreservation. *Ann N Y Acad Sci* 1988; **541:** 541–519.
9. Al-Hasani S, Diedrich K, van der Ven H, *et al.* Cryopreservation of human oocytes. *Hum Reprod* 1987; **2:** 695–700.
10. Tucker M, Wright G, Morton P, *et al.* Preliminary experience with human oocyte cryopreservation using 1,2-propanediol and sucrose. *Hum Reprod* 1996; **11:** 1513–1515.
11. Porcu E, Fabbri R, Seracchioli R, *et al.* Birth of a healthy female after intracytoplasmic sperm injection of cryopreserved human oocytes. *Fertil Steril* 1997; **68:** 724–726.
12. Noyes N, Porcu E, Borini A. Over 900 oocyte cryopreservation babies born with no apparent increase

in congenital anomalies. *Reprod Biomed Online* 2009; **18**: 769–777.
13. Chian R-C, Huang JYJ, Tan SL, *et al.* Obstetric and perinatal outcome in 200 infants conceived from vitrified oocytes. *Reprod Biomed Online* 2008; **16**: 608–610.
14. Porcu E, Fabbri R, Ciotti PM, *et al.* Cycles of human oocyte cryopreservation and intracytoplasmic sperm injection: results of 112 cycles. *Fertil Steril* 1999; **72**(Suppl 1): S2.
15. Borini A, Bonu MA, Coticchio G, *et al.* Pregnancies and births after oocyte cryopreservation. *Fertil Steril* 2004; **82**: 601–605.
16. Tucker MJ, Morton PC, Wright G, *et al.* Clinical application of human egg cryopreservation. *Hum Reprod* 1998; **13**: 3156–3159.
17. Mandelbaum J, Belaïsch-Allart J, Junca AM, *et al.* Cryopreservation in human assisted reproduction is now routine for embryos but remains a research procedure for oocytes. *Hum Reprod* 1998; **13**(Suppl 3): 161–177.
18. Kuleshova LL, Lopata A. Vitrification can be more favorable than slow cooling. *Fertil Steril* 2002; **78**: 449–454.
19. Wininger JD, Kort HI. Cryopreservation of immature and mature human oocytes. *Sem Reprod Med* 2002; **20**: 45–49.
20. Yang DS, Blohm PL, Winslow KL, *et al.* A twin pregnancy after microinjection of human cryopreserved oocyte with a specially developed oocyte cryopreservation regime. *Fertil Steril* 1998; **70**(Suppl 3): S86.
21. Fabbri R, Porcu E, Marsella T, *et al.* Human oocyte cryopreservation: new perspectives regarding oocyte survival. *Hum Reprod* 2001; **16**: 411–416.
22. Yang DS, Blohm PL, Winslow KL, *et al.* Oocyte donation using cryopreserved donor oocytes. *Fertil Steril* 2002; **78**(Suppl 3): S14.
23. Winslow KL, Yang DS, Blohm PL, *et al.* Oocyte cryopreservation: a three year follow up of sixteen births. *Fertil Steril* 2001; **76**(Suppl 3): S120.
24. Chen SU, Lien YR, Tsai YY, *et al.* Successful pregnancy occurred from slowly freezing human oocytes using the regime of 1.5 mol/l 1,2-propanediol with 0.3 mol/l sucrose. *Hum Reprod* 2002; **17**: 1412.
25. Fosas N, Marina F, Torres PJ, *et al.* The births of five Spanish babies from cryopreserved donated oocytes. *Hum Reprod* 2003; **18**: 1417–1421.
26. Chen SU, Lien YR, Chen HF, *et al.* Observational clinical follow-up of oocyte cryopreservation using a slow-freezing method with 1,2-propanediol plus sucrose followed by ICSI. *Hum Reprod* 2005; **20**: 1975–1980.
27. Li XH, Chen SU, Zhang X, *et al.* Cryopreserved oocytes of infertile couples undergoing assisted reproductive technology could be an important source of oocyte donation: a clinical report of successful pregnancies. *Hum Reprod* 2005; **20**: 3390–3394.
28. Borini A, Sciajno R, Bianchi V, *et al.* Clinical outcome of oocyte cryopreservation after slow cooling with a protocol utilizing a high sucrose concentration. *Hum Reprod* 2006; **21**: 512–517.
29. Levi Setti PE, Albani E, Novara PV, *et al.* Cryopreservation of supernumerary oocytes in IVF/ICSI cycles. *Hum Reprod* 2006; **21**: 370–375.
30. Tjer GC, Chiu TT, Cheung LP, *et al.* Birth of a healthy baby after transfer of blastocysts derived from cryopreserved human oocytes fertilized with frozen spermatozoa. *Fertil Steril.* 2005; **83**: 1547–1549.
31. Borini A, Cattoli M, Bulletti C, Coticchio G. Clinical efficiency of oocyte and embryo cryopreservation. *Ann NY Acad Sci* 2008; **1127**: 49–58.
32. Borini A, Bianchi V, Bonu MA, *et al.* Evidence-based clinical outcome of oocyte slow cooling. *Reprod Biomed Online* 2007; **15**: 175–181.
33. Stachecki JJ, Cohen J, Willadsen SM. Cryopreservation of unfertilized oocytes: the effect of replacing sodium with choline in the freezing medium. *Cryobiology* 1998; **37**: 346–355.
34. Donaldson MJ, Quintans CJ, Rocha M, *et al.* Pregnancies achieved after transfer of embryos obtained by IVF of human oocytes cryopreserved in low sodium: report of two cases. *Hum Reprod* 2000; **15**: 152.
35. Quintans CJ, Donaldson MJ, Bertolino MV, *et al.* Birth of two babies using oocytes that were cryopreserved in a choline-based freezing medium. *Hum Reprod* 2002; **17**: 3149–3152.
36. Boldt J, Cline D, McLaughlin D. Human oocyte cryopreservation as an adjunct to IVF-embryo transfer cycles. *Hum Reprod* 2003; **18**: 1250–1255.
37. Azambuja R, Badalotti M, Teloken C, *et al.* Successful birth after injection of frozen human oocytes with frozen epididymal spermatozoa. *Reprod Biomed Online* 2005; **11**: 449–451.
38. Mukaida T, Wada S, Takahashi K, *et al.* Vitrification of human embryos based on the assessment of suitable conditions for 8-cell mouse embryos. *Hum Reprod* 1998; **13**; 2874–2879.
39. Mukaida T, Nakamura S, Tomiyama T, *et al.* Successful birth after transfer of vitrified human blastocysts with use of a cryoloop containerless technique. *Fertil Steril* 2001; **76**: 618–620.
40. Hong SW, Chung HM, Lim JM, *et al.* Improved human oocyte development after vitrification: a comparison of thawing methods. *Fertil Steril* 1999; **72**: 142–146.
41. Kuleshova L, Gianaroli L, Magli C, *et al.* Birth following vitrification of a small number of human oocytes. *Hum Reprod* 1999; **14**: 3077–3079.
42. Kuleshova LL, Shaw JM. A strategy for rapid cooling of embryos within a double straw to eliminate the risk of

contamination during cryopreservation and storage. *Hum Reprod* 2000; **15:** 2604–2609.
43. Yokota Y, Yokota H, Yokota M *et al.* Birth of healthy twins from in vitro development of human refrozen embryos. *Fertil Steril* 2001; **76:** 1063–1065.
44. Chung HM, Hong SW, Lim JM, *et al.* In vitro blastocyst formation of human oocytes obtained from unstimulated and stimulated cycles after vitrification at various maturational stages. *Fertil Steril* 2000; **73:** 545–551.
45. Chi HJ, Koo JJ, Kim MY, *et al.* Cryopreservation of human embryos using ethylene glycol in controlled slow freezing. *Hum Reprod* 2002; **17:** 2146–2151.
46. Cho HJ, Son WY, Yoon SH, *et al.* An improved protocol for dilution of cryoprotectants from vitrified human blastocysts. *Hum Reprod* 2002; **17:** 2419–2422.
47. Vanderzwalmen P, Bertin G, Debauche CH, *et al.* Vitrification of human blastocysts with the Hemi-Straw carrier: application of assisted hatching after thawing. *Hum Reprod* 2003; **18:** 1504–1511.
48. Son WY, Yoon SH, Yoon HJ, *et al.* Pregnancy outcome following transfer of human blastocysts vitrified on electron microscopy grids after induced collapse of the blastocoele. *Hum Reprod* 2003; **18:** 137–139.
49. Yoon TK, Kim TJ, Park SE, *et al.* Live births after vitrification of oocytes in a stimulated in vitro fertilization-embryo transfer program. *Fertil Steril* 2003; **79:** 1323–1326.
50. Katayama KP, Stehlik J, Kuwayama M *et al.* High survival rate of vitrified human oocytes results in clinical pregnancy. *Fertil Steril* 2003; **80:** 223–224.
51. Kyono K, Fuchinoue K, Yagi A, *et al.* Successful pregnancy and delivery after transfer of a single blastocyst derived from a vitrified mature human oocyte. *Fertil Steril* 2004; **84:** 1017.
52. Chian R-C, Son WY, Huang JW, *et al.* High survival rates and pregnancies of human oocytes following vitrification: preliminary report. *Fertil Steril* 2005; **84**(Suppl 1): S36.
53. Kim TJ, Hong SW, Chung HM *et al.* Pregnancy and delivery after vitrification of human oocytes. *Fertil Steril* 2004; **83**(Suppl 1): S13.
54. Kim T, Hong S, Cha K. Pregnancies from cryopreserved oocytes using vitrification protocol. *Fertil Steril* 2005; **84**(Suppl 1): S179.
55. Kuwayama M, Vajta G, Ieda S, *et al.* Comparison of open and closed methods for vitrification of human embryos and the elimination of potential contamination. *Reprod Biomed Online* 2005; **11:** 608–614.
56. Okimura T, Kato K, Zhan Q, *et al.* Update on clinical efficiency of the vitrification method for human oocytes in an in vitro fertilization program. *Fertil Steril* 2005; **84**(Suppl 1): S174.
57. Lucena E, Bernal DP, Lucena C, *et al.* Successful ongoing pregnancies after vitrification of oocytes. *Fertil Steril* 2006; **85:** 108–111.
58. Cobo A, Kuwayama M, Pérez S, Ruiz A, Pellicer A, Remohí J. Comparison of concomitant outcome achieved with fresh and cryopreserved donor oocytes vitrified by the Cryotop method. *Fertil Steril* 2008; **89:** 1657–1664.
59. Sher G, Keskintepe L, Mukaida T, *et al.* Selective vitrification of euploid oocytes markedly improves survival, fertilization and pregnancy-generating potential. *Reprod Biomed Online* 2008; **17:** 524–529.
60. Chian R-C, Huang JYJ, Gilbert L, *et al.* Obstetric outcomes following vitrification of in vitro and in vivo matured oocytes. *Fertil Steril* 2009; **91:** 2391–2398.
61. Cooper A, Paynter SJ, Fuller BJ, *et al.* Differential effects of cryopreservation on nuclear or cytoplasmic maturation in vitro in immature mouse oocytes from stimulated ovaries. *Hum Reprod* 1998; **13:** 971–978.
62. Isachenko EF, Nayudu PL. Vitrification of mouse germinal vesicle oocytes: effect of treatment temperature and egg yolk on chromosomal normality and cumulus integrity. *Hum Reprod* 1999; **14:** 400–408.
63. Mandelbaum J, Junca AM, Plachot M, *et al.* Cryopreservation of human embryos and oocytes. *Hum Reprod* 1988; **3:** 117–119.
64. Toth TL, Baka SG, Veeck LL, *et al.* Fertilization and in vitro development of cryopreserved human prophase I oocytes. *Fertil Steril* 1994; **61:** 891–894.
65. Toth TL, Lanzendorf SE, Sandow BA, *et al.* Cryopreservation of human prophase I oocytes collected from unstimulated follicles. *Fertil Steril* 1994; **61:** 1077–1082.
66. Son WY, Park SE, Lee KA, *et al.* Effects of 1,2-propanediol and freezing on the in vitro developmental capacity of human immature oocytes. *Fertil Steril* 1996; **66:** 996–999.
67. Cha KY, Chian R-C. Maturation in vitro of immature human oocytes for clinical use. *Hum Reprod Update* 1998; **4:** 103–120.
68. Tucker MJ, Wright G, Morton PC, *et al.* Birth after cryopreservation of immature oocytes with subsequent in vitro maturation. *Fertil Steril* 1998; **70:** 578–579.
69. Shaw JM, Oranratnachai A, Trounson AO. Fundamental cryobiology of mammalian oocytes and ovarian tissue. *Theriogenology* 2000; **53:** 59–72.
70. Cao YX, Xing Q, Zhang ZG, Wei ZL, Zhou P, Cong L. Cryopreservation of immature and in-vitro matured human oocytes by vitrification. *Reprod Biomed Online* 2009; **19:** 369–373.
71. Chian R-C, Gilbert L, Huang JY, *et al.* Live birth after vitrification of in vitro matured human oocytes. *Fertil Steril* 2009; **91:** 372–376.

Chapter 15

Cryopreservation of oocytes by slow cooling

Andrea Borini and Giovanni Coticchio

Introduction

In vitro fertilization (IVF) treatment would benefit immensely from a safe and efficient oocyte freezing method. Embryo freezing, which involves important legal and ethical drawbacks, would no longer be needed. Women facing premature ovarian failure through genetic factors or chemo- or radiotherapies could still pursue the hope of conceiving their own children. Moreover, oocytes from donors could be stored and held in quarantine for an adequate period of time, making treatment with donated oocytes safer and more flexible. In light of this, it is surprising how the IVF community has virtually ignored the necessity of devising efficient oocyte freezing methods for more than 20 years. However, studies conducted in the last few years suggest that oocyte cryopreservation can be applied in a systematic and reproducible fashion, in some cases with success rates that appear to compete with those routinely achieved with embryo freezing. Vitrification techniques, recently introduced in the field of human IVF, have given further emphasis to the hope of developing oocyte storage as a viable assisted reproduction strategy. Nevertheless, most IVF specialists remain reluctant to adopt oocyte cryopreservation. One of the major criticisms raised against oocyte freezing is the lack of information on the safety of this methodology. While this is true in principle, this concern does not seem to consider that the history of IVF is in fact full of such cases, such as pre-implantation genetic diagnosis (PGD), in vitro maturation (IVM), or more typically intracytoplasmic sperm injection (ICSI), in which clinical application was started without preliminary safety studies. This does not absolve the IVF community from the moral and professional imperative of shedding light on possible unwanted effects of the process of freezing and thawing. Several investigations have been conducted to detect possible freezing-induced cellular alterations that might compromise oocyte viability. Other studies have aimed at devising more efficient storage methods. Clinical evidence gained from several hundred babies born from frozen oocytes, although still insufficient and incomplete, has not suggested so far that the process of freezing and thawing is associated with an increase in birth abnormalities. Although the number of published studies is still modest, the number of oocyte cryopreservation treatments is dramatically increasing, although it has not emerged yet as a routine clinical procedure. This will undoubtedly have a significant impact on the practice of human IVF in the near future. This chapter offers an overview of the current status of oocyte cryopreservation by slow-cooling methodology; it discusses recent advances, unresolved matters, and possible future developments.

Basic principles and developments

Biological material undergoes time-dependent loss of viability at temperatures above −135°C. By comparison, data from domestic species have shown that mammalian gametes and embryos can be safely cryopreserved in liquid nitrogen at −196°C for decades, without effects of the storage period on viability. During cooling to ultra-low temperatures and subsequent re-warming, cells are exposed to a number of stresses that often result in cell death. Cooling can directly cause cell injury by affecting the organization of the plasmalemma and intracellular membranes as well as the cytoskeletal elements. It can also induce a variety of phenomena, including intracellular and extracellular ice formation, dehydration, gas bubble formation, and an increase in viscosity and solute and ionic concentration; all these factors are believed to contribute to different forms of cell damage, especially of a mechanical nature. In order to succeed with cryostorage, it is, therefore, crucial to implement some form of cryoprotection to prevent in particular intracellular ice formation and other undesired effects

Fertility Cryopreservation, ed. Ri-Cheng Chian and Patrick Quinn. Published by Cambridge University Press.

that derive directly or indirectly from ice formation. Cryoprotection may be achieved through the use of cryoprotective agents (CPAs), chemicals that interfere with the water–ice transition and interact with biomolecules, acting as "water replacement." Some CPAs, classified as permeating or intracellular, are compounds of relative low toxicity that can enter the cell across the plasmalemma. Other CPAs (non-permeating or extracellular) are unable to cross the plasmalemma and do not diffuse into the intracellular compartment.

The cryopreservation methodology of slow (or controlled rate) cooling requires that relatively low concentrations (typically 1.5 M) of penetrating cryoprotectants, such as propanediol (PROH), dimethyl sulfoxide (DMSO), or ethylene glycol (EG), are applied in combination with very slow cooling rates in the attempt to ensure a fine control over various factors that may contribute to cell damage. The action of the diverse CPAs is rather multifactorial and only partly understood at present, especially when cells are subjected to slow freezing. A major effect produced by CPAs is cell dehydration, which is pursued to minimize intracellular ice formation and the ensuing mechanical damage. This is initially achieved by exposing cells to hypertonic solutions of CPA at supra-zero temperatures. Generally, this initial phase of dehydration involves an exposure to a single permeating CPA. A second phase of dehydration occurs when the cell is subsequently exposed to a mixture of the intracellular CPA used in the initial step and an extracellular CPA, the latter generally sucrose or another oligosaccharide. These conditions re-establish an osmotic disequilibrium and drive a further phase of dehydration. Afterward, the cell is cooled down to subzero temperatures slowly (normally at a rate of 2°C/min) to avoid thermal shock. Once the sample temperature has been lowered to –6 to –8°C (just below the equilibrium freezing point of the mixture), ice nucleation (seeding) is intentionally induced while temperature is kept constant to permit dissipation of latent heat of ice nucleation. Thereafter, extracellular water is slowly converted into ice while the sample is subjected to a slow cooling rate (0.3°/min). During the transition of water into ice, the solutes present in the freezing mixture selectively segregate into the non-frozen fraction. If not controlled properly, the increase in solute concentration (dictated kinetically by the cooling rate) may affect cell viability, having a high salt content has a destabilizing effect on membranes and biomolecules (the so-called solution effect). However, in practice, the novel osmotic gradient draws further water out of the cell, reducing the risk of intracellular ice formation. Therefore, the rate of cooling during the extracellular water–ice transition expresses a fine compromise between the need for sufficient dehydration on the one hand, and the limitation of the detrimental effects of an increase in extracellular solute concentration on the other. At temperatures between –30 and –40°C, almost all extracellular water has been converted into ice, while almost all freezable water has been extracted from the cell, and the mixture achieves a "glassy matrix" of ice and highly viscous components. Under these conditions, the sample temperature can be quickly lowered to the liquid nitrogen temperature, ideally avoiding significant intracellular ice formation.

After storage, re-warming is performed in a fashion that depends on cooling conditions. If a sample has been plunged into liquid nitrogen from a relatively high temperature (–20°C to –30°C), it is possible that minute intracellular ice crystal nuclei have formed as a consequence of incomplete dehydration during conversion of extracellular water into ice. Under such conditions, re-warming should be fast to prevent growth of these intracellular ice crystals to a size that may cause harm to the cell organelles and organization. If, however, the samples were moved to liquid nitrogen from a lower plunge temperature, re-warming is compatible with slow warming rates, because it is likely that the more extended phase of dehydration during freezing has coincided with a complete extraction of freezable water from the intracellular environment. Once samples are thawed, cell rehydration is usually obtained by exposure to decreasing concentrations of the intracellular CPA present in the freezing mixture. Rehydration mixtures may also contain fixed or decreasing amounts of the extracellular CPA, such as sugars which act as osmotic buffers, in order to limit the net flux of water towards the intracellular compartment during the dilution of the intracellular CPA. Once rehydration and CPA dilution is completed, the cell is placed in standard culture conditions.

Developments in human oocyte cryopreservation

The first experiences aimed at cryopreserving human oocytes date back to as early as 1986 [1,2], approximately 10 years after the pioneering experience of Whittingham [3], who proved the feasibility of freeze–thawing mature mouse oocytes, fertilizing them in vitro, and obtaining embryos able to give rise to viable fetuses. It became immediately evident that oocyte cryopreservation was difficult to perform reproducibly and efficiently, in contrast to embryo freezing. In particular, survival rates were very low (generally below 40%) and, as such, incompatible with the adoption of this storage strategy in a clinical context. Being the expression of sporadic experiences, it is not clear to what extent these initial results reflected the actual capabilities of contemporary cryopreservation methodology. However, after a loss of interest in oocyte storage that endured for more than 10 years [4], the disappointing outcome of these experiences was confirmed by the first study describing a more systematic approach to oocyte freezing. In fact, after the cryopreservation of more than 700 oocytes, Borini *et al.* [5] reported a survival rate of less than 38%. Fertilization rates were also rather inadequate, despite ICSI, which was not available at the time of the first oocyte freezing reports, being employed. In fact, it was, and still is, believed that cryopreservation could cause fertilization failure with standard IVF as an effect of cortical granule release and zona hardening. Therefore, it became clear that, before oocyte storage could be considered a viable IVF option, slow-cooling methodology required major improvements in order to guarantee a higher efficiency. Meanwhile, experiments conducted in the early 2000s were starting to clarify and solve the problem of low post-thaw survival rates. As explained above, it was long known that the principal source of cell death in slow-cooling cryopreservation resides in damage to various organelles caused by intracellular ice crystals, which form during freezing–thawing as a consequence of inadequate dehydration.

In 2001, a study by Paynter *et al.* [6] suggested that, in effect, the freezing conditions usually applied to cryopreserved human oocytes were likely to coincide with a condition of insufficient dehydration. In particular, they found that a concentration of 0.1 M sucrose, a non-permeable CPA, in the freezing solution was inadequate to generate, by an osmotic effect, a significant dehydration, especially if the treatment was limited to a few minutes before exposing the oocyte to progressively lower temperatures. On this basis, Fabbri *et al.* [7] in 2001 tested the simple but founded hypothesis that by increasing the concentration of sucrose in the freezing solution, and therefore increasing the degree of cell dehydration, it was possible to achieve higher survival rates as a consequence of a reduced risk of intracellular ice formation. In effect, they found that concentrations of sucrose of 0.1, 0.2, and 0.3 M were able to generate survival rates of 39%, 58%, and 83%, respectively. Nowadays, such protocols consistently guarantee survival rates of over 70% [8–11]. Recently, Paynter *et al.* [12] were able to quantify the dehydration effect of different sucrose concentrations and different exposure times, providing information that has led to more finely designed protocols [8,13.] Analysis of precooling dehydration is only one of the approaches that should be further tested to improve post-thaw survival, especially in consideration that vitrification is emerging as a very competitive alternative, with post-storage recoveries in excess of 90% [14,15]. In a recent study from our group using only moderate pre-freeze dehydration conditions (0.2 M sucrose), which alone are unable to raise survival rates above 50%, it was possible to achieve a post-thaw recovery of more than 75%. This was obtained by maintaining a higher (0.3 M) concentration of sucrose in the thawing solutions, thereby controlling possible osmotic stress during the removal of the intracellular CPA [8]. Also, preliminary results suggests that a more systematic study of the oocyte osmotic behavior during post-thaw rehydration may lead to the identification of conditions able to increase survival rate and reduce the rate of osmotic stress and the overall time of exposure to the intracellular CPA at room temperature, thus decreasing the risks of osmotic and chemical damage (A. Borini *et al.*, unpublished data).

The use of alternative and less toxic CPAs is another potential approach in the development of more efficient slow-cooling protocols. A recent study [16] tested the possibility of achieving better oocyte post-thaw survival and/or viability by replacing PROH, almost universally adopted in slow-cooling protocols, with EG, which has been suggested to be less toxic [17]. Initially, an analysis of oolemma permeability to EG was carried out to simulate the oocyte osmotic response on exposure to stepwise addition of the CPA, and thus design a cryoprotectant addition protocol aimed at minimizing osmotic stress. Unfortunately, this approach did not appear to offer advantages in terms of survival (not exceeding 55%) in comparison with more traditional protocols based on PROH. Also, this protocol was found to cause partial disarrangement of the metaphase II (MII) spindle and extensive ultrastructural damage (see below) [18].

Other studies aimed at improving slow-cooling protocols have challenged the potential problem posed by the solution effect: the accumulation of solutes in the unfrozen phase occurring during extracellular ice formation, which is believed to affect the stability of the oolemma and the intracellular membranes. In initial studies conducted in the mouse, Stachecki *et al.* [19,20] replaced sodium, the most represented solute in freezing mixtures, with equimolar amounts of choline, which does not diffuse through the plasmalemma and is believed to be less toxic, and found dramatic increases in the rates of post-thaw survival, fertilization, and preimplantation development. In the same species, the association between the use of choline-based freezing media and high post-thaw survival and development rates was subsequently validated with other experiments [21]. Recently, low-sodium media were tested on human oocytes, with results that do not convincingly confirm the experience in the mouse. Stachecki *et al.* [22] reported that media based on choline and 0.2 mol/l sucrose guaranteed survival rates as high as 90%. However, these rates were obtained with groups of only 20–30 oocytes and in the absence of controls frozen with sodium-rich media. In addition, they have never been confirmed by experiments involving larger numbers. It raises some concern, also, in that after thawing and fertilization oocytes cryopreserved with choline-based freezing mixtures cleaved with a low rate (78%). In a clinical study carried out by Boldt *et al.* [23], in which choline-based media were formulated in combination with a sucrose concentration of 0.3 M, survival rates were disappointing irrespective of the adoption of phosphate-buffered saline or HEPES as pH buffers in separate treatment groups (61% and 59%, respectively). Other authors have tested the effect of sodium-depleted media on the cryopreservation of human oocytes [24,25]. In all these cases, survival rates remained rather low, generally below 62%, not confirming the beneficial effect of choline.

Oocyte quality before and after cryopreservation

The developmental potential of embryos at the cleavage or blastocyst stage may be predicted to a certain degree according to morphological and dynamic parameters, such as proportion of anucleated cytoplasmic fragments, relative blastomere size, multinucleation, pace of cleavage, and so on [26]. These parameters guide the choice at to whether the embryos are to be replaced in a fresh embryo transfer or whether they are suitable for cryopreservation; embryos which are estimated to possess low developmental capacity are disposed of. Therefore, cryopreserved embryos represent a special selection of a cohort generated from a single treatment cycle. After thawing, again, embryo implantation potential may be reasonably assessed by morphological and dynamic parameters. Rate of blastomere integrity is very informative in this respect. Edgar *et al.* [27] have shown that frozen–thawed fully intact 4-cell embryos implant with a rate of 26%, which is comparable to that for fresh controls. Post-thaw loss of one out of four blastomeres does not affect the implantation ability (27.5%). Instead, loss of a further blastomere (i.e. 50% of the total embryo mass) causes a major decrease in the implantation rate (9.4%). Also, ability to resume cleavage reflects the quality of frozen embryos [27], as shown by the fact that fully intact 4-cell frozen–thawed embryos that resume cleavage during overnight culture implant with higher efficiency (27.4%) than embryos that failed to cleave (16.0%).

Assessment of oocyte quality is one of the most crucial, intriguing and, yet, unresolved questions in IVF and gamete biology. The paradigm that identifies a "good quality" MII oocyte (i.e. spherical shape, a regular zona, an intact first polar body and a translucent, homogeneously colored cytoplasm), is by no means a guarantee of high developmental potential. Equally, evidence which suggests that different types of morphological anomaly (irregular zona pellucida, fragmented first polar body, refractile bodies, dark or pitted cytoplasm, small vacuoles) possess a predictive value with respect to oocyte implantation ability is controversial and certainly not conclusive [28]. Furthermore, in contrast to the case of embryos, mature oocytes are in static condition, although transiently, from the cell cycle standpoint, making even narrower the range of possibilities for the functional evaluation of these cells. Non-invasive methodologies for the assessment of oocyte quality based on non-morphological criteria are still in their infancy. In a recent study, Nagy *et al.* [29] have shown that biospectroscopy-based technology can discriminate characteristic profiles of biomarkers of oxidative metabolism released in the culture medium by human oocytes of different maturation stages (germinal vesicle, metaphase I, or MII). This represents the proof of principle that alternative approaches can open novel routes for an objective estimation of oocyte quality, but further progress is still required before developmentally competent oocytes may be selected, irrespective of the meiotic stage. Assessment of oocyte quality after cryopreservation appears even more problematic. By standard microscopic observation, frozen–thawed oocytes may survive and show no signs of widespread cell damage, such as broken zona pellucida, irregular cytoplasmic granularity, vacuolization, shrinkage, or swelling. Yet, under particular conditions, non-routine microscopy techniques have evidenced various forms of cell damage that are suggestive of a compromised developmental ability. Unfortunately, these techniques require methods of preparation (fixation and staining) that are incompatible with the preservation of cell viability and, therefore, cannot be adopted for oocyte selection in a clinical context. Nevertheless, extensive information has been generated by electron microscopy studies as a method to evaluate the performance of different freezing protocols from a non-clinical standpoint.

Nottola *et al.* [30] analyzed human oocytes frozen with two slow-cooling protocols involving different sucrose concentrations, 0.1 M [31] or 0.3 M [7], in the freezing mixture. They found that, overall, oocytes belonging to both study groups had a well preserved and homogeneous cytoplasm. Organelles (mainly mitochondria–smooth endoplasmic reticulum aggregates and mitochondria–vesicle complexes) were abundant and uniformly dispersed in the ooplasm. However, the amount and density of cortical granules appeared to be abnormally reduced in some frozen–thawed samples, independently of the sucrose concentration in the freezing solution. A reduction in the cortical granule population in frozen–thawed oocytes has been confirmed also by other studies [32,33]. Furthermore, slight to moderate microvacuolization was revealed in the ooplasm of some frozen–thawed oocytes, particularly in those treated with 0.3 M sucrose. Ooplasmic vacuolization is frequently detected in mammalian oocytes treated with different cryopreservation protocols or exposed to CPA alone [34,35]. It is interesting to note how the degree of microvacuolization of the oocytes frozen with the 0.1 and 0.3 M sucrose protocols is inversely associated with the implantation rates of the ensuing embryos [5,9] (5–6% and 16%, respectively). This suggests that microvacuolization, a phenomenon that often accompanies degenerative processes in the intracellular environment, may represent a specific form of cryodamage. Massive increases in microvacuoles and secondary lysosomes were found also in human oocytes frozen by an EG-based slow-cooling protocol [18]. In a preliminary study, Nottola *et al.* [30] have recently analyzed oocytes cryopreserved with a slow-cooling protocol involving differential sucrose concentrations at freezing and thawing (0.2 and 0.3 M), which had been optimized to ensure adequate pre-freeze dehydration while controlling osmotic stress during post-thaw rehydration. These oocytes give rise to embryos able to implant with a relatively high rate (above 13%) and are only marginally affected by the presence of microvacuoles [36]. It is, therefore, tempting to speculate that microvacuoles represent a specific form of cryodamage and that freezing conditions that prevent or limit the formation of microvacuoles coincide with those that better preserve oocyte implantation potential. Electron microscopy evidence on vitrified material is scarce, but preliminary data suggest that the high survival and developmental performance of oocytes vitrified with the Cryotop method may be associated with a low incidence of microvacuolization [37].

As a highly dynamic and sensitive structure that depends on the finely regulated process of tubulin polymerization and depolymerization, it is not surprising that the oocyte MII spindle may be affected by the physical stresses occurring during dehydration–rehydration and the phase transitions of extracellular water. In a landmark study as early as 1990, Pickering *et al.* [38] used epiflorescence microscopy to observe human mature oocytes cooled at room temperature for 10–30 minutes; they showed that the meiotic spindle suffered major structural alterations, which often persisted upon re-warming to physiological temperature. For many years, this evidence has generated the concern that cryopreservation is incompatible with maintenance of the MII spindle, discouraging the introduction of oocyte freezing in clinical IVF routine. In effect, partial disruption of the MII spindle was found in association with certain slow-cooling conditions – low sucrose concentration in the freezing solution (0.1 M) [39] or the use of EG as an intracellular CPA [16] – that are known to be particularly inadequate for oocyte storage [5,16]. However, in oocytes frozen with a protocol adopting a higher sucrose concentration (0.3 M) in the freezing solution, an intact chromosome segregation apparatus was found with an incidence comparable to that for freshly collected oocytes [39]. Integrity of the MII spindle has been shown also in oocytes frozen with slow-cooling protocols involving differential sucrose concentration in the freezing and thawing solutions (0.2 and 0.3 M, respectively), replacement of sodium with choline, or Cryotop vitrification [40]. Collectively, these data indicate that disruption of the MII spindle is not an unavoidable consequence of oocyte cryopreservation but that, in fact, the spindle may be found unaltered by using recently developed storage protocols.

Advances in polarized light microscopy have offered the opportunity to visualize the meiotic spindle non-invasively and in a dynamic fashion, an opportunity particularly attractive for frozen–thawed oocytes, which are especially exposed to the risk of spindle damage. In brief, the highly orderly structure of spindle microtubules generates the phenomenon of birefringence, which decomposes a single incident beam of polarized light into two orthogonal rays. This creates a difference in contrast between the spindle and the rest of the cell that may be detected by imaging methods (e.g. the Polscope) that digitally amplify birefringence signals; after computational manipulations, this allows quantifiable assessment of the degree of microtubule orientation. Numerous studies have explored the possibility of predicting oocyte developmental ability by monitoring MII spindle presence, position, or birefringence intensity (referred to as retardance). The majority of these studies indicated that absence of the spindle compromises the ability of the oocyte to fertilize and undergo normal pre-implantation development [41–49]. This has led to the adoption by many IVF laboratories of the Polscope as a tool for non-invasive oocyte assessment, before and/or after cryopreservation [50,51]. However, a recent study in which MII spindles of frozen–thawed oocytes were visualized by the Polscope and confocal microscopy is not consistent with the assumption that qualitative detection of spindle birefringence is indicative of normal spindle organization and chromosome organization [52]. In particular, spindles with normal (bipolar) or highly disarranged conformation are indistinguishable by Polscope analysis. The same study also showed that retardance measurements were unable to predict the degree of order or microtubule polymerization. This suggests that the Polscope may still be a rather inefficient method for assessing the MII spindle and, as a result, for non-invasive oocyte selection, especially after cryopreservation.

Clinical performance after oocyte cryopreservation

Assessment of the clinical performance of an IVF treatment is a very challenging task because of the large number of factors, classifiable as extrinsic (general) on intrinsic (specific), that can have important effects on the final outcome but cannot always be governed or even recognized. Furthermore, controversy surrounds the fundamental concept of clinical endpoint, which in the North American IVF community tends to be identified with the achievement of a term pregnancy, while in Western Europe it has been recently interpreted as synonymous with full-term single pregnancy. Assessment of clinical efficiency is particularly arduous in the case of oocyte cryopreservation because of the impact of specific factors, such as the lack of consensus on a methodological standard, especially from the laboratory standpoint; the absence of a systematic approach to the problem; or inconsistencies in the way in which IVF is offered as a form of treatment dependent on diverse legislative frameworks in different countries. Another factor that makes it difficult to appraise oocyte cryopreservation is that despite the general interest in oocyte cryopreservation, which has increased considerably in the last few years, paradoxically original work is still rather rare (Figure 15.1).

The effect of female age on oocyte developmental potential is probably the single most important factor capable of affecting the outcome of IVF treatment. This has been confirmed also for interventions involving embryo cryopreservation, in which day-2 frozen–thawed embryos implanted with rates of 18.7%, 14.0%, and 7.1% depending on whether female age at the time of storage was < 36, 36–39, or > 39 years, respectively [27]. On this basis, it is very difficult to compare the clinical outcome of oocyte cryopreservation studies that include women of very different ages. For example, by using the cryopreservation protocol developed by Fabbri *et al.* [7], Barritt *et al.* [53] reported an implantation rate of 26.1% in thawing cycles performed with oocytes derived from young women (mean age 28.3 years). However, other studies based on the same protocol but involving patients of rather older age (34–35 years) described much lower implantation rates

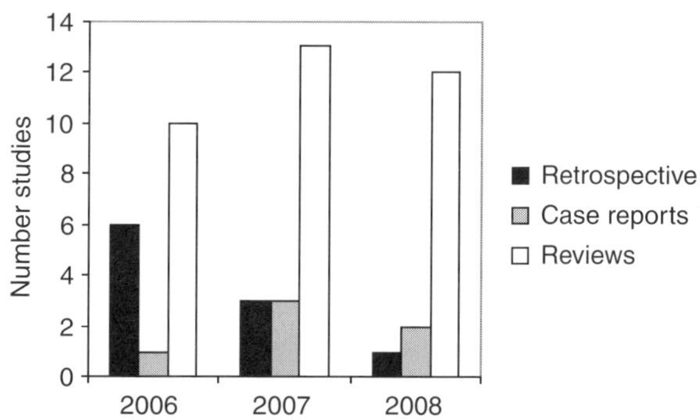

Figure 15.1. Number of clinical publications, retrospective analyses, case reports, and reviews on oocyte cryopreservation in the period 2006–2008.

(5.2–5.7%) [9–11]. Likewise, Cobo *et al.* [14] obtained an implantation rate of more than 40% after the transfer of embryos developed from vitrified oocytes. This rate is much higher than any of those obtained with slow-cooling protocols. Irrespective of the relative merit of vitrification, which may well perform better than slow cooling, it is difficult to imagine that female age factors (mean 26.7 years) did not influence the results of this study. The obvious solution to this problem consists in the stratification of treatments according to patient age, but so far this has been hindered by the small size of oocyte cryopreservation studies. Clearly, female age must have an effect also on the progression of a pregnancy, once it has been established. In general, data concerning the incidence of abortion in oocyte cryopreservation treatments are very scarce and do not pertain to comparisons between different age groups. Rates have been reported to vary between 14.2% and 33.3%, but in the absence of appropriate controls their significance is doubtful, especially in the case of very small studies. Whether, in older women, embryos derived from frozen oocytes are especially susceptible to developmental failure after implantation still remains an unanswered question.

The methodology implemented for using the stored material can profoundly influence the clinical outcome of oocyte freezing, complicating the comparison between different studies. In some cases, the possibility to generate more embryos than those strictly needed for an embryo transfer is precluded by various factors, especially of an ethical and legal nature. In cryopreserved cycles, to avoid the production of "surplus" embryos, only a few oocytes may be thawed at each cycle, with the aim of obtaining two or three survived oocytes suitable for insemination [5]. Since the introduction in Italy of the IVF law in 2004, this thawing scheme has been adopted in various studies [8–11,54]. In other circumstances, oocyte thawing cycles were performed without such limitations [55]. Clearly, by thawing only a few oocytes per cycle, the risks of premature interruption of the treatment as a consequence of increased fertilization failure or cleavage arrest are enhanced [9]. Furthermore, embryo selection is inapplicable and sometimes the number of transferred embryos may be inadequately low. Instead, when an excess of oocytes are thawed in single attempts, embryo selection becomes feasible and, as a consequence, clinical outcome in terms of pregnancy rate per thawing cycle and per transfer, as well as implantation rate, can increase significantly. Therefore, it would be problematic to compare pregnancy and implantation rates of studies in which the mean number of embryos transferred was as different as 1.1 [5] and 4.6 [56]. In light of this, perhaps the concept of implantation rate, intended as the proportion of fetal sacs in relation to the number of embryos transferred, which is considered to be one of the most informative parameters expressing the clinical efficiency of a given form of treatment, should be re-considered.

Assessment of implantation should take into account attrition, which may occur at different stages. This is particularly important in oocyte cryopreservation studies, in which the number of viable oocytes suitable for insemination, fertilized eggs, and cleaved embryos suitable for transfer may be lower than in fresh cycles. In a final analysis, this would allow an answer to the question "How many implantation can we expect from 100 oocytes?" [57]. Such a concept is well explained by a study including a series of 68 oocyte freezing treatments based on the use of the Lassalle protocol [58] and in which thawings were conducted with the aim of obtaining only three to four surviving oocytes suitable for insemination. The implantation rate per embryo transferred was relatively high (16.4%), considering the limitation of the number of oocytes used in each thawing cycle [5]. In reality, survival and fertilization rates were very poor (37% and 45%, respectively) and the overall implantation rate per thawed oocyte used was unacceptably low (2.3%). Under these terms, what implantation per oocyte should we expect from oocyte cryopreservation cycles? Gook and Edgar [57] estimated a rate of four detectable fetal hearts per 100 oocytes subjected to the process of IVF and embryo cryopreservation.

In the last few years, it is possible that improvements in techniques and laboratory skills may have raised the efficiency of embryo freezing to 5–6%. Therefore, oocyte cryopreservation should achieve similar rates in order to become a competitive strategy of preservation. Protocols tested in previous years are clearly inadequate, as described above. With other methods, the achievement of implantation rates in excess of 5% per oocyte used appears realistic. By using a sodium-depleted protocol, Boldt *et al.* [23] reported a remarkable implantation rate of 5.3% per oocyte used. However, this result derived from the treatment of only 23 patients and so far it has not yet been confirmed by a larger series of treatments. A similar value of implantation rate (5.9%) has been reported after the treatment of 62 patients, following the application of

Table 15.1. Rates of survival, pregnancy, and implantation (per embryo transferred and thawed oocyte) in two representative studies in which oocytes where stored by either slow cooling or vitrification

	Slow freezing[a]	Vitrification[b]
No. patients	62 (general)	30 (donors)
Patient age (years [SD])	33.7 (3.4)	26.7 (3.6)
Survival (%)	75	97
Pregnancies per embryo transfer (%)	26	65
Implantation per transferred embryo (%)	17	41
Implantation per thawed oocyte (%)	7.3	8.6

Source: Bianchi *et al.* (2007)[a] and Cobo *et al.* (2007)[b].

a protocol based on differential concentration of sucrose in the freezing (0.2 M) and thawing (0.3 M) solutions [8]. Recently, by using a protocol involving high sucrose concentration in the freezing solution (0.3 M), Parmegiani *et al.* [59] obtained an implantation rate per thawed oocyte of 8.1%. This is the highest rate ever reported for a slow-cooling protocol, but it should be noted that it was generated from only 26 thawing cycles. Despite such a limitation, this work offers other elements for reflection, because it also suggests that the pregnancy rate is higher when oocytes are cultured for less than 2 hours from pick up to freezing. In effect, oocytes may undergo a process of aging in vitro, a phenomenon consisting of alterations in key oocyte factors (cell cycle kinases, intracellular calcium stores, cytoskeleton) that are still compatible with an apparently normal fertilization but that at the same time may have profound detrimental consequences on post-implantation development [60].

The findings of Parmegiani *et al.* [59] require independent confirmation, but it appears entirely possible that the times of culture before and after freezing and thawing may influence oocyte developmental ability, irrespective of the cryopreservation procedure. Uncertainties remain also concerning the relative performance of the slow-freezing and vitrification methodologies. By adopting the Cryotop vitrification method in cycles involving young donors (mean age 26.7 years), Cobo *et al.* [14] achieved an implantation rate per embryo transferred of more than 40%. Nevertheless, when this study is analyzed considering the original number of oocytes used, the implantation rate corresponds to a value of 8.6%. Such a rate is not very dissimilar from the one (7.3%) resulting from a study conducted by a slow-cooling method and including patients with a mean age of 33.7 years (Table 15.1). Overall, the number of oocyte cryopreservation studies is still very small and cannot be considered conclusive. In comparison, the observations conducted on frozen embryos are numerically and analytically much more reliable. For example the cryopreservation data described in the study of Edgar *et al.* [27] originate from the thawing of more than 5000 embryos. Large sets of data concerning frozen–thawed embryos were recently reported also by Borini *et al.* [61].

Health of children from cryopreserved oocytes

Several concerns have been raised concerning the possibility of introducing oocyte cryopreservation into routine clinical IVF, assuming that cryodamage is a frequent event caused by freezing conditions and that its occurrence exposes the conceptus to an increased risk of developmental anomalies. A growing number of births from frozen oocytes have been reported. In 2004, Borini *et al.* [5] described 11 births from frozen oocytes. These children had a mean weight of 3.2 kg, normal karyotype, and no signs of malformations. Shortly afterwards, Chen *et al.* [55] found normal karyotypes in five children born from frozen–thawed oocytes. Other authors have reported a total of 65 healthy births [8–11,23,59,62], but in those studies information on karyotype was only sporadically provided. However, in the 18 pregnancies described by Levi Setti *et al.* [11], it was found that the mean gestational age at delivery was 37.1 weeks and the mean weight was 2807 g. So far, the largest series of babies born from frozen oocyte has been presented in a preliminary study by Borini *et al.* [63] who ascertained two cases of anomalies (Rubinstein–Taiby syndrome, and choanal atresia) in 146 births. Several other births have been described mainly in case reports. Tur-Kaspa *et al.* [64] produced an analysis of more than 37 publications on children born from cryopreserved oocytes. Of 555 live births, including those reported above, five abnormalities (three major) were found. This corresponds to an abnormality rate similar to that of natural pregnancies. The reliability of these data has been questioned [65] on the basis that the authors may have failed to find overlaps between studies and, as a consequence, overestimated the actual number of births. The dispute around the safety of oocyte freezing remains open. For instance, no exhaustive data are available on the number of spontaneous abortions. However, the evidence currently available does not point toward a dramatic increase in the incidence of anomalies at birth. This appears to legitimize further clinical studies on oocyte cryopreservation. Future studies will need to be more analytical and systematic, including also long-term follow-up.

Conclusions

Oocyte cryopreservation has long been envisaged as the ideal solution to the need to capitalize the reproductive potential derived from a cycle of ovarian stimulation, circumventing the ethical and legal problems posed by embryo cryopreservation. The first attempts in that direction were conducted with an inappropriate cryopreservation methodology. This led to rather inadequate results and, as a consequence, a lack of confidence and interest. After a period of eclipse lasting more than 10 years, oocyte cryopreservation has been re-proposed following some methodological modifications, which have improved some parameters of efficiency but not conclusively optimized the freezing procedures. This has made possible the application of oocyte cryopreservation as a reproducible strategy of treatment. Clinical data are progressively emerging, suggesting that in the near future oocyte cryopreservation could represent a valid alternative to embryo cryopreservation. However, several important aspects have not yet been clarified, especially in relation to the objective evaluation of oocyte implantation potential after cryopreservation. Meanwhile, non-clinical studies have established that cell damage from cryostorage may occur under different forms and specific conditions, but is not inevitable. Current knowledge of the health of children from cryopreserved oocytes is still rather limited but does not support the notion of an increased developmental risk for the conceptus. This lends credit to the suggestion that clinical experience in oocyte cryopreservation should be expanded in order to achieve a high and safe standard of treatment.

References

1. Chen C. Pregnancy after human oocyte cryopreservation. *Lancet* 1986; **i:** 884–886.
2. Al-Hasani S, Diedrich K, van der Ven H, Krebs D. [Initial results of the cryopreservation of human oocytes]. *Geburtshilfe Frauenheilkd* 1986; **46:** 643–644.
3. Whittingham DG. Fertilization in vitro and development to term of unfertilized mouse oocytes previously stored at −196 degrees C. *J Reprod Fertil* 1977; **49:** 89–94.
4. Porcu E, Fabbri R, Seracchioli R, *et al.* Birth of a healthy female after intracytoplasmic sperm injection of cryopreserved human oocytes. *Fertil Steril* 1997; **68:** 724–726.
5. Borini A, Bonu MA, Coticchio G, *et al.* Pregnancies and births after oocyte cryopreservation. *Fertil Steril* 2004; **82:** 601–605.
6. Paynter SJ, O ' Neil L, Fuller BJ, Shaw RW. Membrane permeability of human oocytes in the presence of the cryoprotectant propane-1,2-diol. *Fertil Steril* 2001; **75:** 532–538.
7. Fabbri R, Porcu E, Marsella T, *et al.* Human oocyte cryopreservation: new perspectives regarding oocyte survival. *Hum Reprod* 2001; **16:** 411–416.
8. Bianchi V, Coticchio G, Distratis V, *et al.* Differential sucrose concentration during dehydration (0.2 mol/l) and rehydration (0.3 mol/l) increases the implantation rate of frozen human oocytes. *Reprod Biomed Online* 2007; **14:** 64–71.
9. Borini A, Sciajno R, Bianchi V, *et al.* Clinical outcome of oocyte cryopreservation after slow cooling with a protocol utilizing a high sucrose concentration. *Hum Reprod* 2006; **21:** 512–517.
10. De Santis L, Cino I, Rabellotti E, *et al.* Oocyte cryopreservation: clinical outcome of slow-cooling protocols differing in sucrose concentration. *Reprod Biomed Online* 2007; **14:** 57–63.
11. Levi Setti PE, Albani E, Novara PV, Cesana A, Morreale G. Cryopreservation of supernumerary oocytes in IVF/ICSI cycles. *Hum Reprod* 2006; **21:** 370–375.
12. Paynter SJ, Borini A, Bianchi V, *et al.* Volume changes of mature human oocytes on exposure to cryoprotectant solutions used in slow cooling procedures. *Hum Reprod* 2005; **20:** 1194–1199.
13. Borini A, Bianchi V, Bonu MA, *et al.* Evidence-based clinical outcome of oocyte slow cooling. *Reprod Biomed Online* 2007; **15:** 175–181.
14. Cobo A, Kuwayama M, Perez S, *et al.* Comparison of concomitant outcome achieved with fresh and cryopreserved donor oocytes vitrified by the Cryotop method. *Fertil Steril* 2008; **89:** 1657–1664.
15. Cobo A, Bellver J, Domingo J, *et al.* New options in assisted reproduction technology: the Cryotop method of oocyte vitrification. *Reprod Biomed Online* 2008; **17:** 68–72.
16. De Santis L, Coticchio G, Paynter S, *et al.* Permeability of human oocytes to ethylene glycol and their survival and spindle configurations after slow cooling cryopreservation. *Hum Reprod* 2007; **22:** 2776–2783.
17. Kasai M, Mukaida T. Cryopreservation of animal and human embryos by vitrification. *Reprod Biomed Online* 2004; **9:** 164–170.

18. Nottola SA, Coticchio G, de Santis L, *et al.* Ultrastructure of human mature oocytes after slow cooling cryopreservation with ethylene glycol. *Reprod Biomed Online* 2008; **17:** 368–377.
19. Stachecki JJ, Cohen J, Willadsen S. Detrimental effects of sodium during mouse oocyte cryopreservation. *Biol Reprod* 1998; **59:** 395–400.
20. Stachecki JJ, Cohen J, Willadsen SM. Cryopreservation of unfertilized mouse oocytes: the effect of replacing sodium with choline in the freezing medium. *Cryobiology* 1998; **37:** 346–354.
21. Stachecki JJ, Willadsen SM. Cryopreservation of mouse oocytes using a medium with low sodium content: effect of plunge temperature. *Cryobiology* 2000; **40:** 4–12.
22. Stachecki JJ, Cohen J, Garrisi J, *et al.* Cryopreservation of unfertilized human oocytes. *Reprod Biomed Online* 2006; **13:** 222–227.
23. Boldt J, Tidswell N, Sayers A, Kilani R, Cline D. Human oocyte cryopreservation: 5-year experience with a sodium-depleted slow freezing method. *Reprod Biomed Online* 2006; **13:** 96–100.
24. Quintans CJ, Donaldson MJ, Bertolino MV, Pasqualini RS. Birth of two babies using oocytes that were cryopreserved in a choline-based freezing medium. *Hum Reprod* 2002; **17:** 3149–3152.
25. Petracco A, Azambuja R, Okada L, *et al.* Comparison of embryo quality between sibling embryos originating from frozen or fresh oocytes. *Reprod Biomed Online* 2006; **13:** 497–503.
26. Ziebe S, Petersen K, Lindenberg S, *et al.* Embryo morphology or cleavage stage: how to select the best embryos for transfer after in-vitro fertilization. *Hum Reprod* 1997; **12:** 1545–1549.
27. Edgar DH, Archer J, McBain J, Bourne H. Embryonic factors affecting outcome from single cryopreserved embryo transfer. *Reprod Biomed Online* 2007; **14:** 718–723.
28. Coticchio G, Sereni E, Serrao L, *et al.* What criteria for the definition of oocyte quality? *Ann New York Acad Sci* 2004; **1034:** 132–144.
29. Nagy ZP, Chang CC, Shapiro DB, *et al.* Clinical evaluation of the efficiency of an oocyte donation program using egg cryo-banking. *Fertil Steril* 2009; **92:** 520–526.
30. Nottola SA, Macchiarelli G, Coticchio G, *et al.* Ultrastructure of human mature oocytes after slow cooling cryopreservation using different sucrose concentrations. *Hum Reprod* 2007; **22:** 1123–1133.
31. Gook DA, Osborn SM, Johnston WI. Cryopreservation of mouse and human oocytes using 1,2-propanediol and the configuration of the meiotic spindle. *Hum Reprod* 1993; **8:** 1101–1109.
32. Ghetler Y, Skutelsky E, Ben Nun I, *et al.* Human oocyte cryopreservation and the fate of cortical granules. *Fertil Steril* 2006; **86:** 210–216.
33. Gualtieri R, Iaccarino M, Mollo V, *et al.* Slow cooling of human oocytes: ultrastructural injuries and apoptotic status. *Fertil Steril* 2009; **91:** 1023–1034.
34. Fuku E, Xia L, Downey BR. Ultrastructural changes in bovine oocytes cryopreserved by vitrification. *Cryobiology* 1995; **32:** 139–156.
35. Hochi S, Kozawa M, Fujimoto T, *et al.* In vitro maturation and transmission electron microscopic observation of horse oocytes after vitrification. *Cryobiology* 1996; **33:** 300–310.
36. Coticchio G, Distratis V, Borini A, *et al.* Reduced ultrastructural damage in human oocytes cryopreserved after dehydration involving single-step propanediol exposure. *Hum Reprod* 2008; **23**(Suppl 1): i150.
37. Nottola SA, Coticchio G, Sciajno R, *et al.* Ultrastructural changes in human metaphase II oocytes cryopreserved by vitrification. *Hum Reprod* 2008; **23**(Suppl 1): i34.
38. Pickering SJ, Braude PR, Johnson MH, Cant A, Currie J. Transient cooling to room temperature can cause irreversible disruption of the meiotic spindle in the human oocyte. *Fertil Steril* 1990; **54:** 102–108.
39. Coticchio G, de Santis L, Rossi G, *et al.* Sucrose concentration influences the rate of human oocytes with normal spindle and chromosome configurations after slow-cooling cryopreservation. *Hum Reprod* 2006; **21:** 1771–1776.
40. Cobo A, Perez S, de los Santos MJ, Zulategui J, Domingo J, Remohi J. Effect of different cryopreservation protocols on the metaphase II spindle in human oocytes. *Reprod Biomed Online* 2008; **17:** 350–359.
41. Wang WH, Meng L, Hackett RJ, Keefe DL. Developmental ability of human oocytes with or without birefringent spindles imaged by Polscope before insemination. *Hum Reprod* 2001; **16:** 1464–1468.
42. Wang WH, Meng L, Hackett RJ, Odenbourg R, Keefe DL. The spindle observation and its relationship with fertilization after intracytoplasmic sperm injection in living human oocytes. *Fertil Steril* 2001; **75:** 348–353.
43. Cooke S, Tyler JP, Driscoll GL. Meiotic spindle location and identification and its effect on embryonic cleavage plane and early development. *Hum Reprod* 2003; **18:** 2397–2405.
44. Moon JH, Hyun CS, Lee SW, *et al.* Visualization of the metaphase II meiotic spindle in living human oocytes using the Polscope enables the prediction of embryonic developmental competence after ICSI. *Hum Reprod* 2003; **18:** 817–820.
45. Rienzi L, Ubaldi F, Martinez F, *et al.* Relationship between meiotic spindle location with regard to the polar body position and oocyte developmental potential after ICSI. *Hum Reprod* 2003; **18:** 1289–1293.
46. de Santis L, Cino I, Rabellotti E, *et al.* Polar body morphology and spindle imaging as predictors of oocyte quality. *Reprod Biomed Online* 2005; **11:** 36–42.

47. Rama Raju GA, Prakash GJ, Krishna KM, Madan K. Meiotic spindle and zona pellucida characteristics as predictors of embryonic development: a preliminary study using Polscope imaging. *Reprod Biomed Online* 2007; **14:** 166–174.
48. Shen Y, Stalf T, Mehnert C, *et al.* Light retardance by human oocyte spindle is positively related to pronuclear score after ICSI. *Reprod Biomed Online* 2006; **12:** 737–751.
49. Madaschi C, de Souza Bonetti TC, de Almeida Ferreira Braga DP, *et al.* Spindle imaging: a marker for embryo development and implantation. *Fertil Steril* 2008; **90:** 194–198.
50. Bianchi V, Coticchio G, Fava L, Flamigni C, Borini A. Meiotic spindle imaging in human oocytes frozen with a slow freezing procedure involving high sucrose concentration. *Hum Reprod* 2005; **20:** 1078–1083.
51. Rienzi L, Martinez F, Ubaldi F, *et al.* Polscope analysis of meiotic spindle changes in living metaphase II human oocytes during the freezing and thawing procedures. *Hum Reprod* 2004; **19:** 655–659.
52. Coticchio G, Sciajno R, Hutt KJ, *et al.* Comparative analysis of the metaphase II spindle of human oocytes through polarized light and high performance confocal microscopy. *Fertil Steril* 2009; epub ahead pf print.
53. Barritt J, Luna M, Duke M, *et al.* Report of four donor-recipient oocyte cryopreservation cycles resulting in high pregnancy and implantation rates. *Fertil Steril* 2007; **87:** e13–17.
54. La Sala GB, Nicoli A, Villani MT, *et al.* Outcome of 518 salvage oocyte-cryopreservation cycles performed as a routine procedure in an in vitro fertilization program. *Fertil Steril* 2006; **86:** 1423–1427.
55. Chen SU, Lien YR, Chen HF, *et al.* Observational clinical follow-up of oocyte cryopreservation using a slow-freezing method with 1,2-propanediol plus sucrose followed by ICSI. *Hum Reprod* 2005; **20:** 1975–1980.
56. Lucena E, Bernal DP, Lucena C, *et al.* Successful ongoing pregnancies after vitrification of oocytes. *Fertil Steril* 2006; **85:** 108–111.
57. Gook DA, Edgar DH. Cryopreservation of the human female gamete: current and future issues. *Hum Reprod* 1999; **14:** 2938–2940.
58. Lassalle B, Testart J, Renard JP. Human embryo features that influence the success of cryopreservation with the use of 1,2-propanediol. *Fertil Steril* 1985; **44:** 645–651.
59. Parmegiani L, Cognigni GE, Bernardi S, *et al.* Freezing within 2 h from oocyte retrieval increases the efficiency of human oocyte cryopreservation when using a slow freezing/rapid thawing protocol with high sucrose concentration. *Hum Reprod* 2008; **23:** 1771–1778.
60. Ducibella T. Biochemical and cellular insights into the temporal window of normal fertilization. *Theriogenology* 1998; **49:** 53–65.
61. Borini A, Cattoli M, Bulletti C, Coticchio G. Clinical efficiency of oocyte and embryo cryopreservation. *Ann New York Acad Sci* 2008; **1127:** 49–58.
62. Porcu E, Fabbri R, Damiano G, *et al.* Clinical experience and applications of oocyte cryopreservation. *Mol Cell Endocrinol* 2000; **169:** 33–37.
63. Borini A, Cattoli M, Mazzone S, *et al.* Survey of 105 babies born after slow-cooling oocyte cryopreservation. *Fertil Steril* 2007; **88:** S13–S14.
64. Tur-Kaspa I, Gal M, Horwitz A. Genetics and health of children born from cryopreserved oocytes. *Fertil Steril* 2007; **87:** S14.
65. Maher B. Little consensus on egg freezing. *Nature* 2007; **449:** 958.

Chapter 16

Vitrification of human oocytes with different tools

Patrick Quinn

Introduction

The primary focus of this chapter will be the effects of using different types of a physical device, the carrier tool, to carry or enclose the cellular sample in the process of vitrification of human oocytes. To broaden this topic, consideration will also be given to other devices used for different stages of human pre-implantation embryo development and the oocytes and embryos of other mammalian species, as these will most likely be applicable to the vitrification of human oocytes. A brief mention will also be made of some of the differences in media, or more precisely solutions, that have been used in this process.

Interest in the topic of vitrification has increased exponentially in academic and applied science fields since the end of the 1990s [1]. There are several excellent reviews of the history of its development, of its current status, and of areas of current potential research, as well as texts on vitrification methodology. Several of these publications are presented in other chapters of this publication (Chapters 14 and 17). Other excellent publications on these topics include those by Kuwayama [2] and Tucker and Liebermann [3].

The traditional definition of vitrification is the solidification of a liquid brought about not by crystallization but by the extreme elevation in viscosity during cooling [4]. A simpler description is that of Vatja *et al.* [5]: "Vitrification is a physical phenomenon describing solidification of water or water-based solutions without ice crystal formation." As a working model, the following equation has been proposed by Yavin & Arav [6], which predicts the probability of successful vitrification based upon three major factors: (1) the viscosity of the sample that can be modulated by cryoprotectant (CPA) concentration; (2) cooling and warming rates; and (3) sample volume:

$$\text{Probability of vitrification} = \frac{\text{Cooling and warming rates} \times \text{Viscosity (CPA concentration)}}{\text{Volume}}$$

Aspects of this equation will be discussed in more detail later in this chapter and were also considered in Chapter 2.

The role of vitrification in an assisted reproductive technology (ART) setting is gradually replacing traditional slow cooling primarily because of its increased efficiency in terms of its success, its increased speed for preservation of oocytes, and the lack of any requirement for purchase and maintenance of a controlled rate programmable freezer. The issue of success is discussed more fully in Chapter 15 and by Homberg *et al.* [7], but it should be noted that some fertility programs have reported exceptionally good clinical results with slow-freezing cryopreservation of human oocytes [8]. There is an advantage in increased speed in terms of the time required to vitrify a sample of oocytes. However, there are time constraints when large numbers (e.g. ≥ 10) of oocytes from a single patient or oocytes from multiple patients need to be processed around the same time. A programmed slow-cooling device can process multiple samples at the same time but, with experience, it is possible to process considerable numbers of oocytes (and embryos) for vitrification using samples processed in parallel [5].

The reasons for cryopreserving oocytes have been enumerated many times previously [9] and are summarized by Chian in Chapter 14. Briefly, the primary reasons are as follows. First, excess oocytes can be cryopreserved directly, rather than as embryos, thus circumventing some legal, ethical, and societal concerns. Second, oocytes can be salvaged when there are no sperm available from a male partner. Third, oocytes can be collected and stored for later use from patients threatened with loss of fertility from cancer therapy, pelvic disease, surgical needs, and so on. Fourth, women can effectively stop their biological clock by cryopreserving oocytes when they are young and using them later in life: collect and store now, use later. Finally,

Fertility Cryopreservation, ed. Ri-Cheng Chian and Patrick Quinn. Published by Cambridge University Press.

cryopreserved oocytes from donors can be used to create egg banks in the same way that donor sperm are processed and cryostored in sperm banks [10].

The first clinical pregnancy and subsequent live birth from cryopreserved human oocytes was reported in the 1980s by Chen [11,12] using a slow-cooling regimen. In fact, the oocytes had been kept submerged in liquid nitrogen (LN_2) for only 3 hours before being thawed, inseminated, and returned to the uterus of the mother in the same cycle in which they had been collected. In the subsequent decade, there were very few further successes with only approximately 15 babies born [13]. Nearly all of the initial attempts used slow cooling, but there were some instances of using ultra-rapid cooling and vitrification.

The first reported live birth from vitrified human oocytes was by Kuleshova *et al.* [15], with other reports relatively soon thereafter. Reports began to appear slowly at first, with several further live births [16, 17], and then was followed since 2003 by increasing numbers. Some of the more impressive publications included the breakout reports of Kuwayama and colleagues [18,19] together with those of Lucena *et al.* [20], Antinori *et al.* [21], Cobo *et al.* [22], and Chian *et al.* [23] (Homburg *et al.* [7] and Kuwayama [2] reference further studies). There does not appear to be any increased risk of adverse obstetric and perinatal outcomes of infants conceived from vitrified oocytes [24]. Despite the considerable progress in the development and application of the vitrification of human oocytes in a clinical setting [2,25], including the establishment of cryopreserved egg banks and the transport of oocytes internationally [10], there are still some obstacles that need to be overcome. One of the main obstacles, in the opinion of the author and others [2,5], including the major proponent on the issue of microbial contamination in mammalian germplasm cryobiology [26], is that safety and regulatory issues regarding closed and open vitrification devices, that is those that do not and those that do allow direct contact of LN_2 with the oocyte, are causing a road block, hopefully temporarily, to the continued and increased use of this technology. More discussion on this topic is included in the section below on safety.

Vitrification of human oocytes with different tools

In this section, the effectiveness and safety of various tools (also referred to as carriers) used in vitrification to hold the oocytes during cooling, storage, and warming will be discussed, followed by a brief mention of the composition of some of the solutions and how they are used. Here we have a conundrum. Do we talk about the solutions first or the tools? In reality, both are interdependent, so it does not really matter in which order they are discussed. The choice here is to describe first some of the tools themselves and then their effectiveness and safety, and then to move on to aspects of some of the solutions used for cooling and warming.

Carrier tools

A range of carrier tools used for vitrification in human ART are listed in Table 16.1 and examples are shown in Figure 16.1. Pictures and diagrams of these tools occur elsewhere in this book and in many other sources (e.g. searching on the Internet for oocyte vitrification pictures). The carrier tools fall primarily into three types, the primary versions of which are the open pulled straw, Cryotop, and Cryoloop. The electron microscopy (EM) grid was the first carrier tool in which small sample volume and direct contact with LN_2 achieved the very high cooling rates required in vitrification. Considerations of convenience and safety led to the replacement of the EM grid by the Cryotop and Cryoloop by the middle of the 2000s. The open pulled straw was first introduced into mammalian oocyte and embryo vitrification in 1998 [29] but, while remaining popular for domestic animal oocyte and embryo vitrification, it has not gained much of a foothold in human ART vitrification applications. One of its derivatives, the Cryotip, was heavily promoted by its commercial producer, especially as it was the first such vitrification tool to obtain FDA 510k clearance in the USA, but apart from a few enthusiasts, its appeal has been limited. The major concern is the long learning curve required to load and handle the tool correctly [33] and to avoid breakage of a loaded carrier during handling and storage [34]. The Cryoloop has some aficionados in human ART and is marketed by a major ART supply company but its market penetration so far is not widespread. The use of both the open pulled straw and Cryoloop has been modified to enable them to be used as closed systems [35,36]. The most popular carrier tool so far is the Cryotop and several of its derivatives, especially the hemi-straw [31], Cryolock [20], and Cryoleaf (Chapter 17).

Other devices that have been involved in vitrification are the Vitmaster [37], which lowers the temperature of LN_2 by a further 10–15°C to approximately 210°C, and a device that uses pre-cooled metal surfaces

Table 16.1. Widely used carrier tools in human assisted reproductive technology[a]

Carrier tool	Derivative	Reference
Electron microscope (EM) grid		Martino *et al.* (1996) [27]
Standard cryopreservation straw		Mukaida *et al.* (1998) [28]
Open pulled straw		Vajta *et al.* (1998) [29]
	Various micropipette style tips	Vajta and Nagy (2006) [25]
	Cryotip	Kuwayama *et al.* (2005) [19]
Cryotop		Kuwayama and Kato (2000) [30]
	Hemi-straw	Vanderzwalmen *et al.* (2000) [31]
	Cryolock	Lucena *et al.* (2006) [20]
	Cryoleaf	Chapter 17
Cryoloop		Lane *et al.* (1999) [32]

[a] Vatja and Nagy (2006) [25] give a more complete list.

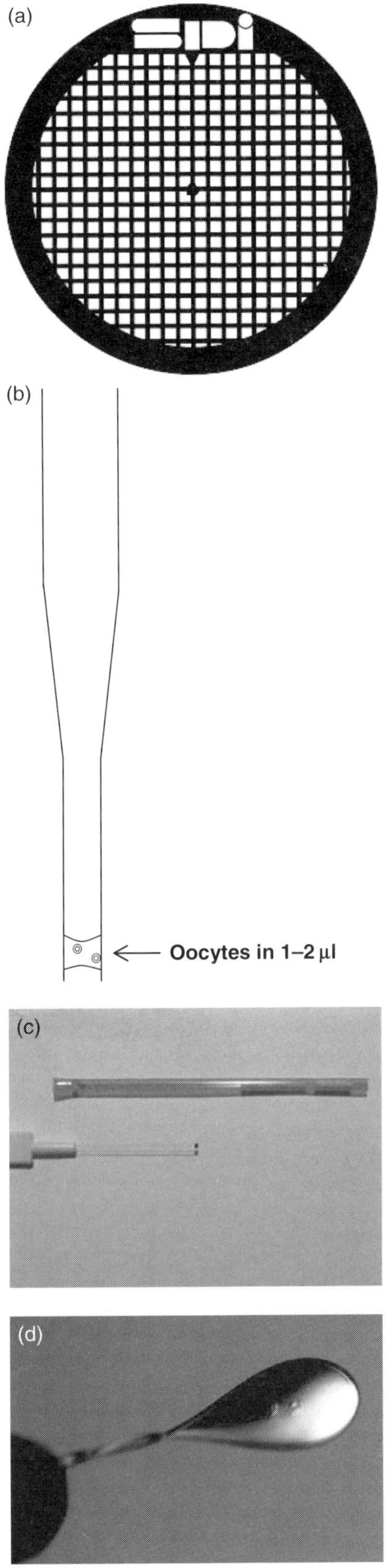

Figure 16.1 Carrier tools for vitrification of mammalian oocytes: (a) electron microscopy grid; (b) open pulled straw; (c) Cryotop; (d) Cryoloop.

in place of LN_2 for cooling; this latter device is now available in a commercial form (CMV; Cryologic, Mulgrave, Australia). For both of these devices, there is very little comparative evidence indicating their superiority over more commonly used vitrification procedures. In an experimental precursor to the LN_2 slush device, there was no significant difference in results whether bovine oocytes were vitrified on EM grids in LN_2 or in LN_2 slush [27]. The inventors of the commercial product (Vitmaster) reported that the rate of cooling of solution in sealed pulled straws obtained with their device when the carrier was placed in LN_2 slush was 32 200°C/min between 25°C and −140°C, below which there is no spontaneous ice nucleation, and only 8100°C/min when the same carrier tool was plunged into LN_2. There were no differences in the in vitro development parameters of mouse blastocysts subjected to these two different cooling rates [38]. This is similar to the observation reported for bovine oocytes [27] and indicates that although the cooling rates obtained with LN_2 slush are suitable for vitrification they are of no greater effectiveness than those obtained when the carrier devices are plunged into LN_2. There is, of course, a considerable cost savings in not requiring the Vitmaster equipment. The other aspect of the technique described by Yavin *et al.*2009 [38] is the rather tedious steps required in their warming procedure,which may also affect success rates compared with the more commonly used combined release of the cellular specimen and warming action obtained by direct plunging of specimens into the first warming solution at 37°C.

Effectiveness

Based on the proposal of Yavin and Arav [6], mentioned above, the volume of the vitrification solution plays a critical role in the probability of achieving satisfactory vitrification in a system. Essentially, if the volume is small enough, the main direct influence is increased cooling and warming rates, all other things being equal. As is mentioned in the Safety section below, direct contact of the sample with LN_2 will achieve very high cooling rates whereas a closed system with an intervening protective barrier to heat transfer will lessen cooling rates. Warming rates are less affected because the sample is usually placed within a protective sheath, secondary larger straw, or vial for storage after or during the vitrification procedure; it is then withdrawn from this protective storage chamber while the chamber is still surrounded by LN_2 and quickly transferred to the first warming solution, which is usually 1 M sucrose at 37°C. The smaller the volume in which the oocyte has been vitrified, the faster the warming rate, but there must be a threshold warming rate, as there must be a threshold for cooling (Figure 16.2) beyond which no further increase in success rates will be achieved. An added benefit to higher rates of both cooling and probably warming is that it is also possible to use lower CPA concentrations,

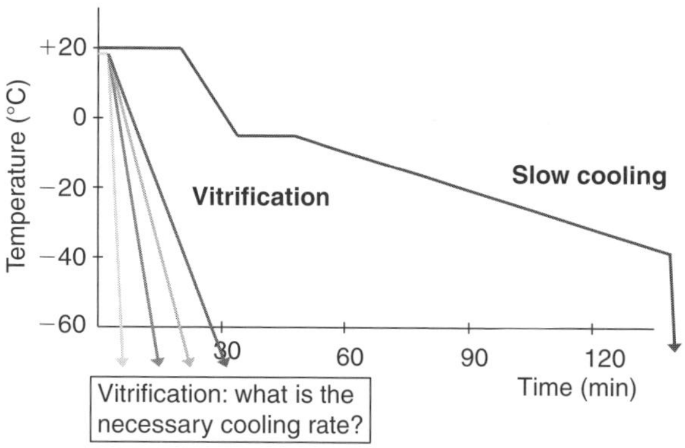

Figure 16.2. Cooling rate for vitrification. The lines for vitrification show variation in possible cooling rate.

thus reducing the detrimental effect of the inherent toxicity of CPAs and increasing the overall success of the procedure. A summary of selected results of human oocyte vitrification over the past decade is given in Table 16.2 and Figure 16.3. In 12 publications covering 1999 to 2009, 355 cases were reported by the authors listed in Figure 16.3, with over half of these cases being performed with the Cryotop, a quarter used the Cryoleaf, and the remaining studies used the Cryolock, the EM grid, or the open pulled straw. All of the carrier tools listed in Table 16.1 can be used with a volume of vitrification solution of 0.5 μl or less, which gives more than adequate rates of cooling and warming, as attested by the very good success rates noted in Figure 16.3. The highest survival rates for vitrified oocytes after warming were with the Cryotop, followed closely by the Cryoleaf; the lower rates were seen with the remaining tools. The EM grid and open pulled straw have not been widely used to vitrify human oocytes so it is not surprising that the success rates with these devices do not compare all that well with the more popular Cryotop and Cryoleaf. However, there have been no randomized, controlled trials comparing the different tools and they all seem to produce satisfactory results when used properly. As with most products in the ART field, choice will be governed primarily by effectiveness, ease of use, customer (both technical and patient customers) satisfaction, and price. It should also be kept in mind that other tools such as the hemi-straw and Cryoloop have been used very successfully to vitrify human embryos, and there is no reason why these tools would not be just as effective if used for human oocytes. Effectiveness of the tools listed in Table 16.1 in terms of pregnancy parameters show that all of them gave overall similar success. Regression analysis also showed that there were no significant changes in the four parameters, three of which are pregnancy outcome parameters, displayed in Figure 16.3. This may indicate that the use of these carrier tools may indeed have been optimized when they were first used and that they continue to perform very well. It should be noted that the live birth and ongoing pregnancy rates for oocyte vitrification listed in Figure 16.3 are actually significantly better than the 2007 US national live birth rates reported by the Society for Assisted Reproductive Technology [43] for autologous fresh and frozen rates and for donor oocyte frozen rates. I believe this is more than adequate evidence that the effectiveness of the currently used carrier tools is satisfactory. As has been pointed out (B. Behr, personal communication), the results with vitrified human oocytes compared with

Table 16.2. Survey of vitrified human oocyte success rates

Study	Carrier tool	No. cases	Survival (%)	Embryos/ET	No. ET	ET/cases (%)	No. pregnancies	Pregnancies/ET (%)	CPR (%)	IR (%)	Live births	No. ongoing	Live birth + ongoing/ET (%)	Comments
Kuleshova *et al.* (1999) [15]	OPS	4	65	1.0	3	75	1	33	33	33	1	NAP	33	Embryo biopsied
Yoon *et al.* (2000) [16]	EM grid	7	63	4.6	7	100	3	43	43	9	2	1	43	
Katayama *et al.* (2003) [17]	Cryotop	6	94	NA	6	100	2	33	33	NA	1	1	33	
Yoon *et al.* (2003) [39]	EM grid	34	69	4.5	28	82	6	21	21	6	6	NAP	21	Probably includes cases from [16]
Kim *et al.* (2005) [40]	EM grid	13	71	3.8	12	92	7	58	58	24	2	3	42	
Oktay *et al.* (2006) [41] (update of data from Chian)	Cryoleaf	25	94	3.6	25	100	11	44	44	20	9	9	36	
Kuwayama *et al.* (2005) [18]	Cryotop	29	91	2.2	29	100	12	41	34	NA	7	3	34	
Selman *et al.* (2006) [42]	OPS	6	34	2.3	6	100	2	33	33	21	NA	2	NA	
Lucena *et al.* (2006) [20]	Cryotop (now Cryolock)	23	75	4.6	23	100	13	57	NA	NA	NA	NA	NA	
Antinori *et al.* (2007) [21]	Cryotop	120	99	2.5	120	100	39	33	33	13	3	28	26	
Cobo *et al.* (2008) [22]	Cryotop	30	97	2.1	23	77	15	65	52	41	NA	11	48	
Chian *et al.* (2009) [23]	Cryoleaf	58	78	3.4	58	100	23	40	36	15	19	NAP	33	38 IVF 20 IVM

Table 16.2 *(cont.)*

Study	Carrier tool	No. cases	Survival (%)	Embryos/ ET	No. ET	ET/ cases (%)	No. pregna- ncies	Pregna- ncies/ET (%)	CPR (%)	IR (%)	Live births	No. ongoing	Live birth + ongoing/ ET (%)	Comments
Total from studies		355			340		134				50	58		
Mean from studies		30	87	3.1	28	96	11	42	38	20	6	7	40	
Society for Assisted Reproductive Technology (2007) [43]														
Autologous, fresh		93 792		2.5	83 020			40		24			33	$p < 0.0001$
Autologous, frozen	NAP			2.2	19 329								30	$p < 0.0001$
Donor, fresh				2.2	9 575								55	$p < 0.0001$
Donor, frozen				2.3	5 087								32	$p < 0.003$

ET, embryo transfer; CPR, clinical pregnancy rate; IR, inplantation rate; OPS, open pulled straw; EM, electron microscopy; IVF, in vitro Fertilization; IVM, in vitro maturation; NAP, not applicable; NA, not available.

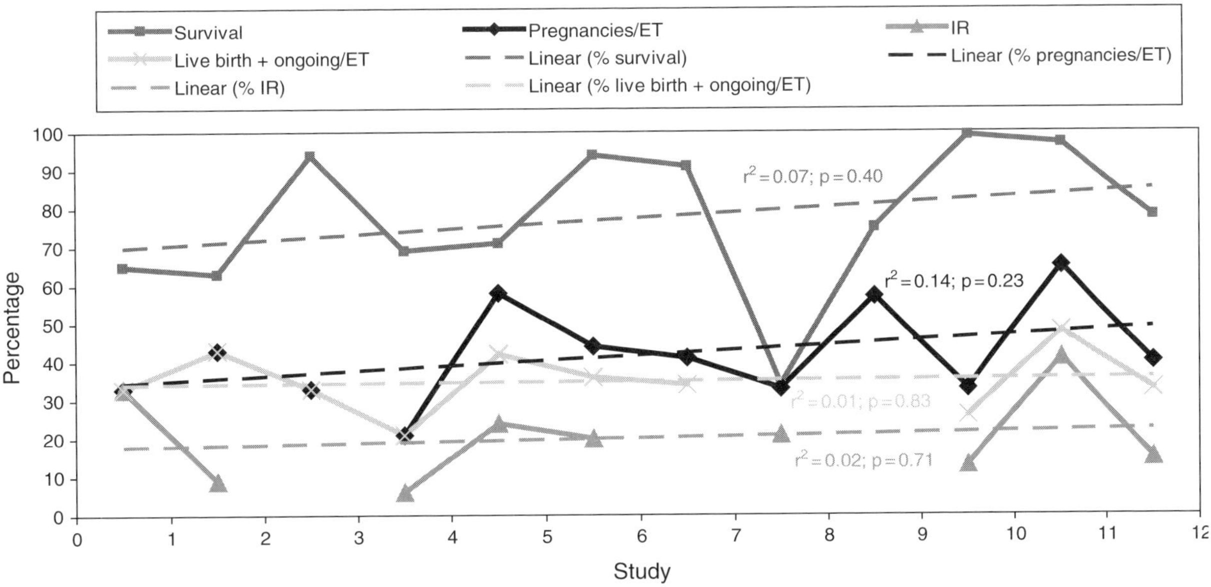

Figure 16.3. Success rates of human oocyte vitrification since 1999.: 1, Kuleshova *et al.* (1999) [15]; 2, Yon *et al.* (2000) [16]; 3, Katayama *et al.* (2003) [17]; 4, Yoon *et al.* (2003) [39]; 5, Kim *et al.* (2005) [40]; 6, Chian updated by Oktay *et al.* (2006) [41]; 7, Kuwayama *et al.* (2005) [18]; 8, Selman *et al.* (2006) [42]; 9, Lucena *et al.* (2006) [20]; 10, Antinori *et al.* (2007) [21]; 11, Cobo *et al.* (2008) [22]; 12, Chian *et al.* (2009) [23]. ET, embryo transfer.

fresh autologous transfers have to be viewed with some caution as several of the trials with vitrified oocytes have been conducted with donor oocytes [22] and, quite often, large numbers of oocytes were warmed for a single procedure [23]. Obviously, this leads to some bias toward the vitrification results obtained so far and we must await a prospective, randomized trial before we can reliably compare the results of oocyte vitrification with those with fresh or frozen autologous oocytes. The observation in Table 16.2 that the pregnancy results with frozen donor oocytes in the Society for Assisted Reproductive Technology data from 2007 (55% live birth per transfer) are significantly higher than those with vitrified oocytes (40% live birth plus ongoing pregnancies per transfer) attest to the need for caution in the interpretation of the results in this table.

Cooling and warming rates

As is mentioned in various sections of this chapter and in other parts of this book, cooling and warming rates play a critical role in the success of vitrification in ART and, in particular, with human oocytes, which appear to be more sensitive to cryopreservation than preimplantation embryonic stages. Because of the widespread discussion of this topic, suffice it to say that the current cooling and warming rates used appear to be adequate and are summarized in Table 16.3. As has been mentioned before and is illustrated in Figure 16.2 (cooling rates), there must be threshold rates of cooling and warming beyond which there are no direct added improvements if no other parameters are changed. The rate of cooling for vitrification appears relatively unimportant as long as it is sufficiently rapid to prevent ice crystallization. It may be possible to further lower CPA concentrations, however, if the cooling rates are fast enough. Another approach is to utilize a lower rate of cooling and/or larger volumes of vitrification solution in a more robust closed carrier tool protocol by making sure the oocyte is pre-loaded with adequate concentrations of CPA before initiating cooling. This can be done by leaving the oocyte or embryo in lower concentrations of the equilibration solution for an adequate time and then passing the cells through increasing concentrations of equilibration solution before transferring them to the vitrification solution for loading on or into the carrier tool and plunging them into LN_2. Adequate success rates using such a protocol have been recently reported [48] and it is most likely to be applied to human oocytes in the near future.

As has been mentioned earlier in this chapter, protocols for warming appear to be almost optimized by removing the carrier tool from storage in LN_2 and transferring it directly to the first warming solution as quickly as possible. As discussed further below in the section on vitrification solutions, it is important to use an adequate volume of this first warming solution and

Table 16.3. Cooling and warming rates with various carrier tools

Tool	Volume of solution (μL)	Cooling rate (°C/min)	Warming rate (°C/min)
0.25 ml straw	100–200	<100[a] – 1540[b]	2000–2500
0.25 ml straw[c]	25	4460	1300
OPS[c]	0.5	16 340–17 700	13 000–13 900
Cryotop[c]	< 0.1	22 800–23 000	18 000–42 100
Hemi-straw[b]	0.5	1 600	3,000 (carrier not removed from protective outer straw
Cut Standard Straw[d]	0.5	600	30 000–90 000
EM grid[e]	NA	9 000	NA
Cryoloop[b]	NA	~15 000	> 48 000

NA, not available.
From: [a] Stachecki & Cohen (2008) [44]; [b] Camus *et al.* (2006) [45]; [c] Kuwayama *et al.* [18]; [d] Isachenko *et al.* (2007) [46]; [e] Shaw & Jones (2003) [47].

to have at a temperature of at least 37°C to optimize the warming rate for best results. Avoiding devitrification and the formation of ice crystals during warming is critical (see Chapter 2). Some researchers have even transferred vitrified specimens to a water bath at 100°C to optimize warming rates [49]. Obviously, this strategy would require precise timing, and perhaps a lower temperature, between 37°C and 100°C, may give more leeway for variation in timing and a more robust system to be used in a clinical setting.

Safety

A thorough review of safety has recently been written by two of the main proponents of cryosafety and vitrification [26]. Cryostorage is the only situation in ART where numerous samples from multiple patients are pooled together in a common liquid environment. If incorrectly sealed, transmission of infective agents between samples is possible, as is infection from environmental microorganisms that might find their way into the storage vessel by various routes. Bielanski and Vajta [26] admit that transfection between samples of sperm/semen or embryos in humans and domestic animals cannot be absolutely attributed to the cryopreservation procedure or cryostorage, but as the possibility of such transfection can be shown experimentally, this justifies taking measures to negate such disease transmission via cryopreserved germplasm. Yavin *et al.* [38] erroneously stated that the reported contamination of cryo-stored blood products by hepatitis B virus [50] involved contamination of straws, whereas the actual storage devices were blood bags, which were prone to leakage.

Disease transmission risk related to cryopreservation can be viewed from the following perspectives [25].

1. The collection, processing, and cryopreservation of gametes and embryos are not wholly sterile procedures.
2. The LN_2 can also be contaminated by contact with the surfaces of straws, racks, and other tools not handled in an aseptic manner.
3. Containers such as some vials and straws are prone to leakage.
4. It is difficult to decontaminate LN_2 storage tanks.

The potential risk of disease transmission via LN_2 in an ART setting exists, but there are no documented cases of this happening. As pointed out by Vajta and Nagy [25], the female reproductive tract may be capable of eliminating infectious agents in the quantity that might be transferred during embryo transfer or insemination.

Because many ART procedures breach the zona pellucida (e.g. biopsy, intracytoplasmic sperm injection [ICSI], assisted hatching, and cryopreservation of hatching/hatched blastocysts), the cells of such embryos are more susceptible to contamination than embryos with an intact zona pellucida. Consequently, it is imperative to screen providers (that means all patients, donors, or otherwise) of germplasm for blood-borne diseases prior to cryopreservation and storage of their gametes or embryos in LN_2. Efficient, multiple washing of oocytes and embryos prior to and after cryopreservation will most likely, as has been shown in many animal models, decrease the risk of cross contamination between samples in a cryo-storage tank. Patient and donor samples should be stored in separate LN_2 tanks until the providers and/or their samples have been tested for the presence of infectious agents. It is also necessary to store germplasm from a patient with infectious microorganisms separately from samples known not to be contaminated. The necessity for sterile LN_2 is questioned because it is very unlikely that commercially produced LN_2 would contain viral agents of concern such as the human immunodeficiency, hepatitis, and herpes viruses, which are not air borne, but there have been no published reports on this topic [26]. Although possible, it is somewhat difficult and expensive to obtain a commercial supply of sterile LN_2 or to produce it effectively in an ART laboratory. It has been reported [26] that no viral agents were isolated from LN_2 and ice sediments in storage tanks with long-term cryostorage for over 35 years, and that most of the bacteria and fungi found were ubiquitous, environmental species. Therefore, long-term cryostorage of gametes and embryos should be fundamentally safe as long as the specimen containers, including the carrier devices used in vitrification, were properly sealed upon storage. Similarly, consideration has been given to approaches using open, direct contact between the specimen carrier tool and LN_2 during the cooling phase of vitrification, but the use of sealed containers for storage [2,25]. Support for this approach comes from the report [26] that current closed systems such as the CryoTop, CBS HSV kits, and the solid surface vitrification device Cryohook (Cryologic) have not been as effective in successfully vitrifying human oocytes as their open system counterparts. One can assume, therefore, that after vitrification in an open system, the specimen should be cryo-stored in a closed, sealed container, preferably with hermetic seals. Although storage of gametes and embryos in the vapor phase of LN_2 is possible, there are problems with long-term storage and handling of specimens in this manner and this has prevented this process from becoming popular in many ART laboratories [26]. Bielanski [51] has shown that dry shippers that use LN_2 vapor are effective for transportation of germplasm, with no evidence of infection with bacterial or viral agents in previously contaminated shippers. In contrast, bacteria and fungi have been detected in the vapor phase of long-term cryostorage tanks and this is probably the result of aerolization of these microbes by boiling LN_2 when samples are transferred to the tank or when it is refilled with LN_2.

Table 16.4. Permeating cryoprotectants used in mammalian gamete and embryo cryopreservation

Parameter	Ethylene glycol	Dimethyl sulfoxide	Propane-diol	Glycerol
Abbreviation	EG	DMSO	PROH	Gly
Molecular weight	62.07	78.13	76.09	92.09
Density at 25°C (g/ml)	1.113	1.10	1.036	1.25
Molality of a 10% (v/v) solution	1.79	1.41	1.36	1.36
Percentage (v/v) of a 1 M solution	5.6	7.1	7.4	7.4

Vitrification solutions

The four major permeating CPAs used in cryopreservation are listed in Table 16.4. The role of media in the effectiveness of vitrification has been less well studied than the effects of cooling rate. For example, no specific permeating CPA or mixture of CPAs has been significantly superior in assessments of success rates. Mixtures of dimethyl sulfoxide plus ethylene glycol and ethylene glycol plus propanediol, and ethylene glycol by itself, all in combination with sucrose, have all provided acceptable survival, fertilization, cleavage rates, and subsequent pregnancy and implantation rates. In addition, the inclusion of components such as Ficoll or polyvinylpyrrolidone may enhance the effectiveness of the permeating CPAs; the reason(s) for this is (are) unknown. The physiological solutions to which the CPAs are added have ranged from phosphate-buffered saline (PBS) to HEPES-buffered human tubal fluid to MOPS-buffered media with, again, no one solution showing superiority over any others. A potential problem that arises when using PBS-based vitrification solutions is that the pH of such solutions becomes acidic during cooling, whereas that of organic-based buffered solutions (e.g. HEPES or MOPS) does not [27]. This can easily be seen by placing 0.25 ml straws filled with either PBS or HEPES-buffered human tubal fluid, both of which contain phenol red, in LN_2. The PBS straw will be yellow, indicating a shift to acidic pH, whereas the HEPES straw will remain rose-pink, in the pH range 7.2–7.4. In a study with slow-freezing cryopreservation of mouse oocytes and their subsequent thawing, fertilization, and development to blastocysts in vitro, the HEPES-buffered medium used for cryopreservation gave significantly better results compared with PBS-buffered medium, but the differences were not as dramatic as expected [52]. This reinforces the need for prospective, randomized trials to see if the buffer system used in vitrification solutions has any impact on outcomes. In 2004 [53], a brief report showed higher success rates with MOPS-buffered solutions than with HEPES-buffered medium for the vitrification of day-3 human embryos, and two commercial producers use MOPS-buffered vitrification solutions. It is becoming evident that a physiological salt solution buffered by either HEPES or MOPS and containing the complete range of amino acids at physiological concentrations may be the best approach to maintain oocyte and embryo homeostasis during the stressful cryopreservation process, whether it be vitrification or slow freezing. In fact, a mixture of MOPS, HEPES, and another zwitterionic buffer, DIPSO (3-[*N*-bis(hydroxyethyl)-amino]-2-hydroxypropane sulfonic acid), may prove superior to any one of the buffering systems alone [54]. Another component of CPA solutions is the type of non-permeating CPA that is used in both the CPA solution and in the dilution solutions upon thawing. Traditionally, sucrose has been used in cryopreservation solutions at concentrations around 0.5 M. In the dilution solutions, again, sucrose has been the saccharide of choice. However, other sugars such as galactose have been just as effective and overcome mixing problems associated with the high densities of solutions containing sucrose [55].

Stepwise addition of CPAs during the equilibration phase of the cooling process is now a standard procedure in vitrification [25]. This first solution, usually called the equilibration solution, contains between 25 and 50% (usually 50%) of the final permeating CPA concentration and can be added in increasing concentrations, for example 25% and then 50% of the final permeating CPA concentration [48]. A number of different methods can be used to pass an oocyte through increasing concentrations of CPA prior to cooling, or through lower concentrations of sucrose after warming. To the best of my knowledge, there are no comparative trials that show that any one procedure is superior, so it is mainly dependent on the choice of embryologists as to which procedure they feel the most comfortable with in terms of ease of use and success rates. Quantal changes in concentrations of the cooling and warming solutes can be achieved by physically transferring an oocyte from one definitive solution to another with minimal carry over of one solution to the next. It is now thought that a more gradual mixing of the different solutions is a better technique. This can be achieved by adding increasing volumes of the second solution to the first solution over time, as is recommended by Kitazato for exposing oocytes to increased concentrations of the CPAs in equilibration solution, or by transferring some of the first solution along with the oocyte into the second solution, for example when diluting oocytes through decreasing concentrations of sucrose upon warming [56].

A variation of the above procedure is to place the oocytes into smaller volume drops, typically 20 μl, and then to merge the drops, again in increasing or decreasing concentrations depending on whether it is the cooling or warming stages [2, 57]. I am among others [56] who are not great supporters of drop merging during warming, because upon immediate transfer of the oocyte from the carrier in LN_2 to the first warming solution, usually 1 M sucrose, a large volume (1 to 4 ml) of the warming solution is recommended to optimize warming rates and also to give an increased rate of diffusion of CPAs out of the cell down the greater concentration gradient created by the larger volume of the first warming solution. Smaller volumes of subsequent dilutions of sucrose and the washing solutions can be used as the concentration gradient will then be less because of exodus of the CPAs from within the cell; typical volumes for these subsequent solutions range from 0.3 to 1 ml (Figure 16.4) [1,58]. Another cause for concern when using small volume drops of solutions, especially at a higher temperature and with no oil overlay, is excessive evaporation if the drops are left for too long under these conditions.

One aspect of reporting solution and media composition in the scientific literature is the increasing entanglement of open, scientific disclosure versus guarded or no disclosure based on proprietary information or "for commercial reasons." I have commented on this previously [59]. Suffice it to say that the response from Dr. James Stachecki [60] regarding his reticence to reveal the full formulation of his cryopreservation solutions still does not meet the requirement for full scientific disclosure, in my opinion. One other aspect of describing ingredient concentrations in solutions is the use of percentages. One of the most common examples of this is when the concentration of protein is described as, for example, 20% [60]. Traditionally, 20% means 20 g/100 ml or 200 mg/ml [61]. So, does an author mean this, or rather that they added two

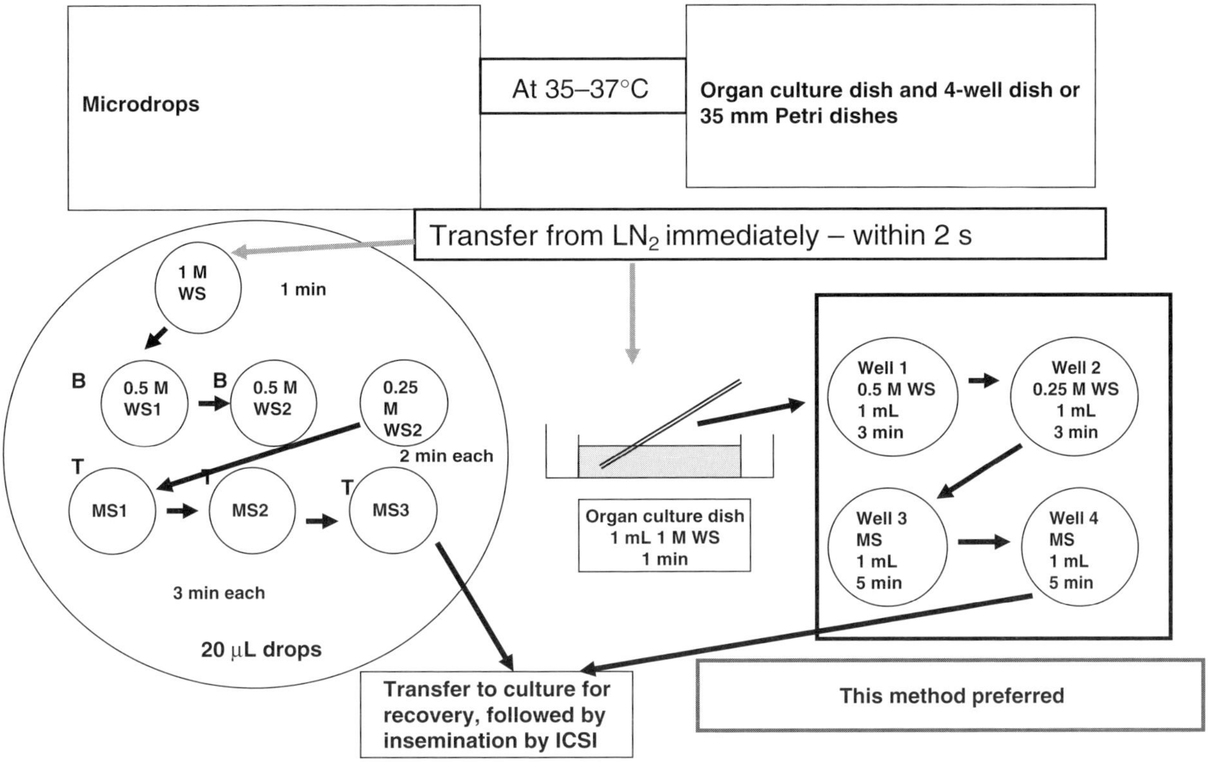

Figure 16.4. Warming and dilution procedure using Sage IVF Vitrification Warming Kit. WS, sucrose warming solution; MS, MOPS solution; T, top of drop; B, bottom of drop; black arrow indicates transfer of oocyte.

volumes of a stock solution containing 100 mg/ml of protein, a common concentration in stock solutions of human serum albumin used in ART, to eight volumes of a medium solution? In the latter, the final protein concentration would be 20 mg/ml, a 10-fold lesser concentration than the example above and likely to have a profound effect on the performance of the product. To solve this problem, concentrations of ingredients should always be expressed as SI units [62].

In summary, now that the physical requirements for vitrification appear close to optimization, with the minimal volume cooling approach, the opportunity is available to conduct meaningful comparisons of the composition of the CPA solutions being used in cryopreservation and dilution after thawing. The manner in which oocytes and embryos are passed through solutions (i.e. by quantal transfer from one solution to another by pipetting or by fusion of two or more drops with different concentrations of solutes) should also be amenable to more rigorous investigation. Ethylene glycol is a standard part of all present vitrification protocols. Combinations of CPAs have been tested, and finally a mix of ethylene glycol and dimethyl sulfoxide seems to be the most popular choice; the permeability of the mixture seems to be higher than the individual parts [25]. Among the non-permeable CPAs, sucrose has become the most used component, with some preference for trehalose. Other strategies such as replacing penetrating CPAs with polymers, use of antifreeze proteins, and intracellular injection of trehalose or its use as an extracellular dehydrating agent have not become routine.

Conclusions

It is evident from the work summarized in this chapter and in other parts of this book that vitrification of human oocytes and embryos is here to stay. My déjà vu experience is that this technology has now reached a similar jumping off point to that for ICSI in the early 1990s. In other words, oocytes and embryos cryopreserved by vitrification will provide a broad vista for application in many areas of ART as we know it now and perhaps in other areas that are only just emerging, such as vitrification of other important cells, tissue, and organs. Two areas pertaining to the application of human oocyte vitrification seem particularly set to become a "must have" technology in society. These are cryostorage of oocytes by younger women who will use them later in life when they feel the time has come to start their family. The second application that is partially linked to this is the creation of cryopreserved oocyte banks. Obviously there has and will be much societal and regulatory discussion of these applications of vitrification technology, but, as others have discussed [7], it is this author's opinion that women and couples seeking effective use of modern ART will embrace this philosophy.

References

1. Fahy GM, Rall WF. Vitrification: an overview. In Tucker MJ, Liebermann J, eds. *Vitrification in Assisted Reproduction. A User's Manual and Trouble-Shooting Guide*. London: Informa Healthcare, 2007, pp. 1–20.
2. Kuwayama M. The human oocyte: vitrification. In Gardner DK, Weissman A, Howles CM, Shoham Z, eds. *Textbook of Asssisted Reproductive Technologies. Laboratory and Clinical Perspectives,* 3rd edn. London: Informa Healthcare, 2009, pp. 267–273.
3. Tucker MJ, Liebermann J (eds.). *Vitrification in Assisted Reproduction. A User's Manual and Trouble-Shooting Guide*. London: Informa Healthcare, 2007.
4. Fahy GM, MacFarlane DR, Angell CA, *et al.* Vitrification as an approach to cryopreservation. *Cryobiology* 1984; **21:** 407–426.
5. Vajta G, Nagy ZP, Cobo A, *et al.* Vitrification in ART: myths, mistakes, disbeliefs and confusion. *Reprod Biomed Online* 2009; in press.
6. Yavin S, Arav A. Measurement of essential physical properties of vitrification solutions. *Theriogenology* 2007; **67:** 81–89.
7. Homburg R, van der Veen F, Silber SJ. Oocyte vitrification: women's emancipation set in stone. *Fertil Steril* 2009; **91:** 1319–1320.
8. Diaz DG, La A-TH, Rodriguez K, *et al.* Human oocyte cryopreservation: outcome from 70 frozen oocyte cycles using a new modified slow-freeze protocol. *Fertil Steril* 2008; **90**: S287.
9. Quinn P. Cryopreservation. In Marrs RP, ed. *Assisted Reproductive Technologies*. Oxford: Blackwell Scientific, 1993, pp. 89–107.
10. The World Egg Bank. 2009. http://www.theworldeggbank.com/tweb2/Home/Default.aspx (accessed July 23, 2009).
11. Chen C. Pregnancy after human oocyte cryopreservation. *Lancet* 1986; **19:** 884–886.
12. Chen C. Pregnancies after human oocyte cryopreservation. *Ann N Y Acad Sci* 1988; **541:** 541–549.
13. Kuleshova LL, Lopata A. Vitrification can be more favorable than slow cooling. *Fertil Steril* 2002; **78:** 449–454.
14. Quinn P. Cryopreservation of embryos and oocytes. In Keye WR, Chang RJ, Rebar RW, Soules MR, eds. *Infertility. Evaluation and Treatment*. Philadelphia, PA: Saunders, 1995, pp. 821–840.
15. Kuleshova L, Gianaroli L, Magli C, *et al.* Birth following vitrification of a small number of human oocytes. *Hum Reprod* 1999; **14:** 3077–3079.
16. Yon TK, Chung HM, Lim JM, *et al.* Pregnancy and delivery of healthy infants developed from vitrified oocytes in a stimulated in vitro fertilization–embryo transfer program. *Fertil Steril* 2000; **74:** 180–181.
17. Katayama KP, Stehlik J, Kuwayama M, *et al.* High survival rate of vitrified human oocytes results in clinical pregnancy. *Fertil Steril* 2003; **80:** 223–224.
18. Kuwayama M, Vajta G, Kato O, *et al.* Highly efficient vitrification method for cryopreservation of human oocytes. *Reprod Biomed Online* 2005; **11:** 300–308.
19. Kuwayama M, Vajta G, Ieda S, *et al.* Comparison of open and closed methods for vitrification of human embryos and the elimination of potential contamination. *Reprod Biomed Online* 2005; **11:** 608–614.
20. Lucena E, Bernal DP, Lucena C, *et al.* Successful ongoing pregnancies after vitrification of oocytes. *Fertil Steril* 2006; **85:** 108–111.
21. Antinori M, Licata E, Dani G, *et al.* Cryotop vitrification of human oocytes results in high survival rate and healthy deliveries. *Reprod Biomed Online* 2007; **14:** 72–79.
22. Cobo A, Kuwayama M, Perez S, *et al.* Comparison of concomitant outcome achieved with fresh and cryopreserved donor oocytes vitrified by the Cryotop method. *Fertil Steril* 2008; **89:** 1657–1664.
23. Chian R-C, Huang JHJ, Gilbert L, *et al.* Obstetric outcomes following vitrification of in vitro and in vivo matured oocytes. *Fertil Steril* 2009; **91:** 2391–2398.
24. Chian R-C, Huang JYJ, Tan SL, *et al.* Obstetric and perinatal outcome in 200 infants conceived from vitrified oocytes. *Reprod Biomed Online* 2008; **16:** 608–610.
25. Vajta G, Nagy ZP. Are programmable freezers still needed in the embryo laboratory? Review on vitrification. *Reprod Biomed Online* 2006; **12:** 779–796.
26. Bielanski A, Vajta G. Risk of contamination of germplasm during cryopreservation and cryobanking in IVF units. *Hum Reprod* 2009; 24 : 2457–2467.
27. Martino A, Songsasen N, Leibo SP. Development into blastocysts of bovine oocytes cryopreserved by ultra-rapid cooling. *Biol Reprod* 1996; **54:** 1059–1069.
28. Mukaida T, Wada S, Takahashi K, *et al.* Vitrification of human embryos based on the assessment of suitable conditions for 8-cell mouse embryos. *Hum Reprod* 1998; **13:** 2874–2879.
29. Vajta G, Lewis IM, Kuwayama M, *et al.* Sterile application of the open pulled straw (OPS) vitrification method. *Cryo Letters* 1998; **19:** 389–392.
30. Kuwayama M, Kato O. All-round vitrification method for human oocytes and embryos. *J Assist Reprod Genet* 2000; **17:** 477.
31. Vanderzwalmen P, Bertin G, Debauche CH, *et al.* 'In vitro' survival of metaphase II oocytes (MII) and

blastocysts after vitrification in an Hemi Straw (HS) system. *Fertil Steril* 2000; **74**: S215–S216.

32. Lane M, Schoolcraft WB, Gardner DK. Vitrification of mouse and human blastocysts using a novel cryoloop container-less technique. *Fertil Steril* 1999; **72:** 1073–1078.
33. Boldt J. CryoTip discussion. *EmbryoMail List*. 2009. http://embryomail.net/mhonarchive/em/msg00341.html (accessed 21 May, 2009).
34. Athayde K. CryoTip breakage. *EmbryoMail List*. 2009. http://embryomail.net/mhonarchive/em/msg00329.html (accessed July 23, 2009).
35. Bielanski A, Hanniman A. Non-cross-contamination of bovine embryos with microbes using the OPS vitrification system. *Reprod Fertil Dev* 2007; **19:** 232.
36. Larman MG, Sheehan CB, Gardner DK. Vitrification of mouse pronuclear oocytes with no direct liquid nitrogen contact. *Reprod BioMed Online* 2006; **12:** 66–69.
37. Arav A, Zeron Y, Ocheretny A. A new device and method for vitrification increases the cooling rate and allows successful cryopreservation of bovine oocytes. *Theriogenology* 2000; **53:** 248.
38. Yavin S, Aroyo A, Roth Z, *et al.* Embryo cryopreservation in the presence of low concentration of vitrification solution with sealed pulled straws in liquid nitrogen slush. *Hum Reprod* 2009; **24**: 797–804.
39. Yoon TK, Kim TJ, Park SE, *et al.* Live births after vitrification of oocytes in a stimulated in vitro fertilization–embryo transfer program. *Fertil Steril* 2003; **79:** 1323–1326.
40. Kim T, Hong S, Cha K. Pregnancies from cryopreserved oocytes using vitrification protocol. *Fertil Steril* 2005; **84**: S179.
41. Oktay K, Cil AP, Bang H. Efficiency of oocyte cryopreservation: a meta-analysis. *Fertil Steril* 2006; **86:** 70–80.
42. Selman H, Angelini A, Barnocchi N, *et al.* Ongoing pregnancies after vitrification of human oocytes using a combined solution of ethylene glycol and dimethyl sulfoxide. *Fertil Steril* 2006; **86:** 997–1000.
43. Society for Assisted Reproductive Technology. *SART Clinical Summary Report 2007*. Birmingham, AL: Society for Assisted Reproductive Technology, https://www.sartcorsonline.com/rptCSR_PublicMultYear.aspx?ClinicPKID=0 (accessed August 2, 2009).
44. Stachecki JJ, Cohen J. S³ vitrification system: a novel approach to blastocyst freezing. *J Clin Embryol* 2008; **11:** 5–14.
45. Camus A, Clairaz P, Ersham A, *et al.* Comparison of the process of five different vitrification devices. *Gynecol Obstet Fertil* 2006; **34:** 737–745.
46. Isachenko V, Katkov II, Yakavenko S, *et al.* Vitrification of human laser treated blastocysts within cut standard straws (CSS): novel aseptic packaging and reduced concentrations of cryoprotectants. *Cryobiology* 2007; **54:** 305–309.
47. Shaw JM, Jones GM. Terminology associated with vitrification and other cryopreservation procedures for oocytes and embryos. *Hum Reprod Update* 2003; **9:** 583–605.
48. Vanderzwalmen P, Ectors F, Grobet L, *et al.* Aseptic vitrification of blastocysts originating from infertile patients, egg donors and after IVM. *Reprod Biomed Online* 2009; **19**: 700–707.
49. Isachenko V, Isachenko E, Reinsberg J, *et al.* Cryopreservation of human ovarian tissue: effect of spontaneous and initiated ice formation. *Reprod Biomed Online* 2008; **16:** 336–345.
50. Tedder RS, Zuckerman MA, Goldstone AH, *et al.* Hepatitis B transmission from contaminated cryopreservation tank. *Lancet* 1995; **346:** 137–140.
51. Bielanski A. Non-transmission of bacterial and viral microbes to embryos and semen stored in the vapor phase of liquid nitrogen in dry shippers. *Cryobiology* 2005; **50:** 206–210.
52. Quinn P. Cryopreservation of mouse oocytes using sodium-depleted media: comparison of HEPES-HTF and PBS-based formulations. *Fertil Steril* 2005; **83:** S24–S25.
53. El-Danasouri I, Selman H, Strehler E, *et al.* Comparison of MOPS and HEPES buffers during vitrification. *Hum Reprod* 2004; **19**: i136.
54. Swain JE, Pool TB. New pH-buffering system for media utilized during gamete and embryo manipulations for assisted reproduction. *Reprod Biomed Online* 2009; **18:** 799–810.
55. McWilliams RB, Gibbons WE, Leibo SP. Osmotic and physiological responses of mouse zygotes and human oocytes to mono- and disaccharides. *Hum Reprod* 2005; **10:** 1163–1171.
56. Kitazato. *Kitazato Cryotop Safety Kit Protocol*. 2009; http://www.kitazato-biopharma.com/images/cryotop/Cryotop_En.pdf (accessed July 21, 2009).
57. Irvine. *Scientific Vit Kit Thaw package insert*. 2009. http://www.irvinesci.com/techinfo/docs/40793-Booklet-Rev5.pdf (accessed July 21, 2009).
58. Sage IVF. *Directions for Use for Vitrification Warming Kit*. 2009. http://www.coopersurgical.com/Documents/ART-8030%20DFU.pdf (accessed July 22, 2009).
59. Quinn P. The impact of culture media on success rate in ART: where have we gone in the last decade? In Gurgan T, Demirol A, eds. *Proceedings of the 13th World Congress: In Vitro Fertilization, Assisted Reproduction and Genetics*, Istanbul, Turkey, 2005, pp. 221–225.
60. Stachecki J. Response to Letter to the JCE editor. *J Clin Embryol* 2009; **12:** 5.
61. Wikipedia. *Concentration*. 2009. http://en.wikipedia.org/wiki/Concentration (accessed July 22, 2009).
62. Wikipedia. *International System of Units*. 2009. http://en.wikipedia.org/wiki/SI_units (accessed July 22, 2009).

Chapter 17

Vitrification of human oocytes using the McGill Cryoleaf protocol

Jack Yu Jen Huang, Seang Lin Tan, and Ri-Cheng Chian

Introduction

In recent years, awareness of the possibilities for fertility preservation has increased. The American Society of Clinical Oncology and the American Society of Reproductive Medicine have endorsed gonadotropin stimulation with in vitro fertilization (IVF) and embryo cryopreservation as the only established method of female fertility preservation [1,2]. However, this strategy may not be applicable to young women without a male partner and those who object to cryopreservation of embryos for personal, financial, religious, or moral reasons.

Cryopreservation of an entire ovary potentially allows the greatest number of follicles to be preserved [3], but this has not been successfully performed in humans. Ovarian tissue cryopreservation with orthotopic transplantation is a promising option [4] but requires two operations, has produced only three published live births [5–7], despite numerous attempts, and in cancer patients carries a small, but finite, risk of re-introducing malignant cells [8].

Oocyte cryopreservation represents an attractive and the least invasive option of fertility preservation strategy for patients wishing to retain their choice of a male partner. Conventional slow cooling of oocytes is considered an experimental procedure because of the inconsistent survival rates and limited number of live births achieved [1,9]. The percentage of live births per thawed egg ranges from 1 to 10% using slow-freezing protocols [9–11].

Recent advances in vitrification techniques have markedly improved the efficacy of oocyte cryopreservation [10–13], demonstrating that vitrification may be more effective than the conventional slow-cooling method [10]. Several groups including the McGill Reproductive Center (MRC) have reported survival rates over 80% [14–18]. To date, most reports of oocyte cryopreservation have been in oocytes matured in vivo and derived from ovarian stimulation protocols; these protocols require 4 to 6 weeks to complete the ovarian stimulation cycle and produce relatively high estradiol levels, which may be deleterious in certain cancers, notably estrogen receptor-positive breast cancer, the most common malignancy in women referred for fertility preservation [1]. Therefore, there is a pressing need for the development of fertility preservation options applicable to young women facing the risk of premature ovarian failure from gonadotoxic treatment, which do not require male partner participation, gonadotropin ovarian stimulation, or delay in treatment.

A potential strategy to avoid spindle depolymerization is to cryopreserve oocytes at the germinal vesicle (GV) stage. The oocytes are arrested in diplotene state of prophase I. Theoretically, the use of immature GV stage eggs circumvents the risk of polyploidy and aneuploidies because the chromatin is diffuse and surrounded by a nuclear membrane [19,20]. However, poor in vitro maturation (IVM) and fertilization have been reported as the major problems associated with cryopreservation of immature oocytes [21–23]. To date, only one human live birth has been reported following cryopreservation of a GV stage oocyte and IVM using a slow-freezing method [24].

A novel strategy of fertility preservation involves retrieval of immature oocytes in an unstimulated menstrual cycle by transvaginal ultrasound guidance within days of initial consultation [25] or from ovarian tissue biopsies [26], followed by IVM and vitrification of oocytes [25,27]. The option of IVM has become an effective treatment for many infertile women, including those with polycystic ovaries or polycystic ovary syndrome and those at increased risk of developing ovarian hyperstimulation syndrome [28–32]. Over 1500 healthy infants have been born [33] and are not associated with any increase in fetal abnormality rates compared with those from IVF or

Fertility Cryopreservation, ed. Ri-Cheng Chian and Patrick Quinn. Published by Cambridge University Press.

spontaneous conceptions [34] (R-C Chian *et al.*, personal communication).

The combination of IVM and vitrification of the oocyte has several advantages including (1) eliminating the cost of drugs and the need for close monitoring; (2) allowing minimal delay in treatment, as it may be completed in as few as 2 days [25]; (3) eliminating the risk of stimulating hormone-sensitive tumors, as in estrogen receptor-positive breast cancer; and (4) allowing the possibility of retrieving oocytes regardless of the phase of the menstrual cycle [35].

Vitrification

Vitrification is glass-like solidification of a solution at low temperature resulting from an extreme increase in viscosity during the cooling process. In simpler terms, vitrification refers to ice crystal-free solidification of an aqueous solution. In 1937, Luyet [36] first proposed the advantages of achieving an ice-free, glass-like state for cryopreservation of cells and tissues. However, it was not until the late 1980s that Fahy [37] and MacFarlane and Forsyth [38] investigated the occurrence and applications of vitrification in several fundamental studies.

The proposed mechanism of vitrification uses a high concentration of cryoprotectant (CPA) and extremely rapid cooling and warming rates in order to avoid intra- and extracellular ice formation. Successful vitrification depends on three factors: (1) extremely high cooling and warming rates (up to 20 000°C/min), achieved by plunging the cells suspended in CPA solution directly into liquid nitrogen (LN_2); (2) high concentration of CPAs to inhibit ice crystallization; and (3) a very small volume of CPA solution (< 1 μl) to optimize the cooling and warming rates.

Cryoprotectants

In addition to the physical injuries caused by the formation of ice crystals, a major cause of injury to the oocytes relates to osmotic dehydration and the toxicity of CPA when they are added to the suspending solution. The commonly used CPAs for cryopreservation of oocytes and embryos are small neutral solutes such as ethylene glycol (EG), 1,2-propanediol (PROH), dimethyl sulfoxide (DMSO), and glycerol. In general, rapidly permeating CPAs are preferable because rapid permeation shortens the exposure time, reduces the toxic injury, and minimizes osmotic swelling during the removal of the CPAs. Furthermore, the permeation of CPAs is largely influenced by temperature and high temperature accelerates the permeation of CPAs. Therefore, it is important to select suitable CPA with low cytotoxicity for oocyte vitrification.

Ethylene glycol is widely used for vitrification because of its low molecular weight, high permeation, and low toxicity [39,40]. However, the use of EG alone required higher concentrations of the CPA (≥ 5.5 M) [41]. Both DMSO and PROH have higher membrane permeability than glycerol [42,43]; PROH is a less toxic and more permeable CPA than DMSO [44,45]. Dimethyl sulfoxide has been shown to cause spindle polymerization in oocytes, resulting in an increased potential for polyploidy [46,47]. Moreover, cryopreservation using PROH did not increase the aneuploidy rates in 1-cell rabbit embryos [48] and mature mouse or human oocytes [49,50].

Oocyte microstructures, such as meiotic spindles, microtubules, and microfilaments, may be damaged by cooling and exposure to CPAs [51]. As a consequence of CPA exposure and freezing–thawing, the spindles of oocytes cannot hold the chromosomes correctly at the metaphase plate prior to polar body extrusion [52], leading to chromosomal dispersion, failure of normal fertilization, increased incidence of aneuploidy or polyploidy, and termination of embryonic development [53–55].

We have shown in mouse model experiments that exposure of oocytes for 3 minutes to a 2.0 M concentration of the five commonly used CPAs (EG, PROH, DMSO, glycerol, and sucrose) significantly reduces fertilization and embryonic development [56]. In fact, exposure to 2.0 M PROH, glycerol, and sucrose also leads to abnormal meiotic spindle morphology and increased incidence of aneuploidy.

Numerous groups, including the MRC, have attempted to minimize the toxicity of vitrification solutions, evaluating various combinations of permeable CPAs and macromolecules [56–58]. A common approach to reduce CPA toxicity is the use of a mixture of CPAs and pre-equilibrating the oocytes or embryos in a mixture of CPAs at low concentration transferring them to a high concentration mixture.

We have shown that exposure of oocytes to a combination of two CPAs, such as 1.0 M EG and 1.0 M PROH, which has the same osmolality as a single 2.0 M CPA, significantly reduced the meiotic spindle malformation rate and improved embryonic developmental potential [56]. Another possibility for minimizing CPA toxicity is replacing permeable CPAs with polymers such as sucrose molecules and polyvinylpyrrolidone [59].

Advantages and disadvantages of vitrification

Vitrification represents an attractive cryopreservation strategy compared with conventional slow-cooling methods [60]. In contrast to slow-cooling techniques, the vitrification procedure is precise and every step can be visualized. More importantly, vitrification minimizes the duration of exposure to a subphysiological environment. The vitrification procedure requires less than 10 minutes to perform, compared with 2 hours for the slow-freezing methods. Also, vitrification procedures are simpler to perform and do not require the use of expensive programmable freezing equipment. In the particular case of oocytes, fracture of zona pellucida and chilling injury can also be prevented by vitrification methods.

The only major drawback of the vitrification procedure is the requirement for a higher and potentially cytotoxic concentration of CPAs in order to prevent ice crystallization. Early vitrification protocols involved pre-equilibrating embryos and oocytes with mixtures of highly toxic concentration of CPAs (up to 12.0 M final concentration) for up to 60 minutes before immersion in LN_2. In order to reduce the permeation and minimize the toxicity of the vitrification solution, the pre-equilibration steps were performed at a low temperature (4°C).

Devices for vitrification

Different carriers have been designed to minimize the volume of CPA solution and to allow the sample to be submerged quickly in LN_2. These devices include the McGill Cryoleaf (Medicult, Jyllinge, Denmark) (Figure 17.1) [13], Cryotip [61], Cryotop [16], nylon loop or Cryoloop [62,63], thin capillary or open pulled straws [64], hemi-straws [65], and electron microscope copper/gold grids [66]. Using the McGill Cryoleaf and the Cryotop, it has been estimated that the freezing speed can be increased up to 20 000°C/min when plunging the device into LN_2.

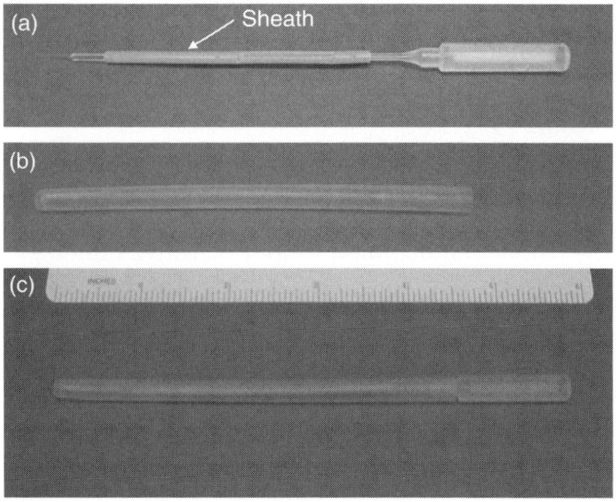

Figure 17.1. Actual view of Cryoleaf. (a) The core part of Cryoleaf; the arrow indicates the loading portion, which is made of thin polyethylene stick. The sheath can slide down to protect the loading stick. (b) The protective straw covers the core part for storage. (c) The Cryoleaf assembled with the core within the protective straw.

The McGill Cryoleaf protocol

The vitrification protocol

A common protocol for vitrification is to first equilibrate the oocytes in a solution containing a lower concentration of permeable CPA or CPA mixture before transferring them to a solution containing the full-strength permeable CPA and a non-permeable CPA such as a disaccharide or macromolecule. All of the cumulus–oocyte complexes are stripped of cumulus cells prior to the vitrification procedure using a finely drawn glass pipette, following 1 minute of exposure to a hyaluronidase solution. The mature, metaphase II (MII) oocytes are then subjected to vitrification.

Preparation of solutions

Equilibration medium, containing 7.5% (v/v) EG plus 7.5% (v/v) PROH (Medicult), and vitrification medium, containing 15% (v/v) EG plus 15% (v/v) PROH plus 0.5 M sucrose (Medicult) in the base medium with phosphate-buffered saline or human tubal fluid supplemented with 20% (v/v) human serum albumin (HSA) solution (Coopersurgical/SAGE, Trumbull, USA), should be prepared at least 1 hour before use and be kept at room temperature. Briefly, two Petri dishes (Falcon, 35 mm × 10 mm) can be prepared for each patient, one containing 1.5 ml of equilibration medium and the other 1.5 ml of vitrification medium. Alternatively, the two media can be prepared in the form of droplets in the same dish (Falcon, 60 mm × 10 mm). The volume of each droplet is 20–50 μl.

Vitrification

The MII oocytes are first suspended in equilibration medium for 5 minutes at room temperature and then transferred to vitrification medium (at room temperature for 45–60 seconds. The oocytes in the vitrification medium are then loaded on the tip of the McGill Cryoleaf in the form of a 2–3 μl droplet (Figure 17.2a) and plunged immediately into LN_2 for

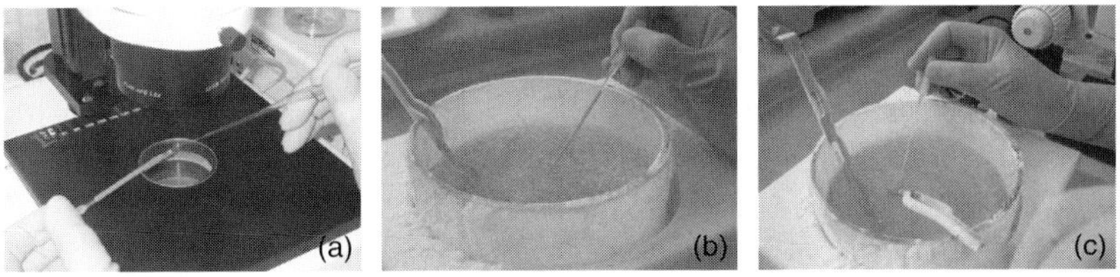

Figure 17.2. The vitrification procedure. (a) Eggs or embryos are loaded on to the McGill Cryoleaf. (b) The Cryoleaf is immersed directly into LN_2. (c) The Cryoleaf is capped under LN_2 for storage.

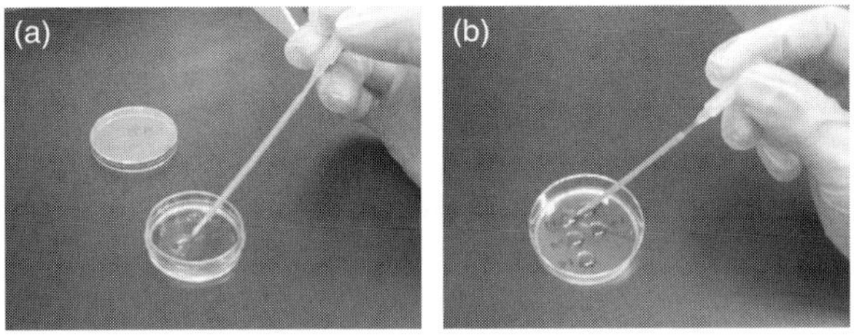

Figure 17.3. The thawing procedure. The tip of the Cryoleaf can be directly immersed into 1.5 ml thawing medium contained in a Petri dish (a) or inserted into a droplet in a Petri Dish (b). The oocytes will slide away from the Cryoleaf within 1 minute and can then be transferred to diluent medium 1.

storage (Figure 17.2b). After vitrification, it is important to store the oocytes safely. The McGill Cryoleaf must be capped under LN_2 in order to avoid exposing the vitrified oocytes to room temperature (Figure 17.2c).

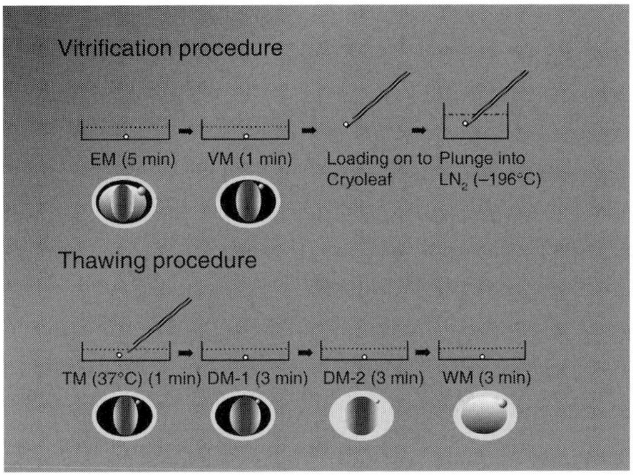

Figure 17.4. Oocyte vitrification and thawing procedures using the McGill Cryoleaf. EM, equilibration medium; VM, vitrification medium; TM, thawing medium; DM, diluent medium; LN_2, liquid nitrogen.

The thawing protocol

Thawing media preparation

The thawing medium should be warmed at 37ºC for at least 30 minutes before being used for thawing the stored material. Diluent medium 1 and 2 (Medicult) and washing medium 1 and 2 (Medicult) should be prepared at least 30 minutes before use and be kept at room temperature. These solutions are prepared in separate petri dishes (Falcon, 35 mm × 10 mm), each containing 1.5 ml of the solution, or as separate droplets (50–100 μl) within in a single larger dish (Falcon, 60 mm × 10 mm).

Oocyte thawing

For thawing, the cap of the McGill Cryoleaf is first removed under LN_2. The Cryoleaf is then directly inserted into thawing medium containing 1.0 M sucrose for 1 minute at 37ºC (Figure 17.3a,b). The thawed oocytes are then transferred into diluent medium 1 (containing 0.5 M sucrose) and then into diluent medium 2 (containing 0.25 M sucrose), for 3 minutes each. Oocytes are washed twice, in washing medium 1 and 2 for 3 minutes in each solution. The key steps of the vitrification and thawing procedures are summarized in Figure 17.4.

Assessment of survival and fertilization

Oocyte survival after thawing can be evaluated microscopically based on the morphology of the oocyte membrane integrity. As our animal model experiments suggested hardening of the zona pellucida of the oocyte following cryopreservation [67,68], viable oocytes should be inseminated by intracytoplasmic sperm injection (ICSI), and fertilized zygotes further cultured for 2–3 days before embryo transfer.

Embryo transfer

The embryos produced from vitrified oocytes are transferred on either day 2 or day 3, depending on the number and quality of the embryos, under ultrasound guidance using a Wallace catheter (SIMS Protex, Hyth, UK).

The endometrium is prepared using 6 mg estradiol (Estrace, Roberts Pharmaceutical, Mississauga, Canada) daily for 10 days, starting on day 2 of the menstrual cycle. Once ultrasound scan confirmed endometrial thickness of 6–8 mm, and 2 days before embryo transfer, vaginal progesterone 200 mg (Prometrium, Schering, Pointe-Claire, Canada) three times daily, or progesterone 50 mg intramuscular once daily, is administered for 14 days. A pregnancy test is done 14 days after embryo transfer and an ultrasound scan is performed 2 weeks later to confirm the presence of a clinical pregnancy; if positive, both estradiol and progesterone are continued until the 12th week of pregnancy for luteal support.

Efficacy of the McGill Cryoleaf protocol

Animal model studies

Before introducing oocyte vitrification using the Cryoleaf for routine use in humans at the assisted reproductive technology clinic, the safety and efficacy of the Cryoleaf vitrification system was evaluated in murine and bovine model studies. In the murine study, vitrification of oocytes using the Cryoleaf was shown to be superior to the choline-supplemented, sodium-depleted slow-freezing method, leading to improved survival of oocytes (92% versus 73%), their fertilization (64% versus 40%), and their in vitro embryonic development (31% versus 20% blastocyst formation rate) [67]. The fertilization, 2-cell cleavage, and blastocyst formation rates of vitrified oocytes remained lower compared with those of fresh oocytes.

Analysis of meiotic spindle integrity and chromosome alignment indicates that less damage is detectable in vitrified compared with slow-frozen oocytes, but the incidence of aneuploidy is similar in both oocytes preserved by both processes (both 9%) [67], raising further questions as to whether aneuploidy is the main cause of reduced in vitro embryonic development. The combined effect of IVM and vitrification was also evaluated on mouse and bovine oocytes in order to improve our understanding of the efficacy of this novel strategy of fertility preservation [68,71]. In the murine model study, 80% of GV stage oocytes matured following IVM and were cryopreserved by vitrification [68]. There was no significant difference in the post-warming survival of oocytes matured in vitro and in vivo (94% and 92%, respectively). The majority of oocytes matured by both methods maintained normal meiotic spindle morphology and chromosome alignment (88% and 87%, respectively) following vitrification, and the incidence of aneuploidy was not increased (11% and 9%, respectively). However, oocytes matured in vitro showed a higher incidence of DNA fragmentation following vitrification–thawing compared with those matured in vivo. Following vitrification–thawing, the cleavage and blastocyst formation rates of the oocytes matured in vitro were significantly lower than those matured in vivo (37% versus 60% and 5% versus 19%, respectively).

Although aneuploidy is a known cause of reduced embryonic development potential and embryonic loss, the above study further suggests that it may not be the primary factor in the reduced embryonic developmental competence of immature mouse oocytes following IVM and vitrification. The efficacy of the Cryoleaf for vitrification of oocytes matured in vitro was also evaluated in bovine model experiments that compared the mixture of EG and PROH with the combination of EG and DMSO, both also containing 0.5 M sucrose [71]. The survival rate of bovine oocytes after warming was 98% when the oocytes were vitrified with 15% (v/v) EG plus 15% (v/v) PROH and 92% when vitrified with 15% (v/v) EG plus 15% (v/v) DMSO. Vitrification using the combination of EG and PROH, rather than EG plus DMSO, resulted in significantly higher rates of embryos developing to the blastocyst stage (7% versus 2%) and reaching the expanded or hatched blastocyst stage (3% versus 1%).

The same study also showed that oocyte survival rates following vitrification can be affected by the presence or absence of cumulus cells. Survival rates after thawing were significantly higher for bovine oocytes without cumulus cells (93%) than for those with cumulus cells (84%). However, pre-incubation of the oocytes before insemination did not improve subsequent fertilization rates and embryonic developmental potential. The results from these studies indicate that murine and bovine oocytes can be successfully vitrified using CPA concentrations that are comparable to those used in the slow-cooling protocol. Furthermore, the risk of CPA toxicity is reduced by using a combination of EG and PROH mixture and by shortening the total exposure time to the CPA solutions. In addition to improvement in the survival rate, vitrification leads to higher fertilization and early embryonic development rates.

Clinical trials

A prospective study was conducted at the MRC to evaluate the pregnancy rates and obstetrical outcomes following vitrification of oocytes matured in vivo or in vitro between October 2003 and April 2007 [13]. The study comprised two groups. The first group included patients undergoing superovulation and intrauterine insemination treatment, who over-responded to ovarian stimulation. Instead of canceling their treatment cycle to avoid high-order multiple pregnancies, this group underwent oocyte retrieval and vitrification of oocytes (OS group). The second group consisted of women who had failed cycles of intrauterine insemination treatment. In this group, immature oocytes were retrieved in a natural unstimulated menstrual cycle and underwent IVM. The in vitro matured oocytes were vitrified (IVM group).

In the OS group, a total of 399 MII and 91 GV oocytes were retrieved. The mean maturation rate was 70.3 ± 20.0%. A total of 463 oocytes were vitrified. After thawing, a mean survival rate of 81.4 ± 22.6% was achieved. Following ICSI, a mean fertilization rate of 75.6 ± 22.5% was achieved. Of the 133 embryos transferred (mean embryo transfer of 3.5 ± 1.1), 17 clinical pregnancies were achieved (44.7% per cycle started). The implantation rate was 19.1 ± 25.8%.

In the IVM group, a total of 290 GV and 6 MII oocytes were retrieved. Following IVM, the mean maturation rate was 67.3 ± 19.3%. A total of 215 MII oocytes were vitrified. The mean survival rate was 67.5 ± 26.1%. The fertilization rate following ICSI was 64.2 ± 19.9%. Of 64 embryos transferred (mean embryo transfer of 3.2 ± 1.5), four clinical pregnancies were achieved, resulting in a 20% clinical pregnancy per cycle started. The implantation rate was 9.6 ± 24.1%.

The mean numbers of MII oocytes vitrified per patient were comparable in the two groups (12.2 ± 5.1 for the OS group and 10.8 ± 5.9 for the IVM group). The clinical efficacy of the OS group was superior to that of the IVM group in terms of oocyte survival after thawing, fertilization rate, and embryo quality. Although the implantation per embryo, pregnancy per cycle started, clinical pregnancy per cycle started, and live birth rate per cycle started were higher in OS group, these differences were not statistically significant.

It is reassuring that the clinical pregnancy and live birth rates achieved by vitrification of mature oocytes are comparable to those achieved using standard IVF treatment, as reported by the American, Canadian, and European IVF registries [72–74] and are much higher than the results achieved by the conventional slow-cooling methods [9]. This study also demonstrates that pregnancies and live births can be achieved by vitrification of oocytes matured in vitro.

Neonatal outcomes following oocyte vitrification

Any new development in IVF treatment must be accompanied by data concerning obstetric and perinatal outcomes. Few data have been reported on the obstetric and perinatal outcome for the infants conceived with vitrified oocytes. In our OS group, there have been nine singleton and six multiple gestation live births (five twins, one triplet), resulting in 22 healthy newborns to date. All newborns were examined for the presence of congenital anomalies by neonatologists from tertiary, university-based hospitals. All singleton pregnancies resulted in term deliveries. Four of the six multiple gestations (67%) delivered at 34 to 37 weeks of gestation. The mean gestation age at delivery was 39 weeks and 1 day for singleton and 36 weeks and 4 days for multiple gestations. The mean birthweight for singletons and twins were 3193.7 ± 376.8 g and 2277.9 ± 395.7 g, respectively. Among singletons, none of the nine newborns weighed less than 2500 g. In the 13 newborns from multiple gestation pregnancies, nine (69%) had low birthweight (1500–2500 g).

In the IVM group, there have been four healthy singleton live births at term gestation. The world's first baby from vitrification of in vitro matured oocytes was born by Cesarean section for breech presentation at 39 weeks and 1 day of gestation on June 6, 2006, weighing 3480 g [27].

We recently reported the obstetric and perinatal outcomes in 165 pregnancies conceived following oocyte vitrification from the MRC in Canada, the Instituto Mexicano de Infertilidad in Mexico, and the CECOLFES in Colombia [75]. The multiple pregnancy rate was 17% (26 twin and 2 triplet pregnancies). In 137 singleton pregnancies, 51 patients underwent cesarean section delivery (37%). The median gestational age at delivery for singletons was 37 weeks. In 28 multiple pregnancies, 27 underwent cesarean section delivery (96%). The mean gestation age at delivery for multiple gestation was 35 weeks and 5 days. A total of 200 babies were born. The mean birthweight was 2920 ± 37 g for singletons and 2231 ± 55 g for multiple births. The median Apgar scores at 1 and 5 minutes were similar between singletons and multiple gestations (9 and

8 at 1 minute and 8 and 10 at 5 minutes, respectively). The incidence of congenital anomalies in this cohort of newborns was 2.5% (two ventricular septal defects, one biliary atresia, one club foot, one skin hemangioma).

The McGill Cryoleaf protocol for preservation of fertility

Over 600 000 women are diagnosed in the USA with cancer each year; approximately 8% are under the age of 40 [76]. Although with modern treatment protocols involving multidrug chemotherapy and/or radiotherapy, coupled with bone marrow transplantation, more than 90% of teenage girls and young women will survive [77], infertility is a frequent consequence [78]. It has been estimated that, in the near future, approximately 1 in 250 young adults will be a long-term survivor of cancer [79].

At the MRC, a full range of fertility preservation options, including oophoropexy [80] and embryo, oocyte, and ovarian tissue cryopreservation, are available to women who are facing the risk of premature ovarian failure. The most appropriate fertility preservation strategy is determined by the time available and the availability or not of a committed male partner (Figure 17.5). Patients who present with time constraints or an objection to receive hormonal stimulation are advised to undergo oocyte collection without prior ovarian stimulation followed by IVM of oocytes. In the absence of a male partner, the in vitro matured oocytes can be cryopreserved by vitrification. In the presence of a male partner, the in vitro matured oocytes are fertilized by ICSI and the resulting embryos are vitrified.

When their treatments are not imminent and there is no contraindication to hormonal stimulation, patients undergo ovarian stimulation with gonadotropins, oocyte collection, followed by oocyte vitrification in the absence of a male partner or embryo vitrification. Whenever feasible or appropriate, patients are also offered the option of laparoscopic ovarian wedge resection biopsy followed by cryopreservation of the ovarian cortex to preserve the possibility of future ovarian tissue transplantation, or in vitro growth of oocytes from primordial follicles in the ovarian tissue.

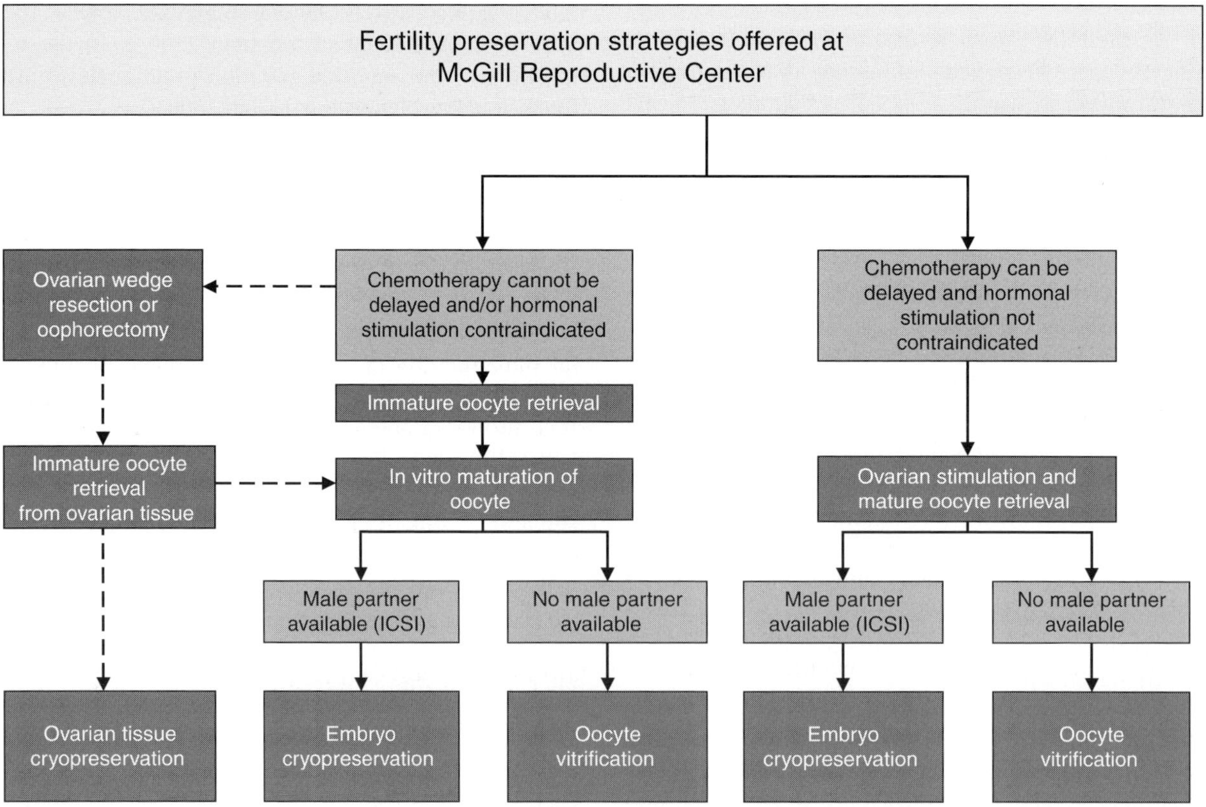

Figure 17.5. Fertility preservation strategies at McGill Reproductive Center. ICSI, intracytoplasmic sperm injection.

Oncological indications for fertility preservation

To date, the MRC has provided fertility preservation to 123 cancer patients, including 46 with breast cancer [25,81], 35 with hematological cancer, 9 with brain cancer, 10 with soft tissue cancer, and 9 with gynecologic cancer.

Breast cancer

We recently reported the use of IVM and oocyte vitrification for young patients with breast cancer who presented with time constraints or concerns regarding hormonal stimulation. Eighteen women of reproductive age (mean age 33.1 ± 5.0 years; range 24–45) with breast cancer were referred for fertility preservation. Because of time constraints, chemotherapy planned to start within a short period, or concerns about the use of gonadotropin ovarian stimulation, these patients underwent immature oocyte retrieval from unstimulated ovaries in a natural menstrual cycle followed by IVM and vitrification of oocytes. The median delay in cancer treatment was 7 days. The median number of vitrified oocytes per retrieval was seven (range, 1–22). The mean estradiol level was physiological, averaging 270.6 ± 90.5 pmol/l on the day of immature oocyte retrieval. Therefore, this novel strategy is not associated with increased estrogen exposure or delay in cancer treatment, and thus represents an attractive fertility preservation option for many breast cancer patients.

Another advantage of IVM is the possibility to retrieve oocytes regardless of the phase of the menstrual cycle. Unlike conventional ovarian stimulation protocols, which are dependent upon the phase of the menstrual cycle and can only be initiated at monthly intervals, it is possible to perform immature oocyte retrieval sequentially in both luteal and follicular phase of the menstrual cycle without affecting the quantity and maturation rate of the oocytes [35].

This strategy may also be used in selected breast cancer patients undergoing conventional IVF with ovarian stimulation [81]. Oktay *et al.* [81] reported the case of a patient with breast cancer who underwent stimulation with follicle-stimulating hormone and letrozole with the intention of embryo cryopreservation. Unfortunately, a premature luteinizing hormone surge resulted in ovulation prior to the oocyte retrieval. As her chemotherapy was scheduled to start in a week and the patient did not wish to delay her cancer treatment, the patient was referred to the MRC. On the day of the consultation, immature oocytes were retrieved, underwent IVM, and fertilized, successfully generating two embryos for cryopreservation

Hematological malignancies

We recently reported a series of 30 patients with hematological malignancies who were referred for fertility preservation, including 17 patients with Hodgkin's lymphoma, five with non-Hodgkin's lymphoma, three with acute myelogenous leukemia, three with myelodysplasia syndrome, one with Burkitt's lymphoma, and one with aplastic anemia. Owing to time constraints, 12 patients underwent immature oocyte retrieval from unstimulated ovaries, followed by IVM and vitrification of oocytes in the absence of a male partner. A median of 10 oocytes was vitrified (range, 2–40). When the cancer therapy was not imminent, 10 patients underwent ovarian stimulation with gonadotropins and mature oocyte retrieval followed by vitrification of the matured oocytes. A total of 124 mature oocytes were vitrified (median of 12 oocytes per retrieval; range, 3–25).

Ovarian neoplasms

We have reported the possibility of fertility preservation for patients with borderline ovarian tumors [82]. This novel strategy involves aspiration of all visible follicles on the surface of the removed ovary using an 18-gauge needle attached to a 10 ml syringe containing oocyte washing medium (Sage/Cooper Surgical, Trumbull, CT, USA). Four immature oocytes were retrieved and underwent IVM. Three oocytes matured after 48 hours and were cryopreserved. Interestingly, the salpingooophorectomy procedure was performed on day 18 of her cycle, indicating that oocytes can be collected, matured in vitro, and cryopreserved regardless of the day of menstrual cycle.

This novel strategy of direct aspiration of all visible follicles can also be combined with ovarian tissue cryopreservation [26]. In a series of four patients who underwent oophorectomy or ovarian wedge resection for the purpose of ovarian tissue cryopreservation, the mean number of immature oocytes recovered was three (one, three, four, and three, respectively). The mean maturation rate following IVM was 79% (100%, 100%, 50%, and 67%, respectively). In total, eight mature oocytes were vitrified.

Non-oncological indications for fertility preservation

Fertility preservation should also be considered in patients undergoing gonadotoxic therapy for other non-oncologic conditions [83], including systemic lupus erythematosus (SLE) or other autoimmune disorders [84], those who have undergone extensive ovarian surgery for endometriosis [85] and ovarian neoplasm, and those with mosaic Turner syndrome.

Systemic lupus erythematosus or other autoimmune disorders

We recently reported a case series of seven women with SLE and other systemic autoimmune rheumatic diseases who required cyclophosphamide therapy and underwent fertility preservation treatments. Five women had SLE with nephritis; one suffered from immune thrombocytopenia purpura, and one had microscopic polyangiitis with renal involvement. All women were nulliparous and younger than 35 years old. Patients with SLE underwent IVM of immature oocytes aspirated during a natural menstrual cycle, followed by vitrification of the matured oocytes if a male partner was not available or vitrification of embryos if one was available. The patient with immune thrombocytopenia purpura and the patient with microscopic polyangiitis underwent gonadotropin ovarian stimulation followed by oocyte or embryo vitrification. There were no complications associated with this treatment and cytotoxic therapy was initiated as scheduled in all cases. Therefore, treatment consideration should include fertility preservation in young women with systemic autoimmune rheumatic diseases who face imminent gonadotoxic treatment. In patients, where gonadotropin ovarian stimulation is deemed unsafe, IVM followed by vitrification represents a safe and feasible option.

Endometriosis

A new indication for fertility preservation includes young women undergoing extensive ovarian surgery for endometriosis [85]. We recently reported a case of a young woman at risk of losing her remaining ovary owing to severe and symptomatic endometriosis. As she had no male partner, she was consulted about the possibility of oocyte cryopreservation before further treatment. With the approval of the Hospital Research Ethics Board, she underwent three cycles of ovarian stimulation and had 21 mature oocytes cryopreserved by vitrification.

Turner syndrome

Women with Turner syndrome are at risk of premature ovarian failure. We recently conducted a retrospective study to identify patients with Turner syndrome who could be potential candidates for fertility preservation and to determine their present reproductive and fertility status [86]. Criteria for fertility preservation included: (1) spontaneous menarche, (2) confirmation by ultrasound examination of the presence of at least one normal ovary, and (3) serum follicle-stimulating hormone levels below 40 IU/l. Using the Montreal Children's Hospital Cytogenetic Database from 1990 to 2006, 28 patients were identified: 13 (46%) were 45X; nine (32%) had mosaic karyotypes; and six (21%) had karyotypes containing isochromosome or ring X chromosome. Six patients (21%) had spontaneous pubertal development and four (14%) were identified as potential candidates for fertility preservation. One underwent an ovarian stimulation protocol of gonadotropin-releasing hormone agonist downregulation followed by recombinant follicle-stimulating hormone and human menopausal gonadotropin stimulation. Two MII stage oocytes were collected and vitrified using the McGill Cryoleaf vitrification system. Another patient conceived spontaneously at the age of 24 years.

We also reported the combination of ovarian tissue cryobanking and immature oocyte collection from the tissue followed by IVM and vitrification of in vitro matured oocytes in a young woman with mosaic Turner syndrome [87]. A 16-year-old female with 20% 45X and 80% 46XX karyotype underwent laparoscopic ovarian wedge resection. Before performing ovarian tissue cryopreservation, all visible follicles on the ovarian surface were aspirated. 11 immature GV stage oocytes were recovered and subjected to IVM. Eight oocytes that matured (73% maturation rate) were cryopreserved by vitrification.

In the case of non-mosaic Turner syndrome, the only option for fertility has been oocyte donation [88]. However, the demand for oocyte donors exceeds supply for third-party conception in many countries. Moreover, in many countries, including Canada, remuneration for donors either through financial gain or benefits is prohibited, which has worsed the shortage of oocyte donors.

We recently reported the first case of mother-to-daughter oocyte donation using oocyte vitrification [89]. A 33-year-old healthy mother of three children requested to undergo ovarian stimulation in order to cryopreserve oocytes for the purpose of donating to her 6-year-old daughter, who was recently diagnosed with Turner syndrome. After three cycles of ovarian stimulation, 30 oocytes were cryopreserved for the daughter's possible future use. This strategy demonstrates the feasibility for the banking of a mother's oocytes as a possible donation to a young daughter with a medical condition that leads to infertility.

While, fertility preservation may not be feasible for most patients with Turner syndrome, after careful consideration of increased pregnancy-associated risks, fertility preservation may be offered to young females with mosaic Turner syndrome. The combination of ovarian tissue cryobanking and immature oocyte collection from the tissue followed by IVM and vitrification of matured oocytes represents a promising approach to fertility preservation for young women with mosaic Turner syndrome. Oocyte cryopreservation allows for mother-to-daughter oocyte donation.

Social indications

Fertility declines with increasing age [90]. Many professional women wishing to delay motherhood may find themselves facing potential childlessness because of irreversible loss of viable oocytes, which is inevitable with advancing age [90]. Oocyte vitrification represents an attractive strategy for these women to bypass their biological clock.

Conclusions

Primary care physicians and oncologists need to be made aware of the fertility preservation options for young female patients that do not entail male partner participation, gonadotropin ovarian stimulation, or delay in gonadotoxic treatment. Early discussion with the patient should be undertaken and, if desired, the woman should be referred to an IVF center that offers the full range of fertility preservation options.

As with any new assisted reproductive technology procedure in humans, it will be necessary to study oocyte vitrification in larger prospective clinical trials for a sufficient length of time in order to determine whether the development of the resulting children is healthy; but we believe this technique offers a realistic hope of fertility preservation for women without partners. Whether this strategy should be offered to any woman of advancing reproductive age anxious to preserve her fertility but whose current circumstances preclude pregnancy is debatable. However, the window of opportunity for fertility preservation in young women who must undergo gonadotoxic treatment for life-threatening diseases such as cancer is small, and once treatment is initiated, fertility loss is often irreversible.

References

1. Lee SJ, Schover LR, Partridge AH, *et al.* American Society of Clinical Oncology recommendations on fertility preservation in cancer patients. *J Clin Oncol* 2006; **24:** 2917–2931.
2. Ethics Committee of the American Society of Reproductive Medicine. Fertility preservation and reproduction in cancer patients. *Fertil Steril* 2005; **83:** 1622–1628.
3. Wang X, Chen H, Yin H, *et al.* Fertility after intact ovary transplantation. *Nature* 2002; **415:** 385.
4. Oktay K, Buyuk E, Veeck LL, *et al.* Embryo development after heterotopic transplantation of cryopreserved ovarian tissue. *Lancet* 2004; **363:** 837–840.
5. Donnez J, Dolmans MM, Demylle D, *et al.* Livebirth after orthotopic transplantation of cryopreserved ovarian tissue. *Lancet* 2004; **364:** 1405–1410.
6. Meirow D, Levron J, Eldar-Geva T, *et al.* Pregnancy after transplantation of cryopreserved ovarian tissue in a patient with ovarian failure after chemotherapy. *N Engl J Med* 2005; **353:** 318–321.
7. Demeestere I, Simon P, Emiliani S, Delbaere A, Englert Y. Fertility preservation: successful transplantation of cryopreserved ovarian tissue in a young patient previously treated for Hodgkin's disease. *Oncologist* 2007; **12:** 1437–1442.
8. Meirow D, Hardan I, Dor J, *et al.* Searching for evidence of disease and malignant cell contamination in ovarian tissue stored from hematologic cancer patients. *Hum Reprod* 2008; **23:** 1007–1013.
9. Practice Committee of the American Society of Reproductive Medicine. Ovarian tissue and oocyte cryopreservation. *Fertil Steril* 2004; **82:** 993–998.
10. Kuleshova LL, Lopata A. Vitrification can be more favorable than slow cooling. *Fertil Steril* 2002; **78:** 449–454.
11. Oktay K, Cil AP, Bang H. Efficiency of oocyte cryopreservation: a meta-analysis. *Fertil Steril* 2006; **86:** 70–80.
12. Huang JY, Tan SL, Chian R-C. Fertility preservation for female. *J Reprod Contracept* 2006; **17:** 109–128.
13. Chian R-C, Huang JYJ, Gilbert L, *et al.* Obstetric outcomes following vitrification of in-vitro and in-vivo matured oocytes. *Fertil Steril* 2009; **91:** 2391–2398.
14. Katayama KP, Stehlik J, Kuwayama M, Kato O, Stehlik E. High survival rate of vitrified human oocytes results in clinical pregnancy. *Fertil Steril* 2003; **80:** 223–224.
15. Kuwayama M, Vajta G, Kato O, Leibo SP. Highly efficient vitrification method for cryopreservation of human oocytes. *Reprod Biomed Online* 2005; **11:** 300–308.
16. Kuwayama M. Highly efficient vitrification for cryopreservation of human oocytes and embryos: the Cryotop method. *Theriogenology* 2007; **67:** 73–80.

17. Lucena E, Bernal DP, Lucena C, *et al.* Successful ongoing pregnancies after vitrification of oocytes. *Fertil Steril* 2006; **85:** 108–111.
18. Cobo A, Kuwayama M, Perez S, *et al.* Comparison of concomitant outcome achieved with fresh and cryopreserved donor oocytes vitrified by the Cryotop method. *Fertil Steril* 2008; **89:** 1657–1664.
19. Cooper A, Paynter SJ, Fuller BJ. Differential effects of cryopreservation on nuclear or cytoplasmic maturation in vitro in immature mouse oocytes from stimulated ovaries. *Hum Reprod* 1998; **13:** 971–978.
20. Isachenko EF, Nayudu PL. Vitrification of mouse germinal vesicle oocytes: effect of treatment temperature and egg yolk on chromosomal normality and cumulus integrity. *Hum Reprod* 1999; **14:** 400–408.
21. Toth TL, Baka SG, Veeck LL, *et al.* Fertilization and in vitro development of cryopreserved human prophase I oocytes. *Fertil Steril* 1994; **61:** 891–894.
22. Toth TL, Lanzendorf SE, Sandow BA, *et al.* Cryopreservation of human prophase I oocytes collected from unstimulated follicles. *Fertil Steril* 1994; **61:** 1077–1082.
23. Son WY, Park SE, Lee KA, *et al.* Effects of 1,2-propanediol and freezing–thawing on the in vitro developmental capacity of human immature oocytes. *Fertil Steril* 1996; **66:** 995–999.
24. Tucker MJ, Wright G, Morton PC, Massey JB. Birth after cryopreservation of immature oocytes with subsequent in vitro maturation. *Fertil Steril* 1998; **70:** 578–579.
25. Rao GD, Chian R-C, Son WS, Gilbert L, Tan SL. Fertility preservation in women undergoing cancer treatment. *Lancet* 2004; **363:** 1829–1830.
26. Huang JY, Tulandi T, Holzer H, Tan SL, Chian R-C. Combining ovarian tissue cryobanking with retrieval of immature oocytes followed by in vitro maturation and vitrification: an additional strategy of fertility preservation. *Fertil Steril* 2008; **89:** 567–572.
27. Chian R-C, Gilbert L, Huang JYJ, *et al.* Live birth after vitrification of in vitro matured human oocytes. *Fertil Steril* 2009; **91:** 372–376.
28. Chian R-C, Buckett WM, Tan SL. In-vitro maturation of human oocytes. *Reprod Biomed Online* 2004; **8:** 148–166.
29. Chian R-C, Lim JH, Tan SL. State of the art in in-vitro oocyte maturation. *Curr Opin Obstet Gynecol* 2004; **16:** 211–219.
30. Jurema MW, Nogueira D. In vitro maturation of human oocytes for assisted reproduction. *Fertil Steril* 2006; **86:** 1277–1291.
31. Al-Sunaidi M, Tulandi T, Holzer H, *et al.* Repeated pregnancies and live births after in vitro maturation treatment. *Fertil Steril* 2007; **87:** 1212.e9–e12.
32. Son W-Y, Chung J-T, Chian R-C, *et al.* A 38 h interval between hCG priming and oocyte retrieval increases in vivo and in vitro oocyte maturation rate in programmed IVM cycles. *Hum Reprod* 2008; **23:** 2010–2016.
33. Edwards RG. Foreword. In Tan SL, Chian R-C, Buckett WM, eds. *In Vitro Maturation of Human Oocytes Basic Science to Clinical Application.* London: Informa Healthcare, 2006, pp. xv–xx.
34. Buckett WM, Chian R-C, Holzer H, *et al.* Obstetric outcomes and congenital abnormalities after in vitro maturation, in vitro fertilization, and intracytoplasmic sperm injection. *Obstet Gynecol* 2007; **110:** 885–891.
35. Demirtas E, Elizur S, Holzer H, *et al.* Immature oocyte retrieval in the luteal phase to preserve fertility in women with cancer facing imminent gonadotoxic therapy: it is worth a try. *Reprod Biomed Online* 2008; **17:** 520–523.
36. Luyet B. The vitrification of organic colloids and protoplasm. *Biodynamica* 1937; **1:** 1–14.
37. Fahy G. Prospect for vitrification of whole organs. *Cryobiology* 1981; **18:** 617–625.
38. MacFarlane D, Forsyth M. Recent insights on the role of the cryoprotection against vitrification. *Cryobiology* 1990; **27:** 345–358.
39. Sommerfeld V, Niemann H. Cryopreservation of bovine in vitro produced embryos using ethylene glycol in controlled freezing or vitrification. *Cryobiology* 1999; **38:** 95–105.
40. Emiliani S, Bergh M, Vannin A, Biramane J, Englert Y. Comparison of ethylene glycol, 1,2-propanediol and glycerol for cryopreservation of slow-cooled mouse zygotes, 4-cell embryos and blastocysts. *Hum Reprod* 2000; **15:** 905–910.
41. Shaw J, Oranratnachai A, Trounson A. Fundamental cryobiology of mammalian oocytes and ovarian tissue. *Theriogenology* 2000; **53:** 59–72.
42. Mazur P. Cryobiology: the freezing of biological systems. *Science* 1970; **168:** 939–949.
43. Kasai M. Advances in the cryopreservation of mammalian oocytes and embryos: development of ultrarapid vitrification. *Reprod Med Biol* 2002; **1:** 1–9.
44. Boutron P, Kaufmann A. Stability of the amorphous state in the system water–1,2-propanediol. *Crybiology* 1979; **16:** 557–568.
45. Renard J, Babinet C. High survival of mouse embryos after rapid freezing and thawing inside plastic straws with 1,2-propanediol as cryoprotectant. *J Exp Zool* 1984; **230:** 443–448.
46. Glenister P, Wood M, Kirby C, Whittingham D. Incidence of chromosome anomalies in first-cleavage mouse embryos obtained from frozen–thawed oocytes fertilized in vitro. *Gamete Res* 1987; **16:** 205–216.
47. Kola I, Kirby C, Shaw J, Davey A, Trounson A. Vitrification of mouse oocytes results in aneuploidy zygotes and malformed fetuses. *Teratology* 1988; **38:** 467–474.
48. Vincent C, Preliere G, Pajot-Augy E, *et al.* Effects of cryoprotectants on actin filaments during the

cryopreservation of one-cell rabbit embryos. *Cryobiology* 1990; **27:** 9–23.
49. Gook D, Osborn S, Bourne H, Johnston W. Fertilization of human oocytes following cryopreservation; normal karyotypes and absence of stray chromosome. *Hum Reprod* 1994; **9:** 684–691.
50. van Blerkom J, Davis P. Cytogenic, cellular, and developmental consequences of cryopreservation of immature and mature mouse and human oocytes. *Micro Res Tech* 1994; **27:** 165–193.
51. Vincent C, Johnson MH. Cooling, cryoprotectants, and the cytoskeleton of the mammalian oocyte. *Oxford Rev Reprod Biol* 1992; **14:** 73–100.
52. Gook D, Osborn S, Johnson W. Cryopreservation of mouse and human oocytes using 1,2-propanediol and the configuration of the meiotic spindle *Hum Reprod* 1993; **8:** 1101–1109.
53. Sathananthan AH, Trounson A, Freeman L. Morphology and fertilization of frozen human oocytes. *Gamete Res* 1987; **16:** 343–354.
54. Eroglu A, Toner M, Leykin L, Toth TL. Cytoskeleton and polyploidy after maturation and fertilization of cryopreserved germinal vesicle-stage mouse oocytes. *J Assist Reprod Genet* 1998; **15:** 447–454.
55. Eroglu A, Toth TL, Toner M. Alterations of the cytoskeleton and polyploidy induced by cryopreservation of metaphase II mouse oocytes. *Fertil Steril* 1998; **69:** 944–957.
56. Huang JY, Chen HY, Tan SL, Chian R-C. Effects of osmotic stress and cryoprotectant toxicity on mouse oocyte fertilization and subsequent embryonic development in vitro. *Cell Preserv Tech* 2006; **4:** 149–160.
57. Ali J, Shelton J. Vitrification of preimplantation stages of mouse embryos. *J Reprod Fertil* 1993; **98:** 459–465.
58. Mukaida T, Wada S, Takahashi K, *et al.* Vitrification of human embryos based on the assessment of suitable conditions for 8-cell mouse embryos. *Hum Reprod* 1998; **13:** 2874–2879.
59. Kasai M, Komi J, Takakamo A, *et al.* A simple method for mouse embryo cryopreservation in a low toxicity vitrification solution, without appreciable loss of viability. *J Reprod Fertil* 1990; **89:** 91–97.
60. Vajta G, Nagy ZP. Are programmable freezers still needed in the embryo laboratory? Review on vitrification. *Reprod Biomed Online* 2006; **12:** 779–796.
61. Kuwayama M, Vajta G, Ieda S, Kato O. Comparison of open and closed methods for vitrification of human embryos and the elimination of potential contamination. *Reprod Biomed Online* 2005; **11:** 608–614.
62. Lane M, Bavister B, Lyons E, Forest K. Container-less vitrification of mammalian oocytes and embryos. *Nat Biotechnol* 1999; **17:** 1234–1236.
63. Lane M, Schoolcraft W, Gardner D. Vitrification of mouse and human blastocysts using a novel cryoloop container-less technique. *Fertil Steril* 1999; **72:** 1073–1078.
64. Vajta G, Holm P, Kuwayama M, *et al.* Open pulled straw (OPS) vitrification: a new way to reduce cryoinjuries of bovine ova and embryos. *Mol Reprod Dev* 1998; **51:** 53–58.
65. Vanderzwalmen P, Bertin G, Debauche C, *et al.* Vitrification of human blastocysts with the Hemi-Straw carrier: application of assisted hatching after thawing. *Hum Reprod* 2003; **18:** 1504–1511.
66. Martino A, Songsasen N, Leibo S. Development into blastocysts of bovine oocytes cryopreserved by ultra-rapid cooling. *Biol Reprod* 1996; **54:** 1059–1069.
67. Huang JYJ, Chen HY, Tan SL, Chian R-C. Effect of choline-supplemented sodium-depleted slow freezing versus vitrification on mouse oocyte meiotic spindles and chromosome abnormalities. *Fertil Steril* 2007; **88:** 1093–1100.
68. Huang JYJ, Chen HY, Park JYS, Tan SL, Chian R-C. Comparison of spindle and chromosome configuration in in vitro- and in vivo-matured mouse oocytes after vitrification. *Fertil Steril* 2008; **90:** 1424–1432.
69. Steer CV, Mills CL, Tan SL, Campbell S, Edwards RG. The cumulative embryo score: a predictive embryo scoring technique to select the optimal number of embryos to transfer in an in-vitro fertilization and embryo transfer programme. *Hum Reprod* 1992; **7:** 117–119.
70. Child TJ, Abdul-Jalil AK, Tan SL. Embryo morphology, cumulative embryo score, and outcome in an oocyte in vitro maturation program. *Fertil Steril* 2002; **77:** 424–425.
71. Chian R-C, Kuwayama M, Tan L, Tan J, Kato O, Nagai T. High survival rate of bovine oocytes matured in vitro following vitrification. *J Reprod Dev* 2004; **50:** 685–696.
72. Donnez J, Dolmans MM, Demylle D, *et al.* Restoration of ovarian function after orthotopic (intraovarian and periovarian) transplantation of cryopreserved ovarian tissue in a woman treated by bone marrow transplantation for sickle cell anaemia: case report. *Hum Reprod* 2006; **21:** 183–188.
73. Gunby J, Daya S. Assisted reproductive technologies (ART) in Canada: 2003 results from the Canadian ART Register. *Fertil Steril* 2007; **88:** 550–559.
74. Andersen AN, Gianaroli L, Felberbaum R, de Mouzon J, Nygren KG. Assisted reproductive technology in Europe, 2002. Results generated from European registers by ESHRE. *Hum Reprod* 2006; **21:** 1680–1697.
75. Chian R-C, Huang JYJ, Tan SL, *et al.* Obstetric and perinatal outcome in 200 infants conceived from vitrified oocytes. *Reprod Biomed Online* 2008; **16:** 608–610.
76. American Cancer Society. *Cancer Facts and Figures, 2006*. Atlanta, GA: American Cancer Society, 2006.
77. Ries L, Percy C, Bunin G. Introduction. In Gurney J, Linet M, Tamra T, Young J, Bunin G, eds. *Cancer*

Incidence and Survival among Children and Adolescents: United States SEER Program 1975–1995. [NIH Pub No 99–4649.] Bethesda, MD: National Cancer Institute, 1999, pp. 1–15.

78. Lobo RA. Potential options for preservation of fertility in women. *N Engl J Med* 2005; **353:** 64–73.
79. Bleyer W. The impact of childhood cancer on the United States and the world. *Cancer* 1990; **40:** 355–367.
80. Tulandi T, Al-Took S. Laparoscopic ovarian suspension before irradiation. *Fertil Steril* 1998; **70:** 381–183.
81. Oktay K, Demirtas E, Son WY, *et al.* In vitro maturation of germinal vesicle oocytes recovered after premature luteinizing hormone surge: description of a novel approach to fertility preservation. *Fertil Steril* 2008; **89:** 228.e19–e22.
82. Huang JY, Buckett WM, Gilbert L, Tan SL, Chian R-C. Retrieval of immature oocytes followed by in vitro maturation and vitrification: a case report on a new strategy of fertility preservation in women with borderline ovarian malignancy. *Gynecol Oncol* 2007; **105:** 542–544.
83. Gidoni Y, Holzer H, Tan SL, Tulandi T. Fertility preservation in non-oncologic patients. *Reprod Biomed Online* 2008;**16:** 792–800.
84. Elizur SE, Chian R, Pineau CA, *et al.* Fertility preservation treatment for young women with autoimmune disease facing treatment with gonadotoxic agents. *Rheumatology* 2008; **47:** 1506–1509.
85. Elizur SE, Chian R-C, Holzer HEG, *et al.* Cryopreservation of oocytes in a young woman with severe and symptomatic endometriosis: a new indication for fertility preservation. *Fertil Steril* 2009; **91:** 293. e1–e3.
86. Lau NM, Huang JYJ, MacDonald S, *et al.* Feasibility of fertility preservation in young females with Turner syndrome. *Reprod Biomed Online* 2008; **17:** 520–523.
87. Huang JY, Tulandi T, Holzer H, *et al.* Cryopreservation of ovarian tissue and in-vitro matured oocytes in a female with mosaic Turner syndrome *Hum Reprod* 2008; **23:** 336–339.
88. Huang JY, Tulandi T, Holzer H, *et al.* Increased maternal cardiovascular mortality associated with pregnancy in women with Turner syndrome. *Fertil Steril* 2006; **86**: S127–S128.
89. Gidoni YS, Takefman J, Holzer HEG, *et al.* Cryopreservation of a mother's oocytes for possible future use by her daughter with Turner syndrome: case report. *Fertil Steril* 2008; **90:** e9–e12.
90. Heffner LJ. Advanced maternal age: how old is too old? *N Engl J Med* 2004; **351:** 1927–1929.

Chapter 18

Cryopreservation of human oocytes and embryos either by direct plunging into liquid nitrogen or by using an aseptic approach

Evgenia Isachenko, Vladimir Isachenko, Jurgen M. Weiss, and Rolf Kreienberg

Introduction

The cryopreservation of human oocytes and blastocysts is an important topic in assisted reproduction. First, cryopreservation of germinal vesicle (GV) stage oocytes allows the elimination or reduction of the need for medication to stimulate folliculogenesis and allows oocyte cryobanking (e.g. for young women who wish to delay motherhood until a later date) [1]. Second, it is illegal in some countries to cryopreserve oocytes after fusion of the pronuclei. Third, the blastocyst is a very favorable stage for embryo transfer, as this can achieve live birth rates >40% for the fresh transfer and a cumulative healthy baby rate of >65% per retrieval once additional cryostored blastocysts have been transferred [2–4]. Additionally, during blastulation, the number of cells increases from 10 to more than 100, accompanied by certain developmental processes, such as mitochondrial-dependent nucleic acid synthesis [5], epigenomic revision plus chromosome X inactivation [6], and increased genetic transcription [7]; these allow a process of self-selection that will reduce the prevalence of the more lethal monosomic aneuploidies [8].

The first births from cryopreserved human oocytes were reported almost 20 years ago by Chen [9], van Uem *et al.* [10], and Al-Hasani *et al.* [11]. These, as well as others [12–15], have used conventional (programmed or slow) freezing methods. However, the results obtained with this slow-freezing mode of cryopreservation of oocytes are quite variable [15,16]. However, conventional slow freezing is a widely used method for pronuclear zygotes and embryos [17–24], and numerous babies have been born after the transfer of embryos derived from frozen pronuclear zygotes with the slow-freezing method. Nevertheless, the low efficacy of the zygote freezing technique is indicated by the pregnancy rates from this technique, which are lower than those resulting from the use of fresh pronuclear zygotes.

There have been recent reports of successful cryopreservation by direct plunging of human metaphase II (MII) ooccytes [25–28], pronuclear zygotes [29–36], and blastocysts [37–46] into liquid nitrogen, a process known as vitrification. This method is currently under intensive investigation in numerous laboratories. Vitrification has the following major advantages over slow freezing:

- speed: the complete procedure requires only a few minutes
- economy: it does not need special equipment.

Glass formation during the cooling phase of vitrification and stability of the amorphous state of the solution during warming have been reported [47]. It was reported that the critical cooling rate of a 40% dimethyl sulfoxide (DMSO) solution (which is a better glass former than ethylene glycol) to avoid ice formation was 500°C/min, and the calculated critical warming rate to avoid ice formation (devitrification) was over one billion degrees per minute [47]. Despite the fact that in the solution described by Baudot *et al.* [47] the base medium and serum solutes provided additional stability against ice formation, a concentration of 30% penetrating cryoprotectants was not able to prevent ice forming during the cooling and, particularly, during the described warming conditions. This explains why these protocols do not involve "real" vitrification, and in this chapter we use the term "rapid freezing" rather than vitrification and "thawing" instead of warming.

Initially, the standard 0.25 ml insemination straws were almost exclusively used as the carrier devices for the cryopreservation of embryos or oocytes by vitrification [48], which allowed a cooling rate of approximately 2500°C/min [49]. New methods are based on the immersion of very small amounts (0.5–1.0 μl) of solutions into liquid nitrogen and most authors have attributed the improved developmental rate

Fertility Cryopreservation, ed. Ri-Cheng Chian and Patrick Quinn. Published by Cambridge University Press.

for cells after cryopreservation using these techniques to the increased speed of freezing and thawing (> 10 000°C/min) that can be achieved [50–55]. These newer methods all

- expose the biological material to a high concentration of vitrification solution
- have direct contact of the biological material with liquid nitrogen during cooling.

There is a potential risk of cross-contamination during the short time of direct contact with liquid nitrogen, and during the long-term banking of cells if specimens are not properly sealed [56–61]. Even vapor from liquid nitrogen can be contaminated by microorganisms [62]. However, if the specimens are isolated from liquid nitrogen in order to avoid such potential problems, there is a consequent decrease in the speed of cooling and most authors consider that this will decrease the efficacy of the vitrification protocol. Because of this issue, we have developed an aseptic vitrification system, the cut standard straws (CSS), which completely prevents contact with liquid nitrogen during any of the steps [63].

Currently the evaluatation of the quality of both oocytes and embryos before or during in vitro culture and after thawing is subjective [64,65]. To improve or develop techniques it is necessary to have a system of scoring the quality of biological material with strict criteria. We have paid special attention to the quality of pronuclei before and after vitrification. The morphology of cells in both oocyte and blastocyst and, in our opinion, the morphological integrity rate of the pronuclei of zygotes and the nuclei of embryos can be valuable criteria for assessing cryostability, developmental potential, and/or the effectiveness of a cryopreservation protocol. However, there are few data that correlate the post-thawing integrity of pronuclei with the potential for embryos to develop and implant. Consequently, our aim has been to assess:

- the viability of human oocytes, pronuclear zygotes, and blastocysts subjected to either a non-aseptic vitrification using decreased concentrations of permeable cryoprotectants in a process that directly submerges a CSS in liquid nitrogen or an aseptic vitrification with cooling of the CSS within a closed 0.5 ml straw
- the integrity rate of pronuclei after cryopreservation of pronuclear zygotes as a possible predictor of future embryo development and implantation.

Aseptic vitrification

The cooling protocol

When developing the aseptic CSS packaging system, we considered aspects of effectiveness and simplicity of handling. As a prototype for the CSS [67], the open pulled straw was fitted within a standard 0.25 ml insemination straw and hermetically closed by metal balls at both ends (Figure 18.1). Any contact between the metal ball and the vitrification solution holding the oocytes was prevented by the meniscus of the vitrification solution. The CSS was made from a standard 0.25 ml insemination straw cut at an angle of approximately 45° (Figure. 18.2). After appropriate exposure to equilibration solution, one or two oocytes or embryos in 0.5–0.75 μl of the final vitrification solution were placed in the cut part of the straw (Figure 18.2). The rate of cooling during direct immersion of the CSS into liquid nitrogen was approximately 15 000°C/min whereas it was approximately 600°C/min with the aseptic version of the CSS ("straw in straw") [63,66,67].

The cooling and warming techniques are described below. The vitrification solution that was tested with these package systems contained DMSO and ethylene glycol at a combined concentration of 40%. While we obtained relatively high maturation rates for GV oocytes after warming [67], and there was no statistical difference between open and closed ("straw in straw") systems (71% and 72%, respectively), we considered it was important to develop a new CSS system because we did not consider that the closed system could be

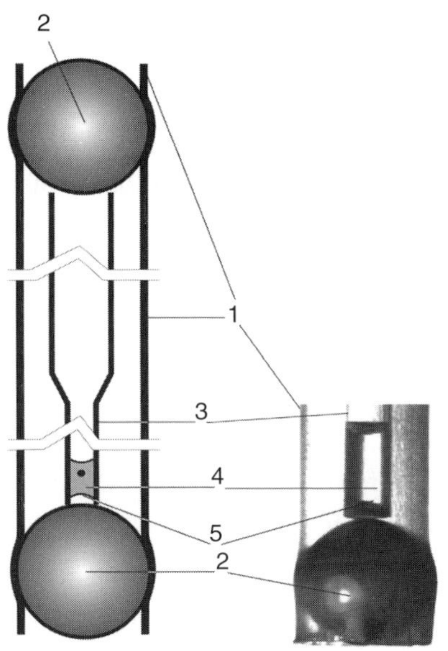

Figure 18.1. The aseptic packaging system using a 0.5 ml standard insemination straw (1) hermetically sealed by balls (2) as a package for a standard open pulled straw (3). A drop of cryopreservation solution with cells (4) can be seen and the meniscus of the vitrification medium (5).

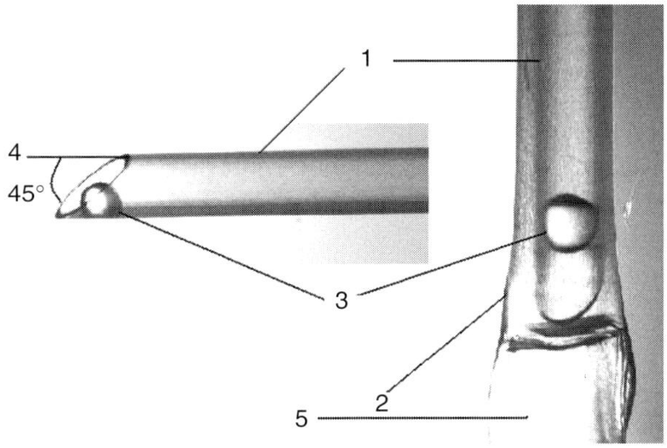

Figure 18.2. Aseptic packaging using a cut standard straw (1) placed within the 0.5 ml standard insemination (packaging) straw (2) and containing a drop of cryopreservation solution with cells (3). The insemination straw is cut at an angle (4) and is hermetically sealed (5).

considered as really closed. The contact between the metal ball and the plastic tube wall was not a complete seal and any micro-cracks formed in this contact area could allow penetration of the liquid nitrogen and eventually contamination of the sample.

The warming protocol

The warming process used involved partially removing the packaging tube from the liquid nitrogen at the opposite end to the oocyte/embryo location. This end of sealed packaging straw was then cut and the open pulled straw or CSS was quickly removed from the packaging and submerged into a tube containing 1.5 ml of dilution solution at 40°C. This procedure produces a warming rate of approximately 30 000–90 000°C/min. This is then followed by stepwise removal of cryoprotectants. The rate of warming can be calculated from the Biot–Fourier equation for heat transfer in a thermal conductor. In a general form for an isotropic material with no internal heat sources [68], the rate of warming ($\partial T/\partial t$) is given by

$$\partial T/\partial t = D_T \nabla^2 T$$

where T is temperature; t is time; D_T is the temperature diffusivity ($\kappa/c\rho$, where κ is the thermal conductivity, c is the specific heat capacity, and ρ is the density of the conductor), and $\nabla^2 T$ is the Laplace operator.

For simplicity, the pellet is considered to be warmed in a CSS as a homogeneous sphere with initial temperature T_0 immersed into a highly thermoconductive medium with temperature T_f. The heat flow distribution is then dependent only on the distance from the center to the position in consideration (r), and is independent of the spherical angles θ and φ. This is effectively a one-dimensional case [69]. The heat transfer can then be expressed as [68]:

$$T(r,t) = \left(\frac{4}{\pi}\right)\left(T_f - T_0\right)\sum_{m=1}^{\infty} \frac{\sin(2m+1)\pi\left(\frac{r}{R}\right)}{2m+1} e^{-[(2m+1)\pi]^2\left(\frac{t}{\tau}\right)}$$

where d is the thickness of the film and $\tau = d^2/D_T$ is the characteristic time after which all the processes are practically equilibrated.

According to our calculations [69], nearly the whole droplet is in equilibrium with the warming surrounding at time $q = 0.4\tau$, so even the center at $\lambda = 0$ is warmed to approximately 268K (−5°C) at that time. Consequently, it is safe to assume that the system is in full equilibrium at approximately 0.45τ. After that, the droplet devitrifies, detaches from the surfaces, and dissolves in the medium. The rate of warming (B) can be estimated as:

$$B \approx \frac{T_f - T_0}{0.45\tau}$$

Taking into the account that for ice $\kappa = 0.005$ cal/s per cm per degree K, $c = 0.49$ cal/g per degree K, and $\rho = 0.92$ g/cm^3 [70], this gives $D_T = 0.011$ cm^2/s. A spherical droplet of volume 0.75 µl has radius of 0.056 cm, so the characteristic time for heat equilibration (τ) can be estimated as aproximately 0.3 s. That means that the rate of warming will be approximately 90 000°C/min. The presence of sucrose and DMSO will affect viscosity and vitrification kinetics but the value for the rate of warming will be in same range [69]. Most authors credit the high effectiveness of protocols of vitrification of oocytes and embryos using decreased volumes of samples to the higher rates of cooling. Our results with human oocytes do not support this view. The survival and development rates for human GV oocytes and pronuclear zygotes were as efficient with the relatively slow cooling rate as with the rapid cooling rates of "conventional" vitrification. It should be remembered that rapid warming has always been a crucial point for successful vitrification [67,71].

Vitrification of specific stages

The discussion will now move on to considerations of the vitrification procedure for different stages of oocytes during maturation, including fertilized embryos and blastocysts.

Vitrification of germinal vesicle oocytes

The potential of vitrification as a method of cryopreservation was shown for the first time in 1985 [72] when vitrification was successfully applied to immature oocytes. Usually the vitrification protocol contained DMSO. However, there are no data regarding the use of DMSO for the vitrification of GV oocytes and, therefore, we performed a series of experiments to investigate the role of DMSO during the vitrification of GV oocytes. This cryoprotectant has been reported to affect the organization of microfilaments in mouse oocytes [73] as well as to induce chromosomal abnormalities leading to an increase in the rates of degeneration and digenic polyploid embryos after cryopreservation [74]. Consequently, we also examined the possibility of cryopreserving GV oocytes using a solution completely free of DMSO (40% ethylene glycol plus 0.75 M sucrose). If DMSO is not present in the vitrification medium, there is a significant decrease in maturation rates (51%) compared with GV oocytes vitrified in the presence of DMSO (85%). However, the long contact period (5 minutes) of oocytes with the vitrification solution containing 20% DMSO at 37°C in both "direct" and "straw in straw" vitrification was enough to cause spontaneous oocyte activation and parthenogenetic development. The protocol that we now recommend for use in medical practice is a compromise between avoiding use of DMSO in the vitrification medium and the parthenogenetic activation that it causes. Based on our results we propose the following protocol.

1. Exposure in three steps to a pre-warming solution (37°C) containing 20%, 33%, and 50% DMSO (in 40% ethylene glycol plus 0.75 M sucrose) for 2, 1, and 1 minute, respectively.
2. One-step exposure to a vitrification solution with 20% DMSO in 20% ethylene glycol plus 0.75 M sucrose for 1 minute at room temperature, with subsequent cooling in liquid nitrogen.

This protocol has a short (1 minute) period of contact with a high DMSO concentration, in the last of the stepped portion of the protocol, followed by contact with DMSO at room temperature, which in theory can decrease the negative effects on oocytes. The high maturation rates and the absence of parthenogenesis seen support the use of DMSO with decreasing time and temperature of contact for vitrification of human GV oocytes.

The use of DMSO in a vitrification medium for human reproductive cells is supported by studies by Vanderzwalmen *et al.* [38], Huang *et al.* [75], and Isachenko *et al.* [67], who have all used DMSO for vitrification of blastocysts. These authors all reported high pregnancy rates after warming of blastocysts (41% [38] and 54% [75]) as well as evidence of the efficiency of a vitrification media containing 20% DMSO, 20% ethylene glycol, sucrose, and other compounds. These pregnancies resulted in the birth of healthy babies: P. Vanderzwalmen (personal communication) reported 98 healthy births including 28 twins from 414 warmed and transferred embryos; C. C. Huang and T. H. Lee (personal communication) reported 10 healthy births from 14 implantations, with three spontaneous abortions and one reduction from triplet. Using DMSO for vitrification of oocytes was also successful, with a high survival rate of warmed oocytes, ongoing clinical pregnancy [28], and later birth of healthy babies after embryo transfers (K. P. Katayama, personal communication).

Our studies also examined if vitrification of GV oocytes could be performed using the aseptic technology that we had initially developed for human and mouse pronuclear zygotes, embryos, and human spermatozoa [71,76,77]. Aseptic vitrification using a "straw in straw" system leads to decreased cooling rates. Rall [78] reported in 1987 that cooling rates of 10°C/min were sufficient for vitrification of mouse embryos. The speed of warming is a very important parameter in a vitrification procedure. All combinations of "slow" or "quick" cooling with "slow" warming have resulted in decreased viability of vitrified mouse embryos [79]. Elevated warming rates and the absence of visible crystal formation during thawing of oocytes was shown to be most effective when the proportion of "speed of warming to speed of cooling" was higher than 1.3 [80,81]. These observations about the lesser importance of the speed of cooling for the vitrification of human pronuclear oocytes can probably be applied to all human reproductive cells, including spermatozoa. We recently reported that vitrification of human spermatozoa by fast (20 000°C/min) or relatively slow (600°C/min and 200°C/min) cooling resulted in similar post-thaw characteristics [82] and that slow cooling/rapid warming can also be applied to human GV oocytes. In fact, this approach allowed maturation rates for GV oocytes after vitrification of around 85%. This high rate is promising for future applications of cryopreservation of GV oocytes for reproductive purposes.

Vitrification of fertilized (pronuclear) zygotes: integrity rate of pronuclei as a criterion of effectiveness

The following cryopreservation protocol has been tested for vitrification of pronuclear zygotes using the CSS packaging system. The rapid freezing solution contained 15% ethylene glycol, 15% DMSO, and 0.2 M sucrose. Pre-cooling treatment of the zygotes consisted of stepwise exposure to 12%, 25%, 50%, and 100% (v/v) of the vitrification solution for 2 minutes, 1 minute, 1 minute, and 30–50 seconds, respectively, before placing them in the CSS packaging system. Although the term vitrification is used for this protocol, at the relatively slow speed of cooling (600°C/min), an ice-free state of vitrification medium is not maintained through cooling and warming.

The quality of pronuclei was examined 17–18 hours after fertilization. Zygotes and pronuclear morphology were scored visually on an inverted microscope at magnification of 400×. The *Z*-score of zygotes was derived as described by Scott *et al.* [83]. Grades Z1, Z2, Z3, and Z4 corresponded to *Z*-scores of 6%, 37%, 47%, and 10%, respectively (Figure 18.3). Photographic records were taken at the time of pronucleus assessment and during subsequent in vitro development after 8, 24, 48, 72, 80, 92, 100, and 120 hours in both fresh and vitrified zygotes [84]. A satisfactory integrity rate of pronuclei was detected in 85% of the zygotes (Figure 18.3). There was a correlation between the scoring group and the post-thawing pronuclear integrity rate. Only one zygote from seven in the Z2 group and one zygote from eight in the Z3 group had low post-thawing integrity rate. In contrast, approximately half of the zygotes in the Z1 group had poor pronuclear integrity rate. Cryostability in the mid range was observed in zygotes from the Z4 group: one of five zygotes had a low post-thaw integrity rate for pronuclei (Figure 18.3).

The integrity rate of zygote pronuclei after thawing could be distributed into two groups, high and low [84]. The appearance of the membrane and nucleoli of the two pronuclei was assessed. In the initial planning, it was intended to determine post-thawing integrity rate based on the these two elements, membrane and nucleoli, separately, allowing distribution of zygotes into four groups: (1) high integrity rate for pronuclear membranes and nucleoli in both pronuclei; (2) high integrity rate for pronuclear membranes plus a low rate for nucleoli in both pronuclei; (3) a low integrity rate for both pronuclear membranes and a high one for nucleoli in both pronuclei; and (4) a low integrity rate for pronuclear membranes and nucleoli in both pronuclei. After 10 minutes of thawing, the zygotes would be assessed to see if they had a clearly observable border of pronuclear membrane and at least half of the chromatin in a condensed form as nucleoli; this was considered as a high integrity rate (Figure 18.4a–e). If it was not possible to clearly observe any structure in these two elements in the pronuclei, the integrity rate was denoted as low (Figures 18.5a–d and 18.6a–d). However, it became clear that it was not necessary to evaluate these two elements separately, because if the integrity rate of a nuclear membrane was high, the rate of at least half of the nucleoli was also high.

We have noted that, as a rule, the integrity rate is high soon after thawing for the pronuclear membrane but not for the appearance of pronuclei. It is only 10 minutes after thawing and washing that the nucleoli can be clearly seen [66]. We have established a direct correlation between the post-thawing integrity rates of the pronuclear membrane and nucleoli. Our data indicate that zygote in vitro developmental rates up to the expanded blastocyst stage were 39% (291 from 732 zygotes) if the integrity rate of pronuclei was high, and 4% (5 from 130) if the integrity rate was low (Figure 18.7). Figures 18.4–18.6, illustrate different cases of

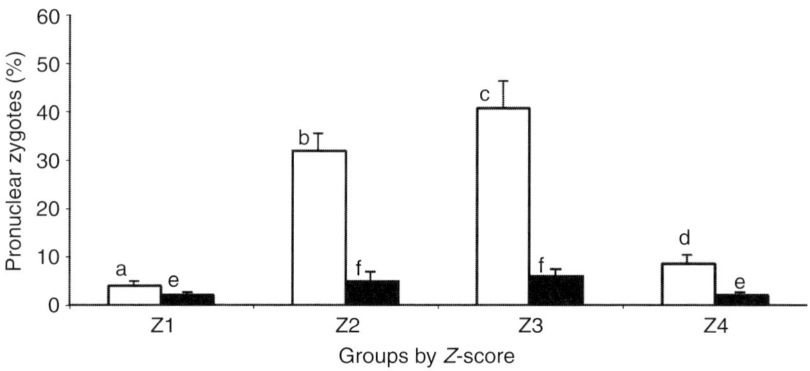

Figure 18.3. Scoring of cryopreserved pronuclear zygotes and their post-thaw integrity rates: 732 zygotes had a high integrity rate (white columns) and 130 had a low rate (black columns). The groups Z1–Z4 correspond to Z-score groups, see text [83]. Different letters above the columns indicate significant differences ($p < 0.05$); the same letters indicate no significant differences ($p > 0.1$).

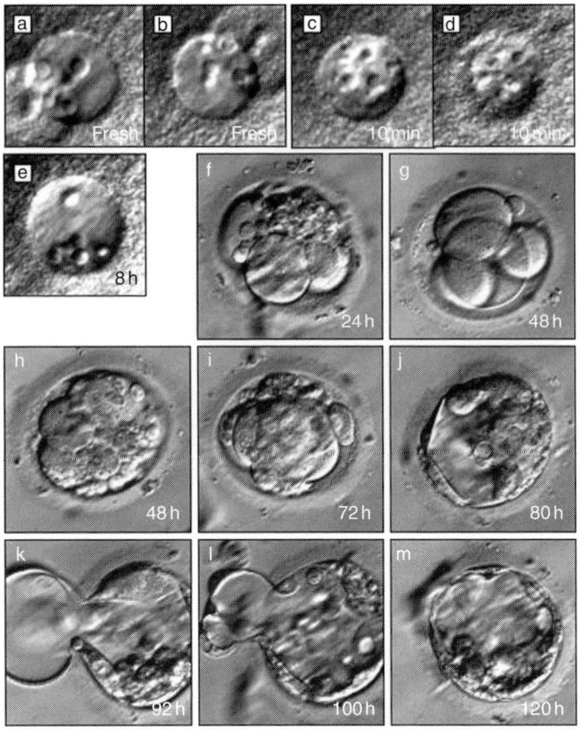

Figure 18.4. Two two-pronuclear zygotes scored as Z2: development dependent on the post-thaw integrity rate of the pronuclei. (a,b) Fresh pronucleus; (c,d) pronucleus after thawing; (e–m) embryos after the given times in in vitro culture; (g,h) the same embryo at 48 h photographed with a different focus, demonstrating fragmentation; (m) the 5 day blastocyst transferred.

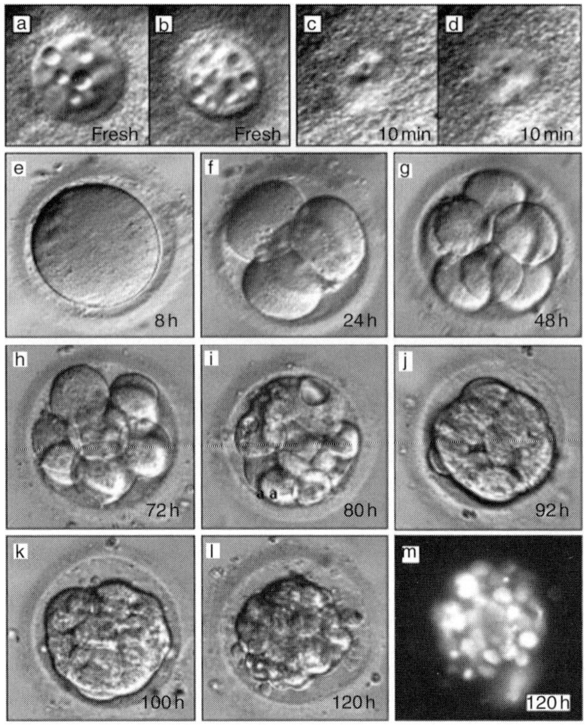

Figure 18.5. Two two-pronuclear zygotes scored as Z3: development dependent on the post-thaw integrity rate of the pronuclei. (a,b) Fresh pronucleus; (c,d) pronucleus after thawing; (e–m) embryos after the given times in in vitro culture; (m) stained by Hoechst 33342, which indicates normal cleavage and the location of nuclear chromatin.

pronuclei post-thawing integrity rate and the subsequent development of zygotes. Good pronuclear integrity rate resulted in the development of embryos to blastocysts with a high implantation rate after transfer (Figure 18.4). Based on these observations, we consider that the regularity of the integrity rate of the pronuclei after thawing of zygotes plays an important role as a predictor of future development

The protocol in a number of laboratories is to presuppose transfer of a single blastocyst and the decision on quality of thawed zygotes, usually one or two pronuclear zygotes, is only made after they have been in culture for 5 days. If at this point these zygotes do not demonstrate development to blastocyst stage, then their transfer is probably useless. We suggest that assessment of the integrity rate of the pronuclei should be considered immediately after thawing of zygotes. If this rate is high in at least one zygote, the zygotes can then be cultured for 5 days. If the integrity rate is low, then the developmental prognosis is extremely low and more zygotes should be thawed.

The initial zygote score (Z1–Z4) appears to have less of an impact on both development and implantation ability after freezing and thawing than does the recovery of the integrity of the pronuclei. Post-warming pronuclear integrity rate refers more generally to cellular integrity. However, it is possible that the use of a more detailed zygote scoring may allow for a greater correlation between scoring of zygotes and cryostability of pronuclei. For example, it has been reported that a cumulative pronuclear score might be used as a single prognostic tool for predicting the implantation potential of both fresh and frozen–thawed zygotes [85].

Osmosis plays a central role in all the negative effects of the cryopreservation process for human pronuclear embryos [86–88]. We have shown that, in contrast with zygotes of animal species, human pronuclear zygotes that were vitrified, warmed, and directly rehydrated with intense osmotic processes were completely destroyed [86]. As exposure to cryoprotectants is also accompanied by osmotic processes, our aseptic technology includes a stepwise method of addition of

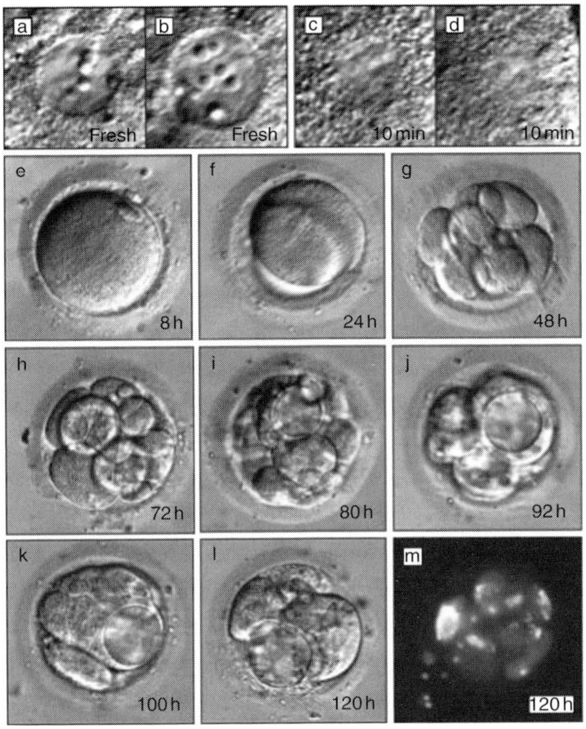

Figure 18.6. Two two-pronuclear zygotes scored as Z4: development dependent on the post-thaw integrity rate of pronuclei. (a,b) Fresh pronucleus; (c,d) pronucleus after thawing; (e–m) embryos after the given times in in vitro culture; (m) stained by Hoechst 33342 shows defective cleavage and abnormal dispersion of nuclear chromatin.

cryoprotectants [66]. The results from these studies clearly show that the membranes of nuclei are more sensitive to osmotic stress than the membrane of nucleoli, and that the integrity rate of these nucleoli membranes is the most informative criteria for the integrity rate of human pronuclear zygotes after cryopreservation.

The photographs of cryopreserved fertilized oocytes and developing embryos were analyzed for other potential prognostic criteria and their relationship to post-thawing integrity rate of the cells and their subsequent development, including the appearance of blastomere fragmentation and vacuolization of the developing embryos. We concluded that fragmentation was an "automatic" process and not connected with the cryostability of pronuclear zygotes. In zygotes with a high integrity rate of pronuclei after thawing and good developmental rate to blastocysts, intensive fragmentation was often observed (Figure 18.4f–i). Zygote in vitro developmental rates up to the expanded blastocyst stage were 39% if the integrity rate of pronuclei was high, and 4% if the integrity rate was low (Figure 18.7). In contrast to fragmentation, vacuolization was associated with low developmental potential of the zygotes. Morphology of the developing embryos (Figures 18.5e–h and 18.6e–h) at 72 hours of culture looked good. Later, however, the appearance of vacuoles (Figures 18.5i and 18.6i) predicted defective development.

Disruption of chromatin was not connected directly with defective cleavage of embryos, reflected in non-development to the blastocyst stage. For example, some zygotes with a low post-thawing integrity rate developed to compacted morula (Figure 18.5) or early blastocyst but then stopped developing. Serious chromatin abnormalities in such embryos were not detected. In contrast, deformation of chromatin was detected in embryos with intensive vacuolization (Figure 18.6). Immunofluorescent staining of some embryos, which had not developed to blastocysts, indicated normal cleavage in the absence of nuclear chromatin deformation (Figure 18.5). In contrast, staining of some embryos that had intensive vacuolization of cytoplasm and also defective cleavage showed deformation of nuclear chromatin (Figure 18.6). In both cases of degenerative development of cultured embryos, the post-warming pronuclear integrity rate of the zygotes was low. After transfer of 296 5-day blastocysts to 296 recipients, 126 patients (43%) became pregnant. The pregnancy rate was dependent on the pronuclear integrity rate after transfer, being 43% with a high rate and 13% with a low rate (Figure 18.8) [63].

Vitrification of blastocysts

It is already known that the embryo is less affected by low temperatures than the various stages of oocytes. However, among the different developmental stages of pre-implantation embryos, the blastocyst stage is the more sensitive to the influences of low temperatures because it comprises two different phases: the liquid contained in the blastocele and the cellular component. Theoretically, as the GV oocytes and pronuclear zygotes can tolerate the vitrification procedure when using "slow" cooling and very "fast" warming in the presence of decreased concentrations of permeable cryoprotectants, then the CSS packaging system could be used in these stages.

The usefulness of DMSO for the vitrification of blastocysts has been reported. A 33% pregnancy rate and birth of a healthy baby have been obtained when blastocysts were vitrified using ethylene glycol and DMSO [89]. Subsequently, the same clinic vitrified two

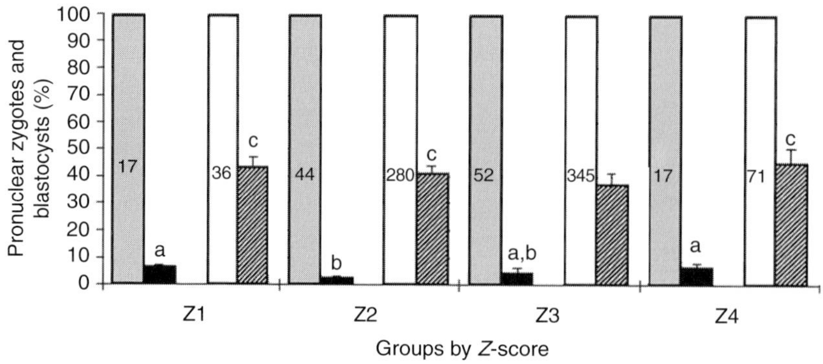

Figure 18.7. Blastocyst formation from cryopreserved pronuclear zygotes is dependent on the quality of pronuclei (Z-scoring [83]; see text) and their post-thaw integrity rate: zygotes with low pronuclei integrity rates (130; gray columns); zygotes with high pronuclei integrity rates (732; white columns); blastocysts from zygotes with low pronuclei integrity rates (5; black columns); blastocysts from zygotes with high pronuclei integrity rates (291; hatched columns). Numbers on the columns indicate the number in that group. Different letters above the columns indicate significant differences ($p < 0.05$).

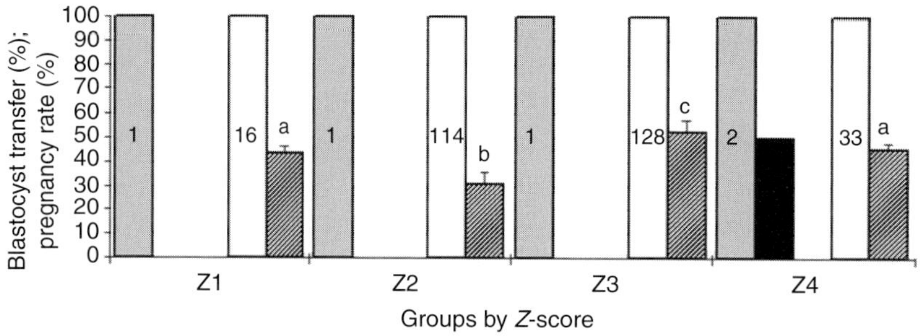

Figure 18.8. Pregnancy rate after transfer of blastocysts is dependent on the quality of the pronuclei (Z-scoring [83]; see text)and their post-thaw integrity rate: blastocysts from zygotes with low pronuclei integrity rates (5; gray columns); blastocysts from zygotes with high pronuclei integrity rates (291; white columns); pregnancies after transfer of blastocysts from zygotes with low pronuclei integrity rates (1; black columns); pregnancies after transfer of blastocysts from zygotes with high pronuclei integrity rates (125; hatched columns). Numbers on the columns indicate the number in that group. Different letters above the columns indicate significant differences ($p < 0.05$).

embryos at the morula stage using the same protocol, resulting in the birth of healthy twins [90]. Up to March 2005, 86 healthy babies have been born after the transfer of 332 embryos (birth rate 26%) using the vitrification solution containing ethylene glycol and DMSO (Y. Yokota, personal communication).

We found that developmental rates for vitrified blastocysts after cryopreservation with the non-packaged CSS (direct contact with liquid nitrogen) were very similar with either increased (20% DMSO, 20% EG, sucrose) or decreased (15% DMSO, 15% EG, sucrose) concentrations of permeable cryoprotectants with subsequent in vitro culture: 85% and 86%, respectively [84]. We have also tested two different packaging systems [84], one that does not prevent contact with liquid nitrogen and one that completely prevents contact. Both systems showed the same rate of re-expansion after in vitro culture: 81% and 80%, respectively. The re-expansion (the blastocele) of viable embryos usually begins 2 to 6 hours after warming. The collapse of a blastocyst (when its appearance is similar to that of a compact morula) is a sign of viability of the embryo after warming, and embryos were not viable after vitrification if the collapse of the blastocysts did not occur in the first 10 minutes after warming.

We know that embryos with a laser-opened zona pellucida are more difficult to cryopreserve than early blastocysts or blastocysts with an intact zona pellucida. An early report found that the survival rate of expanded blastocysts after vitrification was relatively low. The authors attributed this to the large volume of water in the blastocele and its lethal crystallization during cooling [91]. Laser opening of the zona pellucida can also decrease the cryosurvival of blastocysts; however, the reports on vitrification of laser-treated blastocysts are limited [43].

We have tried the new CSS method of vitrification on laser-hatched blastocysts that had been chosen for embryo transfer. Clinical pregnancies using CSS vitrification with direct contact with liquid nitrogen and the aseptic CSS "straw-in-straw" method were established in 6 of 18 patients (33%) in both groups, as determined by the presence of a fetal sac by ultrasound 6 weeks after embryo transfer. The implantation rates were similar in both groups (22% and 28%, respectively).

Conclusions

The placement of human oocytes, zygotes, and embryos inside an hermetically closed container before plunging into liquid nitrogen for vitrification permits a reliable isolation of the cells from the liquid nitrogen and avoids the potential for contamination by microorganisms. Although this technique is associated with a relatively slow cooling rate, the developmental potential of these oocytes and embryos is not compromised if the thawing process involves rapid warming and simultaneous removal of cryoprotectants. Efficient aseptic vitrification of oocytes and embryos can be performed with decreased concentrations of permeable cryoprotectants and complete isolation of embryos from liquid nitrogen.

Acknowledgements

The authors would like to thank Dr. Igor I. Katkov for the mathematical calculations of the speed of oocyte warming in the CSS methodology.

References

1. Leibo SP. Cryopreservation of mammalian oocytes. In Tulandi T, Gosden R, eds. *Preservation of Fertility*. London: Taylor & Francis, 2004; pp. 141–154.
2. Catt J, Wood T, Henman M, *et al.* Single embryo transfer in IVF to prevent multiple pregnancies. *Twin Res* 2003; **6:** 536–539.
3. Henman M, Catt JW, Wood T, *et al.* Elective transfer of single fresh blastocysts and later transfer of cryostored blastocysts reduces the twin pregnancy rate and can improve the in vitro fertilization live birth rate in younger women. *Fertil Steril* 2005; **84:** 1620–1627.
4. de Boer KA, Catt JW, Jansen RP, *et al.* Moving to blastocyst biopsy for preimplantation genetic diagnosis and single embryo transfer at Sydney IVF. *Fertil Steril* 2004; **82:** 295–298.
5. Jansen RP, Burton GJ. Mitochondrial dysfunction in reproduction. *Mitochondrion* 2004; **4:** 577–600.
6. Taylor DM, Handyside AH, Ray PF, *et al.* Quantitative measurement of transcript levels throughout human preimplantation development: analysis of hypoxanthine phosphoribosyl transferase. *Mol Hum Reprod* 2001; **7:** 147–154.
7. Telford NA, Watson AJ, Schultz GA. Transition from maternal to embryonic control in early mammalian development: a comparison of several species. *Mol Reprod Dev* 1990; **26:** 90–100.
8. Clouston HJ, Herbert M, Fenwick J, *et al.* Cytogenetic analysis of human blastocysts. *Prenat Diagn* 2002; **22:** 1143–1152.
9. Chen C. Pregnancy after human oocytes cryopreservation. *Lancet* 1986; **11:** 884–886.
10. van Uem JFHM, Siebzehnrübl ER, Schuh B, *et al.* Birth after cryopreservation of unfertilized oocytes. *Lancet* 1987; **8535:** 752–753.
11. Al-Hasani S, Diedrich K, van der Ven, *et al.* Cryopreservation of human oocytes *Hum Reprod* 1987; **2:** 695–700.
12. Tucker M, Wright G, Morton F, *et al.* Preliminary experience with human oocytes cryopreservation using 1,2-propanediol and sucrose. *Hum Reprod* 1996; **11:** 1513–1515.
13. Porcu E, Fabbri R, Seracchioli, *et al.* Birth of a healthy female after intracytoplasmic sperm injection of cryopreserved human oocytes. *Fertil Steril* 1997; **68:** 724–726.
14. Young E, Kenny A, Puigdomenech E, *et al.* Triplet pregnancy after intracytoplasmic sperm injection of cryopreserved oocytes: case report. *Fertil Steril* 1998; **70:** 360–361.
15. Boldt J, Cline D, McLaughlin D. Human oocytes cryopreservation as an adjunct to IVF-embryo transfer cycles. *Hum Reprod* 2003; 18: 1250–1255.
16. Kuleshova LL, Lopata A. Vitrification can be more favourable than slow cooling. *Fertil Steril* 2002; **78:** 449–454.
17. Mohr LR, Trounson AO, Freeman L. Deep freezing and transfer of human embryos. *J In Vitro Fertil Embryo Transfer* 1985; **2:** 1–10.
18. Siebzehnrübl ER. Cryopreservation of gametes and cleavage stage embryos. *Hum Reprod* 1989; **4**(Suppl): 105–110.
19. Testart J, Lassale B, Forman R, *et al.* Factors influencing the success of human embryo freezing in an in vitro fertilization and embryo transfer program. *Fertil Steril* 1987; **48:** 107.
20. Veeck LL, Amudson CH, Brothman LJ, *et al.* Significantly enhanced pregnancy rates per cycle through cryopreservation and thaw of pronuclear stage oocytes. *Fertil Steril* 1993; **59:** 1202–1207.
21. Van den Abbeel E, Campus M, van Waesberghe L, *et al.* A randomised comparison of the cryopreservation of one cell human embryos with a slow controlled cooling procedure or a rapid cooling procedure by direct plunging into liquid nitrogen. *Hum Reprod* 1997; **12:** 1554–1560.
22. Al-Hasani S, Demirel LC, Schöpper B, *et al.* Pregnancies achieved after frozen-thawed pronuclear oocytes obtained by intracytoplasmic sperm injection with spermatozoa extracted from frozen–thawed testicular tissues from non-obstructive azoospermic men. *Hum Reprod* 1999; **14:** 2031–2035.
23. Damario MA, Hammitt DG, Galantis TM, *et al.* Pronuclear stage cryopreservation after intracytoplasmic sperm injection and conventional

IVF: implication for timing of the freeze. *Fertil Steril* 1999; **72:** 1049–1054.
24. Borini A, Cattoli M, Bulletti C, Coticchio G. Clinical efficiency of oocyte and embryo cryopreservation. *Ann N Y Acad Sci* 2008; **1127:** 49–58.
25. Kuleshova LL, Gianaroli L, Magli C, *et al.* Birth following vitrification of a small number of human oocytes. *Hum Reprod* 1999; **14:** 3077–3039.
26. Yoon TK, Chung HM, Lim JM, *et al.* Pregnancy and delivery of healthy infants developed from vitrified oocytes in a stimulated in vitro fertilization-embryo transfer program. *Fertil Steril* 2000; **74:** 180–181.
27. Yoon TK, Kim TJ, Park SE, *et al.* Live birth after vitrification of oocytes in a stimulated in vitro fertilization-embryo transfer programm. *Fertil Steril* 2003; **79:** 1323–1326.
28. Katayama KP, Stehlik J, Kuwayama M, *et al.* Huge survival rate of vitrified human oocytes results in clinical pregnancy. *Fertil Steril* 2003; **80:** 223–224.
29. Park SP, Kim EY, Oh JH, *et al.* Ultra-rapid freezing of human multipronuclear oocytes using electron microscope grids. *Hum Reprod* 2000; **15:** 1787–1790.
30. Selman HA, El-Danasouri I. Pregnancies derived from vitrified human oocytes. *Fertil Steril* 2002; **77**, 422–423.
31. Liebermann J, Tucker MJ, Graham JR, *et al.* Blastocyst development after vitrification of multipronuclear oocytes using the Flexipet denuding pipette. *RBM Online* 2002; **4:** 148–152.
32. Liebermann J, Nawroth F, Isachenko V, *et al.* Potential importance of vitrification in reproductive medicine. *Biol Reprod* 2002; **67:** 1671–1680.
33. Jelinkova L, Selman HA, Arav A, *et al.* Twin pregnancy after vitrification of 2-pronuclei human embryos. *Fertil Steril* 2002; **77:** 412–414.
34. Ciotti PM, Porcu E, Notarangelo L, *et al.* Meiotic spindle recovery is faster in vitrification of human oocytes compared to slow freezing. *Fertil Steril* 2009; **91**: 2399–2407.
35. Bagchi A, Woods EJ, Critser JK. Cryopreservation and vitrification: recent advances in fertility preservation technologies. *Expert Rev Med Devices* 2008; **5:** 359–370.
36. Al-Hasani S, Ozmen B, Koutlaki N, *et al.* Three years of routine vitrification of human zygotes: is it still fair to advocate slow-rate freezing? *RBM Online* 2007; **14:** 288–293.
37. Reed ML, Lane M, Gardner DK, *et al.* Vitrification of human blastocysts using the cryoloop method: successful clinical application and birth of offspring. *J Assist Reprod Genet* 2002; **19:** 304–306.
38. Vanderzwalmen P, Bertin G, Debauche CH, *et al.* Vitrification of human blastocysts with the Hemi-Straw carrier: application of assisted hatching after thawing. *Hum Reprod* 2003; **18:** 1504–1511.
39. Mukaida T, Nakamura S, Tomiyama T, *et al.* Vitrification of human blastocysts using cryoloops: clinical outcome of 223 cycles. *Hum Reprod* 2003; **18:** 384–391.
40. Son WY, Yoon SH, Park SJ, *et al.* Ongoing twin pregnancy after vitrification of blastocysts produced by in-vitro matured oocytes retrieved from a woman with polycystic ovary syndrome: case report. *Hum Reprod* 2002; **17:** 2963–2966.
41. Son WY, Lee SY, Chang MJ, *et al.* Pregnancy resulting from transfer of repeat vitrified blastocysts produced by in-vitro matured oocytes in patient with polycystic ovary syndrome. *RBM Online* 2005; **10:** 398–401.
42. Takahashi K, Mukaida T, Goto T, *et al.* Perinatal outcome of blastocyst transfer with vitrification using cryoloop: a 4-year follow-up study. *Fertil Steril* 2005; **84:** 88–92.
43. Zech NH, Lejeune B, Zech H, *et al.* Vitrification of hatching and hatched human blastocysts: effect of an opening in the zona pellucida before vitrification. *RBM Online* 2005; **11:** 355–361.
44. Liebermann J, Tucker MJ. Comparison of vitrification and conventional cryopreservation of day 5 and day 6 blastocysts during clinical application. *Fertil Steril* 2006; **86:** 20–26.
45. Hiraoka K, Hiraoka K, Kinutani M, *et al.* Vitrification of human hatched blastocysts: a report of 4 cases. *J Reprod Med* 2007; **52:** 413–415.
46. Lee SY, Son WY, Yoon SH, *et al.* Clinical-pregnancy outcome after vitrification of blastocysts produced from in vitro maturation cycles. *Fertil Steril* 2007; **88:** 1449–1451.
47. Baudot A, Alger L, Boutron P. Glass-forming tendency in the system water–dimethyl sulfoxide. *Cryobiology* 2000; **40:** 151–158.
48. Kuleshova LL, Shaw JM. A strategy for rapid cooling of mouse embryos within a double straw to eliminate the risk of contamination during storage in liquid nitrogen. *Hum Reprod* 2000; **15:** 2604–2609.
49. Palasz AT, Mapletoft RJ. Cryopreservation of mammalian embryos and oocytes: recent advances. *Biotechnol Adv* 1996; **14:** 127–149.
50. Martino A, Songansen N, Leibo SP. Development into blastocysts of bovine oocytes cryopreserved by ultra-rapid cooling. *Biol Reprod* 1996; **54:** 1059–1069.
51. Vajta G, Kuwayama M, Holm P, *et al.* Open pulled straw (OPS) vitrification: a new way to reduce cryoinjuries of bovine ova and embryos. *Mol Reprod Dev* 1998; **51:** 53–58.
52. Lane M, Bavister BD, Lyons EA, *et al.* Containerless vitrification of mammalian oocytes. *Nat Biotechnol* 1999; **17:** 1234–1236.
53. Lane M, Gardner DK. Vitrification of mouse oocytes using a nylon loop. *Mol Reprod Dev* 2001; **58:** 342–347.
54. Dinnyes A, Dai Y, Jiang S, *et al.* High developmental rates of vitrified bovine oocytes following

parthenogenetic activation, in vitro fertilization, and somatic cell nuclear transfer. *Biol Reprod* 2000; **63:** 513–518.

55. Kuwayama M, Kato O. Successful vitrification of human oocytes. *Fertil Steril* 2000; **74:** 549.
56. Berry ED, Dorsa WJ, Siragusa GR, *et al.* Bacterial cross-contamination of meat during liquid nitrogen immersion freezing. *J Food Prot* 1998; **61:** 1103–1108.
57. Khuu HM, Cowley H, David-Ocampo V, *et al.* Catastrophic failures of freezing bags for cellular therapy products: description, cause, and consequences. *Cytotherapy* 2002; **4:** 539–549.
58. Bielanski A, Nadin-Davis S, Sapp T, *et al.* Viral contamination of embryos cryopreserved in liquid nitrogen. *Cryobiology* 2000; **40:** 110–116.
59. Bielanski A, Bergeron H, Lau PC, *et al.* Microbial contamination of embryos and semen during long term banking in liquid nitrogen. *Cryobiology* 2003; **46:** 146–152.
60. Bielanski A. Experimental microbial contamination and disinfection of dry (vapour) shipper dewars designed for short-term storage and transportation of cryopreserved germplasm and other biological specimens. *Theriogenology* 2005; **63:** 1946–1957.
61. Morris GJ. The origin, ultrastructure, and microbiology of the sediment accumulating in liquid nitrogen storage vessels. *Cryobiology* 2005; **50:** 231–238.
62. Fountain D, Ralston M, Higgins N, *et al.* Liquid nitrogen freezers: a potential source of microbial contamination of hematopoietic stem cell components. *Transfusion* 1997; **37:** 585–591.
63. Isachenko V, Katkov II, Yakovenko S, *et al.* Vitrification of human laser treated blastocysts within cut standard straws (CSS): novel aseptic packaging and reduced concentrations of cryoprotectants. *Cryobiology* 2007; **54:** 305–309.
64. Veeck, LL. *An Atlas of Human Gametes and Concepts.* London: Parthenon, 1998; p. 215.
65. Veeck, LL, Zaninovic N. *An Atlas of Human Blastocysts.* London: Parthenon, 2003; p. 286.
66. Isachenko V, Montag M, Isachenko E, *et al.* Aseptic technology of vitrification of human pronuclear oocytes using open-pulled straws. *Hum Reprod* 2005; **20:** 492–496.
67. Isachenko V, Montag M, Isachenko E, *et al.* Aseptic vitrification of human germinal vesicle oocytes using dimethyl sulfoxide as a cryoprotectant. *Fertil Steril* 2006; **85:** 741–747.
68. Aramanovich IG, Levin VI. Equations of thermal conductivity. In *Equations of Mathematical Physics.* Moscow: Nauka, 1969, pp. 145–216.
69. Katkov II, Isachenko V, Isachenko E. Vitrification in small quenched volumes with a minimal amount of or without vitrificants: biophysics and thermodynamics in vitrification in assisted reproduction. In Tucker MJ, Liebermann J, eds. *A User's Manual and Troubleshooting Guide.* Oxford: Informa Healthcare, 2007, pp. 21–32.
70. Nave CR. *HyperPhysics.* 2005:// hyperphysics. phy-astrastr.gsu.edu/hbase/hph.html (accessed October 5, 2009).
71. Isachenko V, Montag M, Isachenko E, *et al.* Aseptic technology of vitrification of human pronuclear oocytes using open-pulled straws. *Hum Reprod* 2005; **20:** 492–496.
72. Rall WF, Fahy GM. Ice-free cryopreservation of mouse embryos at −196°C by vitrification. *Nature* 1985; **313:** 573–575.
73. Vincent C, Pickering SJ, Johnson MH, *et al.* Dimethyl sulphoxide affects the organization of microfilaments in the mouse oocytes. *Mol Reprod Dev* 1990; **26:** 227–235.
74. Bouquet M, Selva J, Auroux M. Effect of cooling and equilibration in DMSO, and cryopreservation of mouse oocytes, on the rates of in vitro fertilization, development and chromosomal abnormalities. *Mol Reprod Dev* 1995; **40:** 110–115.
75. Huang CC, Lee TH, Chen SU, *et al.* Successful pregnancy following blastocyst cryopreservation using super-cooling ultra-rapid vitrification. *Hum Reprod* 2005; **20:** 122–128.
76. Isachenko V, Isachenko E, Katkov II, *et al.* Cryoprotectant-free cryopreservation of human spermatozoa by vitrification and freezing in vapor: effect on motility, DNA integrity, and fertilization ability. *Biol Reprod* 2004; **71:** 1167–1173.
77. Isachenko V, Montag M, Isachenko E, *et al.* Vitrification of mouse pronuclear embryos after polar body biopsy without direct contact with liquid nitrogen. *Fertil Steril* 2005; **84:** 1011–1016.
78. Rall WF. Factor affecting the survival of mouse embryos cryopreserved by vitrification. *Cryobiology* 1987; **24:** 387–402.
79. Rall WF, Wood MJ. High in vitro and in vivo survival of day 3 mouse embryos vitrified in a non-toxic solution of glycerol and albumin. *J Reprod Fertil* 1994; **101:** 681–688.
80. Isachenko V, Perez-Sanchez F, Isachenko E, *et al.* Vitrification of GV-porcine oocytes with intact intracellular lipids: effect of the cryoprotectant saturation/dilution stepping, elevated temperature and cytoskeletal inhibitor. *Cryobiology* 1998; **36:** 250–253.
81. Isachenko V, Gorbunov L, Isachenko E, *et al.* Some physical and technological aspects of GV porcine oocyte vitrification. *Cryobiology* 1999; **39:** 35.
82. Isachenko V, Isachenko E, Montag M, *et al.* Clean technique of cryoprotectant-free vitrification of human spermatozoa. *RBM Online* 2005; **10:** 350–354.

83. Scott L, Alvero R, Leondires M, *et al.* The morphology of human pronuclear embryos is positively related to blastocyst development and implantation. *Hum Reprod* 2000; **15:** 2394–2403.
84. Isachenko V, Todorov P, Dimitrov Y, *et al.* Integrity rate of pronuclei after cryopreservation of pronuclear-zygotes as a criteria for subsequent embryo development and pregnancy. *Hum Reprod* 2008; **23:** 819–826.
85. Senn A, Urner F, Chanson A, *et al.* Morphological scoring of human pronuclear zygotes for prediction of pregnancy outcome. *Hum Reprod* 2006; **21:** 234–239.
86. Isachenko V, Montag M, Isachenko E, *et al.* Developmental rate and ultrastructure of vitrified human pronuclear oocytes after stepwise versus direct rehydration. *Hum Reprod* 2004; **19:** 660–665.
87. Isachenko V, Selman H, Isachenko E, *et al.* Effect of cryoprotectants on the ultrastructure of cooled human pronuclear oocytes. *Fertil Steril* 2004; **81:** 720–722.
88. Isachenko V, Selman H, Isachenko E, *et al.* Modified vitrification of human pronuclear oocytes: efficacy and effect on ultrastructure. *RBM Online* 2003; **7:** 211–216.
89. Yokota Y, Sato S, Yokota M, Araki Y. Birth of a healthy baby following vitrification of human blastocysts. *Fertil Steril* 2001; **75:** 1027–1029.
90. Yokota Y, Yokota H, Yokota M, *et al.* Birth of healthy twins from in vitro development of human refrozen embryos. *Fertil Steril* 2001; **76:** 1063–1065.
91. Cho HJ, Son WY, Yoon SH, *et al.* An improved protocol for dilution of cryoprotectants from vitrified human blastocysts, *Hum Reprod* 2002; **17:** 2419–2422.

Chapter 19

Vitrification of human oocytes for a donor program

Elkin Lucena, Carolina Lucena, and Sandra Mojica

Introduction

The demand for oocyte donation (OD) has increased substantially over recent years. This has imposed the need for centers for assisted reproductive therapy (ART) to set up their own banks of donor eggs in order to meet the needs of patients participating in in vitro fertilization (IVF) programs. The main clinical indications for entering the donor egg program are premature ovarian failure, failed embryo implantations after several rounds of ART [1], and advanced maternal age. Premature ovarian failure is characterized by hyperandrogenic amenorrhea before 35 years of age. Women of advanced maternal age may decide to resort to OD because of low ovarian response after ovarian stimulation treatment. A further indication for OD is for patients with genetic abnormalities, in particular X-linked abnormalities such as Turner syndrome and gonadal dysgenesis [2]. It is also important to highlight other factors that have resulted in changes in reproductive expectations, such as the changing role of women in society, their professional development, and their financial position in the household. In other words, women in the 21st century are delaying motherhood and this has detrimental implications for a successful natural pregnancy as their biological clocks do not stop. A high percentage of women complaining of infertility belongs to this older age group, 38–45 years of age, and are considered candidates for OD.

Cryopreservation of human oocytes is of significant clinical value in reproductive medicine, although it does not yet play a critical role in these treatments. It is also a solution to the ethical, religious, and legal issues associated with embryo storage. The application of the technique in standard ART procedures, aside from giving rise to a bank of donor oocytes, allows for the preservation of supernumerary eggs. This makes it easier to attempt a new pregnancy in the event that the ovarian stimulation cycle fails or for a further child without the need for additional stimulation. Moreover, it is an important method for preserving fertility in women undergoing radiotherapy, chemotherapy, or surgical removal of the ovaries [3]. Cryopreservation of human oocytes also impacts certain practical aspects of routine IVF, giving rise to the possibility of freezing oocytes when a semen sample cannot be obtained (e.g. when the partner is unavailable on the day when the sample is required) or when testicular or epididimal samples are required and the two procedures cannot be synchronized.

In the absence of vitrification, there are several options for OD in various programs. "Shared egg donation" is where the donor is an infertile patient willing to donate a given number of eggs in exchange for a subsidy for IVF treatment. This program is limited by the number of available eggs for donation and the quality of the oocytes, which depends on the age of the donor patient and the etiology of her infertility [4]. Donor–recipient synchronization for fresh transfer results in higher pregnancy and implantation rates than achieved if embryos are frozen [5]. Gamete donation by friends or relatives is also an option, but in the case of relatives there may be future problems with consanguinity affiliation.

Vitrification has enabled the creation of a bank of cryopreserved donor eggs as a solution for the growing demand of OD in fertility clinics. However, not many centers are using this option, mainly because of the variability in survival, fertilization, pregnancy, and implantation rates [6,7]. Since the first live birth from a frozen egg in 1986 using slow freezing [8], advances in cryopreservation techniques for oocytes have not been as effective as those achieved with other biological entities such as sperm and embryos. This has been explained on the basis of the size and morphology of the pre-ovulation egg, a lower permeability of the oolemma membrane, and temperature-sensitive

Fertility Cryopreservation, ed. Ri-Cheng Chian and Patrick Quinn. Published by Cambridge University Press.

spindle and metaphase zone. These characteristics result in high susceptibility to cryodamage. A meta-analysis conducted at Cornell University assessed the efficiency of oocyte cryopreservation and concluded that pregnancy rates are lower with frozen eggs than with fresh eggs. However, vitrification shows better results than seen with other oocyte cryopreservation techniques [9]. In recent years, a higher percentage of pregnancies has been achieved in a small group of IVF centers using cryopreserved oocytes [10–12], creating the need for more clinical trials that can provide evidence regarding the effects of vitrification techniques on pregnancy, implantation, and the production of healthy offspring.

Donor selection

Although donor recruitment is a limiting factor in any OD program, relevant selection has made it possible to offer a pool of donors to meet the needs of a program in high demand. Each center establishes the parameters considered relevant for the selection in accordance with the criteria defined by the institution's ethical and medical committee, and in accordance with any existing government regulations [13,14]. In general terms, these parameters include a medical, family, social, reproductive, and psychological history [15]. Once donors are selected, they are required to sign an informed consent before entering the program. Donors are placed under the care of a group of professionals, and the program director is in charge of maintaining permanent communication with them throughout the selection process and the ovarian stimulation treatment.

The OD program is directed by a health professional in charge of screening potential candidates, conducting interviews, and collecting data on the selected donors. Donors come to the institution by referral from other donors, prompted by their own research, or because of direct contact with the program director through the surveys conducted among university students. It is accepted practice to offer financial compensation to the donors to cover for their time, physical effort, commuting, and dedication during the treatment.

The selection process begins with a survey designed to determine personal information such as age, civil status, sexual orientation, education, and occupation. As far as reproductive history goes, information is gathered regarding the number of children (if applicable), miscarriages or abortions, and the desire for more children in the future. The interview also focuses on determining psychological and emotional stability

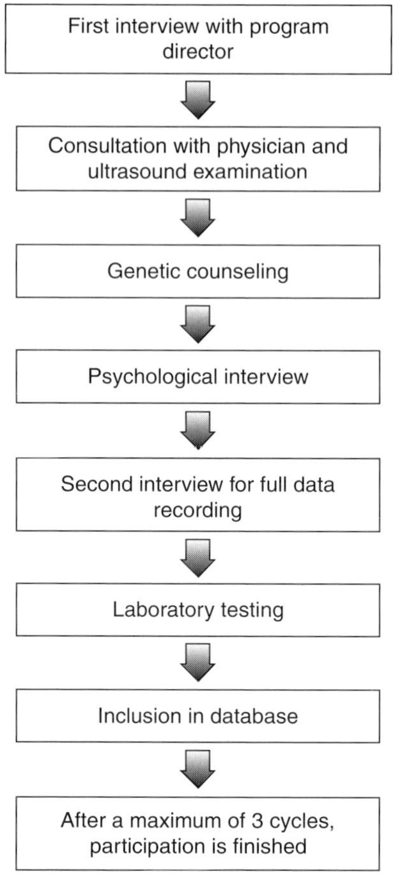

Figure 19.1. Donor selection scheme.

on the basis of certain aspects of the past. The purpose and potential risks of the program are explained, and the level of commitment, availability, and responsibility toward the treatment is determined. The donor selection scheme is illustrated in Figure 19.1.

Inclusion criteria include:

- age between 19 and 29 years
- already having healthy children
- physical characteristics: assessed and recorded, including: eye, skin and hair color, height (a picture is attached to the database)
- medical examination and transvaginal ultrasound: assessing the ovaries (structure, size, volume, and position), uterus (size, morphology, ultrasound patterns, and position), endometrial cavity (appearance and consistency with cycle phase aside from potential diseases such as polyps and submucosal miomas), and transvaginal accessibility to the ovary for oocyte retrieval
- genetic consultation based on the family history in order to rule out heritable diseases, thus protecting

recipient couples from the risk of having children with genetic diseases
- psychological consultation.

The physician writes a complete clinical record from the medical assessment that is analyzed together with all the other relevant information.

Exclusion criteria include

- recurrent miscarriages
- undesirable family history
- habits involving the use of toxic substances such as alcohol, tobacco, and other drugs
- participation in previous OD programs where, after initial stimulation and follicular aspiration, abnormal oocyte characteristics were observed such as intracytoplasmatic vacuoles, thick zona pellucida, etc.

A number of tests are performed:

- hormone levels: follicle-stimulating hormone (FSH), luteinizing hormone (LH), prolactin, estradiol, total testosterone, progesterone
- infections: IgG and IgM for herpes types I and II; IgG and IgM for cytomegalovirus; IgG and IgM for Epstein–Barr virus; specific tests for human immunodeficiency virus 1 and 2; surface antigen for hepatitis B virus; antibodies against hepatitis C virus; antibody testing using the VDRL (Venereal Disease Research Laboratory) test for syphilis
- blood group
- Karyotype: ΔF508 for cystic fibrosis.

Stimulation protocols

Ovarian stimulation of donors is based on the same criteria used in young healthy patients entering the IVF program for male factor infertility. The protocol of choice includes gonadotropin-releasing hormone (GnRH) agonists and recombinant FSH or human menopausal gonadotropin (HMG). Courses of treatment that were less aggressive for the ovary and more patient friendly were introduced in 2008 as a second choice, with better effects on egg quality and a lower risk of inducing ovarian hyperstimulation [16,17]. The protocol includes the use of low-dose gonadotropins, clomiphene citrate, and indometacin to delay follicular rupture and thus avoiding the premature effect of LH and early ovulation [18]. In both protocols, induction (Figure 19.2) is initiated after a 21 day preparation period with oral contraceptive pills. Stimulation is started 4–5 days after menses using the most suitable protocol according to the age of the donor and the characteristics of the ovary in the ultrasound performed on the first menstruation day.

Protocol 1

Pituitary desensitization is started on the first day of the menstrual cycle using leuprolide acetate 0.5 mg subcutaneously until day 11. Gonadotropins (HMG 150 IU or recombinant FSH 200 IU) are started on day 3 and continued for a period of 8 days. Ultrasound follow-up is performed on days 7, 9, and 11; once follicular size is between 17 and 19 mm, 10 000 IU of human chorionic gonadotropin (HCG) is administered and transvaginal follicular aspiration follows 36 hours later.

Protocol 2

A daily dose of 100 mg clomiphene citrate is started on day 3 together with 150 IU HMG for 6 days. Ultrasound follow-up is done on day 6, and once follicles are 14 mm in size, 50 mg of indometacin is given three times daily in order to stop the endogenous LH peak until 1 day after the administration of 10 000 IU HCG, which is injected when the follicles reach 17 mm in size. Follicular aspiration is performed 36 hours later.

Vitrification of donor eggs

Clinical trials designed to assess the application of different techniques were started in the mid 1990s. Trials have covered cooling technique, slow freezing to vitrification (rapid freezing); changes in timing and cryoprotectant concentrations; use of new devices that allow submicroliter volumes to be stored; warming technique; and the rates of cooling and warming, increasing to more than −20 000°C/min. These advances have

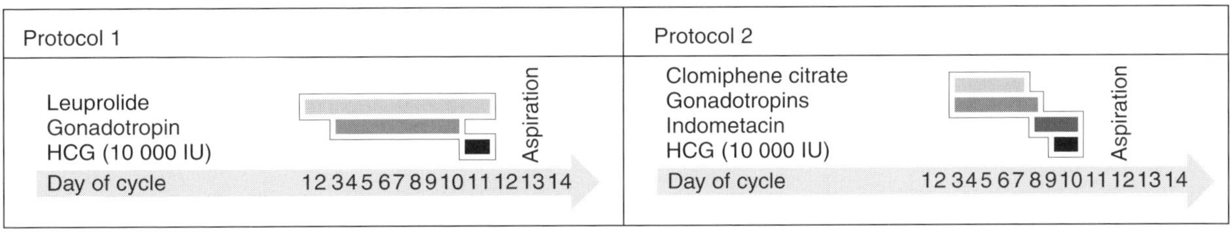

Figure 19.2. Donor stimulation protocols. HCG, human chorionic gonadotropin.

enabled routine application of these technical advances in ART laboratories [6,19,20].

It has not been easy to apply cryopreservation to human eggs because of their structural and physiological characteristics, and in particular because of the susceptibility of the meiotic spindle to low temperatures, which cause depolymerization of the microtubules and the disappearance of the microtubule organizing core [21]. While it seems that this effect is reversible in mouse oocytes, in human oocytes the reorganizing ability of the spindle is compromised [22], especially in slow-freezing protocols. In contrast, vitrification is a valuable option that reduces the effects on the stability of the meiotic spindle and the chromosomes and has, in general, a lower impact on cell physiology. It is a process in which vitreous solidification of a solute occurs without ice crystals forming inside the cells during the cooling and warming balance, thus avoiding the main cause of cell damage under slow-freezing conditions [23]. In vitrification, cooling speed increases as eggs are directly submerged in liquid nitrogen, and high cryoprotectant concentrations lead to high-speed cell dehydration, indicating that there is a strong correlation between cryoprotectant concentrations and the cooling–warming rates during the vitrification process [24]. Several studies have shown the efficiency of vitrification in terms of the high survival rates of devitrified oocytes [6,25,26], highlighting its advantages over slow freezing in terms of short duration, absence of zona ruptures, and cost reduction (because there is no need for sophisticated equipment) [23]. Moreover, permeable cryoprotectant mixes have been replaced by ethylene glycol, because of its low toxicity and rapid diffusion through the oocyte membrane, plus a non-permeable cryoprotectant (sucrose) that helps to regulate intracellular ethylene glycol concentration during the balance process [10,27].

The routine implementation of vitrification in 2004 at our center led to the creation of the donor egg bank. Advantages of having a bank include not having to synchronize with the recipient, eliminating month-long waiting lists, the availability of varying phenotypes, and reducing the costs for the recipient, considering that oocytes retrieved from a single donor may be used in several recipients. As mentioned above, demand for donor eggs has been increasing and, at our center, close to 40% of bank eggs are for recipients living abroad, mainly Colombian women living in the USA or women who come from Peru, Ecuador, Central America, and, to a lesser extent Europe, particularly the UK.

Vitrification protocol

In the modified vitrification protocol [25], cooling and warming rates are increased by reducing cryoprotectant concentrations (Kitazato, Tokyo, Japan) to 15% dimethyl sulfoxide, 15% ethylene glycol, and 0.5 M sucrose in minimum volume cooling solution. This mixture reduces the osmotic stress and the toxic effect that is linked to the high concentrations of cryoprotectants required to avoid the formation of ice crystals in the cytoplasm. We have developed our own "cryolock" crystal polystyrene device for holding the eggs (Figure 19.3). Two hours following oocyte aspiration, hyaluronidase is used to remove cumulus cells and the following steps are performed at room temperature. All the solutions are prepared in Medium 199 and contain 20% Serum Substitute Supplement (forming the basic washing solution [WS]); to this is then added the cryoprotectants as listed below.

1. One 50 μl drop of WS and two 50 μl drops of equilibrium solution (ES; 7.5% ethylene glycol, 7.5% dimethyl sulfoxide) are prepared. Oocytes are then placed on the WS drop and immediately a bridge is made to join it with the ES drop. After 2 minutes, the second ES drop is brought into the

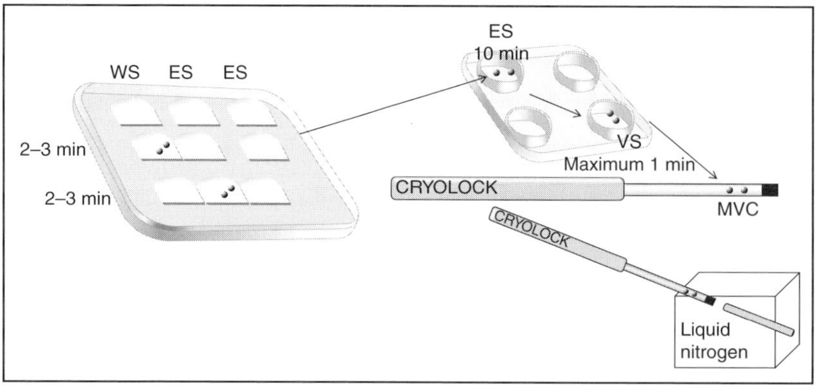

Figure 19.3 Egg vitrification protocol. See the text for the details of the protocol. WS, washing solution; ES, equilibrium solution; VS, vitrification solution; MVC, minimum volume cooling solution.

mix, where the oocytes are allowed to remain for an additional 2 minutes.

2. Using a four-well plate, 500 µl of ES is placed in one well and 500 µl of vitrification solution (VS; 15% ethylene glycol, 15% dimethyl sulfoxide, 0.5 M sucrose) is placed in a second well.
3. Oocytes are placed in the ES solution for 10 minutes.
4. Oocytes are then placed in the VS and two oocytes are mounted in the cryolock in a minimum volume (approximately 2 µl) of VS solution and submerged immediately in liquid nitrogen before closing the cryolock lid. Not more than 1 minute may pass between the moment in which the egg is placed in the VS solution and the moment in which the cryolock is submerged in liquid nitrogen. The cooling rate is approximately 23 000°C/min.

Recipient preparation

Perhaps the most important factor for achieving the desired result is the endometrial preparation of the recipients in order to allow a synchronized dialogue between the embryo and the endometrium. Synchronization refers to the right timing for embryo transfer during the "implantation window." Most of the schemes proposed include an initial estrogen phase to simulate the natural menstrual cycle, followed by the use of a fixed dose of estrogen and progesterone. Flexibility in the length of administration of estradiol allows synchronization to occur between days 17 and 19 of the artificial cycle in order to perform the transfer within an appropriate receptivity window, with good clinical results [28].

Endometrial preparation of the recipient is done before the hormonal replacement course, consisting of 21 days of oral contraceptive, one tablet every 24 hours from day 1 of the cycle. Vaginal progesterone 200 mg three times a day is started on day 14. After finishing the oral contraceptive tablets on day 22 of the cycle, 2 mg estradiol valerate (Progynova) is taken every 8 hours for 3 days, and menstruation is expected 2 to 3 days after the course is finished.

Hormone supplementation with 2 mg estradiol valerate twice daily is started on the first day of menstruation in the conceptional cycle. A biophysical uterine profile is performed on day 13 of the cycle in order to assess endometrial thickness, morphology and blood flow, miometrial echogenicity, contractions and blood flow, and arterial pulsatility index [29]. If the score is between 17 and 20, the IVF laboratory is informed in order to initiate thawing of the donor eggs that have been previously assigned on the basis of the recipient–donor phenotype. On the same day, the recipient is started on 100 mg intramuscular progesterone per day. For all OD patients, transfer is performed on day 16 of the cycle under transabdominal ultrasound using an Ultrasoft Frydman Set Echo (Laboratoire CCD, Paris, France) catheter. Hormone supplementation is maintained until the pregnancy test and the confirmation of fetal heart beats.

The program is 100% anonymous and the selection of the donor phenotype profile for each recipient is determined by a committee consisting of the treating physician and the program director in charge of the database of selected donors and recipient applications.

Oocyte thawing

Egg thawing depends on the biophysical profile score of the recipient obtained on day 13 of the cycle. Four oocytes in metaphase II per recipient are devitrified and intracytoplasmic sperm injection (ICSI) is performed 2 hours later. Fertilization is determined on the basis of the presence of pronuclei 16–18 hours after ICSI and the in vitro culture is maintained for an additional 72 hours at 37°C and 6% carbon dioxide, using sequential Vitrolife media. The thawing protocol is shown in Figure 19.4.

Thawing protocol

The thawing protocol uses the WS as in the vitrification protocol. This is then modified as below.

1. Oocyte thawing is performed by immersion of the cryolock in thawing solution (TS; 1 M sucrose) at 37°C for 1 minute.
2. Using a 4-well plate, 500 µl of dilution solution (DS; 0.5 M sucrose) is added to one well and 500 µl of WS solution is placed in each of two wells at room temperature.
3. The oocytes are then placed in the DS well for 3 minutes.
4. The oocytes are rinsed twice in WS for 5 minutes each wash.
5. Oocytes are then placed in G1 medium (Vitrolife) for 2–4 hours at 37°C and 5% carbon dioxide. After this time, viability is assessed and ICSI is performed.

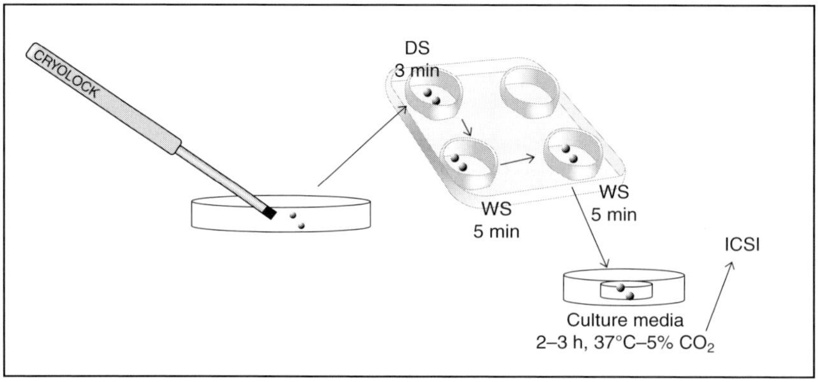

Figure 19.4. Thawing protocol. See the text for the details of the protocol. WS, washing solution; DS, dilution solution; TS, thawing solution; ICSI, intracytoplasmic sperm injection.

Results using cryopreserved oocytes in a donation program

The assessment of the first OD vitrification program in Latin America has shown positive results and significant benefits for the recipients. These results are measured on the basis of the survival rate after thawing, fertilization, cleavage, pregnancy, losses, and birth of healthy babies. Some observations have been made regarding the behavior of the egg during the process of vitrification and warming: less than 1% of the eggs are affected during vitrification, perhaps by technical problems during the process. In contrast, a larger number do not survive thawing, and there are many ongoing research studies on the effects of the technique on the organelles, cytoplasm, and zona pellucida [30]. It is yet to be determined whether this loss on thawing can be reduced through additional adjustments to cryoprotectant concentrations and protocol timing, or by means of new devices that can ensure the integrity of the meiotic spindle and hence the normal chromosome distribution in the cryopreserved oocyte.

One of the potential changes on thawing is the development of vacuoles, which are thought to be associated with other ultrastructural abnormalities leading to oocyte degeneration [31]. Formation of vacuoles is considered an important ooplasm characteristic associated with fertilization failure, or embryo arrest in those rare cases in which cleavage occurs [30]. It has also been demonstrated that zona hardening is an effect of the technique resulting from an increase in intracellular calcium, which causes exocytosis of the cortical granules located just under the plasma membrane; the enzymes contained in these granules prevent polyspermia as a calcium-dependent event [31]. This fertilization control system could be activated prematurely during freezing, preventing normal fertilization [32]. The percentage of losses is also associated in certain instances with high hormone levels in response to the stimulation regimen. For this reason, stimulation protocols are being reassessed with the idea of reducing dosages or the days of stimulation. This might result in a lower number of better quality "competent" eggs capable of tolerating the freezing–thawing process and of resulting in embryo development and successful pregnancies.

Table 19.1 shows results from 4 years of experience with vitrified oocytes used in the OD program as well as in supernumerary eggs after stimulation treatments. To date, 3232 eggs have been vitrified. Of these, 810 are donor eggs. The number of OD transfers is higher compared with the supernumerary oocytes vitrified from patients, considering that patients' eggs are thawed only in the event that there is no pregnancy or the couple wishes to come back for a second pregnancy after initial success.

So far, 185 donors have entered the program. Of them, 30% are active and the rest have completed the three donor cycles, have become pregnant, or have left the program voluntarily for personal reasons. Four to five donors are scheduled every month in order to maintain approximately 40 eggs in stock in the bank.

Social and cultural effects

Oocyte freezing can be used either by women who wish to postpone reproduction and enter the Mother of the Future program or for egg donation. In the former situation, women may want to postpone reproduction for medical reasons, such as radio- or chemotherapy or bilateral oophorectomy, or personal reasons, when they do not want to run the risk of genetic abnormalities of their offspring because of aging oocytes.

Table 19.1. Oocyte vitrification results

	Oocyte donation	Autologous egg use[a]	Total
Transfer number	328	202	530
No. vitrified oocytes	810	2422	3232
Post-thawing viability (%)	81	76	78
Fertilization (%)	78	68	73.2
Embryo development (%)	82	78	80
Pregnancy rate (%)	42	38	40
Losses (%)	15	17	16
Births (37 weeks)	115	67	182
Abnormal birth	0	0	0

[a] Autologous egg use is a patient using their own supernumerary oocytes.

Women may also want to avoid embryo freezing as part of an ART program. In the past, demand for ART came mainly from infertile heterosexual couples, but societal changes have created a demand for donor eggs from single women and homosexual couples.

Within the context of ART, donation is understood as a "voluntary and free action." The financial reward concept was introduced several years ago. However, the American Fertility Society formally opposes egg sale, although it accepts that "donors may be compensated for the inconvenience and their time" [33].

Restrictions vary from country to country. In Colombia and Spain, among others, anonymous donation is allowed. In the UK, for example, a change in the legislation now allows children born through the use of these methods to know the identity of the donors. This has led to a sharp reduction in the number of donors. Differences in legislations and prices have created a significant movement of women who travel outside their own countries in search of safer and lower-cost treatments.

The main objections to egg donation are physical and psychological, in particular regarding the risk of ovarian hyperstimulation syndrome. However, with the newer and milder stimulation schemes, this complication can be avoided . Moral objections include objections against the trade of human body products. Although legitimate, these concerns do not justify banning egg donation, because the aim is to promote individual freedom and to benefit donors, recipients, and future children born after ART [34].

For some couples, the only option for pregnancy is egg donation. Vitrified donor egg programs (cryobanks) offer a wide range of phenotypical and timing options, especially for couples living far from the cities where the centers are located. A successful egg donor program must be based on strong resources, interest, and commitment and depends on an interdisciplinary approach from doctors and mental health counselors to guide the entire process and help couples to cope and make decisions.

At present, it is not clear what the real effects of this approach will be upon individuals, families, and society. Though the OD option allows many to experience the joys of parenthood, real social implications will only be seen in the future. While a more in-depth debate is desirable, an informed democratic social debate is essential in order to ensure that legislation is implemented that is not simply based on the expert opinions of health professionals and scientists. Informed consents must be very explicit and detailed. Couples or single women contemplating the use of donor egg programs should be fully aware and informed of the legal issues and regulations that exist in their community.

Conclusions

The demand for donor eggs from ART centers has been increasing steadily for several reasons, including premature ovarian failure, low response to ovarian stimulation treatments, genetic abnormalities (to a lesser extent), and women with advanced maternal age. For this reason, it is important to have a donor egg program to meet current demand and to ensure that recipients can have access to good-quality eggs from a selection of donors who meet a range of medical and psychological criteria and who have no family history of genetic diseases. Oocyte vitrification has emerged as a valuable tool in ART since it circumvents the ethical issues of embryo freezing. Moreover, it is an excellent option for women undergoing chemo- or radiotherapy for cancer, and also for supernumerary eggs after ovarian stimulation treatments. In OD programs, oocyte vitrification is an important breakthrough because of the ease of cryopreserving donor eggs with different phenotypes without the need for donor–recipient synchronization. This chapter summarizes 4 years of experience with an OD program using vitrified oocytes, including a description of the routine management of the program and the results obtained.

Acknowledgements

We are grateful to Abby Moran, director of the Bio-Psychology Department, Angela Saa, embryologist and IVF laboratory in chief, and Zulma Suarez, microbiologist and director of the donor egg program at our institution for their valuable contributions to this chapter, based on their experience with the management and organization of the program.

References

1. Vegetti W, Marozzi A, Manfredini E, *et al.* Premature ovarían failure. *Mol Cell Endocrinol* 2000; **161:** 53–57.
2. Portnoi MF, Aboura A, Tachdjian G, *et al.* Molecular cytogenetic studies of Xq critical regions in premature ovarian failure patients. *Hum Reprod* 2006; **21:** 2329–2334.
3. Li XH, Chen SU, Zhang X, *et al.* Cryopreserved oocytes of infertile couples undergoing assisted reproductive technology could be an important sourse of oocyte donation: a clinical report of successful pregnancies. *Hum Reprod* 2005; **20:** 3390–3394.
4. Shulman A, Frenkel Y, Dor Jehoshua, *et al.* The best donor. *Hum Reprod* 1999; **14:** 2493–2499.
5. Check JH, Choe JK, Nazari, A, *et al.* Fresh embryo transfer is more effective than frozen for donor oocyte recipients but not for donor. *Hum Reprod* 2001; **16:** 1403–1408.
6. Fabbri R, Porcu E, Marsella T, *et al.* Human oocyte cryopreservation: new perspectives regarding oocyte survival. *Hum Reprod* 2001; **16:** 411–416.
7. Ghetler Y, Skutelsky E, Ben Nun I, *et al.* Human oocyte cryopreservation and the fate of cortical granules. *Fertil Steril* 2006; **86**: 210–215.
8. Chen C. Pregnancy after human oocyte cryopreservation. *Lancet* 1986; **i:** 884–886.
9. Okay K, Pelin C, Bang H . Efficiency of oocyte cryopreservation: a meta-analysis. *Fertil Steril* 2006; **86**: 70–79.
10. Chen SU, Lien YR, Chen HF, *et al.* Observational clinical follow-up of oocyte cryopreservation using a slow-freezing method with 1,2-propanediol plus sucrose followed by ICSI. *Hum Reprod* 2005; **20:** 1975–1980.
11. Katayama KP, Stehlik J, Kuwayama M, *et al.* High survival rate of vitrified human oocytes results in clinical pregnancy. *Fertil Steril* 2003; **80:** 223–224.
12. Kuleshova L, Gianaroli L, Magli C, *et al.* Birth following vitrification of a small number of human oocytes. *Hum Reprod* 1999; **14:** 3077–3079.
13. Lindheim SR, Frumovitz MV, Sauer M. Recruitment and screening policies and procedures used to establish a paid donor oocyte registry. *Hum Reprod* 1998; **13:** 2020–2024.
14. Birminghan A. Guidelines for gamete and embryo donation. *Fertil Steril* 2006; **86**:S39-S50.
15. Marina S, Expósito R, Marina F, *et al.* Oocyte donor selection from 554 candidates. *Hum Reprod* 1999; **14**: 2770–2776.
16. Højgaard A, Ingerslev HJ, Dinesen J. Friendly IVF: patient opinions. *Hum Reprod* 2001; **16:** 1391–1396.
17. Inge GB, Brinsden PR, Elder KT. Oocyte number per live birth in IVF: were Steptoe and Edwards less wasteful? *Hum Reprod* 2005; **20:** 588–592.
18. Kadoch IJ. Spontaneous ovulation rate before oocyte retrieval in modified natural cycle IVF with and without indomethacin. *Reprod Bio Med Online* 2008; **16:** 245–249.
19. Tucker MJ, Morton PC, Wright G, *et al.* Clinical application of human egg cryopreservation. *Hum Reprod* 1998; **13:** 3156–3159.
20. Porcu E, Fabbri R, Seracchioli R, *et al.* Birth of a healthy female after intracytoplasmatic sperm injection of cryopreserved human oocytes. *Fertil Steril* 1997; **68:** 724–726.
21. Mullen SF, Agca Y, Broermann DC, *et al.* The effects of osmotic stress on the metaphase II spindle of human oocytes, and the relevance to cryopreservation. *Hum Reprod* 2004; **5:** 1148–1154.
22. Pickering SJ, Braude PR, Johnson MH, *et al.* Transient cooling to room temperature can use irreversible disruption of the meiotic spindle in the human oocyte. *Fertil Steril* 1990; **54:** 102–108.
23. Kuleshova LL, Lopata A. Vitrification can be more favourable than slow cooling. *Fertil Steril* 2002; **78:** 449–454.
24. Chian R-C, Kuwayama M, Tan L, *et al.* High survival rate of bovine oocyte matured in vitro following vitrification. *J Reprod Develop* 2004; **50:** 685–696.
25. Kuwayama M. High efficient vitrification method for cryopreservation of human oocytes. *Reprod Biomed Online* 2005; **11:** 300–308.
26. Lucena E, Bernal D, Lucena C, *et al.* Successful ongoing pregnancies after vitrification of oocytes. *Fertil Steril* 2006; **85:** 108–111.
27. Hong SW, Chung HM, Lim JM, *et al.* Improved human oocyte development after vitrification: a comparison of thawing methods. *Fertil Steril* 1999; **72:** 142–146.
28. Michalas S, Loutradis D, Drakakis P, *et al.* A flexible protocol for the induction of recipient endometrial cycle in an oocyte donation programme. *Hum Reprod* 1996; **11:** 1063–1066.
29. Applebaum M. The uterine biophysical profile. *Ultrasound Obstet Gynecol* 1995; **5:** 67–68.

30. Nottola SA, Macchiarelli, Coticchio G, *et al.* Ultrastructure of human mature oocyte after slow cooling cryopreservation using different sucrose concentrations. *Hum Reprod* 2007; **22:** 1123–1132.

31. Larman MG, Katz-Jaffe MG, Sheehan CB, Gardner DK. 1,2-Propanediol and the type of cryopreservation procedure adversely affect mouse oocyte physiology. *Hum Reprod* 2007; **22:** 250–259.

32. Ludwing M, Al-Hasani S, Felberbaum R, *et al.* New aspects of cryopreservation of oocyte and embryos in assisted reproduction and future perspectives. *Hum Reprod* 1999; **14:** 162–168.

33. American Fertility Society. Guidelines for oocyte donation. *Fertil Steril* 1993; **58:** 55–75.

34. Resnik DB. The commodification of human reproductive materials. *J Med Ethics* 1998; **24:** 338–339.

Chapter 20

Obstetric and perinatal outcomes in pregnancies conceived following oocyte cryopreservation

William Buckett and Ri-Cheng Chian

Introduction

Assisted reproductive technologies (ART) are practiced all over the world, with clinics offering these services in all developed countries and many parts of the developing world too. Results generated from the European registries by the European Society of Human Reproduction and Embryology (ESHRE) show that over 350 000 ART cycles every year are performed in a total of 28 different countries [1]. With a live birth rate of approximately 20% across Europe, this accounts for 70 000 deliveries per year. In the USA alone, over 120 000 cycles ART are performed each year, resulting in over 35 000 deliveries per year [2,3]. With an incidence of 20% for twin pregnancies in ART, this means that approximately 200 000 babies are born per year as a result of ART. Since the advent of in vitro fertilization (IVF), well over 1 million babies have been born using this technology [4].

All this is a far cry from the scepticism and concerns that accompanied the early days of IVF, both in the lay press [5,6] and the medical literature [7]. However, this is exactly the position again now, with much written and many concerns expressed about fertility preservation in general and oocyte cryopreservation in particular [8,9].

Concerns are primarily two-fold. First, there are the unknown risks to any child or pregnancy conceived following oocyte cryopreservation. The process of oocyte freezing (whether by conventional slow cryopreservation or by vitrification) is known to result in the loss of some oocytes and in meiotic spindle and chromosome configuration abnormalities in the oocytes that survive [10]. Furthermore, the process of vitrification, where the oocytes may be directly exposed to liquid nitrogen, also raises theoretical concerns of transmission of infective disease [11]. Second, there are increased pregnancy risks to the mother by virtue of her own status, whether age or having survived cancer and cancer treatment, that will also, by extension, have an effect on the child. Examples include increased risk of preterm delivery (and its associated complications), pregnancy-induced hypertension, gestational diabetes, and cesarean delivery [12].

Therefore, it is paramount that data on pregnancy, pregnancy outcome (including miscarriages or terminations of pregnancy for congenital or chromosomal abnormalities), pregnancy complications, and neonatal outcomes are reported and collected. In October 2007, the American Society for Reproductive Medicine stated: "Oocyte cryopreservation, or egg freezing, remains an experimental procedure that should not be offered or marketed as a means to defer reproductive aging. Currently available data are too limited to allow egg freezing to be considered an established medical treatment. Because of the experimental nature of egg freezing, the ASRM recommends comprehensive counseling" [13]. This further highlights the importance of disseminating all available information.

This chapter will discuss the current state of knowledge regarding pregnancy outcomes in ART in general and then, more specifically, detail the current evidence regarding pregnancy and perinatal outcomes in pregnancies conceived following oocyte cryopreservation. How these data, which come usually from short-term oocyte cryopreservation programs, may be applied to women undergoing these treatments for more long-term elective social reasons or for women who have undergone sterilizing chemotherapy and/or radiotherapy for cancer treatment will be discussed.

Pregnancy outcomes following assisted reproduction in general

Miscarriage

Relatively early in the development of ART, workers became aware of the early pregnancy loss – termed

Fertility Cryopreservation, ed. Ri-Cheng Chian and Patrick Quinn. Published by Cambridge University Press.

chemical beta-human chorionic gonadotropin (β-hCG) abortion or biochemical pregnancy – as opposed to "later" clinical first trimester miscarriage [14]. Ideally, ART programs should report clinical pregnancy rates where a clinical pregnancy is defined using the World Health Organization/ESHRE definition of ultrasound evidence of an intrauterine pregnancy. Biochemical pregnancies are, therefore, pregnancies lost before this stage.

Because very early pregnancy losses may occur following spontaneous conception before awareness of pregnancy, it is impossible to determine the rate of biochemical pregnancy in the population as a whole. However, biochemical pregnancy loss rates following ART are typically around 15–20% [15,16], although rates from as low as 11% to as high as 35% have been reported [17–19]. The reasons for biochemical pregnancy loss are unclear. However, maternal age (particularly over 40 years), smoking, and poor embryo quality at transfer have been shown to be associated with an increased risk of biochemical pregnancy loss following ART [15].

Clinical miscarriage rates amongst spontaneously conceived pregnancies are reasonably consistent at 10–15% pregnancies [20–22]. However, there are many confounding variables that may affect couples undergoing ART, predominantly maternal age [22,23], which is higher in women undergoing ART than in non-ART pregnancies. Also, other risks for miscarriage, such as polycystic ovary syndrome, are over-represented in couples undergoing ART. Polycystic ovary syndrome is associated with an increased risk of miscarriage, typically reported at approximately 25%, either following spontaneous conception [24] or following ovulation induction [25,26]. Following ART, the clinical miscarriage rate is typically around 15% [1,2,16,27], although it ranges from 10% to 45% depending on maternal age [27]. In women with polycystic ovary syndrome or in those who are overweight or obese, the clinical miscarriage rate is higher [28,29].

In conclusion, clinical miscarriage rates seem to be similar following ART as in spontaneously conceived pregnancies, around 15%, although the higher maternal age and higher incidence of polycystic ovary syndrome seen in women undergoing ART are associated with an increased risk of miscarriage. Biochemical loss is impossible to ascertain following spontaneously conceived pregnancies; however, rates of 15–20% are typical following ART. Overall, therefore, approximately 30% of women with positive pregnancy tests following ART will lose their pregnancies before the end of the first trimester. This high loss rate highlights the importance of reporting live birth rates following ART rather than pregnancy rates or clinical pregnancy rates [30,31].

Ectopic pregnancy

Ectopic pregnancy rates have risen since the mid 1990s, although the reasons are unclear; improved and earlier diagnosis certainly has an effect. Currently, estimates are that ectopic pregnancy affects approximately 2% of all pregnancies. Although some earlier case series showed a higher incidence of ectopic pregnancy (at approximately 4%) following ART [32,33], most large prospective studies show a rate of 2.0–2.2%, which is similar to that of the general population [34,35]. This change is probably because tubal disease was the major indication for ART early in the development of ART.

Late pregnancy loss

The incidence of late pregnancy loss (after 12 weeks of gestation) after ART, through mid-trimester miscarriage, fetal death, or termination of pregnancy for chromosomal or other abnormality, is typically between 2 and 4% [27,36]. This is higher than that of spontaneously conceived pregnancies (typically around 1%) [37,38].

One reason for this is advancing maternal age, which is associated with a higher incidence of chromosomal and other abnormalities and may result in mid-trimester termination of pregnancy. However, with the exception of case reports and case series, there are no comparative data for mid-trimester termination of pregnancy following ART. Maternal age is also associated with a higher spontaneous late pregnancy loss rate, both following spontaneous conceptions and following ART [27].

Congenital abnormality

Initial studies comparing babies born following IVF or intracytoplasmic sperm injection (ICSI) with spontaneously conceived controls suggested no increase in the incidence of congenital abnormalities [39–41], although the magnitude of these were in the hundreds rather than the thousands or tens of thousands that are needed in order to determine any genuine difference. However, since the beginning of this century, some two decades after the beginnings of IVF, an increasing number of papers have compared ART babies with spontaneously conceived controls [42,43] and there have been several systematic reviews [44]; these show an increase in the risk of congenital abnormality associated with ART. Current

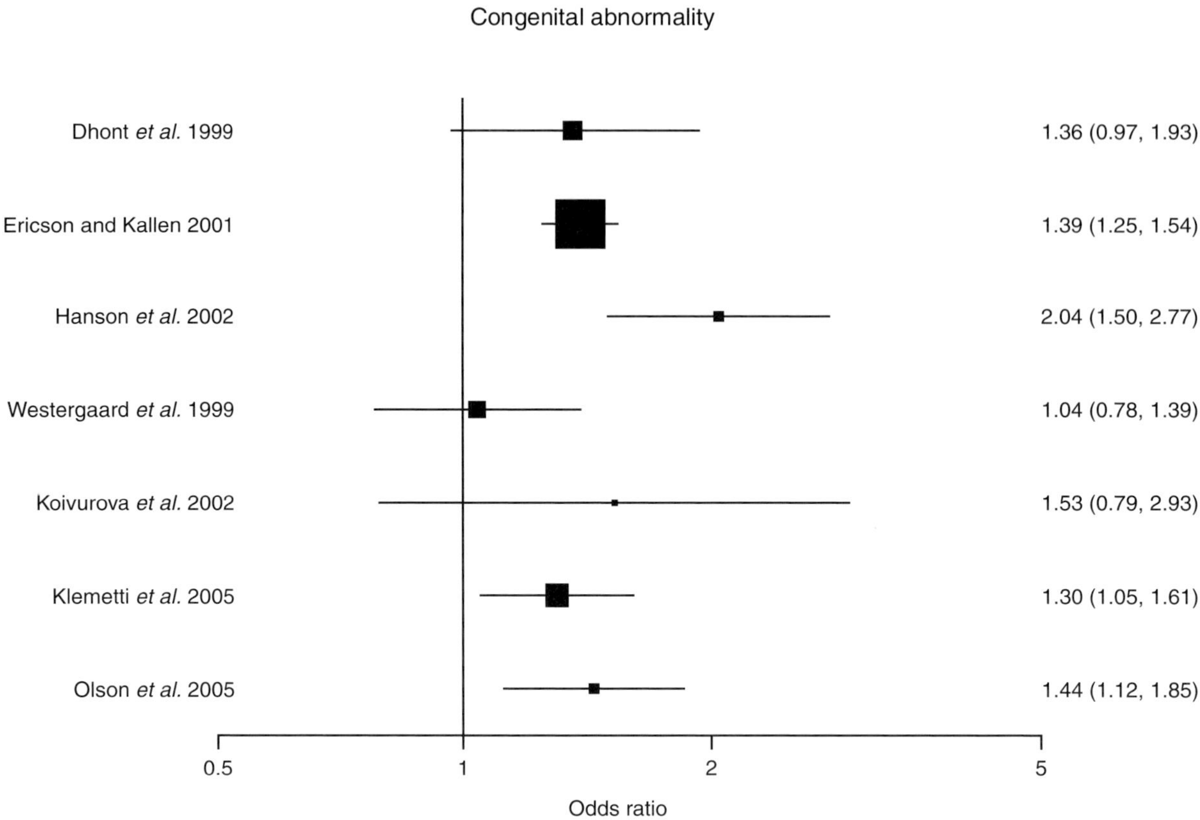

Figure 20.1. Odds ratio estimates (95% confidence intervals) from major studies comparing major congenital abnormalities in babies born following assisted reproductive therapy with spontaneously conceived controls [42,43,45–49].

information, therefore, shows that ART is associated with a 1.5 times increased risk of congenital abnormality when compared with spontaneously conceived controls (Figure 20.1) [45–49].

Subgroup analyses from the major published systematic reviews shows a persistently elevated odds ratio when singleton deliveries are compared. Similarly, there is no difference when IVF without ICSI is compared with that with ICSI [44]. Furthermore, a number of studies have compared congenital abnormality risk in babies born following IVF without ICSI and babies born following ICSI and have not found significant differences. Therefore, it would appear that other mechanisms apart from ICSI or multiple pregnancy account for this increase in congenital abnormality [50,51].

Some studies have attempted to determine whether any particular abnormalities are associated with ART. Musculoskeletal abnormalities [42] and urogenital abnormalities [42,47] have been found to be increased in babies born following ART, particularly male babies. Some studies have also found heart malformations to be increased in babies born following ART, although multiple pregnancy is a confounding variable for this, and subgroup analysis of singleton and multiple gestations has not shown any difference [42].

Chromosomal abnormalities have not been shown to be increased in the babies born following ART compared with spontaneously conceived controls. This may, of course, be as a result of mid-trimester termination of pregnancy. As noted above, few data concerning mid-trimester termination of pregnancy for chromosomal or other major abnormalities are available. It is already well established that chromosomal abnormalities are more frequent in men with severe male factor infertility who are referred for IVF/ICSI [52]. More recently, it has become apparent that chromosomal abnormalities amongst the "normal" female partners of men who are referred for IVF/ICSI are also increased and indeed is higher with less severe degrees of male factor infertility [53]. These data imply that unexplained female subfertility also confers a higher risk of chromosomal abnormality.

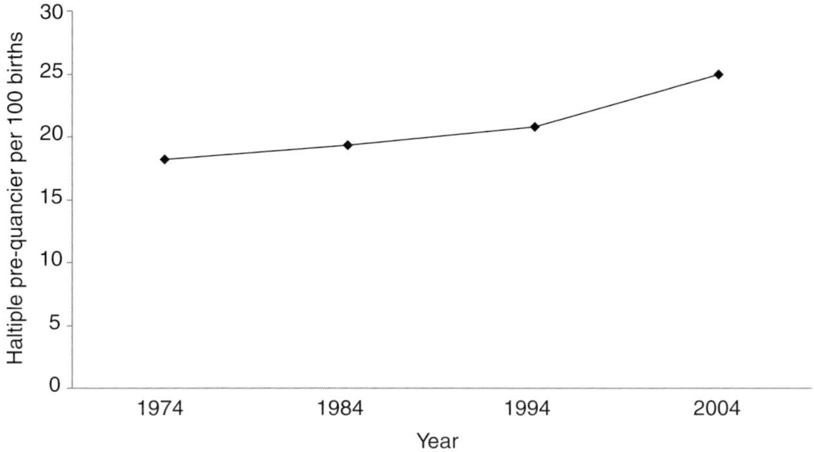

Figure 20.2. Multiple pregnancy rates (per 1000 births) in Canada 1974–2004.

Furthermore, since the association of imprinting disorders and ART [54,55], more recent evidence has suggested that spontaneous conceptions, with and without ovarian stimulation in the absence of ART, is also associated with imprinting disorders [56].

In conclusion, there is a genuine – albeit small (1.5-fold) – increase in the risk of congenital abnormality amongst children born to couples who conceived following ART. However, it appears that couples with infertility may have an a priori increased risk for congenital abnormality. Whether any of the myriad features of ART also have a role to increase this risk remains unclear. Research to answer these questions needs careful planning, prospective surveillance, imaginative use of possible control groups, and enough time to generate the data. In the meantime, couples electing to undergo ART should be counseled concerning the small increased risk of congenital abnormality associated with ART, although it is unclear whether this is related to their infertility itself or its treatment.

Multiple pregnancy

Early in the development of ART, following the advent of ovarian hyperstimulation to produce multiple oocytes and the practice of transferring multiple embryos in order to improve pregnancy and live birth rates, there has been an increase in the rate of multiple pregnancies [57,58]. It is the single most common complication of ART pregnancies and is associated with the huge increase in the multiple pregnancy rate seen over the last two decades [59] (Figure 20.2).

Despite the 5–10 time increase in the risk of perinatal death and cerebral palsy multiple conceptions, over 20% of pregnancies following ART in Europe are twin pregnancies and over 1% are triplet pregnancies [1]. In the USA, over 25% pregnancies following ART are twin pregnancies and approximately 5% are triplet pregnancies [2]. Therefore, around 50% of all babies born following ART belong to a set of multiples. A full discussion concerning the appropriate way to address this issue, the commonest risk associated with all types of ART (including oocyte cryopreservation), is beyond the scope of this chapter.

Pregnancy outcome in singleton pregnancies

Not unreasonably, most earlier descriptive studies presumed that the poorer obstetric outcome associated with ART resulted from the increased multiple pregnancy rates [57,58]. However, only relatively recently have sufficiently sized and appropriately performed studies and meta-analyses been available to explore the effect of ART in singleton gestations [60,61]. Although the great majority of singleton ART pregnancies are uncomplicated, there is recent evidence of higher rates of adverse pregnancy outcomes in singleton ART pregnancies compared with spontaneously conceived singleton gestations.

Women with IVF-conceived singletons are at increased risk of pre-eclampsia, gestational diabetes, placenta previa, and perinatal mortality (Table 20.1). Singleton pregnancies from ART also have higher relative risks of having induction of labour and both emergency and elective cesarean deliveries [62]. It is not possible to separate ART-related risks from those secondary to the underlying reproductive pathology at this time. In addition, patients undergoing ART are

Table 20.1. Adverse obstetric outcomes in singleton pregnancies following assisted reproductive therapy

	Absolute risk (%)	Odds ratio (95% confidence interval)
Perinatal risks		
Preterm birth	11.5	2.0 (1.7–2.2)
Low birthweight (< 2500 g)	9.5	1.8 (1.4–2.2)
Very low birthweight (< 1500 g)	2.5	2.7 (2.3–3.1)
Small for gestational age	14.6	1.6 (1.3–2.0)
Admission to neonatal intensive care unit	17.8	1.6 (1.3–2.0)
Stillbirth	1.2	2.6 (1.8–3.6)
Neonatal mortality	0.6	2.0 (1.2–3.4)
Cerebral palsy	0.4	2.8 (1.3–5.8)
Maternal risks		
Pre-eclampsia	10.3	1.6 (1.2–2.0)
Placenta praevia	2.4	2.9 (1.5–5.4)
Placental abruption	2.2	2.4 (1.1–5.2)
Gestational diabetes	6.8	2.0 (1.4–3.0)
Cesarean delivery	26.7	2.1 (1.7–2.6)

older than average, and age is an independent contributory risk factor for most of these complications. Although evidence of an effect is convincing, questions remain about whether this is a treatment effect or relates to any of the factors causing the underlying infertility.

Neonatal development

Babies conceived with ART also have increased neonatal morbidity [42]. One study demonstrated an increased frequency of intraventricular hemorrhage following IVF even when controlling for multiple birth, gestational age, and birthweight [63]. Other studies also have suggested an increase in morbidity and mortality but do not sufficiently address the effect of confounders such as birthweight and gestational age.

A review of the long-term developmental outcomes in children conceived by ART has been reassuring, demonstrating that the great majority of children are developing normally [64]. However, these evaluations suffer from major methodological limitations, including limited statistical power, selection bias, inadequate or inappropriate comparison groups, and high loss to follow-up. Of concern is a recent study with improved methodology (stratification by gestational age, birthweight, and plurality) that demonstrated an overall increased relative risk of cerebral palsy (odds ratio 3.7) and suspected developmental delay (odds ratio 4) [65].

Pregnancy outcomes following oocyte cryopreservation

Evaluation of current data

Unlike IVF and ICSI, where decades of data and millions of pregnancies have allowed genuine comparative analyses to be carried out with spontaneously conceived pregnancies, other ART pregnancies, and pregnancies conceived following other infertility treatments, data from oocyte cryopreservation (whether slow freezing or vitrification) is limited to case series. These range from single case reports [66–68] to case series of over 100 pregnancies [69–71].

All these reports are uncontrolled and, therefore, accurate comparison with pregnancies conceived spontaneously, or those following ART in general, is difficult. Furthermore, particularly in the small series, there is a risk of selection bias, where adverse outcomes are not submitted for publication (or not accepted). Despite these caveats, over 500 pregnancies have been reported in the literature and, worldwide, over 1000 babies have been born from cryopreserved protocols. Therefore, an appraisal of the current data is appropriate. The remainder of this chapter will present current data regarding pregnancies conceived following oocyte cryopreservation and compare these with the same outcomes as above.

Although there are methodological differences between the slow-cryopreservation protocols and the vitrification protocols (and indeed even within these different modalities), all pregnancy outcome data will be pooled. This is because with such small numbers it is impossible to control for all the laboratory differences.

Miscarriage

To date, 11 published studies have reported miscarriage rates amongst the pregnancy outcomes for a total of over 400 reported pregnancy outcomes [68,69,72–80]

Table 20.2. Pregnancy loss following oocyte cryopreservation

	No. pregnancies	No. pregnancy losses	Miscarriage rate (%)
Quintans *et al.* [72]	6	3	50
Konc *et al.* [73]	7	1	14
De Geyter *et al.* [68]	3	1	33
Borini *et al.* [69]	267	37	14
Borini *et al.* [74]	18	3	17
Sher *et al.*[75]	14	2	14
Kim *et al.* [76]	16	3	19
Chang *et al.* [77]	16	2	13
Chian *et al.* [78]	17	2	12
Chian *et al.* [78]	5	1	20
Yoon *et al.* [79]	13	2	15
Antinori *et al.* [80]	39	8	21
Total	**421**	**65**	**15**

(Table 20.2). The overall miscarriage rate is 15%, which, as noted above, is comparable with both the rate of clinical miscarriage following spontaneous pregnancy [20–22] and that following ART [1,2,16,27].

Although these data are uncontrolled and there may be differences in the diagnosis of clinical pregnancy and, therefore, miscarriage rates, it is reassuring that the rate is very similar to that reported following spontaneous conception and following ART. Therefore, based on the reported data, it is unlikely that oocyte cryopreservation is associated with an increase in this risk, although further data need to be collected.

Ectopic pregnancy

So far there have been two cases of ectopic pregnancy reported in pregnancies conceived following oocyte cryopreservation [68,72]. Although a bias in reporting is likely, if all the studies noted above were counted, this would give an ectopic pregnancy rate of 0.5%. This is lower than that normally quoted for rates of ectopic

Table 20.3. Congenital abnormalities in pregnancies following oocyte cryopreservation

	Absolute risk (%)
Total babies	200
Abnormalities	
Biliary atresia	1
Club foot	1
Skin hemangioma	1
Ventriculoseptal defect	2
Abnormality rate	2.5%

Source: adapted from Chian *et al.* [71].

pregnancy in spontaneously conceived pregnancies and ART pregnancies in general [33,34]. However, rates of 0.5% have been reported in some groups undergoing ART, such as recipients of oocyte donation [27], so it could represent a true incidence.

Late pregnancy loss and oocyte cryopreservation

There has only been one report of a late pregnancy loss (at 16 weeks of gestation) in a pregnancy conceived by oocyte cryopreservation [81]. There was another single case of miscarriage where the karyotype of the fetus was abnormal (45XO), although the gestational age of the miscarried fetus is not given [72]. Whether these cases represent a genuine incidence of this, already rare, outcome of pregnancy is unclear at present.

Congenital abnormality

Although many of the case reports and case series have stated that the live birth was a healthy infant, only one study has specifically presented data concerning congenital abnormalities in pregnancies following oocyte cryopreservation [71]. In this study, 200 children from 165 pregnancies (28 sets of twins and 137 singleton pregnancies) were examined (Table 20.3). A total of five congenital abnormalities in five different infants were reported (two ventriculoseptal defect, one club foot, one skin haemangioma, and one congenital biliary atresia). This gives an incidence of congenital abnormality affecting 2.5% pregnancies, which is in the same order of magnitude as spontaneously conceived pregnancies and pregnancies conceived following ART [42–44].

As noted above under ART, there are multiple confounding variables when rates of congenital abnormality are compared, and continued surveillance and registration of all infants born following oocyte cryopreservation, such as that proposed by the HOPE registry [82], are needed.

Multiple pregnancy

As noted above, twin and higher-order multiple pregnancy is the most frequent complication associated with ART in general [1,2], and pregnancies conceived following oocyte cryopreservation are no different [66–80, 83–85]. In reported series, multiple pregnancy rates range from 0% to over 50% [68,83]. Most series of pregnancies following oocyte cryopreservation that report multiple pregnancy [31,68,69,72–75,79–80, 83, 84] have twin pregnancy rates at between 15 and 30%. This is comparable to that reported in the large ART registries.

The risks and consequences of multiple pregnancy are beyond the scope of this chapter. However, as cryopreservation techniques improve and pregnancy and implantation rates increase, just as in ART using fresh oocytes, the number of embryos transferred will decrease and the incidence of multiple pregnancy following oocyte cryopreservation will fall.

Obstetric outcomes

As twin pregnancies are associated with an increase in preterm delivery and low-birthweight babies, these outcomes should be analyzed only in singleton pregnancies. Only one study so far has presented these outcomes [71]. This study presents data from 137 singleton pregnancies delivered in three different countries (Canada, Columbia, and Mexico). When the data were pooled, the incidence of delivery before 34 weeks was 4% (6/137) and the incidences of low birthweight (< 2500 g) and very-low birthweight (< 1500 g) babies were 17% (24/137) and 1% (1/137), respectively. This is similar to the rates of these outcomes reported in singleton pregnancies following ART [60,61,62].

Although these limited data are encouraging, it is difficult to draw definitive conclusions as the "background" rates of preterm delivery and low-birthweight babies vary greatly amongst different populations. As noted above, registration, either separately or within existing ART registries, will allow continued monitoring of the incidence of these and other risks.

Neonatal and child development

As yet, no data have been reported concerning neonatal and child development following oocyte cryopreservation. The primary reason for this is that the number of babies born, until recently has been very small. Therefore, these data will become available over the coming years.

Interpretation of outcomes after oocyte cryopreservation

As this review of obstetric and perinatal outcomes in pregnancies conceived following oocyte cryopreservation has shown, broadly speaking, the risks are very similar to ART in general. This is not surprising for several reasons. First, the process of oocyte cryopreservation involves similar hormonal treatments (leading to increased estrogen levels in the follicular phase and supraphysiological progesterone levels in the luteal phase and early pregnancy), similar laboratory conditions for fertilization of the thawed oocytes and culture of the resultant embryos, and similar physical interventions (such as ICSI, assisted hatching, and the number of embryos transferred). Consequently, if any of these interventions have an effect on pregnancy in ART they will have a similar impact in oocyte cryopreservation. Second, most series reported so far in the literature have included oocyte cryopreservation for various reasons for couples undergoing infertility treatment. Therefore any a priori increased risk will be the same or similar to that in couples undergoing ART with fresh oocytes. Finally, the history of oocyte cryopreservation is still young and much, much more data are needed if small differences are to be identified.

As noted elsewhere in this volume, oocyte cryopreservation is indicated for preserving fertility in women who will undergo potentially sterilizing treatment, often to cure fatal diseases such as breast cancer or lymphoma. Therefore, pregnancy outcome in these women may differ from that in women who present with infertility. Although there are many reports of pregnancies following oocyte cryopreservation, there have been few in cancer survivors and some have used gestational surrogates [85].

Furthermore, there has been an increasing trend for women to cryopreserve oocytes as "an insurance" against failing ovarian function. These situations are likely to involve cryopreservation for several years. Again, it is difficult to predict pregnancy outcome in otherwise fertile women who may have had oocytes cryopreserved for over 5 years. As yet, there are only a few published cases of live birth after such long-term oocyte cryopreservation [86]. As noted above, there may also be differences in laboratory/freezing protocols that could affect obstetric and perinatal outcome. However, well-designed long-term trials are needed to answer this and, in fact, many other questions regarding ART in general.

Conclusions

Certainly the data from over 500 pregnancies following oocyte cryopreservation presented in the world literature are reassuring. Pregnancy outcomes and congenital abnormalities are similar to those reported following spontaneous conceptions and following ART in general.

Obviously, the dataset is still too small to determine small differences, and couples should be counseled that, although the data so far are reassuring, there may be small increases in the risk of poor pregnancy outcome that cannot be detected at present. Similarly, some abnormalities or complications may become apparent at a much later date. However, the likelihood of either of these outcomes is small.

National or international registries (either within established ART registries or as stand-alone registries) for oocyte cryopreservation should be established and continue to collect treatment, pregnancy outcome, and childhood data over the next several decades.

References

1. Andersen AN, Goosens V, Gianaroli L, *et al.* Assisted reproductive technology in Europe, 2003. Results generated from European registries by ESHRE. *Hum Reprod* 2007; **22**: 1513–1525.
2. Society for Assisted Reproductive Technology; American Society for Reproductive Medicine. Assisted reproductive technology in the United States: 2001 results generated from the American Society for Reproductive Medicine/Society for Assisted Reproductive Technology Registry. *Fertil Steril* 2007; **87**: 1253–1256.
3. Society for Assisted Reproductive Technology. *SART Clinical Summary Report 2005*. Birmingham, AL: Society for Assisted Reproductive Technology, www.sartcorsonline.com/rpt.
4. Adamson GD, de Mouzon J, Lancaster P, for the International Committee for Monitoring Assisted Reproductive Technology, . World collaborative report on in vitro fertilization, 2000. *Fertil Steril* 2006; **85**: 1586–1622.
5. Auerbach S. Fears aired in test tube baby debate. *Washington Post* 1974; **Jul 21**: A1.
6. Wright P. Less risk of test-tube baby being born with brain damage, doctor says. *The Times* 1974; **Sept 7**: 4.
7. Fitzgerald J. Veto in vitro, or turn off the tube. *Can Fam Physician* 1978; **24**: 816.
8. Harwood K. Egg freezing: a breakthrough for reproductive autonomy? *Bioethics* 2009; **23**: 39–46.
9. Goold I, Savalescu J. In favour of freezing eggs for non-medical reasons. *Bioethics* 2009; **23**: 47–58.
10. Cao YX, Xing Q, Li L, *et al.* Comparison of survival and embryonic development in human oocytes cryopreserved by slow-freezing and vitrification. *Fertil Steril* 2009; **92**: 1306–1311
11. Tedder RS, Zukerman MA, Goldstone AH, *et al.* Hepatitis transmission from contaminated cryopreservation tank. *Lancet* 1995; **346**: 137–140.
12. Chan BC, Lao TT. Effect of parity and advanced maternal age on obstetric outcome. *Int J Gynaecol Obstet* 2008; **102**: 237–241.
13. American Society for Reproductive Medicine. *ASRM Urges Caution, Strong Counseling for Women Seeking Egg Freezing*. Washington, DC: American Society for Reproductivve Medicine, October 16, 2007, http://www.asrm.org/Media/Press/AM07urgecautioneggfreezing.html.
14. Jones HW, Jr., Acosta AA, Andrews MC, *et al.* What is a pregnancy? A question for programs of in vitro fertilization. *Fertil Steril* 1983; **40**: 728–733.
15. Winter E, Wang J, Davies MJ, Norman R. Early pregnancy loss following assisted reproductive technology treatment. *Hum Reprod* 2002; **17**: 3220–3223.
16. Buckett WM, Chian R-C, Dean NL, *et al.* Pregnancy loss in pregnancies conceived following in vitro oocyte maturation (IVM), conventional in vitro fertilization (IVF), and intra-cytoplasmic sperm injection (ICSI). *Fertil Steril* 2008; **90**: 546–550.
17. Bellver J, Albert C, Labarta E, Pellicer A. Early pregnancy loss in women stimulated with gonadotropin-releasing hormone antagonist protocols according to oral contraceptive pill pretreatment. *Fertil Steril* 2007; **87**: 1089–1101.
18. European Recombinant LH Study Group. Human recombinant luteinizing hormone is as effective as, but safer than, urinary human chorionic gonadotropin in inducing final follicular maturation and ovulation in in vitro fertilization procedures: results of a multicenter double-blind study. *J Clin Endocrinol Metab* 2001; **86**: 2607–2618.
19. Barlow P, Lejeune B, Puissant F, *et al.* Early pregnancy loss and obstetrical risk after in-vitro fertilization and embryo replacement. *Hum Reprod* 1988; **3**: 671–675.
20. Miller JF, Williamson E, Glue J, *et al.* Fetal loss after implantation: a prospective study. *Lancet* 1980; **ii**: 554–556.
21. Regan L, Braude P, Trembath PL. Influence of past reproductive performance on risk of spontaneous abortion. *Br Med J* 1989; **299**: 541–545.
22. Nybo Andersen AM, Wohlfahrt J, Christens P, *et al.* Maternal age and fetal loss: population based register linkage. *Br Med J* 2000; **320**: 1708–1712.
23. Buckett W, Regan L. Sporadic and recurrent miscarriage. In Shaw RA, Soutter WP, Stanton SL, eds. *Gynaecology*, 3rd edn. London: Churchill Livingstone, 2003, pp. 343–360.

24. Rotterdam ESHRE/ASRM-sponsored PCOS Consensus Workshop Group. Revised 2003 consensus on diagnostic criteria and long-term health risks related to polycystic ovary syndrome. *Fertil Steril* 2004; **81**: 19–25.
25. Homburg R. Pregnancy complications in PCOS. *Best Pract Res Clin Endocrinol Metab* 2006; **20**: 281–292.
26. MacGregor AH, Johnson JE, Bunde CA. Further clinical experience with clomiphene citrate. *Fertil Steril* 1968; **19**: 616–622.
27. Farr SL, Schieve LA, Jamieson DJ. Pregnancy loss among pregnancies conceived through assisted reproductive technology, United States, 1999–2002. *Am J Epidemiol* 2007; **165**: 1380–1386.
28. Wang JX, Davies MJ, Norman RJ. Polycystic ovarian syndrome and the risk of spontaneous abortion following assisted reproductive technology treatment. *Hum Reprod* 2001; **16**: 2606–2609.
29. Maheshwari A, Stofberg L, Bhattacharya S. Effect of overweight and obesity on assisted reproductive technology: a systematic review. *Hum Reprod Update* 2007; **13**: 433–444.
30. Centers for Disease Control and Prevention. Current trends in ectopic pregnancy-United States, 1990–1992. *MMWR Surveill Summ* 1995; **44**: 46–48.31. Fosas N, Marina F, Torres PJ, *et al.* The births of five Spanish babies from cryopreserved donated oocytes. *Hum Reprod* 2003; **18**: 1417–1421
31. Fosas N, Marina F, Torres PJ, *et al.* The births of five Spanish babies from cryopreserved donated oocytes. *Hum Reprod* 2003; **18**: 1417–1421.
32. Ribic-Pucelj M, Tomazevic T, Vogler A, Meden-Vrtovec H. Risk factors for ectopic pregnancy after in vitro fertilization and embryo transfer. *J Assist Reprod Genet* 1995; **12**: 594–598.
33. Dubuisson JB, Aubriot FX, Mathieu L, *et al.* Risk factors for ectopic pregnancy in 556 pregnancies after in vitro fertilization: implications for preventive management. *Fertil Steril* 1991; **56**: 686–690.
34. Verhulst G, Camus M, Bollen N, Van Steirteghem A, Devroey P. Analysis of the risk factors with regard to the occurrence of ectopic pregnancy after medically assisted procreation. *Hum Reprod* 1993; **8**: 1284–1287.
35. Clayton HB, Schieve LA, Peterson HB, *et al.* Ectopic pregnancy risk with assisted reproductive technology procedures. *Obstet Gynecol* 2006; **107**: 595–604.
36. Buckett WM, Chian R-C, Dean NL, *et al.* Pregnancy loss in pregnancies conceived after in vitro oocyte maturation, conventional in vitro fertilization, and intracytoplasmic sperm injection. *Fertil Steril* 2008; **90**: 546–550.
37. Brigham SA, Conlon C, Farquharson RG. A longitudinal study of pregnancy outcome following idiopathic recurrent miscarriage. *Hum Reprod* 1999; **14**: 2868–2871.
38. Confidential Enquiry into Maternal and Child Health. *Stillbirth, Neonatal and Post-neonatal Mortality 2000–2003, England, Wales, and Northern Ireland.* London: RCOG Press, 2005.
39. Morin NC, Wirth FH, Johnson DH, *et al.* Congenital malformations and psychosocial development in children conceived by in vitro fertilization. *J Pediatr* 1989; **115**: 222–227.
40. Sutcliffe AG, D'Souza SW, Cadman J, *et al.* Minor congenital anomalies, major congenital malformations and development in children conceived from cryopreserved embryos. *Hum Reprod* 1995; **10**: 3332–3337.
41. Isaksson R, Gissler M, Tiitinen A. Obstetric outcome among women with unexplained infertility after IVF: a matched case-control study. *Hum Reprod* 2002; **17**: 1755–1761.
42. Klemetti R, Gissier M, Sevon T, *et al.* Children born after assisted fertilization have an increased rate of major congenital anomalies. *Fertil Steril* 2005; **84**: 1300–1307.
43. Olson CK, Keppler-Noreuil KM, Romitti PA, *et al.* In vitro fertilization is associated with an increase in major birth defects. *Fertil Steril* 2005; **84**: 1308–1315.
44. Hansen M, Bower C, Milne E, de Klerk N, Kurinczuk JJ. Assisted reproductive technologies and the risk of birth defects: a systematic review. *Hum Reprod* 2005; **20**: 328–338.
45. Dhont M, de Sutter P, Ruyssinck G, Martens G, Bekaert A. Perinatal outcome of pregnancies after assisted reproduction: a case-control study. *Am J Obstet Gynecol* 1999; **181**: 688–695.
46. Hansen M, Kurinczuk JJ, Bower C, Webb S . The risk of major birth defects after intracytoplasmatic sperm injection and in vitro fertilization. *N Engl J Med* 2002; **346**: 725–730.
47. Ericson A, Kallen B. Congenital malformations in infants born after IVF: a population-based study. *Hum Reprod* 2001; **16**: 504–509.
48. Westergaard HB, Johansen AM, Erb K, Andersen AN. Danish national in-vitro fertilization registry 1994 and 1995: a controlled study of births, malformations and cytogenetic findings. *Hum Reprod* 1999; **14**: 1896–1902.
49. Koivurova S, Kartikainen AL, Gissler M, *et al.* Neonatal outcome and congenital malformations in children born after in-vitro fertilization. *Hum Reprod* 2002; **17**: 1391–1398.
50. Bonduelle M, Liebaers I, Deketelaere V, *et al.* Neonatal data on a cohort of 2889 infants born after ICSI (1991–1999) and of 2995 infants born after IVF (1983–1999). *Hum Reprod* 2002; **17**: 671–694.
51. Place I, Englert Y. A prospective longitudinal study of the physical, psychomotor, and intellectual development of singleton children up to 5 years who were conceived by intracytoplasmic sperm injection compared with

children conceived spontaneously and by in vitro fertilization. *Fertil Steril* 2003; **80**: 1388–1397.

52. Buckett W, Aird L, Luckas M, *et al.* Intracytoplasmic sperm injection. Karyotyping should be done before treatment. *Br Med J* 1996; **313**: 1334.
53. Gekas J, Thepot F, Turleau C . For the Association des Cytogeneticiens de Langue Francaise. Chromosomal factors of infertility in candidate couples for ICSI: an equal risk of constitutional aberrations in women and men. *Hum Reprod* 2001; **16**: 82–90.
54. Gosden R, Trasler J, Lucifero D, Faddy M. Rare congenital disorders, imprinted genes, and assisted reproductive technology. *Lancet* 2003; **361**: 1974–1977.
55. Chang AS, Moley KH, Wangler M, Feinberg AP, Debaun MR. Association between Beckwith–Wiedemann syndrome and assisted reproductive technology: a case series of 19 patients. *Fertil Steril* 2005; **83**: 349–354.
56. Ludwig M, Katalinic A, Gross S, *et al.* Increased prevalence of imprinting defects in patients with Angelman syndrome born to subfertile couples. *J Med Genet* 2005; **42**: 2890–2891.
57. Wood C, Trounson A, Leeton JF, *et al.* Clinical features of eight pregnancies resulting from in vitro fertilization and embryo transfer. *Fertil Steril* 1982; **38**: 22–29.
58. Mushin D, Spensley J, Barreda-Hanson M. Children of IVF. *Clin Obstet Gynacol* 1985; **12**: 865–876.
59. Bissonnette F, Cohen J, Collins J, *et al.* Incidence and complications of multiple gestation in Canada: proceedings of an expert meeting. *Reprod Biomed Online* 2007; **14**: 773–790.
60. Helmerhorst FM, Perquin DAM, Donker D, Keirse MJNC. Perinatal outcome of singletons and twins after assisted conception: a systematic review of controlled studies. *Br Med J* 2004; **328**: 261.
61. Jackson RA, Gibson KA, Wu YW, Croughan MS. Perinatal outcomes in singletons following in vitro fertilization: a meta-analysis. *Obstet Gynecol* 2004; **103**: 551–563.
62. Rimm AA, Katayama AC, Diaz M, Katayama KP. A meta-analysis of controlled studies comparing major malformation rates in IVF and ICSI infants with naturally conceived children. *J Assist Reprod Genet* 2004; **21**: 437–443.
63. Linder N, Haskin O, Levit O, *et al.* Risk factors for intraventricular hemorrhage in very low birth weight premature infants: a retrospective case–control study. *Pediatrics* 2003; **111**: 590–595.
64. Olivennes F, Fanchin R, Ledee N, *et al.* Perinatal outcome and developmental studies on children born after IVF. *Hum Reprod Update* 2002; **8**: 117–128.
65. Stromberg B, Dahlquist G, Ericson A, *et al.* Neurological sequelae in children born after in-vitro fertilisation: a population-based study. *Lancet* 2002; **359:** 461–465.
66. De Geyter M, Steimann S, Holzgreve W, De Geyter C. First delivery of healthy offspring after freezing and thawing of oocytes in Switzerland. *Swiss Med Wkly* 2007; **137**: 443–447.
67. Chian R-C, Gilbert L, Huang JY, *et al.* Live birth after vitrification of in vitro matured human oocytes. *Fertil Steril* 2009; **91**: 372–376.
68. Kyono K, Nakajo Y, Nishinaka C, *et al.* A birth from the transfer of a single vitrified-warmed blastocyst using intracytoplasmic sperm injection with calcium ionophore oocyte activation in a globozoospermic patient. *Fertil Steril* 2009; **91**: 931.e7–e11.
69. Borini A, Bianchi V, Bonu M A, *et al.* Evidence based clinical outcome of oocyte slow cooling. *Reprod BioMed Online* 2007; **15**: 175–181.
70. Albani E, Barbieri J, Novara PV, *et al.* Oocyte cryopreservation. *Placenta* 2008; **29**(Suppl B): 143–146.
71. Chian R-C, Huang JY, Tan SL, *et al.* Obstetric and perinatal outcome in 200 infants conceived from vitrified oocytes. *Reprod Biomed Online* 2008; **16**: 608–610.
72. Quintans CJ, Donaldson MJ, Bertolino MV, Pasqualini RS. Birth of two babies using oocytes that were cryopreserved in a choline-based freezing medium. *Hum Reprod* 2002; **17**: 3149–3152.
73. Konc J, Kanyo K, Varga E, Kriston R, Cseh S. Births resulting from oocyte cryopreservation using a slow freezing protocol with propanediol and sucrose. *Syst Biol Reprod Med* 2008; **54**: 205–210.
74. Borini A, Sciajno R, Bianchi V, *et al.* Clinical outcome of oocyte cryopreservation after slow cooling with a protocol utilizing a high sucrose concentration. *Hum Reprod* 2006; **21**: 512–517.
75. Sher G, Keskintepe L, Mukaida T, *et al.* Selective vitrification of euploid oocytes markedly improves survival, fertilization and pregnancy-generating potential. *Reprod Biomed Online* 2008; **17:** 524–529.
76. Kim TJ, Laufer LR, Hong SW. Vitrification of oocytes produces high pregnancy rates when carried out in fertile women. *Fertil Steril* 2010; **93:** 467–474.
77. Chang CC, Shapiro DB, Bernal DP, *et al.* Human oocyte vitrification: in-vivo and in-vitro maturation outcomes. *Reprod Biomed Online* 2008; **17**: 684–688.
78. Chian R-C, Huang JY, Gilbert L, *et al.* Obstetric outcomes following vitrification of in vitro and in vivo matured oocytes. *Fertil Steril* 2009; **91**: 2391–2398.
79. Yoon TK, Lee DR, Cha SK, *et al.* Rate of human oocytes and pregnancy outcome after vitrification using slush nitrogen in assisted reproductive technologies. *Fertil Steril* 2007; **88**: 952–956.
80. Antinori M, Licata E, Dani G, *et al.* Cryotop vitrification of human oocytes results in high survival rate and healthy deliveries. *Reprod Biomed Online* 2007; **14**: 72–79.

81. Li Y, Chen ZJ, Yang HJ, *et al.* Comparison of vitrification and slow-freezing of human day 3 cleavage stage embryos: post-vitrification development and pregnancy outcomes. *Zhonghua Fu Chan Ke Za Zhi* 2007; **42**: 753–755.
82. Ezcurra D, Rangnow J, Craig M, Schertz J. The HOPE Registry: first US registry for oocyte cryopreservation. *Reprod Biomed Online* 2008; **17**: 743–744.
83. Chen SU, Lien YR, Tsai YY, *et al.* Successful pregnancy occurred from slowly freezing human oocytes using the regime of 1.5 mol/l 1,2-propanediol with 0.3 mol/l sucrose. *Hum Reprod* 2002; **17**: 1412.
84. Ding J, Rana N, Dmowski WP. Successful pregnancies after oocyte cryopreservation with slow-freezing method: a report of 3 cases. *J Reprod Med* 2008; **53**: 813–820.
85. Yang D, Brown SE, Nguyen K, *et al.* Live birth after the transfer of human embryos developed from cryopreserved oocytes harvested before cancer treatment. *Fertil Steril* 2007; **87**: 1469.
86. Parmegiani L, Fabbri R, Cognigni GE, *et al.* Blastocyst formation, pregnancy, and birth derived from human oocytes cryopreserved for 5 years. *Fertil Steril* 2008; **90**: 2014.

Section 5 Chapter 21

Cryopreservation of ovarian tissue

Cryopreservation of ovarian tissue: an overview

Jacques Donnez, Pascale Jadoul, Olivier Donnez, Anne-Sophie van Eyck, Jean Squifflet, and Marie-Madeleine Dolmans

Introduction

According to previous reports, around 700 000 new cancers are expected every year in the female population in the USA [1] and 8% of these women will be under 40 years of age. By 2010, it is estimated that 1 in every 250 people in the adult population will be a survivor of childhood cancer [2].

Advances in the diagnosis and treatment of childhood, adolescent, and adult cancer have greatly increased the life expectancy of premenopausal women with cancer. Indeed, aggressive chemotherapy and radiotherapy, and bone marrow transplantation, can cure more than 90% of girls affected by childhood malignancies [3], and this has resulted in a growing population of adolescent and adult long-term survivors of childhood malignancies [2] who may experience infertility problems from induced premature ovarian failure (POF).

Gonadotoxicity

Chemotherapy

The ovaries are very sensitive to cytotoxic treatment, especially to alkylating agents [4]. Table 21.1 lists the main agents used in chemotherapy in terms of the level of their risk for causing gonadal dysfunction.

Cyclophosphamide is the agent most commonly implicated in causing damage to oocytes and granulosa cells in a dose-dependent manner [5,6]. This follicular destruction generally results in loss of both endocrine and reproductive function, depending on the dose and the age of the patient. Indeed, Larsen *et al.* reported a four-fold increased risk of POF in teenagers treated for cancer, and a 27-fold increased risk in women aged 21–25 years [7]. Complete amenorrhea was reported after a dose of 5 g cyclophosphamide in women over 40 years of age, and after doses of 9 g and 20 g in women aged 30–40 and 20–30 years, respectively [8]. A combination of various chemotherapeutic agents further increases gonadal toxicity. After chemotherapy with MOPP/ABV (mechlorethamine, vincristine [Oncovin], procarbazine, prednisone/doxorubicin (adriamycin), bleomycin, and vinblastine [or vincristine]) hybrid chemotherapy, Schilsky *et al.* [9] found that amenorrhea developed in 89% and 20% of patients over and under 25 years of age at the time of treatment, respectively. The median age of patients who became amenorrheic after therapy was significantly higher than that of patients who maintained normal menses (26 years versus 20 years; $p = 0.008$).

Radiotherapy

Abdominal ionizing radiation that is often used in combination with alkylating agents often induces POF, rendering patients infertile in almost 100% of cases. Indeed, for radiotherapy, it has been stated that a dose of 5–20 Gy administered to the ovary is sufficient to completely impair gonadal function [10] whatever the age of the patient. The dose of radiation required to destroy 50% of the oocyte reserve has been found to be < 2 Gy [11]. Moreover, uterine irradiation at a young age reduces adult uterine volume [12]. Radiation doses between 14 and 30 Gy have been reported to result in uterine dysfunction [13,14]. The practitioner should be aware of this effect of radiotherapy on the uterus, which could interfere with the implantation capacity of embryos.

Chemo/radiotherapy

Intensive chemotherapy and total body irradiation required before bone marrow transplantation constitute the treatment combination presenting the greatest risk of POF. Indeed, the high doses of chemotherapy (commonly using the highly cytotoxic cyclophosphamide/busulfan regimen) and/or radiotherapy lead to subsequent ovarian failure in almost all cases, children

Fertility Cryopreservation, ed. Ri-Cheng Chian and Patrick Quinn. Published by Cambridge University Press.

Table 21.1. Cytotoxic agents according to degree of gonadotoxicity

Risk of ovarian dysfunction	Agents
High risk	Cyclophosphamide, busulfan, melphalan, chlorambucil, dacarbazine, procarbazine, ifosfamide, thiotepa, nitrogen mustard
Intermediate risk	Doxorubicin, cisplatin, carboplatin
Low/no risk	Methotrexate, bleomycin, 5-fluorouracil, actinomycin D, mercaptopurine, vincristine

and adults alike [15–17]. The risk of POF was estimated to be 92% in the study by Meirow and Nugent [16], and 100% in an earlier study by Teinturier *et al.* [18]. Teinturier *et al.* [18] actually reported 0% of ovarian recovery after busulfan treatment before bone marrow transplant. A large retrospective survey of pregnancy outcomes after hematopoietic stem cell transplantation (peripheral blood or bone marrow transplant) involving 37 362 patients revealed that only 0.6% of patients conceived after autologous or allogenic stem cell transplantation [19,20].

Consequently, it is clear that high doses of alkylating agents, irradiation, and advancing age all increase the risk of gonadal damage.

Indications for ovarian tissue cryopreservation

Oncological indications for ovarian tissue cryopreservation are summarized in Table 21.2 [21]. In gynecological malignancy, a conservative fertility approach is only valuable if the uterus can be spared during surgery. This includes for early cervical carcinoma, early vaginal carcinoma, early endometrial adenocarcinoma, ovarian tumors of low malignancy, and some selected cases of unilateral ovarian carcinoma (stage IA) [21,22]. The choice of a possible conservative surgical approach in these patients, and the question of implementing such treatment alone, remains controversial, and all the published results have been derived from retrospective studies and/or case reports. The fertility outcome is conditioned by the adjuvant therapy (i.e. local radiotherapy and/or chemotherapy).

Cryopreservation should not be reserved solely for women with malignant disease [4]. Indeed, hematopoietic stem cell transplantation has been increasingly used for non-cancerous diseases such as benign hematological disease (sickle-cell anemia, thalassemia major,

Table 21.2. Indications for cryopreservation of ovarian tissue in those with malignant and non-malignant diseases

	Diseases
Malignant disease	
Extrapelvic	Bone cancer (osteosarcoma, Ewing's sarcoma), breast cancer, melanoma, neuroblastoma, bowel malignancy
Pelvic malignancy: non-gynecological	Pelvic sarcoma, rhabdomyosarcoma, sacral tumors, rectosigmoid tumors
Pelvic malignancy: gynecological	Early cervical carcinoma, early vaginal carcinoma, early vulvar carcinoma, selected cases of ovarian carcinoma (stage IA), borderline ovarian tumors
Systemic malignancies	Hodgkin's disease, non-Hodgkin's lymphoma, leukemia, medulloblastoma
Non-malignant disease	
Uni/bilateral oophorectomy	Benign ovarian tumors, severe and recurrent endometriosis, carriers of *BRCA-1* or *BRCA-2* mutations
Risk of premature menopause	Turner syndrome, family history
Benign diseases requiring chemotherapy	Autoimmune diseases (systemic lupus erythematosus, rheumatoid arthritis, Behçet disease, Wegener's granulomatosis)
Bone marrow transplantation	Benign hematological diseases (sickle-cell anemia, thalassemia major, aplastic anemia), autoimmune diseases unresponsive to immunosuppressive therapy

and anemia) and for autoimmune diseases previously unresponsive to immunosuppressive therapy (systemic lupus erythematosus, autoimmune thrombocytopenia) [4,23–26]. Other benign diseases, such as recurrent ovarian endometriosis or recurrent ovarian mucinous cysts, are also indications for ovarian cryopreservation. Patients undergoing oophorectomy for prophylaxis may potentially benefit from ovarian cryopreservation too. The indications for cryopreservation of ovarian tissue in non-malignant disease are summarized in Table 21.2.

Fertility preservation in women with cancer: cryopreservation options

The only established method of fertility preservation is embryo cryopreservation according to the Ethics Committee of the American Society for Reproductive Medicine [27], but this option requires the patient to be of pubertal age, have a partner or use donor sperm, and be able to undergo a cycle of ovarian stimulation, which is not possible when chemotherapy has to be initiated immediately or when stimulation is contraindicated according to the type of cancer.

Crypreservation of oocytes can be performed in postpubertal patients who are able to undergo a stimulation cycle, but the effectiveness of this technique is still low, with delivery rates from 1 to 5% for frozen–thawed oocytes using the slow-cooling techniques [28]. Since the recent introduction of oocyte vitrification, delivery rates have almost doubled per thawed oocyte [29].

Ovarian tissue cryopreservation

For patients who need immediate chemotherapy, cryopreservation of ovarian tissue is the only possible option [21,30–34]. The main aim of this strategy is to re-implant cortical ovarian tissue into the pelvic cavity (orthotopic site) or a heterotopic site like the forearm or abdominal wall once treatment is completed and the patient is disease free [4,26,34–46].

Lessons from xenografting cryopreserved human ovarian tissue

Human ovarian tissue can be successfully cryopreserved, showing good survival and function after thawing, as indicated by a review of all relevant studies from 1996 to 2005 [47]. The first case of cryopreservation of human ovarian tissue was described in 1996. The choice of a cryoprotectant with maximum permeation capacity but minimum toxicity and ice crystal formation potential is specific to each cell and tissue type [48]. Therefore, in the ovary, it is a compromise between the stroma, follicular cells, and oocytes [47]. On the basis of current knowledge, the standard method for human ovarian cryopreservation is slow freezing in a medium containing human serum albumin, and using propanediol, dimethyl sulfoxide (DMSO), or ethylene glycol as a cryoprotectant, with or without sucrose [47].

All reports on human ovarian tissue grafting to mice [4,49] that have studied the implantation site have shown peritoneal transplantation, either under the peritoneum [50] or under the kidney capsule [51,52], to be better than subcutaneous transplantation in terms of follicular survival and development. After xenografting cryopreserved human ovarian tissue into the kidney capsule of immunodeficient (with severe combined immunodeficiency) mice, Oktay *et al.* [53] achieved follicular development up to the antral stage, and Gook *et al.* [54,55] obtained metaphase II stage oocytes. The ovulatory capacity of frozen–thawed human follicles in xenografts was evidenced by the formation of morphologically normal corpora lutea and elevated progesterone levels in the immunodeficient mice [54,56]. Very few data are available on the final maturation of follicles in xenografts and the quality of oocytes obtained. It has, therefore, not been established whether human oocytes matured in xenografts are ultrastructurally normal and functionally competent.

Experimental studies have indicated a fall in the number of primordial follicles in grafted tissue, which could be caused by hypoxia and the delay before re-implanted cortical tissue becomes revascularized. The loss of primordial follicles in cryopreserved ovarian tissue after transplantation is estimated to be at least 50–65% in some studies [50].

The crucial issue of revascularization

Van Eyck *et al.* [57] recently characterized the oxygen environment in human ovarian xenografts in the early post-grafting period (until day 21) using electron paramagnetic resonance oximetry. This technique allows sensitive, non-invasive, and repeated measurement of the partial pressure of oxygen in vivo. Before day 5, grafts were exposed to hypoxia. From day 5 to day 10, progressive reoxygenation was observed, suggesting an active process of graft revascularization.

Using a combined method of perfusion study and double immunohistochemical staining of human and murine vessels, the same team evaluated the revascularization process of human ovarian tissue in this model (Van Eyck *et al.* [58]). On day 5, reperfusion of ovarian grafts was initiated by host angiogenesis, as evidenced by the appearance of murine neovessels penetrating from the periphery and colocalized with perfused areas. By day 10, the center of the fragments was perfused and ovarian graft angiogenesis contributed to the vascular pattern of the ovarian transplants.

Host and graft angiogenesis, therefore, both appear to contribute to post-transplantation vascular behavior and could be potential targets to improve the mechanisms leading to perfusion of grafts, with the aim of reducing the avascular period.

Autotransplantation of cryopreserved human ovarian tissue

There have been numerous reported cases of autotransplantation of cryopreserved ovarian tissue, either to an orthotopic or heterotopic site [4,25–26,35–46,59,60].

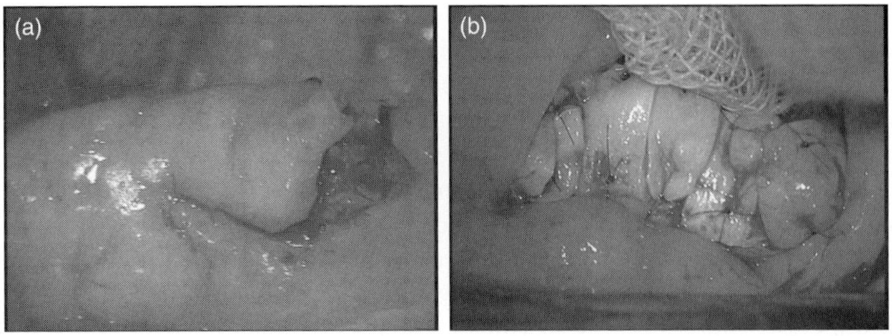

Figure 21.1. Ovarian cortical pieces measuring 4–5 mm to 1 cm in size were grafted on to the remaining ovary after the cortex of this ovary had been removed. (a) The cortex of the remaining ovary was removed; (b) The cortical pieces were sutured with 7-0 thread.

Orthotopic autotransplantation

In theory, natural pregnancy may be achieved via orthotopic tissue transplantation if the fallopian tubes remain intact. Figure 21.1 shows transplantation of ovarian cortical fragments to the remaining ovary.

In 2000, Oktay and Karlikaya reported laparoscopic transplantation of frozen–thawed ovarian tissue in a 29-year-old patient who had undergone bilateral oophorectomy for a non-malignant disease [35]. Follicular development was demonstrated only once by ultrasonography after the patient had been stimulated by gonadotropin 15 weeks after transplantation.

Radford *et al.* [37] have reported on a patient with a history of Hodgkin's disease treated by chemotherapy. Ovarian tissue had been cryopreserved before the woman received high doses of chemotherapy for a third recurrence of disease. Histological section of the ovarian cortical tissue revealed only a few primordial follicles as a consequence of the previous chemotherapy. Eight months after re-implantation, estradiol was detected and plasma concentrations of follicle-stimulating hormone (FSH) and luteinizing hormone (LH) decreased. One month later, LH and FSH concentrations returned definitively to menopausal levels.

We have reported the first successful transplantation of cryopreserved ovarian tissue that resulted in a pregnancy and live birth [38]. In 1997, a 25-year-old woman presented with clinical stage IV Hodgkin's lymphoma. Ovarian tissue cryopreservation was undertaken before chemotherapy. After laparoscopy, the patient received hybrid chemotherapy from August 1997 to February 1998, followed by supradiaphragmatic radiotherapy (38 Gy). In 2003, once the patient had been declared completely disease free, re-implantation of the ovarian tissue was carried out in orthotopic sites [4,40]. From 5 to 9 months after re-implantation, concentrations of FSH, 17β-estradiol, and progesterone showed the occurrence of ovulatory cycles. At 11 months, the patient became pregnant and subsequently delivered a healthy baby. This birth was announced in the *Lancet* in September 2004 [40]. This is particularly pleasing in that the risk of POF after such a regimen in a woman aged 26 years is more than 90% according to Schilsky *et al.* [9], while according to Wallace *et al.* [6] and Lobo [17], the risk of subfertility after Hodgkin's treatment with alkylating agents is more than 80%.

In 2005, Meirow *et al.* [41] also published a live birth after orthotopic autotransplantation of cryopreserved ovarian tissue in a patient with POF after chemotherapy. Eight months after orthotopic transplantation, the patient spontaneously menstruated. Nine months after transplantation, she experienced a second spontaneous menstrual period. After a modified natural cycle, a single mature oocyte was retrieved and fertilized. Two days later, a four-cell embryo was transferred. The patient became pregnant from this embryo transfer and delivered a healthy infant weighing 3000 g.

Demeestere *et al.* [43] have reported a pregnancy after natural conception in a woman who had undergone orthotopic and heterotopic transplantation of cryopreserved ovarian tissue. Unfortunately, this pregnancy, obtained by natural conception, ended in miscarriage at 7 weeks owing to aneuploidy. The same team performed a second re-implantation to an orthotopic site in the same patient after cessation of graft secretion was evidenced [44]. The patient became pregnant and delivered a healthy baby.

Silber *et al.* [45] have reported a pregnancy following re-implantation of cryopreserved ovarian tissue between monozygotic twins. It should be noted, however, that the same woman had already delivered a first healthy baby after re-implantation of fresh tissue [45]. It is, therefore, difficult to know from which grafted tissue the ovulation leading to the pregnancy ensued.

In a very recent paper, Andersen *et al.* [46] described a series of six orthotopic re-implantations

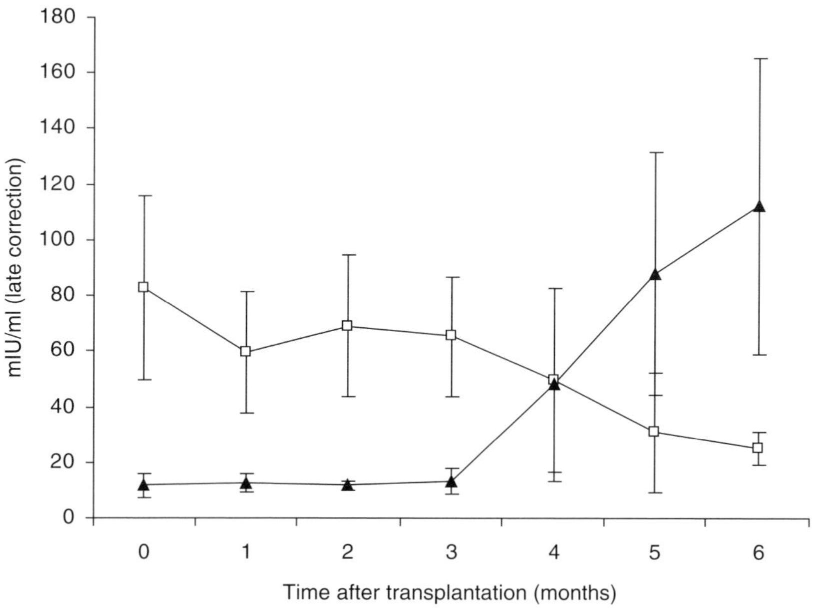

Figure 21.2. Mean follicle-stimulating hormone (squares) and 17β-estradiol (triangles) in seven women with transplantation of frozen–thawed ovarian tissue. It took between 4 and 6.5 months for the change in hormones to become apparent. (NB in four of the women, the hormone values at 1 month post-transplantation were not taken into account, as the patients were taking a gonadotropin-releasing hormone agonist, which would have caused downregulation.) The bars indicate the standard deviation.

of cryopreserved ovarian cortex. In this series, two women became pregnant and delivered healthy babies Single mature oocytes were retrieved during optimized cycles; they were fertilized and transferred on day 3.

We have recently published a series of nine orthotopic transplantations of ovarian tissue in six women, proving restoration of ovarian function in all cases [26]. Analysis of these cases raises some important points for discussion. In three women, it took between 4.5 and 5 months after re-implantation before a follicle could be seen by ultrasonography (Figure 21.2). The process of folliculogenesis takes approximately 4–6 months, during which time the oocyte and surrounding somatic cells undergo a series of changes that eventually result in the development of a large antral follicle, capable of producing a mature oocyte [61]. Therefore, the appearance of the first follicle originating from grafted tissue 5 months after re-implantation, proved by laparoscopy in one woman, is totally consistent with the expected time course. This time interval between implantation of cortical tissue and the first estradiol peak is also consistent with data obtained from sheep [62,63] and humans, although some variations may be observed. Indeed, the delay between transplantation and follicular development was found varying from 6 weeks to 8 months. Such a variation could be explained by a difference in follicular reserve at the time of cryopreservation.

Another very interesting finding in our series was the persistence of relatively high FSH levels during the follicular phase; these remained as high as 25 mIU/ml during the follicular phase until ovulation, and then decreased to less than 15 mIU/ml during the luteal phase. This may constitute an argument against the use of gonadotropin injections. The relatively high FSH levels may be explained by the relatively low number of surviving primordial follicles in the graft. The patient should be considered a poor responder, with reduced inhibin B secretion. These results are in agreement with those obtained in sheep by Campbell *et al.* [64].

A further significant observation was the return to an FSH level of >25 mIU/ml immediately after each menstrual bleed, which supports the theory suggested by Baird *et al.* [63] that some inhibitory mechanisms, such as inhibin B or anti-Müllerian hormones, which are normally produced by developing follicles in intact human ovaries, are probably almost non-existent in transplanted tissue. After transplantation, the patient would have been regarded as a poor responder because, of the 500–1000 primordial follicles that would have been transplanted, more than 50% would have been lost through hypoxia [40].

Heterotopic autotransplantation

There are only a few existing reports on heterotopic autotransplants. Callejo *et al.* [59] have evaluated the long-term function of cryopreserved heterotopic grafts, but no conclusions could be drawn since the patient was perimenopausal at the time of ovarian biopsy for cryopreservation.

In 2004, Kim *et al.* [38] reported a case of a 37-year-old woman who underwent heterotopic (rectus and pectoralis muscle) transplantation of cryopreserved ovarian tissue. By 14 weeks after the transplantation, restoration of endocrine function was demonstrated; however, approximately 28 weeks after transplantation, cessation of ovarian function was evidenced by very high FSH levels (62–99 mIU/ml) and very low estradiol levels.

The same year, Oktay *et al.* [36] reported transplantation of frozen–thawed ovarian tissue to beneath the skin of the abdomen. A four-cell embryo was obtained from 20 oocytes retrieved from an ovarian graft, but no pregnancy occurred after transfer. Oocyte quality might have been compromised by transplantation to a heterotopic site.

Kim *et al.* in 2004 [38] reported heterotopic transplantation of cryopreserved ovarian tissue in a patient cured of squamous cell carcinoma of the cervix. Tissue was transplanted to two heterotopic sites: abdominal (rectus muscle) and breast site (pectoralis muscle). Growing follicles were seen in the abdominal site from 14 weeks after transplantation, but ovarian function ceased around 28 weeks after transplantation.

Wolner-Hanssen *et al.* [25] reported subcutaneous transplantation of frozen–thawed tissue to the forearm in 2005. Two follicles developed, but only to a maximum diameter of 12.6 and 6.7 mm, respectively, and the tissue survived 7 months.

Recently, Kim *et al.* [39] have reported heterotopic autotransplantation of cryopreserved ovarian tissue in four patients (three with cervical cancer and one with breast cancer). Thawed ovarian fragments were transplanted into a space between the rectus muscle and the rectus sheath. Recovery of ovarian function was evidenced in three patients by hormone profiles obtained between 12 and 20 weeks after transplantation, but only lasted 3 to 5 months. These three patients subsequently underwent a second transplantation. Long-term ovarian function (15–36 months) was then established. Ovarian grafts were stimulated daily with FSH until a dominant follicle size of 14 to 16 mm was reached. During a 27 month follow-up period in two patients, six oocytes were retrieved (one germinal vesicle, four in metaphase I, and one in metaphase II). The four oocytes metaphase I were subjected to in vitro maturation and all four then fertilized and developed to cleavage stage embryos (up to six cells on day 3) before being frozen for transfer to a surrogate.

Papers describing heterotopic transplantation have all reported follicular development, but with follicles always less than 16 mm in size [38,43]. As stressed by Wolner-Hanssen [25] and Oktay *et al.* [36], differences in temperature and pressure could interfere with follicular development in heterotopic sites.

Should cryopreservation include the whole ovary with its vascular pedicle?

The main drawback of ovarian tissue cryopreservation followed by avascular transplantation is that the graft is completely dependent on neovascularization and, as a result, a large proportion of follicles are lost during the initial ischemia occurring after transplantation [50,62,65]. Reducing the ischemic interval between transplantation and revascularization is, therefore, essential to maintaining the follicular reserve and extending the lifespan and function of the graft [57]. In theory, the best way to achieve this is by transplantation of an intact ovary with vascular anastomosis, allowing immediate revascularization of the transplant [66] (Figure 21.3).

Successful vascular transplantation of intact frozen–thawed ovaries has been reported in rats [67,68] and sheep [69–72]. Nevertheless, follicular survival after microvascular transplantation could be less than expected, as shown in a sheep study [73]. In humans, the challenge of whole ovary cryopreservation results from the difficulty of achieving adequate cryoprotective agent diffusion into the large tissue masses and the risk of vascular injury caused by intravascular ice formation.

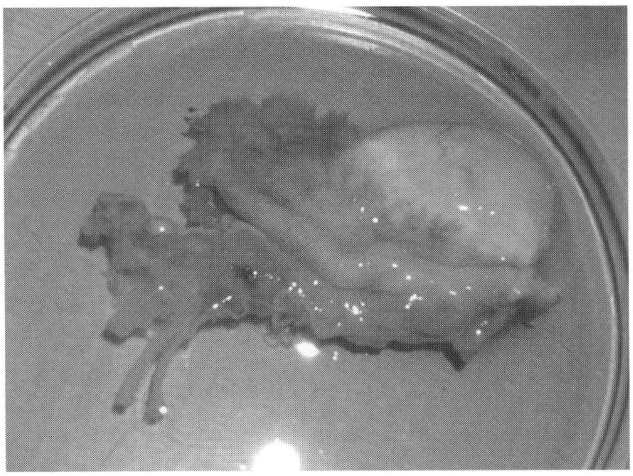

Figure 21.3. The whole ovary with its vascular pedicle is removed by laparoscopy and then perfused with a cryoprotectant.

We have recently described a cryopreservation protocol for intact human ovary with its vascular pedicle and shown high survival rates for follicles (75.1%), small vessels, and stroma, and a normal histological structure in all the ovarian components after thawing [74].

After freeze–thawing the whole human ovaries using this protocol, no induction of apoptosis was observed in any cell types [75]. Transmission electron microscopy confirmed that the majority (96.7%) of primordial follicles were intact after cryopreservation and that 96.3% of the endothelial cells had a completely normal ultrastructure [76].

Our results in humans have led us to seriously consider proposing this option to women in the future where there is a very high risk (> 90%) of POF after therapy, if there is no risk of transmitting malignant cells via the graft. So far, in our department, 11 whole ovaries have been cryopreserved with a view to future re-implantation (grafting) and vascular anastomosis.

Research and development in the technology to cryopreserve whole organs, as well as surgical techniques for the autotransplantation of an entire ovary with its vascular pedicle, should be encouraged. Further studies are also needed to evaluate the risk of thrombosis of the ovarian pedicle after transplantation. If these problems can be overcome, this could lead to the transplantation of intact ovaries with microvascular anastomosis carried out to restore immediate vascularization and minimize post-transplantation ischemia, which is responsible for the reduction in follicular density. One must bear in mind, however, that re-implantation of the ovary cannot be considered if there is a risk of neoplastic cell contamination.

Re-implantation of isolated primordial follicles

Although safe transplantation of ovarian tissue from patients with lymphoma to immunodeficient mice has been reported [77], the possibility of re-introducing tumor cells into cancer patients by autografting of ovarian tissue cannot be excluded [78]. Screening methods must be developed to eliminate the risk of cancer cell transmission with the implantation [79]. In some diseases, other options must be considered.

To avoid transferring malignant cells, ovarian tissue culture with in vitro follicle maturation could be performed. Culturing isolated follicles from the primordial stage is another particularly attractive proposition, since they represent more than 90% of the total follicular reserve and show high cryotolerance [80]. However, isolated primordial follicles do not grow properly in culture and further studies are clearly needed to identify factors sustaining follicular growth and maturation in humans, and to assess the contribution of stromal cells to these processes [80,81]. Encouraging results were achieved by Hovatta and Telfer *et al.* [82,83] when human primordial follicles were grown in organ culture. Follicle isolation, or partial follicle isolation, can severely impair follicular viability, and after isolation, only more advanced multilaminar preantral follicular stages can survive in short-term culture, few reaching the early antral stage.

Another approach could be to transplant a suspension of isolated follicles [84]. As the follicular basal lamina encapsulating the membrana granulosa excludes capillaries, white blood cells, and nerve processes from the granulosa compartment, grafting fully isolated follicles could be considered safer [85]. Transplantation of frozen–thawed isolated primordial follicles has indeed been successfully achieved in mice, yielding normal offspring [86]. For human primordial follicles, however, mechanical isolation is not possible because of their size (30–40 μm) and their fibrous and dense ovarian stroma; therefore, enzymatic digestion has to be used [87] (Figure 21.4). Recent xenotransplantation experiments show encouraging results with development of isolated human follicles to the antral stage [88]. In order to enhance the chances of follicular survival and reproductive function restoration, enzymatic digestion procedures for human ovarian tissue need to be optimized and standardized [87].

Ethical issues and safety

One of the most important ethical issues is ensuring that the intervention does not harm the patient by dangerously delaying cancer treatment and that no remnant malignant cells are re-introduced by subsequent transplantation. Taking these points into account, we agree with Dudzinski [89] that policies to protect the patient's future rights to her gametes should be developed, as well as policies addressing the disposition of the gametes if the patient dies.

Although an adolescent is more vulnerable when consent is sought in the rush to begin chemotherapy, she must be mature enough to understand the risks and benefits of the procedure. Consent must then be discussed extensively, the discussion including both the adolescent and her parents, in order to minimize the risk of conflict of interest or inadvertent caution [90].

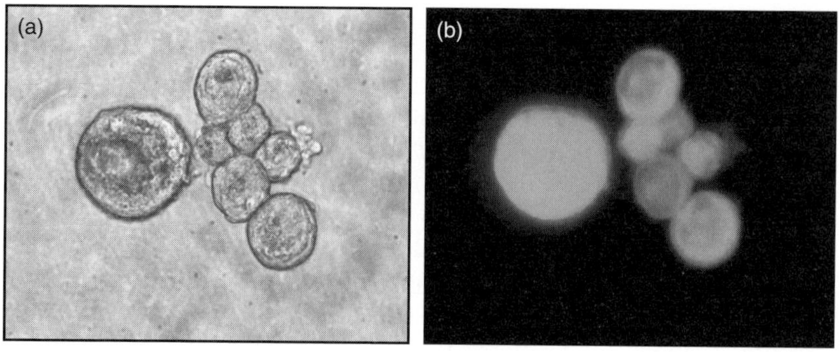

Figure 21.4. Enzymatically isolated follicles (between 30 and 110 μm) are visible under an inverted fluorescence microscope after fluorescent viability staining (calcein-AM and ethidium homodimer-1). Follicles are visible on light microscopy (a) and fluorescence microscopy (b), which show that all are viable.

Respecting the code of good practice, all patients who may become infertile have the right to receive proper consideration of their interests for future possibilities in the field of ovarian function preservation. The selection of cases should be carried out on the basis of multidisciplinary staff discussions, including oncologists, gynecologists, biologists, psychologists, and pediatricians. Counseling should be given and informed consent obtained from the patient. Cancer treatment takes priority over potential restoration of fertility, but offering the chance to preserve fertility may greatly enhance quality of life for cancer survivors and provide support at the time in that it has considerations of hope for the future.

Conclusions

Approximately one third of young women exposed to chemotherapy develop ovarian failure. In 2008, we believe it is our ethical responsibility to propose cryopreservation of ovarian tissue to all adolescents and young women, under local institutional review board guidance, having to undergo chemotherapy with alkylating agents.

The age of the patient should be taken into consideration, since the follicular reserve of the ovary is age dependent. Because a decline in fertility is now well documented after the age of 38 years, the procedure should probably be restricted to patients below this age. In any case, irradiation and chemotherapy appear to be less harmful to the gonads of prepubertal than postpubertal women [15,16,91].

This is why, since 1996, we have systematically proposed cryopreservation to all women under 35 years of age prior to chemotherapy when there is a risk of POF, so far numbering more than 300. We accept that ovarian tissue cryopreservation is a more innovative and invasive procedure than sperm cryopreservation, and that all possible applications in adolescents are ethically complex. However, we believe that ovarian cortex banking should be offered before chemotherapy in all cases where emergency IVF is not possible.

In conclusion, the six live births obtained after transplantation of frozen–thawed ovarian tissue in humans give hope to young cancer patients, but there is still much work to be done. Research programs need to determine whether active angiogenesis can be induced to accelerate the process of neovascularization in grafted tissue, if isolated human follicles can be grafted, or indeed if microvascular reanostomosis of an entire cryopreserved ovary is a valuable option.

References

1. Jemal A, Siegel R, Ward E, *et al.* Cancer statistics, 2006. *CA Cancer J Clin* 2006; **56:** 106–130.
2. Blatt J. Pregnancy outcome in long-term survivors of childhood cancer. *Med Pediatr Oncon* 1999; **33:** 29–33.
3. Ries LAG, Percy CL, Bunin GR. Introduction. In Ries LAG, Smith MA, Gurney JG, *et al.*, eds. *Cancer Incidence and Survival among Children and Adolescents: United States SEER Program 1975–1995.* [NIH Pub. No. 99–4649]. Bethesda, MD: National Cancer Institute, 1999, pp. 1–15.
4. Donnez J, Dolmans MM, Demylle D, *et al.* Restoration of ovarian function after orthotopic (intraovarian and periovarian) transplantation of cryopreserved ovarian tissue in a woman treated by bone marrrow transplantation for sickle cell anaemia: case report. *Hum Reprod* 2006; **21:** 183–188.
5. Meirow D, Lewis H, Nugent D, Epstein N. Subclinical depletion of primordial follicular reserve in mice treated with cyclophosphamide: clinical importance and proposed accurate investigative tool. *Hum Reprod* 1999; **14:** 1903–1907.
6. Wallace WH, Thomson AB, Saran F, Kelsey TW. Predicting age of ovarian failure after radiation to a field that includes the ovaries. *Int J Radiat Oncol Biol Phys* 2005; **62:** 738–744.

7. Larsen EC, Muller J, Schmiegelow K, Rechnitzer C, Andersen AN. Reduced ovarian function in long-term survivors of radiation- and chemotherapy-treated childhood cancer. *J Clin Endocrinol Metab* 2003; **88:** 5307–5314.
8. Shalet SM. Effects of cancer chemotherapy on gonadal function of patients. *Cancer Treat Rev* 1980; **7:** 141–152.
9. Schilsky RL, Sherins RJ, Hubbard SM, *et al.* Long-term follow up of ovarian function in women treated with MOPP chemotherapy for Hodgkin's disease. *Am J Med* 1981; **71:** 552–556.
10. Wallace WH, Anderson RA, Irvine DS. Fertility preservation for young patients with cancer: who is at risk and what can be offered? *Lancet Oncol* 2005; **6:** 209–218.
11. Wallace WH, Thomson AB, Kelsey TW. The radiosensitivity of the human oocyte. *Hum Reprod* 2003; **18:** 117–121.
12. Larsen EC, Schmiegelow K, Rechnitzer C, *et al.* Radiotherapy at a young age reduces uterine volume of childhood cancer survivors. *Acta Obstet Gynecol Scand* 2004; **83:** 96–102.
13. Critchley HO, Wallace GH. Impact of cancer treatment on uterine function. *J Natl Cancer Inst Monogr* 2005; **34:** 64–68.
14. Bath LE, Critchley HO, Chambers SE, *et al.* Ovarian and uterine characteristics after total body irradiation in childhood and adolescence: response to sex steroid replacement. *Br J Obstet Gynaecol* 1999; **106:** 1265–1272.
15. Sanders J, Hawley J, Levy W, *et al.* Pregnancies following high-dose cyclophosphamide with or without high-dose busulfan or total body irradiation and bone marrow transplantation. *Blood* 1996; **87:** 3045–3052.
16. Meirow D, Nugent D. The effects of radiotherapy and chemotherapy on female reproduction. *Hum Reprod Update* 2001; **7:** 534–543.
17. Lobo RA. Potential options for preservation of fertility in women. *N Engl J Med* 2005; **353:** 64–73.
18. Teinturier C, Hartmann O, Valteau-Couanet D, Benhamou E, Bougneres PF. Ovarian function after autologous bone marrow transplantation in childhood: high-dose busulfan is a major cause of ovarian failure. *Bone Marrow Transplant* 1998; **22:** 989–994.
19. Salooja N, Szydlo RM, Socie G, *et al.* for the Late Effects Working Party of the European Group for Blood and Marrow Transplantation. Pregnancy outcomes after peripheral blood or bone marrow transplantation: a retrospective survey. *Lancet* 2001; **358:** 271–276.
20. Lutchman Singh K, Davies M, Chatterjee R. Fertility in female cancer survivors: pathophysiology, preservation and the role of ovarian reserve testing. *Hum Reprod Update* 2005; **11:** 69–89.
21. Donnez J, Bassil S. Indications for cryopreservation of ovarian tissue. *Hum Reprod Update* 1998; **4:** 248–259.
22. Kleine W. Results of fertility preserving operations in malignant ovarian tumors. *Zentralbl Gynakol* 1996; **118:** 317–321.
23. Slavin S, Nagler A, Aker M, *et al.* Non-myeloablative stem cell transplantation and donor lymphocyte infusion for the treatment of cancer and life-threatening non-malignant disorders. *Rev Clin Exp Hematol* 2001; **5:** 135–146.
24. Mattle V, Behringer K, Engert A, Wildt L. Female fertility after cytotoxic therapy-protection of ovarian function during chemotherapy of malignant and non-malignant diseases. *Eur J Haematol* 2005; **75:** 77–82.
25. Wolner-Hanssen P, Hägglund L, Ploman F, *et al.* Autotransplantation of cryopreserved ovarian tissue to the right forearm 4 ½ years after autologous stem cell transplantation. *Acta Obstet Gynecol Scand* 2005; **84:** 695–698.
26. Donnez J, Squifflet J, Van Eyck AS, *et al.* Restoration of ovarian function in orthotopically transplanted cryopreserved ovarian tissue: a pilot experience. *Reprod Biomed Online* 2008; **16:** 694–704.
27. Ethics Committee of the American Society for Reproductive Medicine. Fertility preservation and reproduction in cancer patients. *Fertil Steril* 2005; **83:** 1622–1628.
28. Stachecki JJ, Cohen J. An overview of oocyte cryopreservation. *Reprod Biomed Online 2004*; **9:** 152–163.
29. Cobo A, Domingo J, Pérez S, *et al.* Vitrification: an effective new approach to oocyte banking and preserving fertility in cancer patients. *Clin Transl Oncol* 2008; **10**: 268–273.
30. Gosden RG, Baird DT, Wade JC, Webb R. Restoration of fertility to oophorectomized sheep by ovarian autografts stored at −196°C. *Hum Reprod* 1994; **9:** 597–603.
31. Oktay K, Newton H, Aubard Y, Salha O, Gosden RG. Cryopreservation of immature human oocytes and ovarian tissue: an emerging technology? *Fertil Steril* 1998; **69:** 1–7.
32. Meirow D, Ben Yehuda D, Prus D, *et al.* Ovarian tissue banking in patients with Hodgkin's disease: is it safe? *Fertil Steril* 1998; **69:** 996–998.
33. Donnez J, Godin PA, Qu J, Nisolle M. Gonadal cryopreservation in the young patient with gynaecological malignancy. *Current Opin Obstet Gynecol* 2000; **12:** 1–9.
34. Donnez J, Dolmans MM, Martinez-Madrid B, Demylle D, Van Langendonkt A. The role of cryopreservation for women prior to treatment of malignancy. *Curr Opin Obstet Gynecol* 2005; **17:** 333–338.
35. Oktay K, Karlikaya G. Ovarian function after transplantation of frozen, banked autologous ovarian tissue. *N Engl J Med* 2000; **342:** 1919.

36. Oktay K, Buyuk E, Veeck L, *et al.* Embryo development after heterotopic transplantation of cryopreserved ovarian tissue. *Lancet* 2004; **363:** 837–840.
37. Radford JA, Lieberman BA, Brison D, *et al.* Orthotopic reimplantation of cryopreserved ovarian cortical strips after high-dose chemotherapy for Hodgkin's lymphoma. *Lancet* 2001; **357:** 1172–1175.
38. Kim SS, Hwang I-T, Lee H-C. Heterotopic autotransplantation of cryobanked human ovarian tissue as a strategy to restore ovarian function. *Fertil Steril* 2004; **82:** 930–932.
39. Kim SS, Lee WS, Chung MK, *et al.* Long-term ovarian function and fertility after heterotopic autotransplantation of cryobanked human ovarian tissue: 8-year experience in cancer patients. *Fertil Steril* 2009; **91**: 2349–2954.
40. Donnez J, Dolmans MM, Demylle D, *et al.* Livebirth after orthotopic transplantation of cryopreserved ovarian tissue. *Lancet* 2004; **364**: 1405–1410.
41. Meirow D, Levron J, Eldar-Geva T, *et al.* Pregnancy after transplantation of cryopreserved ovarian tissue in a patient with ovarian failure after chemotherapy. *N Engl J Med* 2005; **353:** 318–321.
42. Schmidt KL, Yding Andersen C, Loft A, *et al.* Follow-up of ovarian function post-chemotherapy following ovarian cryopreservation and transplantation. *Hum Reprod* 2005; **20:** 3539–3546.
43. Demeestere I, Simon P, Buxant F, *et al.* Ovarian function and spontaneous pregnancy after combined heterotopic and orthotopic cryopreserved ovarian tissue transplantation in a patient previously treated with bone marrow transplantation: case report. *Hum Reprod* 2006; **21:** 2010–2014.
44. Demeestere I, Simon P, Emiliani S, Delbaere A, Englert Y. Fertility preservation: successful transplantation of cryopreserved ovarian tissue in a young patient previously treated for Hodgkin's disease. *Oncologist* 2007; **12:** 1437–1442.
45. Silber SJ, DeRosa M, Pineda J, *et al.* A series of monozygotic twins discordant for ovarian failure: ovary transplantation (cortical versus microvascular) and cryopreservation. *Hum Reprod* 2008; **23:** 1531–1537.
46. Andersen CY, Rosendahl M, Byskov AG, *et al.* Two successful pregnancies following autotransplantation of frozen/thawed ovarian tissue. *Hum Reprod* 2008; **23**: 2266–2272.
47. Hovatta O. Methods for cryopreservation of human ovarian tissue. *Reprod Biomed Online* 2005; **10**: 729–734.
48. Fuller B, Paynter S. Fundamentals of cryobiology in reproductive medicine. *Reprod Biomed Online* 2004; **9**: 680–691.
49. Aubard Y. Ovarian tissue xenografting. *Eur J Obst Gynecol Reprod Biol* 2003; **108**: 14–18.
50. Nisolle M, Godin PA, Casanas-Roux F, *et al.* Histological and ultrastructural evaluation of fresh and frozen–thawed human ovarian xenografts in nude mice. *Fertil Steril* 2000; **74**: 122–129.
51. Hernandez-Fonseca H, Bosch P, Sirisathien S, *et al.* Effect of site of transplantation on follicular development of human ovarian tissue transplanted into intact or castrated immunodeficient mice. *Fertil Steril* 2004; **81**: 888–892.
52. Abir R, Orvieto R, Raanani H, *et al.* Parameters affecting successful transplantation of frozen–thawed human fetal ovaries into immunodeficient mice. *Fertil Steril* 2003; **80**: 421–428.
53. Oktay K, Newton H, Mullan J, Gosden RG. Development of human primordial follicles to antral stages in SCID/hpg mice stimulated with follicle stimulating hormone. *Hum Reprod* 1998; **13**: 1133–1138.
54. Gook DA, Edgar DH, Borg J, *et al.* Oocyte maturation, follicle rupture and luteinization in human cryopreserved ovarian tissue following xenografting. *Hum Reprod* 2003; **18**: 1772–1781.
55. Gook DA, Edgar DH, Borg J, Archer J, McBain JC. Diagnostic assessment of the developmental potential of human cryopreserved ovarian tissue from multiple patients using xenografting. *Hum Reprod* 2005; **20:** 72–78.
56. Kim SS, Soules MR, Battaglia DE. Follicular development, ovulation, and corpus luteum formation in cryopreserved human ovarian tissue after xenotransplantation. *Fertil Steril* 2002; **78:** 77–82.
57. Van Eyck AS, Jordan BF, Gallez B, *et al.* Electron paramagnetic resonance as a tool to evaluate human ovarian tissue reoxygenation after xenografting. *Fertil Steril* 2009; **92**: 374–381.
58. Van Eyck AS, Bouzin C, Feron O, *et al.* Both host and graft vessels contribute to revascularization of xenografted human ovarian tissue in a murine model. *Fert Steril* 2010; in press.
59. Callejo J, Salvador C, Miralles A, *et al.* Long-term ovarian function evaluation after autografting by implantation with fresh and frozen–thawed human ovarian tissue. *J Clin Endocrinol Metab* 2001; **86:** 4489–4494.
60. Oktay K. Spontaneous conceptions and live birth after heterotopic ovarian transplantation: is there a germline stem cell connection? *Hum Reprod* 2006; **21:** 1345–1348.
61. Gougeon A. Regulation of ovarian follicular development in primates: facts and hypotheses. *Endocrin Rev* 1996; **17:** 121–155.
62. Baird, DT, Webb R, Campbell BK, Harkness LM, Gosden RG. Long-term ovarian function in sheep after ovariectomy and transplantation of autografts stored at −196°C. *Endocrinol* 1999; **140**: 462–471.
63. Baird DT, Campbell BK, Souza C, Telfer EE. Long-term ovarian function in sheep after ovariectomy and autotransplantation of cryopreserved cortical strips. *Eur J Obst Gynecol Reprod Biol* 2004; **113:** 55–59.

64. Campbell BK, Telfer EE, Webb R, Baird DT. Ovarian autografts in sheep as a model for studying folliculogenesis. *Mol Cell Endocrinol* 2000; **163:** 131–139.
65. Liu J, Van der Elst J, van den Broecke R, Dhont M. Early massive follicle loss and apoptosis in heterotopically grafted newborn mouse ovaries. *Hum Reprod* 2002; **17:** 605–611.
66. Jadoul P, Donnez J, Dolmans MM, *et al.* Laparoscopic ovariectomy for whole human ovary cryopreservation: technical aspects. *Fertil Steril* 2007; **87**: 971–975.
67. Wang X, Chen H, Yin H, *et al.* Successful pregnancy after intact ovary transplantation. *Nature* 2002; **415:** 385.
68. Yin H, Wang X, Kim SS, *et al.* Transplantation of intact rat gonads using vascular anastomosis: effects of cryopreservation, ischemia and genotype. *Hum Reprod* 2003; **18:** 1165–1172.
69. Bedaiwy MA, Jeremias E, Gurunluoglu R, *et al.* Restoration of ovarian function after autotransplantation of intact frozen–thawed sheep ovaries with microvascular anastomosis. *Fertil Steril* 2003; **79:** 594–602.
70. Revel A, Elami A, Bor A, *et al.* Whole sheep ovary cryopreservation and transplantation. *Fertil Steril* 2004; **82:** 1714–1715.
71. Arav A, Revel A, Nathan Y, *et al.* Oocyte recovery, embryo development and ovarian function after cryopreservation and transplantation of whole sheep ovary. *Hum Reprod* 2005; **20:** 3554–3559.
72. Imhof M, Bergmeister H, Lipovac M, *et al.* Orthotopic microvascular re-anastomosis of whole cryopreserved ovine ovaries resulting in pregnancy and life birth. *Fertil Steril* 2006; **85:** 1208–1215.
73. Courbiere B, Caquant L, Mazoyer C, *et al.* Difficulties improving ovarian functional recovery by microvascular transplantation and whole ovary vitrification. *Fertil Steril* 2009; **91**: 2697–2706.
74. Martinez-Madrid B, Dolmans MM, Van Langendonckt A, Defrère S, Donnez J. Freeze–thawing intact human ovary with its vascular pedicle with a passive cooling device. *Fertil Steril* 2004; **82:** 1390–1394.
75. Martinez-Madrid B, Camboni A, Dolmans MM, *et al.* Apoptosis and ultrastructural assessment after cryopreservation of whole human ovaries with their vascular pedicle. *Fertil Steril* 2007; **87:** 1153–1165.
76. Camboni A, Martinez-Madrid B, Dolmans MM, *et al.* Preservation of fertility in young cancer patients: contribution of transmission electron microscopy. *Reprod Biomed Online* 2008; **17:** 136–150.
77. Kim SS, Radford J, Harris M, *et al.* Ovarian tissue harvested from lymphoma patients to preserve fertility may be safe for autotransplantation. *Hum Reprod* 2001; **16:** 2056–2060.
78. Shaw JM, Bowles S, Koopman P, Wood EC, Trounson AO. Fresh and cryopreserved ovarian tissue samples from donors with lymphoma transmit the cancer to graft recipients. *Hum Reprod* 1996; **11:** 1668–1673.
79. Meirow D, Hardan I, Dor J, *et al.* Searching for evidence of disease and malignant cell contamination in ovarian tissue stored from hematologic cancer patients. *Hum Reprod* 2008; **23:** 1007–1013.
80. Smitz JE, Cortvrindt RG. The earliest stages of folliculogenesis in vitro. *Reproduction* 2002; **123:** 185–202.
81. Hovatta O, Wright C, Krausz T, Hardy K, Winston RML. Human primordial, primary and secondary ovarian follicles in long-term culture: effect of partial isolation. *Hum Reprod* 1999; **14:** 2519–2524.
82. Hovatta O. Cryopreservation and culture of human ovarian cortical tissue containing early follicles. *Eur J Obstet Gynecol Reprod Biol* 2004; **5**:S50–S54.
83. Telfer EE, McLaughlin M, Ding C, Thong KJ. A two-step serum-free culture system supports development of human oocytes from primordial follicles in the presence of activin. *Hum Reprod* 2008; **23:** 1151–1158.
84. Dolmans MM, Martinez-Madrid B, Gadisseux E, *et al.* Short-term transplantation of isolated human ovarian follicles and cortical tissue into nude mice. *Reproduction* 2007; **134:** 253–262.
85. Motta PM, Nottola SA, Familiari G, *et al.* Morphodynamics of the follicular-luteal complex during early ovarian development and reproductive life. *Int Rev Cytol* 2003; **223:** 177–288.
86. Carroll J, Gosden RG. Transplantation of frozen–thawed mouse primordial follicles. *Hum Reprod* 1993; **8:** 1163–1167.
87. Dolmans MM, Michaux N, Camboni A, *et al.* Evaluation of Liberase, a purified enzyme blend, for the isolation of human primordial and primary ovarian follicles. *Hum Reprod* 2006; **21**: 413–420.
88. Dolmans MM, Yuan WY, Camboni A, *et al.* Development of antral follicles after xenografting of isolated small human preantral follicles. *Reprod Biomed Online* 2008; **16:** 705–711.
89. Dudzinski DM. Ethical issues in fertility preservation for adolescent cancer survivors: oocyte and ovarian tissue cryopreservation. *J Pediatr Adolesc Gynecol* 2004; **17:** 97–102.
90. Bukovsky A. Can ovarian infertility be treated with bone marrow- or ovary-derived germ cells? *Reprod Biol Endocrinol* 2005; **3:** 36.
91. Haie-Meder C, Mlika-Cabanne N, Michel G, *et al.* Radiotherapy after ovarian transposition ovarian function and fertility preservation. *Int J Radiat Oncol Biol Phys* 1993; **25:** 419–424.

Chapter 22

In vitro culture of human primordial follicles

Benoit Schubert and Johan Smitz

Introduction

In vitro culture of ovarian tissue is challenging. The first live births were obtained in the mouse model starting cultures early from preantral follicles [1]. Nearly 10 years later, the same team has achieved live births from in vitro grown oocytes initiated from the earliest stage of development, the primordial follicle [2,3]. Similar results have not yet been reported in any other species.

Interest is focusing on the in vitro growth of human follicles from the earliest stages. Cancer treatment has improved; more young women of reproductive age are surviving, but quite often they will be confronted with infertility as a consequence of radio- and/or chemotherapy. Other diseases such as systemic lupus erythematosus, sickle cell anemia, and rheumatoid arthritis might also need sufficiently intensive chemotherapy to lead to similar consequences for their fertility. It is proposed that ovarian cortical tissue should be removed before administering aggressive therapies. Ovarian cortex containing immature primordial follicles can be successfully cryopreserved. The ultimate aim of ovary cryopreservation is to restore ovarian function, with hormone production and follicular growth. These results have been observed after autotransplantation of frozen–thawed ovarian tissue, and eight pregnancies have been reported to date [4–10]. Some studies have demonstrated a risk of transmitting malignant cells with the cryopreserved tissue [11–14]. In some types of cancer, the risk for transmission of cancer cells can be very high, and in such cases, autotransplantation cannot be proposed. To avoid this risk, follicles could be grown in vitro in order to obtain fully matured oocytes surrounded by the zona pellucida and excluding any other cell type.

In addition, study of follicles during the culture period could also help to improve our understanding of early folliculogenesis in humans and other large mammalian species. Particularly the earliest stages (i.e. those that survive the cryopreservation procedure well) need more attention and study. Other aims such as managing follicular quality after cryopreservation or even making an oocyte cell bank could also profit from observations of in vitro culture.

Among species whose ovaries can be compared with the human in size and structure, culture systems for secondary follicles have been described for sheep [15,16], cattle [17,18], and pigs [19,20]. However, little progress has been made in developing culture systems to grow primordial or primary follicles in these species. This chapter discusses the current achievements obtained with in vitro culture of female germ cells and primordial ovarian follicles and the attempts to improve their development by adding various factors to the culture medium. The established methods for the evaluation of survival and growth in culture are also discussed: follicular counts, immunocytochemical methods, transmission electron microscopy, viability markers, and endocrine assays.

Primordial follicle development in vivo

In fetal life, primordial follicles are formed in the ovary by the organization of oocytes and pre-granulosa cells. Autocrine and/or paracrine signaling involving growth factors from granulosa cells, oocytes, and stromal interstitial cells regulate follicular growth up to the antral stage. As soon as the follicle is formed, growth and atresia of some follicles can already be observed, while other follicles stay quiescent until menopause.

Numerous factors are involved in the growth beyond the primordial stage, and while some are necessary, it does not appear that exit from the resting pool is dependent on any one single factor. Factors from vascular and neuronal origin participate in follicular formation and in the earliest growth processes. These factors can be either stimulatory or inhibitory. Ovarian function is also under the control of the hypothalamic gonadotropin-releasing

Fertility Cryopreservation, ed. Ri-Cheng Chian and Patrick Quinn. Published by Cambridge University Press.

hormone pulse generator, which drives production of follicle-stimulating hormone (FSH) and luteinizing hormone (LH). Gene knockout technology has revealed that oocyte-derived factors (bone morphogenetic protein [BMP] 6 and growth differentiation factors [GDF] 9 and 9B [BMP-15]) of the transforming growth factor [TGF] β superfamily play key roles at the earliest stages of folliculogenesis. Targeted deletion of the gene for GDF-9 in mice [21] or naturally occurring point mutations of the gene for BMP-15 in sheep [22] result in arrest of follicle development at the primary stage. Several lines of evidence point to a role for anti-Müllerian hormone (AMH) as a regulator of primordial follicle activation, inhibiting their recruitment into the growing phase. A mouse knockout model homozygous for AMH showed rapid depletion of the primordial follicle pool [23].

Oocyte growth during early folliculogenesis was shown to be regulated by the Kit ligand (KL) and its receptor c-Kit. Mice with mutations at the white spotting (W locus encoding c-kit) and/or steel locus (Sl locus encoding KL) had a severe or mild defect in early follicular development [24,25]. The multitude of processes and factors involved in follicular formation and early follicle growth stages have been reviewed by Juengel and McNatty [26] and by Matzuk and Lamb [27]. Identification of autocrine/paracrine factors and their receptors involved in the regulation of the earliest stages of folliculogenesis have led to the investigation of their requirements for follicle development in vitro.

Sources of ovarian tissue

Ovarian cortical tissue is mainly populated with primordial and primary follicles and is the major source of immature oocytes for in vitro folliculogenesis. Harvesting ovarian cortical tissue is commonly done through an invasive procedure, and most of the research teams working on human ovarian tissue have retrieved specimens during operations performed for adult consenting patients who have faced pathologies requiring treatment that would affect their fertility (e.g. breast cancer and acute leukemia) [28], during cesarean section [29–33], during gynecological or infertility evaluation [24,34–36], and during sterilizing hysterectomy or oophorectomy [37–39]. Given the limited availability of donated human ovarian tissue, other sources have been investigated. Ovaries removed from female-to-male transsexual patients have also been postulated as a potential source of human ovarian cortical tissue for research [40], as has been ovarian cortex surrounding benign ovarian cysts [41,42].

Taking into consideration both the heterogeneous distribution of primordial follicles within the cortex of adult patients and the decline in follicle density with age, fetal (from second or third trimester aborted fetuses) and prepubertal ovaries are very densely populated and would be considered as the ideal sources of human follicles for comparing different culture conditions in prospective study protocols. Moreover, ovarian cortex from very young patients is already cryopreserved [43,44] for fertility preservation, and study of these tissues is needed to ensure they are available when they are potentially wanted for use in the next 10–20 years. The very high density of follicles in ovarian cortex from very young patients facilitates the interpretation of the outcomes of cultures. However, tissue from fetal or prepubertal patients has a gonadal physiology that differs from that in the adult, and behavior in culture might also be different. Preference has been given to fetal ovarian tissue in some studies [45–47].

Methods of in vitro culture

Basically, three major approaches in follicle culture techniques can be distinguished: culture of ovarian cortical tissue (humans and larger animals), culture of entire ovaries (rodents), and culture of isolated follicles (humans, larger animals, and rodents).

Ovarian cortex samples

The large size of adult human ovaries does not allow their culture as entire organs since nutrients cannot diffuse through the different regions of the ovary and difficulties in gas exchange and accumulation of waste metabolites usually lead to necrosis. For these reasons, follicles are often cultured within small thin pieces of ovarian cortex measuring approximately 1 mm^2 and 0.1–1 mm in thickness [36,38,47–53]. Such a small size is preferred because it offers an increased ratio of surface area to volume and allows better contact with media and gas exchange [33]. Culture of ovarian cortical tissue has the advantage that it allows not only preserving the structural integrity of the tissue but also the physical interaction between the surrounding interstitial tissue and the follicles.

Techniques for isolation of follicles

In vitro follicle culture also involved the use of isolated early-stage follicles. There are two approaches for the isolation of follicles: mechanical (microdissection) and enzymatic. The mechanical approach involves the use of fine needles to detach the follicles from the tough

Table 22.1. Reports of human follicular culture in vitro

Authors	Origin/ nature of ovarian tissue used	Basal medium	Supplements	Follicular isolation technique	Periods of culture (days)	Outcomes
Roy and Treacy, 1993 [37]	Adult/fresh	DMEM	BSA, ITS, FSH	Enzymatic	5	Antral follicle development
Zhang *et al.*,1995 [45]	Fetal/ fresh + frozen	Waymouth	FBS, FSH, insulin	None	25+40	Metaphase II oocytes
Hovatta *et al.*, 1997 [38]	Adult/ fresh + frozen	αMEM/EBSS	Serum, FSH, LH, extracellular matrix	None	21	Follicle survival and growth
Abir *et al.*,1997 [39]	Adult/ fresh	αMEM	Serum, FSH/LH	Mechanical	28	Antral follicle development
Hovatta *et al.*, 1999 [34]	Adult/ fresh	EBSS	Serum, FSH, extracellular matrix	None + enzymatic or mechanical	7–9 + 11–18	Follicle survival and growth
Wright *et al.*, 1999 [59]	Adult/ fresh	αMEM/EBSS/ Waymouth	Serum/HSA-ITS, FSH, extracellular matrix	None	10	Follicle growth
Roy and Terada, 1999 [54]	Adult/ fresh	DMEM	BSA, ITS, FSH/ LH/IGF-1/EGF/ transforming growth factor β_1	Enzymatic	1	Glucose metabolic capacity
Abir *et al.*,1999 [57]	Adult/ fresh	EBSS	FBS, FSH, collagen gel	Enzymatic	1	Secondary follicle development
Louhio *et al.*, 2000 [60]	Adult/ fresh	EBSS	Serum, FSH, insulin, IGF, extracellular matrix	None	14	Follicle growth
Abir *et al.*, 2001 [55]	Adult/ fresh + frozen	EBSS	FBS/serum + FSH, extracellular matrix	Enzymatic	1	Follicle survival and growth
Rahimi *et al.*, 2001 [36]	Adult/ fresh	DMEM	FBS, FSH	None	45	Decrease in apoptosis
Hreinsson *et al.*, 2002 [32]	Adult/ fresh	αMEM	FBS/HSA, ITS, FSH, GDF-9, cyclic guanosine monophosphate	None	7	Follicle survival and growth
Otala *et al.*, 2002 [48]	Adult/ fresh	EBSS	serum, FSH, *N*-acetylcysteine, extracellular matrix	None	21	Inhibition of apoptosis
Isachenko *et al.*, 2003 [49]	Adult/ fresh + frozen	DMEM	FCS, β-mercaptoethanol, FSH	None	21	Follicle survival and steroid production
Biron-Shental *et al.*, 2004 [46]	Fetal/ frozen	Serum-free medium	FBS, FSH	None	28	Follicle survival, PCNA, bromodeoxyuridine incorporation
Otala *et al.*, 2004 [48]	Adult/ fresh	Ham's F10	FSH, insulin, HSA, testosterone, dihydrotestosterone, 17-estradiol	None	1	Follicle survival, androgen receptors expression

Table 22.1. (*Cont.*)

Authors	Origin/ nature of ovarian tissue used	Basal medium	Supplements	Follicular isolation technique	Periods of culture (days)	Outcomes
Scott *et al.*, 2004 [33]	Adult/?	αMEM	HSA, FSH, ITS, extracellular matrix	None	14	Follicle survival and growth
Zhang *et al.*, 2004 [61]	Adult/ fresh	αMEM	Serum, cyclic adenosine monophosphate	None	21	Follicle survival and growth
Schmidt *et al.*, 2005 [62]	Child-adult/ frozen	αMEM	HSA, EGF, ITS, FSH, LH, AMH	None	28	Stimulation of follicle growth initiation
Carlsson *et al.*, 2006 [63]	Adult/ fresh	EBSS	Serum/HSA, FSH, Kit ligand, extracellular matrix	None	14	Follicle survival
Carlsson *et al.*, 2006 [63]	Adult/ fresh	αMEM	HSA, FSH, ITS, AMH, cyclic guanosine monophosphate, extracellular matrix	None	7	Inhibition of follicle growth initiation
Sadeu *et al.*, 2006 [47]	Fetal/ frozen	Serum-free medium	None	None	63	Follicle survival and growth
Isachenko *et al.*, 2006 [50]	Adult/ frozen	IMDM	FCS, EGF, FSH	None	14 or 42	Follicle morphology
Isachenko *et al.*, 2007 [51]	Adult/ fresh + frozen	AIM-V	None	None	14	Follicle survival and steroid production
Telfer *et al.*, 2008 [52]	Adult/ fresh	Mc Coy 5a	BSA, ITS, ascorbic acid	None + mechanical	6 + 4	Follicle morphology
Telfer *et al.*, 2008 [52]	Adult/ fresh	Mc Coy 5a	BSA, ITS, ascorbic acid, activin A	None + mechanical	6 + 4	Follicle morphology and estradiol production
Amorim *et al.*, 2009 [56]	Adult/ frozen	MEM	FBS, ITS, isolated follicles embedded in an alginate matrix	Enzymatic + mechanical	7	Follicle viability and morphology
Garor *et al.*, 2009 [64]	Fetal + child-adult/ frozen	αMEM	Ribonucleotides, FSH, FCS/HSA-ITS, basic fibroblast growth factor	None	28	Follicle morphology, PCNA, bromodeoxyuridine incorporation, estradiol production
Sadeu and Smitz, 2008 [53]	Child-adult/ frozen	Defined keratinocyte serum-free medium	None	None	28	Follicle survival and growth; PCNA, AMH, and GDF-9 staining

AIM-V: Adoptive Immunotherapy Media-V, AMH: anti-Müllerian hormone, BSA: bovine serum albumin, DMEM: Dulbecco's Modified Eagle's Medium, EBSS: Earle's Balanced Salt Solution, IMDM: Iscove's Modified Dulbecco's Medium, EGF: epidermal growth factor, FBS: fetal bovine serum, FCS: fetal calf serum, FSH: follicle-stimulating hormone, GDF-9: growth differentiation factor 9, HSA: human serum albumin, ITS: insulin, transferrin, selenium, IGF: insulin-like growth factor, IMDM: Iscove's Modified Dulbecco's Medium, LH: luteinizing hormone, MEM: Minimum Essential Medium, PCNA: proliferating cell nuclear antigen.

fibrous interstitial tissue [39,52]. Using the enzymatic method, human follicles have been isolated after partial or total disaggregation of ovarian tissue with proteolytic enzymes such as collagenase I, II, or IV [34,54–56], mixtures of collagenase and deoxyribonuclease [37,57], or liberase [58]. Mechanical isolation is often facilitated after enzymatic application for partial digestion. Both enzymatic and mechanical methods have their limitations. Mechanical isolation is a tedious and time-consuming process because of the fibrous nature of ovarian interstitial tissue in larger mammals and in particular in the human. Furthermore, the recovery in terms of number of follicles isolated mechanically is usually very low. Enzymatic isolation generally has a negative effect on follicle integrity. The enzymes often disaggregate the basal membrane and theca cells, leading to disruption of oocyte–granulosa cell communications in culture. These disruptions often result in a poor follicular development in vitro. Therefore, most of the studies using isolated follicles are begun from preantral follicles (Table 22.1), as they are bigger with a basal membrane that is more apparent and easier to isolate.

Regardless of these disadvantages, culture of isolated follicles is of significant importance. Follicle isolation helps to determine the follicular content within the tissue fragment, and culturing "empty" (follicle-free) tissue pieces can be avoided. To prove that the isolation techniques are safe for application in larger animals and humans is not an easy task. The validation of the methods was carried out in the rodent models, where secondary follicles were isolated from mouse ovaries using either enzymatic [2] or mechanical [65] methods. These follicles were proven to be capable of growing in culture and producing developmentally competent oocytes and live offspring.

Basal culture conditions

Several basal culture media have been used to grow follicles from different species either within ovarian cortical tissue or as isolated follicle units. These include balanced salt solution (BSS), Iscove's Modified Dulbecco's Medium (IMDM), AIM-V, minimum essential medium alpha (α-MEM), D-minimum essential medium (D-MEM), and Waymouth's medium for humans (Table 22.1). Insulin, transferrin, and selenium alone or in combination with human serum albumin (HSA) and/or serum have been the major components added as supplements to the media with the aim of supporting metabolic and hormonal activities during follicle growth in vitro. In most of the studies, serum from human or animal origin is used. In others, HSA or bovine serum albumin (BSA) has been used instead of serum with significant results, and a few studies have used albumin-free media [53] (Table 22.1).

The culture containers have also varied, from simple test tubes to plastic culture well plates [45,47]. Well plates have been combined with either uncoated [38,39] or coated tissue culture inserts [32,33,38,45,46]. The extracellular matrix compounds utilized to coat the inserts have included collagen I [55], a mixture of laminin, collagen IV, and proteoglycans [38], and collagen I and collagen III [45]. Low concentration of growth factors (basal fibroblast growth factor [bFGF], epidermal growth factor [EGF], insulin-like growth factor [IGF] 1, platelet-derived growth factor, nerve growth factor, TGF-β) can be included in the composition of some manufactured extracellular matrix systems. These factors may also help the follicular growth. Using isolated follicles, the extracellular matrix is clearly missing; therefore, agar [37], collagen gel overlay [55,57], or calcium alginate droplets [56] have been used as supporting components. The rational is to help to preserve the three-dimensional architecture of the follicles and their environment; the cohesion of follicle cells in vitro in such systems is more likely to approximate the in vivo condition, which is desirable to maintain physiological control mechanisms during culture [66].

Whole ovary organ culture has been the main approach to activate the growth of resting primordial follicles because the growth of these follicles after isolation from the stromal environment has been unsuccessful. Whole ovary culture has been carried out in species with small ovaries, such as the rodents [3,67–70]. Culture of isolated follicles has been confined mostly to the study of primary and secondary follicles. These follicles have been isolated from human [34,37,39,56], goat [71], cow [17,72–75], pig [19,20,76], and rodent [1,3,65,77–81] ovaries, as well as from sheep ovaries at the primordial stage [82] and they have been grown in culture to various endpoint follicle stages.

Supplementation of in vitro culture media

Activation of primordial follicles cultured within tissue slices

Knowledge of the function of the majority of growth factors acting on the activation of resting primordial follicles into the growth phase, with subsequent follicular development to further stages of folliculogenesis, has been mainly obtained from animal models [83]. The development of follicle culture systems for larger mammals has been attempted in several species including goat [84], sheep [85], cow [86,87], and baboon [88]. Several culture media used to grow human follicles in vitro have been supplemented with these growth factors to assess their potential physiological significance in regulating the earliest stages of follicular development in humans.

The beneficial effects of several components added to culture media on the activation and/or regulation of the processes of early folliculogenesis in culture has been experimentally reported in several studies, while the biological pathway remains to be determined. For example, it has been shown that supplementing the medium with FSH reduced follicle atresia and increased follicle diameter [59] (Table 22.1). However, FSH receptors in primordial and primary follicles remain to be shown at these stages. Other factors, such as insulin, IGF-1 and IGF-2 [60], secondary messengers such as 8-bromoguanosine 3′,5′-cyclic monophosphate [33], and cyclic adenosine 3′,5′-monophosphate [61] have also positive effects on the development of the early stages of human follicles. Data from studies on human [32] and goat [89] follicle culture showed that addition of 200 ng/ml GDF-9 enhances activation of primordial follicles and stimulates the transition from primary to secondary follicles. This in vitro observation suggested that GDF-9 might have supportive effects on the earliest stages of ovarian follicles. It was also demonstrated that AMH inhibits the early development of human [90] and mouse [91] follicles in culture. However, the presence of AMH in culture has been shown to increase the development of human follicles in a single study [62].

The addition of KL to the medium supported the survival of human follicles [63] and stimulated the development of rodent primordial follicles into primary stage [69]. Addition of bFGF has been shown to increase primordial follicle transition in neonatal rat ovary organ cultures [69,92] and in adult human ovarian cortex, but at a 10 times higher concentration and this was not observed in fetal tissue [64]. Activin A has shown an enhancement of oocyte development in cultured ovine preantral follicles [93] and the growth of rat preantral follicles [94]. This glycoprotein also promotes antrum formation in rat follicles as well as in human [52,94]. Keratinocyte growth factors [95], leukemia inhibitory factor [96], BMP-4 [97], and BMP-7 [98] have also been shown to enhance the primordial to primary follicle transition in neonatal rat ovary organ cultures, while stromal-derived factor-1 and its receptor CXCR4 [70] inhibited that transition. The development of goat primordial follicles was stimulated by FSH and EGF in cultures of goat ovarian tissue [84]. Factors that had been studied previously in animal models and subsequently used in human confirmed that factors likely had effects that were both species dependent and follicular stage dependent, as was already reported for activin A [52] and bFGF [64]. For example, activin A appeared folliculogenetic in the prepubertal mouse but not in adults [99].

Culture of isolated early-stage follicles

Attempts to grow isolated human follicles in vitro have resulted in follicle development along different stages of folliculogenesis. In vitro culture of isolated follicles has been carried out for larger mammals, and the effect of different growth factors has been investigated. Both EGF and bFGF were shown to sustain oocyte survival during culture of isolated goat preantral follicles, while IGF-1 not only supported follicle survival but also stimulated follicle growth [71]. Insulin, FSH, IGF-1, EGF, IGF-2, and vascular endothelial growth factor were shown to stimulate follicle growth in bovine preantral follicle culture [17,75,100]. In humans, isolated follicles are mostly cultured from the secondary or preantral stage (Table 22.1). Primary follicles have been isolated in a single study [57].

Two-step systems

Ovarian cortex culture followed by isolated follicle culture has been used in rodent species with success, as pups were born. This two-step strategy used intact ovaries from newborn mice, which were organ cultured for 8 days. Oocyte–granulosa cell complexes isolated from these were cultured for a further 14 days [2]. The composition of the media was subsequently also modified during the culture periods with the addition of FSH and insulin, transferrin, selenium [2,3]. Human ovary culture is impossible because of its larger size. However, an adaptation of the previous methods has been used with human follicles [34,52]. Primordial and primary follicles were grown within cortical pieces for 6 to 9 days, and then preantral follicles were dissected from the strips using 25 gauge needles or with collagenase II. Care was taken to include the adherent theca/stromal cells attached to the follicles. The medium was also modified. In the most recent study using this approach, activin A was added during the second step of the culture [52].

Methods for evaluation of follicular culture

Histological analysis still remains the gold standard method in 2008. Several histomorphometric methods can be used to investigate follicular development in vitro. Regardless of the species, the following morphological and morphometric parameters can be analyzed: follicle viability, antral cavity formation, oocyte viability, follicle diameter, and enclosed oocyte diameter. Unlike culture of isolated follicles, which can be quickly monitored and evaluated under an inverted microscope, culture of ovarian cortical tissue can only be analyzed after processing of tissues for histological examination. This approach entails the tissues being fixed either in formalin or in Bouin's solution, paraffin embedded, and serially sectioned at the end of each culture period. The sections are placed in order on glass slides and stained with hematoxylin, eosin, and saffran before being analyzed by light microscope for the presence of follicles and the stages of development. Different approaches have been used for estimating follicle numbers, based on histological analysis of tissue sections [101].

The oocyte nucleolus is commonly used as a central mark to avoid double counting of the same follicle. Follicle viability is determined based upon defined morphological criteria of atresia, such as pyknosis of nuclei, basal membrane integrity, and granulosa cell organization. Follicular development in vitro is assessed by counting the number of follicles of various stages in control (uncultured or cultured in the absence of growth factors under study) versus the number in studied samples throughout the culture period. To assess follicle growth, follicle and oocyte diameters are measured and the number of layers of granulosa cells is counted. Although conventional histological analysis remains an obligatory method in the study of ovarian tissue culture, the major disadvantage of this technique is that it is tedious. As follicles are usually grouped in nests rather than regularly distributed in the cortex, extrapolation from limited tissue pieces to total ovary remains inaccurate.

Transmission electron microscopy provides detailed analysis of follicular ultrastructure and has been used to evaluate intracellular integrity of bovine [74] and human [47] follicles after prolonged culture periods. Signs of intracellular damage include the presence of cytoplasmic vacuoles, swollen mitochondria, lipid droplets, chromatin condensation, and wrinkled or ruptured nuclear membrane. Morphological differences between apoptotic and atretic cells have also been demonstrated by transmission electron microscopy, and its contribution to the study of ovarian tissue has been recently reviewed [102].

Follicular viability and cell death in human ovarian cortex have been evaluated with fluorescent markers using fluorescent microscopy. The polyanionic dye calcein is retained in living cells and the cleavage product induced by cellular esterase activity provides an intense, uniform green fluorescence in the cytoplasm. The nuclei of all cells with damaged membrane are counterstained with ethidium homodimer-1 (red fluorescence) [56,103]. In binding DNA of nuclei, ethidium homodimer-1 increases in fluorescence. Considering the huge volume of the oocyte's cytoplasm compared with that in other cells of the ovarian cortex, the follicles are easily observed within the tissue. The oocyte and the granulosa cells can be detailed within the tissue through confocal microscopy [103] or with isolated follicles [56]. This technique has also been used as a quick method for scoring the density of follicles within human ovarian cortex using simple fluorescent microscopy [41]. Similar results can be obtained with rhodamine staining, which reflects mitochondrial activity. Rhodamine accumulates into active mitochondria with a membrane potential [104].

Evaluation of the adequacy of culture conditions has been investigated by accounting for follicle death through apoptosis. Morphological characteristics of apoptosis at the early stage include chromatin condensation and cell shrinkage. Terminal deoxyribonucleotidyl transferase-mediated deoxyuridine triphosphate nick end labeling (TUNEL) has been used to detect fragmented DNA in nuclei of granulosa cells and oocyte from goat [84]. However, false-positive results with this method have been reported [36]. Apoptosis is an active process that requires expression of specific proteases such as caspases. Cultured ovarian tissue pieces have been stained with anti-caspase-3 or anti-active caspase-3 [36,48]. Furthermore, pyknotic nuclei can be revealed on tissue sections by their incubation with the fluorescent dye SYTOX, which binds with high affinity to the triplex structure of the nucleic acids of dead cells [36]. This DNA staining allows easier nuclei visualization in large areas of tissue, and pictures can be digitalized for computer analysis. Obviously, this staining concerns the follicles and the stromal tissue.

Cell proliferation is a key marker during in vitro culture as evidence that viable follicles are able to grow during the culture period. Granulosa cell expression of proliferating cell nuclear antigen (PCNA) in culture is a valuable marker for cell replication. This is a nuclear protein that plays an essential role in cell cycle regulation, and it is an important mediator of cell proliferation; it can be detected by immunohistochemistry. The correlation between PCNA production and initiation of growth has been shown in fetal bovine and baboon follicles [88]. The granulosa cells were strongly immunostained for PCNA when their shape changed from flattened to cuboidal [86,88]. Positive PCNA immunostaining was also demonstrated in granulosa cells of growing follicles after a few days of culture in human tissue [47]. This finding could indicate some DNA synthesis activity at the early stage of growth initiation. Granulosa cell proliferation has also been demonstrated in cultured follicles using a bromodeoxyuridine incorporation technique. Bromodeoxyuridine can be incorporated into newly synthesized DNA of replicating cells during the S-phase of the cell cycle, and it is, therefore, used as a marker of DNA synthesis in mouse [105], cow [72], and human tissue [46,64]. Classical radioactive thymidine ([^{3}H]-thymidine) uptake has also been used to demonstrate DNA synthesis in granulosa cells of isolated follicles in culture. In other studies, [^{3}H]-thymidine was added to the culture medium and the follicles or oocytes–cumulus complexes were examined after a few hours for [^{3}H]-thymidine incorporation [37,106].

Functional approaches have also been used for the evaluation of follicular growth with expression of stage-specific markers and the measure of secreted proteins such as estradiol. Follicle stage-specific factors such as GDF-9 and AMH are known to be involved in the regulation and initiation of the processes of early folliculogenesis in vivo and have been used as functional markers during follicle culture. Their expression in oocytes and granulosa cells in human cultured follicles has been observed after a 21-day in vitro culture period [53]. A functional approach to evaluation of in vitro cultured follicles can also be achieved using molecular biology techniques. Gene regulation is the basis for cellular differentiation, cell growth, and morphogenesis, and the amount of gene expression has been used to determine the function of the cells. Quantitative real-time polymerase chain reaction can be integrated in the evaluation of cultured follicles. This approach is more appropriate for isolated follicles and was investigated for GDF-9 and AMH in mouse cultured follicles [107].

The conditioned media collected at each time point of culture can provide information as to the degree of somatic cell differentiation in vitro, which should be related to a follicular growth. Several secretion products can be measured to evaluate follicle growth during culture. Absence or low estrogen production could be related either to absence or incomplete aromatization in granulosa cells or to the non-functionality of the theca compartment. The differential analysis can be made by adding androgen (androstenedione) to the culture medium. Estradiol production was observed and measured with radioimmunoanalysis [39] or enzyme-linked immunosorbent assay [52] during in vitro culture of human tissue. A heterogeneous competitive magnetic separation immunoassay analysis was also used to measure estradiol and progesterone in an unchanged medium during the whole 14 day culture period [51].

Outcomes of follicular culture

In vivo, the growth initiation of primordial follicles has an evolution over several months [108]. However, when media supplemented with growth factors were used, massive activation of primordial follicles to initiate growth in vitro within human adult cortical ovarian tissues occurred within the first week of culture [32,34,59,107]. When human fetal ovarian tissues were cultured in growth factor-supplemented media, the growth initiation of primordial follicles took more than 3 weeks [45]. In a simplified long-term culture system using a defined serum-free medium, initiation of follicle growth and progression to subsequent stages of development took almost 2 months [47]. Culture of human ovarian cortical tissue for 1–3 weeks resulted in 30–53% of the surviving follicles developing into the secondary stage [32,34,38]. There was no correlation between the development of secondary follicles and a corresponding increase in oocyte diameter, as described in vivo: oocyte growth was limited or not detectable. The development of secondary follicles in vitro was characterized by an increase in the number of granulosa cells through cell proliferation but a limited increase in oocyte diameter.

Human primary follicles have been isolated and cultured for 1 day. Follicular growth was observed, with the increase of their diameter from approximately

34 μm to approximately 69 μm [55,57]. Human preantral follicles have been cultured as isolated follicles from 5 days [37] to 4 weeks [39]. The starting diameters of cultured follicles ranged between 220 μm [54] and 350 μm [39]. Already after 5 days of culture, the follicles had developed to reach the antral stage, and granulosa cells proliferation in vitro was observed [37]. After 4 weeks of culture, 70% of the isolated preantral follicles had developed an antral cavity (follicular size up to 125 μm). However, atretic cells were observed within the granulosa cells, and follicular development beyond the early antral stage could not be achieved, likely because of suboptimal culture conditions. At the end of culture, only 10–20% of the isolated preantral follicles contained an enclosed oocyte. The missing oocytes in the majority of follicles might have degenerated by atresia before (as a physiological process) or after being cultured [39]. These culture experiments indicate that preantral follicle development can be achieved in vitro, leading to oocyte growth and granulosa cell differentiation, but at a very low yield.

A two-step strategy, with the addition of activin A in the second period, led to antral cavity formation with significantly less atresia (than without activin A). These follicles grew from primordial/primary stage to the antral stage, reaching a size of 143 μm. In these follicles, oocyte growth was also observed: oocyte diameter was 31.9 μm for follicles grown in control medium and 51.3 μm for oocytes grown with activin A supplementation in the second step [52].

Conclusions

Follicle culture systems offer interesting experimental models to address several biological issues that are important for our understanding of human folliculogenesis. The investigation of mechanisms regulating primordial follicle activation and early development are the major points in the studies described here, and several have observed follicular growth up to the early antral stage. This stage appears to be a boundary that is difficult to cross.

Regardless of the final purpose of the study, the culture technique is determined by the size of the ovary (the species), the developmental stage of the follicle of interest, and the duration of folliculogenesis. Success of a culture system will finally be judged by the production of developmentally competent oocytes, able to be fertilized and to produce healthy births. This goal has only been reached in the mouse model so far. The human ovary is very different from that of the rodent in its size, structure, and folliculogenesis duration. Therefore, studies on human tissue are mandatory. We are confronted by several problems when research on human tissue is being planned. The first difficulty is to obtain human material, as ethic and legal considerations differ from one country to another. The second major problem with human tissue is its follicular density, which can be extremely low, and its heterogeneity. This leads to a need for a high number of samples. The stromal tissue in the ovaries of larger mammals is fibrous and dense, preventing the easy isolation of the follicles and the development of a successful culture system. Fetal ovaries could be considered as a first choice of material because of their high follicle density and the softness of their tissue. The few reports with this approach showed that healthy follicles grown in culture are morphologically comparable to those grown in vivo. However, because its function and physiology might differ from the adult ovary, the results obtained with fetal tissue should be ultimately confirmed with adult tissue. Although these difficulties cannot be denied, the number of studies on human ovarian tissue has increased in the last few years and this provides hope that these problems can be solved.

Although the requirements for normal follicle growth at the earliest stages are still unknown and remain to be determined, follicular growth has been shown in several studies and this growth is usually applied to the majority of the follicle types cultured. Follicular atresia is a major concern during in vitro culture, but is also supposed to be at a high level in normal physiology. Considering the long time required for complete follicular development in larger mammals, and the difficulties with long-term maintenance of tissue culture, it is likely that a multistep procedure should be applied to the culture of primordial follicles of larger mammals in order to achieve a successful culture system.

Follicular growth up to the antral stage is obtained after different culture time periods but usually shorter than what is believed to happen in vivo. It is likely that the in vitro conditions cannot mimic the normal physiology, and so this different timing should not be surprising. However, potential side effects of this modification of timing have to be determined. For example, cellular development under culture conditions, and especially for long duration, is more susceptible to genetic modifications. Therefore, the genetic status of in vitro grown oocytes will have to be studied before using them for human fertilization and embryo transfer. Long-term culture might result in unappropriated cellular differentiation and genetic modification. Hence, molecular techniques should be considered to analyze the normal methylation pattern of primary imprints in oocytes.

The final measure of success will be the ability of the in vitro matured oocytes to fertilize and produce healthy offsprings. Combination of cryopreservation of ovarian cortical tissue with successful in vitro culture of follicles will bring a major breakthrough in fertility preservation. The availability of such techniques might increase the demand from a range of women, not just those with cancer.

References

1. Eppig JJ, Schroeder AC. Capacity of mouse oocytes from preantral follicles to undergo embryogenesis and development to live young after growth, maturation, and fertilization in vitro. *Biol Reprod* 1989; **41:** 268–276.
2. Eppig JJ, O'Brien MJ. Development in vitro of mouse oocytes from primordial follicles. *Biol Reprod* 1996; **54:** 197–207.
3. O'Brien MJ, Pendola JK, Eppig JJ. A revised protocol for in vitro development of mouse oocytes from primordial follicles dramatically improves their developmental competence. *Biol Reprod* 2003; **68:** 1682–1686.
4. Donnez J, Dolmans MM, Demylle D, *et al.* Livebirth after orthotopic transplantation of cryopreserved ovarian tissue. *Lancet* 2004; **364:** 1405–1410.
5. Meirow D, Levron J, Eldar-Geva T, *et al.* Pregnancy after transplantation of cryopreserved ovarian tissue in a patient with ovarian failure after chemotherapy. *N Engl J Med* 2005; **353:** 318–321.
6. Meirow D, Levron J, Eldar-Geva T, *et al.* Monitoring the ovaries after autotransplantation of cryopreserved ovarian tissue: endocrine studies, in vitro fertilization cycles, and live birth. *Fertil Steril* 2007; **87:** 418.e7–e15.
7. Demeestere I, Simon P, Buxant F, *et al.* Ovarian function and spontaneous pregnancy after combined heterotopic and orthotopic cryopreserved ovarian tissue transplantation in a patient previously treated with bone marrow transplantation: case report. *Hum Reprod* 2006; **21:** 2010–2014.
8. Demeestere I, Simon P, Emiliani S, *et al.* Fertility preservation: successful transplantation of cryopreserved ovarian tissue in a young patient previously treated for Hodgkin's disease. *Oncologist* 2007; **12:** 1437–1442.
9. Silber SJ, DeRosa M, Pineda J, *et al.* A series of monozygotic twins discordant for ovarian failure: ovary transplantation (cortical versus microvascular) and cryopreservation. *Hum Reprod* 2008; **23:** 1531–1537.
10. Andersen CY, Rosendahl M, Byskov AG, *et al.* Two successful pregnancies following autotransplantation of frozen/thawed ovarian tissue. *Hum Reprod* 2008; **23:** 2266–2272.
11. Shaw JM, Bowles J, Koopman P, *et al.* Fresh and cryopreserved ovarian tissue samples from donors with lymphoma transmit the cancer to graft recipients. *Hum Reprod* 1996; **11:** 1668–1673.
12. Meirow D, Ben Yehuda D, Prus D, *et al.* Ovarian tissue banking in patients with Hodgkin's disease: is it safe? *Fertil Steril* 1998; **69:** 996–998.
13. Meirow D, Hardan I, Dor J, *et al.* Searching for evidence of disease and malignant cell contamination in ovarian tissue stored from hematologic cancer patients. *Hum Reprod* 2008; **23:** 1007–1013.
14. Kyono K, Uto H, Toya M, *et al.* Potential indications for ovarian autotransplantation based on the analysis of 5571 autopsy findings of females with malignant diseases under the age of 40 in Japan. *Fertil Steril* 2008; **90** (Suppl 1): S267.
15. Cecconi S, Barboni B, Coccia M, *et al.* In vitro development of sheep preantral follicles. *Biol Reprod* 1999; **60:** 594–601.
16. Newton H, Picton H, Gosden RG. In vitro growth of oocyte–granulosa cell complexes isolated from cryopreserved ovine tissue. *J Reprod Fertil* 1999; **115:** 141–150.
17. Gutierrez CG, Ralph JH, Telfer EE, *et al.* Growth and antrum formation of bovine preantral follicles in long-term culture in vitro. *Biol Reprod* 2000; **62:** 1322–1328.
18. McCaffery FH, Leask R, Riley SC, *et al.* Culture of bovine preantral follicles in a serum-free system: markers for assessment of growth and development. *Biol Reprod* 2000; **63:** 267–273.
19. Hirao Y, Nagai T, Kubo M, *et al.* In vitro growth and maturation of pig oocytes. *J Reprod Fertil* 1994; **100:** 333–339.
20. Wu J, Emery BR, Carrell DT. In vitro growth, maturation, fertilization, and embryonic development of oocytes from porcine preantral follicles. *Biol Reprod* 2001; **64:** 375–381.
21. Dong J, Albertini DF, Nishimori K, *et al.* Growth differentiation factor-9 is required during early ovarian folliculogenesis. *Nature* 1996; **383:** 531–535.
22. Galloway SM, McNatty KP, Cambridge LM, *et al.* Mutations in an oocyte-derived growth factor gene (BMP15) cause increased ovulation rate and infertility in a dosage-sensitive manner. *Nat Genet* 2000; **25:** 279–283.
23. Durlinger AL, Kramer P, Karels B, *et al.* Control of primordial follicle recruitment by anti-Mullerian hormone in the mouse ovary. *Endocrinol* 1999; **140:** 5789–5796.

24. Huang EJ, Manova K, Packer AI, *et al.* The murine steel panda mutation affects kit ligand expression and growth of early ovarian follicles. *Dev Biol* 1993; **157:** 100–109.
25. Kuroda H, Terada N, Nakayama H, *et al.* Infertility due to growth arrest of ovarian follicles in Sl/Slt mice. *Dev Biol* 1988; **126:** 71–79.
26. Juengel JL, McNatty KP. The role of proteins of the transforming growth factor-beta superfamily in the intraovarian regulation of follicular development. *Hum Reprod Update* 2005; **11:** 1143–1160.
27. Matzuk MM, Lamb DJ. Genetic dissection of mammalian fertility pathways. *Nat Cell Biol* 2002; **4**(Suppl): s41–s9.
28. Gook DA, McCully BA, Edgar DH, *et al.* Development of antral follicles in human cryopreserved ovarian tissue following xenografting. *Hum Reprod* 2001; **16:** 417–422.
29. Newton H, Aubard Y, Rutherford A, *et al.* Low temperature storage and grafting of human ovarian tissue. *Hum Reprod* 1996; **11:** 1487–1491.
30. Oktay K, Nugent D, Newton H, *et al.* Isolation and characterization of primordial follicles from fresh and cryopreserved human ovarian tissue. *Fertil Steril* 1997; **67:** 481–486.
31. Oktay K, Newton H, Mullan J, *et al.* Development of human primordial follicles to antral stages in SCID/hpg mice stimulated with follicle stimulating hormone. *Hum Reprod* 1998; **13:** 1133–1138.
32. Hreinsson JG, Scott JE, Rasmussen C, *et al.* Growth differentiation factor-9 promotes the growth, development, and survival of human ovarian follicles in organ culture. *J Clin Endocrinol Metab* 2002; **87:** 316–321.
33. Scott JE, Carlsson IB, Bavister BD, *et al.* Human ovarian tissue cultures: extracellular matrix composition, coating density and tissue dimensions. *Reprod Biomed Online* 2004; **9:** 287–293.
34. Hovatta O, Wright C, Krausz T, *et al.* Human primordial, primary and secondary ovarian follicles in long-term culture: effect of partial isolation. *Hum Reprod* 1999; **14:** 2519–2524.
35. Nisolle M, Casanas-Roux F, Qu J, *et al.* Histologic and ultrastructural evaluation of fresh and frozen–thawed human ovarian xenografts in nude mice. *Fertil Steril* 2000; **74:** 122–129.
36. Rahimi G, Isachenko E, Sauer H, *et al.* Measurement of apoptosis in long-term cultures of human ovarian tissue. *Reproduction* 2001; **122:** 657–663.
37. Roy SK, Treacy BJ. Isolation and long-term culture of human preantral follicles. *Fertil Steril* 1993; **59:** 783–790.
38. Hovatta O, Silye R, Abir R, *et al.* Extracellular matrix improves survival of both stored and fresh human primordial and primary ovarian follicles in long-term culture. *Hum Reprod* 1997; **12:** 1032–1036.
39. Abir R, Franks S, Mobberley MA, *et al.* Mechanical isolation and in vitro growth of preantral and small antral human follicles. *Fertil Steril* 1997; **68:** 682–688.
40. van den Broecke R, Van Der Elst J, Liu J, *et al.* The female-to-male transsexual patient: a source of human ovarian cortical tissue for experimental use. *Hum Reprod* 2001; **16:** 145–147.
41. Schubert B, Canis M, Darcha C, *et al.* Human ovarian tissue from cortex surrounding benign cysts: a model to study ovarian tissue cryopreservation. *Hum Reprod* 2005; **20:** 1786–1792.
42. Schubert B, Canis M, Darcha C, *et al.* Follicular growth and estradiol follow-up after subcutaneous xenografting of fresh and cryopreserved human ovarian tissue. *Fertil Steril* 2008; **89:** 1787–1794.
43. Poirot C, Vacher-Lavenu MC, Helardot P, *et al.* Human ovarian tissue cryopreservation: indications and feasibility. *Hum Reprod* 2002; **17:** 1447–1452.
44. Sánchez M, Novella-Maestre E, Teruel J, *et al.* The Valencia Programme for Fertility Preservation. *Clin Transl Oncol* 2008; **10:** 433–438.
45. Zhang J, Liu J, Xu KP, *et al.* Extracorporeal development and ultrarapid freezing of human fetal ova. *J Assist Reprod Genet* 1995; **12:** 361–368.
46. Biron-Shental T, Fisch B, van den Hurk R, *et al.* Survival of frozen–thawed human ovarian fetal follicles in long-term organ culture. *Fertil Steril* 2004; **81:** 716–719.
47. Sadeu JC, Cortvrindt R, Ron-El R, *et al.* Morphological and ultrastructural evaluation of cultured frozen–thawed human fetal ovarian tissue. *Fertil Steril* 2006; **85**(Suppl 1): 1130–1141.
48. Otala M, Erkkila K, Tuuri T, *et al.* Cell death and its suppression in human ovarian tissue culture. *Mol Hum Reprod* 2002; **8:** 228–236.
49. Isachenko E, Isachenko V, Rahimi G, *et al.* Cryopreservation of human ovarian tissue by direct plunging into liquid nitrogen. *Eur J Obstet Gynecol Reprod Biol* 2003; **108:** 186–193.
50. Isachenko V, Montag M, Isachenko E, *et al.* Effective method for in-vitro culture of cryopreserved human ovarian tissue. *Reprod Biomed Online* 2006; **13:** 228–234.
51. Isachenko V, Isachenko E, Reinsberg J, *et al.* Cryopreservation of human ovarian tissue: comparison of rapid and conventional freezing. *Cryobiology* 2007; **55:** 261–268.
52. Telfer E, McLaughlin M, Ding C, *et al.* A two step serum free culture system supports development of human oocytes from primordial follicles in the presence of activin. *Hum Reprod* 2008; **23:** 1151–1158.
53. Sadeu JC, Smitz J. Growth differentiation factor-9 and anti-Müllerian hormone expression in cultured human follicles from frozen–thawed ovarian tissue. *Reprod Biomed Online* 2008; **17:** 537–548.
54. Roy SK, Terada DM. Activities of glucose metabolic enzymes in human preantral follicles: in vitro

modulation by follicle-stimulating hormone, luteinizing hormone, epidermal growth factor, insulin-like growth factor I, and transforming growth factor beta1. *Biol Reprod* 1999; **60:** 763–768.

55. Abir R, Fisch B, Nitke S, *et al.* Morphological study of fully and partially isolated early human follicles. *Fertil Steril* 2001; **75:** 141–146.
56. Amorim CA, Van Langendockt A, David A, Dolmans M-M, Donnez J. Survival of human pre-antral follicles after cryopreservation of ovarian tissue, follicular isolation and in vitro culture in a calcium alginate matrix. *Hum Reprod* 2009; **24:** 92–99.
57. Abir R, Roizman P, Fisch B, *et al.* Pilot study of isolated early human follicles cultured in collagen gels for 24 hours. *Hum Reprod* 1999; **14:** 1299–1301.
58. Dolmans MM, Michaux N, Camboni A, *et al.* Evaluation of Liberase, a purified enzyme blend, for the isolation of human primordial and primary ovarian follicles. *Hum Reprod* 2006; **21:** 413–420.
59. Wright CS, Hovatta O, Margara R, *et al.* Effects of follicle-stimulating hormone and serum substitution on the in-vitro growth of human ovarian follicles. *Hum Reprod* 1999; **14:** 1555–1562.
60. Louhio H, Hovatta O, Sjoberg J, *et al.* The effects of insulin, and insulin-like growth factors I and II on human ovarian follicles in long-term culture. *Mol Hum Reprod* 2000; **6:** 694–698.
61. Zhang P, Louhio H, Tuuri T, *et al.* In vitro effect of cyclic adenosine 3′, 5′-monophosphate (cAMP) on early human ovarian follicles. *J Assist Reprod Genet* 2004; **21:** 301–306.
62. Schmidt KL, Kryger-Baggesen N, Byskov AG, *et al.* Anti-Mullerian hormone initiates growth of human primordial follicles in vitro. *Mol Cell Endocrinol* 2005; **234:** 87–93.
63. Carlsson IB, Laitinen MP, Scott JE, *et al.* Kit ligand and c-Kit are expressed during early human ovarian follicular development and their interaction is required for the survival of follicles in long-term culture. *Reproduction* 2006; **131:** 641–649.
64. Garor R, Abir R, Erman A, *et al.* Effects of basic fibroblast growth factor on in vitro development of human ovarian primordial follicles. *Fertil Steril* 2009; **91**(Suppl 5): 1967–1975.
65. Cortvrindt R, Smitz J, Van Steirteghem AC. In-vitro maturation, fertilization and embryo development of immature oocytes from early preantral follicles from prepuberal mice in a simplified culture system. *Hum Reprod* 1996; **11:** 2656–2666.
66. Woodruff TK, Shea LD. The role of the extracellular matrix in ovarian follicle development. *Reprod Sci* 2007; **14**(Suppl): 6–10.
67. Parrott JA, Skinner MK. Kit-ligand/stem cell factor induces primordial follicle development and initiates folliculogenesis. *Endocrinology* 1999; **140:** 4262–4271.
68. Kezele P, Skinner MK. Regulation of ovarian primordial follicle assembly and development by estrogen and progesterone: endocrine model of follicle assembly. *Endocrinology* 2003; **144:** 3329–3337.
69. Nilsson EE, Skinner MK. Kit ligand and basic fibroblast growth factor interactions in the induction of ovarian primordial to primary follicle transition. *Mol Cell Endocrinol* 2004; **214:** 19–25.
70. Holt JE, Jackson A, Roman SD, *et al.* CXCR4/SDF1 interaction inhibits the primordial to primary follicle transition in the neonatal mouse ovary. *Dev Biol* 2006; **293:** 449–460.
71. Zhou H, Zhang Y. Regulation of in vitro growth of preantral follicles by growth factors in goats. *Domest Anim Endocrinol* 2005; **28:** 235–242.
72. Hulshof SC, Figueiredo JR, Beckers JF, *et al.* Effects of fetal bovine serum, FSH and 17beta-estradiol on the culture of bovine preantral follicles. *Theriogenology* 1995; **44:** 217–226.
73. Katska L, Rynska B. The isolation and in vitro culture of bovine preantral and early antral follicles of different size classes. *Theriogenology* 1998; **50:** 213–222.
74. van den Hurk R, Spek ER, Hage WJ, *et al.* Ultrastructure and viability of isolated bovine preantral follicles. *Hum Reprod Update* 1998; **4:** 833–841.
75. Itoh T, Kacchi M, Abe H, *et al.* Growth, antrum formation, and estradiol production of bovine preantral follicles cultured in a serum-free medium. *Biol Reprod* 2002; **67:** 1099–1105.
76. Mao J, Wu G, Smith MF, *et al.* Effects of culture medium, serum type, and various concentrations of follicle-stimulating hormone on porcine preantral follicular development and antrum formation in vitro. *Biol Reprod* 2002; **67:** 1197–1203.
77. Roy SK, Greenwald GS. Hormonal requirements for the growth and differentiation of hamster preantral follicles in long-term culture. *J Reprod Fertil* 1989; **87:** 103–114.
78. Nayudu PL, Osborn SM. Factors influencing the rate of preantral and antral growth of mouse ovarian follicles in vitro. *J Reprod Fertil* 1992; **95:** 349–362.
79. Spears N, Boland NI, Murray AA, *et al.* Mouse oocytes derived from in vitro grown primary ovarian follicles are fertile. *Hum Reprod* 1994; **9:** 527–532.
80. Lenie S, Cortvrindt R, Adriaenssens T, *et al.* A reproducible two-step culture system for isolated primary mouse ovarian follicles as single functional units. *Biol Reprod* 2004; **71:** 1730–1738.
81. Kreeger PK, Deck JW, Woodruff TK, *et al.* The in vitro regulation of ovarian follicle development using alginate-extracellular matrix gels. *Biomaterials* 2006; **27:** 714–723.
82. Muruvi W, Picton HM, Rodway RG, *et al.* In vitro growth of oocytes from primordial follicles isolated from frozen–thawed lamb ovaries. *Theriogenology* 2005; **64:** 1357–1370.

83. Smitz JE, Cortvrindt RG. The earliest stages of folliculogenesis in vitro. *Reproduction* 2002; **123:** 185–202.
84. Silva JR, van den Hurk R, Costa SH, *et al.* Survival and growth of goat primordial follicles after in vitro culture of ovarian cortical slices in media containing coconut water. *Anim Reprod Sci* 2004; **81:** 273–286.
85. Mery L, Lefevre A, Benchaib M, *et al.* Follicular growth in vitro: detection of growth differentiation factor 9 (GDF9) and bone morphogenetic protein 15 (BMP15) during in vitro culture of ovine cortical slices. *Mol Reprod Dev* 2006; **74:** 767–774.
86. Wandji SA, Srsen V, Voss AK, *et al.* Initiation in vitro of growth of bovine primordial follicles. *Biol Reprod* 1996; **55:** 942–948.
87. Braw-Tal R, Yossefi S. Studies in vivo and in vitro on the initiation of follicle growth in the bovine ovary. *J Reprod Fertil* 1997; **109:** 165–171.
88. Wandji SA, Srsen V, Nathanielsz PW, *et al.* Initiation of growth of baboon primordial follicles in vitro. *Hum Reprod* 1997; **12:** 1993–2001.
89. Martins FS, Celestino JJH, Saraiva MVA, *et al.* Growth and differentiation factor-9 stimulates activation of goat primordial follicles in vitro and their progression to secondary follicles. *Reprod Fertil Dev* 2008; **20:** 916–924.
90. Carlsson IB, Scott JE, Visser JA, *et al.* Anti-Mullerian hormone inhibits initiation of growth of human primordial ovarian follicles in vitro. *Hum Reprod* 2006; **21:** 2223–2227.
91. Durlinger AL, Gruijters MJ, Kramer P, *et al.* Anti-Mullerian hormone inhibits initiation of primordial follicle growth in the mouse ovary. *Endocrinol* 2002; **143:** 1076–1084.
92. Nilsson E, Parrott JA, Skinner MK. Basic fibroblast growth factor induces primordial follicle development and initiates folliculogenesis. *Mol Cell Endocrinol* 2001; **175:** 123–130.
93. Thomas FH, Armstrong DG, Telfer EE. Activin promotes oocyte development in ovine preantral follicles in vitro. *Reprod Biol Endocrinol* 2003; **1:** 76.
94. Zhao J, Taverne MA, van der Weijden GC, *et al.* Effect of activin A on in vitro development of rat preantral follicles and localization of activin A and activin receptor II. *Biol Reprod* 2001; **65:** 967–977.
95. Kezele P, Nilsson EE, Skinner MK. Keratinocyte growth factor acts as a mesenchymal factor that promotes ovarian primordial to primary follicle transition. *Biol Reprod* 2005; **73:** 967–973.
96. Nilsson EE, Kezele P, Skinner MK. Leukemia inhibitory factor (LIF) promotes the primordial to primary follicle transition in rat ovaries. *Mol Cell Endocrinol* 2002; **188:** 65–73.
97. Nilsson EE, Skinner MK. Bone morphogenetic protein-4 acts as an ovarian follicle survival factor and promotes primordial follicle development. *Biol Reprod* 2003; **69:** 1265–1272.
98. Lee WS, Yoon SJ, Yoon TK, *et al.* Effects of bone morphogenetic protein-7 (BMP-7) on primordial follicular growth in the mouse ovary. *Mol Reprod Dev* 2004; **69:** 159–163.
99. Yokota H, Yamada K, Liu X, *et al.* Paradoxical action of activin A on folliculogenesis in immature and adult mice. *Endocrinol* 1997; **138:** 4572–4576.
100. Yang MY, Fortune JE. Vascular endothelial growth factor stimulates the primary to secondary follicle transition in bovine follicles in vitro. *Mol Reprod Dev* 2007; **74:** 1095–1104.
101. Tilly JL. Ovarian follicle counts: not as simple as 1, 2, 3. *Reprod Biol Endocrinol* 2003; **1:** 11.
102. Camboni A, Martinez-Madrid B, Dolmans MM, *et al.* Preservation of fertility in young cancer patients: contribution of transmission electron microscopy. *Reprod Biomed Online* 2008; **17:** 136–150.
103. Cortvrindt RG, Smitz JE. Fluorescent probes allow rapid and precise recording of follicle density and staging in human ovarian cortical biopsy samples. *Fertil Steril* 2001; **75:** 588–593.
104. Schotanus K, Hage WJ, Vanderstichele H, *et al.* Effects of conditioned media from murine granulosa cell lines on the growth of isolated bovine preantral follicles. *Theriogenology* 1997; **48:** 471–483.
105. Cortvrindt RG, Hu Y, Liu J, *et al.* Timed analysis of the nuclear maturation of oocytes in early preantral mouse follicle culture supplemented with recombinant gonadotropin. *Fertil Steril* 1998; **70:** 1114–1125.
106. Cecconi S, Capacchietti G, Russo V, *et al.* In vitro growth of preantral follicles isolated from cryopreserved ovine ovarian tissue. *Biol Reprod* 2004; **70:** 12–17.
107. Sadeu JC, Adriaenssens T, Smitz J. Expression of growth differentiation factor 9, bone morphogenetic protein 15, and anti-Müllerian hormone in cultured mouse primary follicles. *Reproduction* 2008; **136:** 195–203.
108. Gougeon A. Regulation of ovarian follicular development in primates: facts and hypotheses. *Endocr Rev* 1996; **17:** 121–155.

Chapter 23

Concept of human ovarian tissue cryobanking

Vladimir Isachenko, Friedrich Gagsteiger, Evgenia Isachenko, Juergen Weiss, and Rolf Kreienberg

Ovarian tissue as a perspective object for cryobanking

It is estimated that a total of around 692 000 women were diagnosed with cancer in the USA alone in 2008 [1]. Because of the increasing effectiveness of oncological treatments [2], young women need a chance to regain their reproductive potential after treatment. This can be achieved by the cryopreservation of ovarian tissue before medical intervention. Therefore, cryopreservation of human ovarian tissue has become one of the main research projects in reproductive medicine.

After thawing, ovarian tissue can be grafted, followed by normal follicular development and ovulation of mature oocytes with or without gonadotropin stimulation [3]. In animals, as well as in humans, live births have been reported [4–7].

Cryobanking ovarian tissue

The concept of cryobanking ovarian tissue is based on two potential approaches.

1. Ovarian tissue itself can be cryopreserved. After thawing, the tissue can be used either for purely therapeutic purposes or for therapeutic plus reproductive purposes. There are reports of patients with premature ovarian failure (POF) after cancer treatment who had restoration of ovarian function after re-implantation of ovarian cortex [3,8–19]. The cryopreserved ovarian tissue can also be used for the restoration of reproductive functions. A review of the literature provides convincing evidence that young women with cancer should have parts of the ovarian cortex removed for cryopreservation before treatment. After thawing and grafting of this cryopreserved tissue, it may serve as a source of oocytes for future pregnancies.
2. Two important cell types can be cryopreserved in addition to ovarian tissue: immature oocytes (germinal vesicle [GV] stage) and ovarian stem cells. The concept of "double-fertility preservation" was put forward by Isachenko *et al.* in 2004 [20]. This concept means that, prior to the freezing of ovarian tissue, immature follicles can be punctured to obtain germinal vesicle [GV] oocytes, which can then be frozen after in vitro maturation to metaphase II (MII) stage.

Technical requirements for the storage of tissue and gametes

For the transportation of specimens to the cryobank, it is normally recommended to transport ovarian tissue or GV oocytes either on ice (0°C) or at 5–6°C. However, after a maximum of 1 hour, GV oocytes die at these temperatures. In contrast, if ovaries are transported at 32–37°C, GV oocytes retain their developmental potential for up to 2 hours. Therefore, we believe that it is necessary to transport ovarian tissue at the higher temperature. This will allow the puncture of small antral follicles to obtain GV oocytes after the tissue has arrived in the laboratory. After in vitro maturation for 28–36 hours, they can be cryopreserved in the MII stage using the aseptic technique of vitrification [21,22]. It is possible to obtain up to 20 good-quality GV oocytes from a 3 cm^3 piece of ovarian cortex (E. Isachenko *et al.*, unpublished data). Figure 23.1 shows a GV oocyte before and after aseptic vitrification and after in vitro maturation up to the MII stage. This immature oocyte was punctured from an antral follicle out of a piece of ovarian cortex that was transported into the laboratory at a temperature of 32°C 2 hours after surgical removal of the tissue.

After thawing, oocytes or the ovarian tissue can also be used as a source of ovarian stem cells [23]. Both

Fertility Cryopreservation, ed. Ri-Cheng Chian and Patrick Quinn. Published by Cambridge University Press.

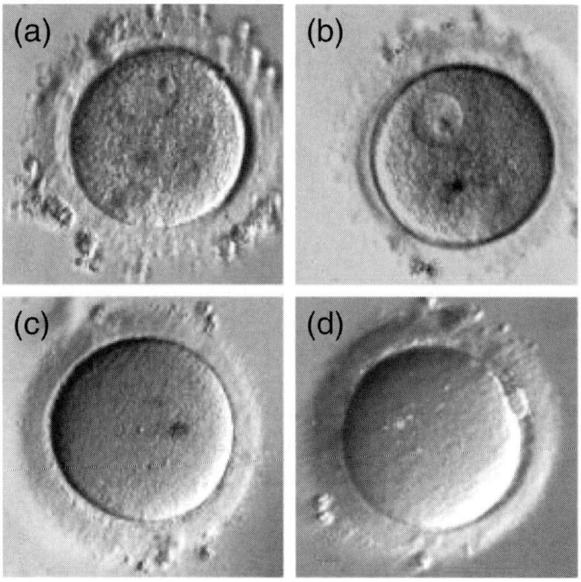

Figure 23.1. A germinal vesicle oocyte punctured from an ovarian fragment. (a) The oocyte before vitrification; (b), 10 minutes after warming; (c) 20 hours after beginning of in vitro maturation; (d) 28 h after beginning of in vitro maturation.

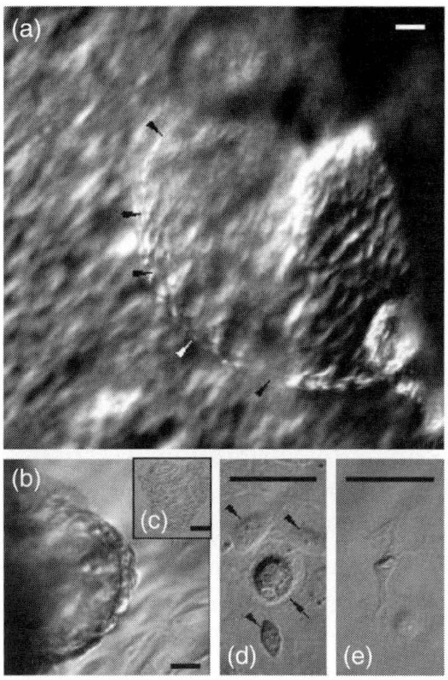

Figure 23.2. Human ovarian surface epithelium cultured in vitro for 12 days after cryopreservation (aseptic vitrification). The protocol was adapted for cell suspension. (a) Monolayer of stem cells (black arrowheads) and vesicles formed from this monolayer (white arrowhead); (b,c) stem cell vesicle and h (b) "seating place" of formed vesicle (c) after swimming up of this vesicle; (d) "large oocytes" (arrows) and fibroblast cells (arrowheads) showing evidence of the presence of germ cells; (e) neuron. This spontaneous differentiation shows evidencesof the presence of stem cells. Bar, 40 μm (a,b,d,e); 100 μm (c).

the use of cryopreserved GV or MII oocytes, which will become a standard procedure in the future, and the employment of ovarian stem cells is ethically acceptable. It is easy to obtain these cells by a technique that simply requires a slight scarification of the ovarian surface. In our experiments, we were able to obtain up to 50×10^6 stem cells from a piece of 3 cm^3 ovarian cortex. The cryostability of these cells is high: it was noted that their capacity to form monolayer and stem cell vesicles (Figure 23.2a,b) originates from so-called "seating places" (Figure 23.2b) after aseptic vitrification by the method of Isachenko *et al.* [21,22]. After these vesicles have developed a certain volume, they loosen from their "seating place" and start to float in the culture medium. The presence of large vesicles (Figure 23.2d) and neurons (Figure 23.2e) in the culture provides evidence that a mixture of stem cells and germ cells has been obtained from the ovarian surface.

In contrast to embryonic stem cells, there is no ethical debate about the use of these adult stem cells. In addition, obtaining these stem cells does not significantly increase the cost of cryobanking of ovarian tissue.

From frozen ovarian tissue to pregnancies

In 1996, the first cryopreservation of human ovarian tissue with good survival of follicles after warming was reported [24]. One of the important aims of ovarian cryobanking is a restoration of reproductive function after oncological treatment [3,4,7,11,25–36]. At present, there are three different pathways to follow for the use of cryopreserved ovarian tissue for reproductive purposes (Figure 23.3).

So far, pregnancies have been reported only after the use of the second and third path. It is recommended that any effort to restore fertility should always be started with the third pathway, which includes a transplantation of frozen/thawed parts of the ovary. There is always a possibility that this tissue will be re-integrated into the ovary, which until then was inefficient, and this may result in pregnancy, with or without the use of hormonal stimulation [5]. If this mode is not realizable or is unsuccessful, the second pathway can be used as an alternative (Figure 23.3).

Methodology of ovarian tissue cryopreservation

Cryopreservation of ovarian tissue can be performed in two ways: conventional slow freezing or by direct

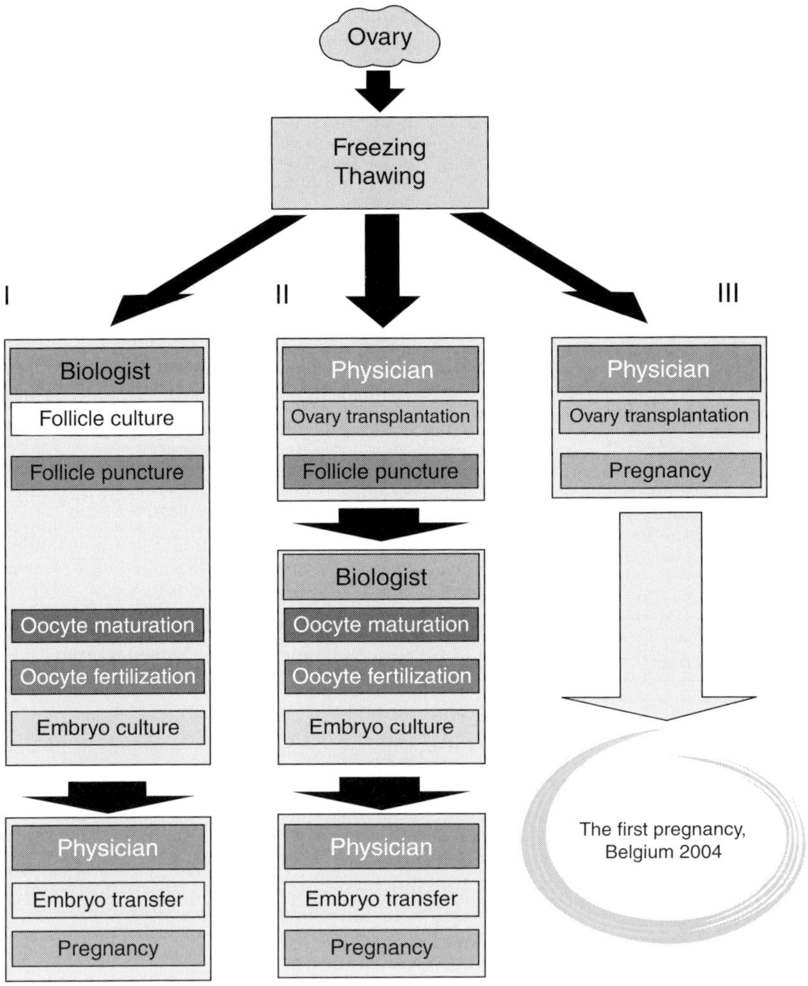

Figure 23.3. Schema of three methodological pathways to pregnancies after cryopreservation and thawing of ovaries. The same shading designates the same stage of manipulations. The first live birth was reported by Donnez *et al.* in 2004 [5].

plunging of the material into liquid nitrogen (rapid freezing, ultra-rapid freezing, vitrification).

Studies have demonstrated the advantage of slow freezing compared with vitrification [37]. Despite the fact that direct plunging of ovarian tissue into liquid nitrogen is also successful, the effectiveness of a slow-freezing program is, at present, greater and this is recommended for use in routine practice [38–40]. However, the potential of vitrification of ovarian tissue has not been exploited so far and must be subject to further intensive studies [38]. It has been shown that rapid thawing of cryopreserved ovarian tissue in boiling water (100°C) significantly improves the survival rate of tissue cells [41].

In the course of tissue cryopreservation, routine histological analysis is mandatory to minimize the risk of re-implantation of cancerous cells and, therefore, parts of the ovarian tissue are used for histology while other parts are cultured in vitro, in order to evaluate the presence of follicles. The appearance and quality of follicles allows a prognosis of the possibility for the woman to restore her reproductive function. Histological micrographs have provided evidence of the developmental capacity of ovarian fragments after slow conventional freezing, fast thawing, and in vitro culture in large volumes of medium under constant agitation [41]. These micrographs indicate whether there is a good possibility of a pregnancy after transplantation of the tissue.

As an example, Figure 23.4 shows images from ovarian tissue taken from the right ovary of a 27-year-old-patient with borderline cancer. These show a high developmental rate in the tissue. Primary follicles (Figure 23.4a) developed to secondary and preantral follicles after freezing–thawing. Although some follicles appeared degenerated (Figure 23.4c,d arrowheads), others developed quite normally. So, the chance of this

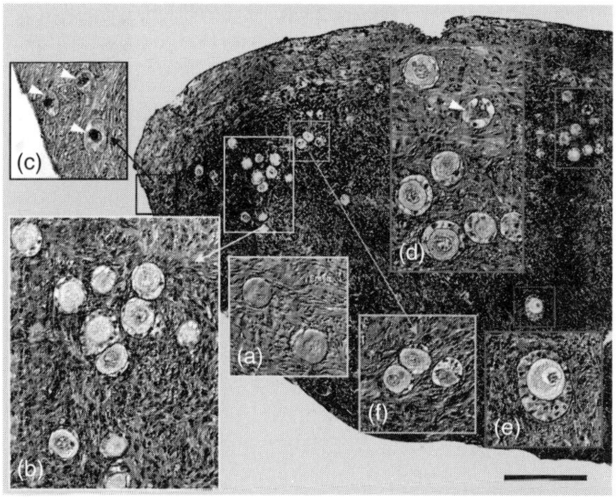

Figure 23.4. Histological micrographs of different areas of an ovarian piece after freezing, warming and in vitro culture for 2 weeks. (a) Fresh control OP. Degenerated follicles can be seen in some sections (c,d; arrowheads). Bar, 300 μm for the main image and 100 μm for the micro-sections (a–f).

patient becoming pregnant after replacing the frozen–thawed ovarian tissue is fairly good.

The likely direction that will be taken for human ovarian tissue cryopreservation is freezing of the whole ovary. It has been established that freezing of intact human ovary with its vascular pedicle is not associated with any signs of apoptosis or ultrastructural alterations in any cell types. Whole organ vascular transplantation may, therefore, be a viable option [42–45].

Conclusions

Cryopreservation of ovarian tissue from cancer patients does not simply provide the potential for restoration of fertility after cancer treatment, it also has certain therapeutic benefits. For reproductive purposes, ovarian tissue can be used in two ways: either the fresh tissue can be used to produce GV oocytes for maturation and then cryopreservation, or the ovarian tissue can be frozen, stored, and then thawed later for transplantation or to be used as a source to generate new GV oocytes (follicles with GV oocytes in the original fresh tissue will not survive freezing and thawing). Whichever pathway, the final step will be standard in vitro fertilization procedure.

References

1. Jemal A, Siegel R, Ward E, *et al.* Cancer statistics, 2008. *CA Cancer J Clin* 2008; **58:** 71–96.
2. Grovas A, Fremgen A, Rauck A, *et al.* The National Cancer Data Base report on patterns of childhood cancers in the United States. *Cancer* 1997; **80:** 2321–2332.
3. Oktay K, Karlikaya G. Ovarian function after transplantation of frozen, banked autologous ovarian tissue. *N Engl J Med* 2000; **342:** 1919.
4. Gosden RG, Baird DT, Wade JC, *et al.* Restoration of fertility to oophorectomized sheep by ovarian autografts stored at −196 degrees C. *Hum Reprod* 1994; **9:** 597–603.
5. Donnez J, Dolmans MM, Demylle D, *et al.* Live birth after orthotopic transplantation of cryopreserved ovarian tissue. *Lancet* 2004; **364:** 1405–1410.
6. Meirow D, Levron J, Eldar-Geva T, *et al.* Pregnancy after transplantation of cryopreserved ovarian tissue in a patient with ovarian failure after chemotherapy. *N Engl J Med* 2005; **353:** 318–321.
7. Meirow D, Baum M, Yaron R, *et al.* Ovarian tissue cryopreservation in hematologic malignancy: ten years' experience. *Leuk Lymphoma* 2007; **48:** 1569–1576.
8. Callejo J, Salvador C, Miralles A, *et al.* Long-term ovarian function evaluation after autografting by implantation with fresh and frozen–thawed human ovarian tissue. *J Clin Endocrinol Metab* 2001; **86:** 4489–4494.
9. Radford JA, Lieberman BA, Brison DR, *et al.* Orthotopic reimplantation of cryopreserved ovarian cortical strips after high-dose chemotherapy for Hodgkin's lymphoma. *Lancet* 2001; **357:** 1172–1175.
10. Schmidt KL, Andersen CY, Loft A, *et al.* Follow-up of ovarian function post-chemotherapy following ovarian cryopreservation and transplantation. *Hum Reprod* 2005; **20:** 3539–3546.
11. Oktay K, Buyuk E, Veeck L, *et al.* Embryo development after heterotopic transplantation of cryopreserved ovarian tissue. *Lancet* 2004; **363:** 9412.
12. Wolner-Hanssen P, Haegglund L, Ploman F, *et al.* Autotransplantation of cryopreserved ovarian tissue to the right forearm 4 1/2 years after autologous stem cell transplantation. *Acta Obstet Gynecol Scand* 2005; **84:** 695–698.
13. Silber SJ, Lenahan KM, Levine DJ, *et al.* Ovarian transplantation between monozygotic twins discordant for premature ovarian failure. *N Engl J Med* 2005; **353:** 58–63.
14. Silber SJ, Gosden R. Ovarian transplantation in a series of monozygotic twins discordant for ovarian failure. *N Engl J Med* 2007; **356:** 1382–1384.
15. Donnez J, Martinez-Madrid B, Jadoul P, *et al.* Ovarian tissue cryopreservation and transplantation: a review. *Hum Reprod Update* 2006; **12:** 519–535.
16. Donnez J, Dolmans MM, Demylle D, *et al.* Restoration of ovarian function after orthotopic (intraovarian and periovarian) transplantation of cryopreserved ovarian tissue in a woman treated by bone marrow

transplantation for sickle cell anaemia: case report. *Hum Reprod* 2006; **21:** 183–188.
17. Donnez J, Squifflet J, Van Eyck A-S, *et al.* Restoration of ovarian function in orthotopically transplanted cryopreserved ovarian tissue: a pilot experience. *Reprod Biomed Online* 2008; **16:** 694–704.
18. Meirow D, Levron J, Eldar-Geva T, *et al.* Monitoring the ovaries after autotransplantation of cryopreserved ovarian tissue: endocrine studies, in vitro fertilization cycles, and live birth. *Fertil Steril* 2007; **87:** 418.e7–e15.
19. Nottola SA, Camboni A, Van Langendonckt A, *et al.* Cryopreservation and xenotransplantation of human ovarian tissue: an ultrastructural study. *Fertil Steril* 2008; **1:** 23–32.
20. Isachenko E, Gohar R, Isachenko V, *et al.* In-vitro maturation of germinal vesicle oocytes and cryopreservation in metaphase I/II: a possible addition option to preserve fertility during ovarian tissue cryopreservation. *Reprod Biomed Online* 2004; **8:** 553–557.
21. Isachenko V, Katkov II, Yakovenko S, *et al.* Vitrification of human laser treated blastocysts with cut standard straw (CSS), aseptic mode and reduction of cryoprotectants. *Cryobiology* 2007; **54:** 305–309.
22. Isachenko V, Todorov P, Dimitrov Y, *et al.* Integrity rate of pronuclei after cryopresrvation of PN-zygotes as a criteria for subsequent embryo development and pregnancy. *Hum Reprod* 2008; **23:** 819–826.
23. Edwards RG. Stem cells today: A. Origin and potential of embryo stem cells. *Reprod Biomed Online* 2004; **8:** 275–306.
24. Hovatta O. Methods for cryopreservation of human ovarian tissue. *Reprod Biomed Online* 2005; **10:** 729–734.
25. Gosden RG. Prospects for oocyte banking and in vitro maturation. *J Natl Cancer I Monogr* 2005; **34:** 60–63.
26. Donnez J, Bassil S. Indications for cryopreservation of ovarian tissue. *Hum Reprod Update* 1998; **4:** 248–259.
27. Oktay K, Newton H, Aubard Y, *et al.* Cryopreservation of immature human oocytes and ovarian tissue: an emerging technology? *Fertil Steril* 1998; **69:** 1–7.
28. Meirow D, Nugent D. The effects of radiotherapy and chemotherapy on female reproduction. *Hum Reprod Update* 2001; **7:** 534–543.
29. Torrents E, Boiso I, Barri PN, *et al.* Applications of ovarian tissue transplantation in experimental biology and medicine. *Hum Reprod Update* 2003; **9:** 471–481.
30. Lobo RA. Potential options for preservation of fertility in women. *N Engl J Med* 2005; **353:** 64–73.
31. Kim SS. Fertility preservation in female cancer patients: current developments and future directions. *Fertil Steril* 2006; **85:** 1–11.
32. Demeestere I, Simon P, Buxant F, *et al.* Ovarian function and spontaneous pregnancy after combined heterotopic and orthotopic cryopreserved ovarian tissue transplantation in a patient previously treated with bone marrow transplantation: case report. *Hum Reprod* 2006; **21:** 2010–2014.
33. Rosendahl M, Loft A, Byskov AG, *et al.* Biochemical pregnancy after fertilization of an oocyte aspirated from a heterotopic autotransplant of cryopreserved ovarian tissue: case report. *Hum Reprod* 2006; **21:** 2006–2009.
34. Bedaiwy M, Falcone T. Harvesting and autotransplantation of vascularized ovarian grafts: approaches and techniques. *Reprod Biomed Online* 2007; **14:** 360–371.
35. Donnez J, Squifflet J, Van Eyck A-S, *et al.* Restoration of ovarian function in orthotopically transplanted cryopreserved ovarian tissue: a pilot experience. *Reprod Biomed Online* 2008; **16:** 694–704.
36. Meirow D, Levron J, Eldar-Geva T, *et al.* Monitoring the ovaries after autotransplantation of cryopreserved ovarian tissue: endocrine studies, in vitro fertilization cycles, and live birth. *Fertil Steril* 2007; **87:** 418.e7–e15.
37. Isachenko V, Isachenko E, Reinsberg J, *et al.*: Cryopreservation of human ovarian tissue: comparison of rapid and conventional freezing. *Cryobiology* 2007; **55:** 261–268.
38. Isachenko V, Isachenko E, Reinsberg J, *et al.* Cryopreservation of human ovarian tissue: comparison of rapid and conventional freezing. *Cryobiology* 2007; **55:** 261–268.
39. Isachenko V, Isachenko E, Reinsberg J, *et al.* Freezing of human ovarian tissue: effect of spontaneous and initiated ice formation. *Reprod Biomed Online* 2008; **16:** 336–345.
40. Isachenko V, Isachenko E, Reinsberg J, *et al.* Simplified technique of human ovarian tissue freezing: quick cooling from −36°C. *CryoLetters* 2008; **29**: 261–268.
41. Isachenko V, Montag M, Isachenko E, *et al.* Effective method for in-vitro culture of cryopreserved human ovarian tissue. *Reprod Biomed Online* 2006; **13:** 228–234.
42. Martinez-Madrid B, Donnez J. Cryopreservation of intact human ovary with its vascular pedicle or cryopreservation of hemiovaries? *Hum Reprod* 2006; **21:** 3258–3269.
43. Martinez-Madrid B, Dolmans MM, Van Langendonckt A, *et al.* Freeze–thawing intact human ovary with its vascular pedicle with a passive cooling device. *Fertil Steril* 2004; **82:** 1390–1397.
44. Martinez-Madrid B, Camboni A, Dolmans M, *et al.* Apoptosis and ultrastructural assessment after cryopreservation of whole human ovaries with their vascular pedicle. *Fertil Steril* 2007; **87:** 1153–1165.
45. Jadoul P, Donnez J, Dolmans MM, *et al.* Laparoscopic ovariectomy for whole human ovary cryopreservation: technical aspects. *Fertil Steril* 2007; **87:** 971–975.

Chapter 24

Transplantation of cryopreserved ovarian tissues

Dror Meirow

Introduction

The concept of transplantation in reproductive medicine has been considered by physicians and scientists for many years and it is now over a century since the first human ovarian graft was performed. The ovary is well suited for transplantation since the most abundant primordial follicles are present in the periphery and are the first to benefit from revascularization. In addition, ovarian follicles may be resistant to ischemia as they normally develop within an avascular epithelium and a relatively hypoxic environment. Ovarian tissue transplantation has become clinically feasible with advances in cryobiology and the effective cryopreservation of ovarian tissue. Today, ovarian tissue harvesting is performed by a simple laparoscopic procedure. In addition, accurate patient monitoring is possible before and after transplantation using endocrine studies and sonography imaging. For patients, transplantation of ovarian tissue has become an attractive option to overcome the risk of pending premature menopause caused by various clinical conditions.

Among these clinical treatments, radiotherapy and curative chemotherapy, used for cancer treatment, often pose a threat to fertility, as ovarian damage is a common long-term side effect. For these patients, harvesting and cryopreservation of ovarian tissue before commencing potentially sterilizing chemotherapy has been practiced since the mid 1990s. In addition, the transplantation of thawed tissue has been shown to successfully restore their fertility. This chapter describes different aspects of ovarian tissue transplantation including history, basic experiments, and the results of clinical studies.

History of ovarian tissue grafting and transplantation

Ovarian grafting has a long history, beginning in 1863 [1]. Early experiments using dog, rabbit, and sheep models showed that graft implants of ovarian tissue slices could survive, relying upon rapid growth of blood vessels into the tissue. In humans, ovarian tissue transplantation studies have been conducted since 1895 [2] as a means to restore fertility and/or as a treatment for menopausal symptoms before the era of hormone therapies. Menstrual cyclicity, pregnancies, and deliveries following ovarian tissue transplantation have been described since [3]. These early works claimed successful pregnancies as a result of autografts; while successes were also reported from ovarian allografts, these claims seem to be exaggerated. It has subsequently become clear that immunosuppressive therapies are essential if ovarian allografts are to survive [4]. It has also been shown that the ovary does not have an immunological privilege, contrary to early reports. Pioneer experiments with ovarian grafts in animal models and selected clinical case reports of ovarian implantation from the early literature are presented in Tables 24.1 and 24.2 [3].

Ovarian tissue can be transplanted back to the original site (orthotopic) or to a large number of alternative sites (heterotopic) [5]. Orthotopic graft transplantation to the broad ligament was the favored procedure for establishing a pregnancy because of the simplicity of the procedure. However, from a fertility standpoint, these human ovarian implants were generally disappointing and better results have been obtained by transposing the ovary with its vascular pedicle either to the uterine cavity or to the uterine horn [6]. As a potential treatment for menopause, and not to restore fertility, the graft site is not considered critical and a large number of potential heterotopic sites have been tested, including the rectus muscle, abdominal skin, omentum, and cervix [3]. Grafts in these heterotopic locations can restore menstrual cycles with the exception of sites connected with the portal vein circulation. This is largely because hepatic clearance of steroid hormones

Fertility Cryopreservation, ed. Ri-Cheng Chian and Patrick Quinn. Published by Cambridge University Press.

Table 24.1. Pioneer experiments with ovarian grafts in animal models

First author (Year)	Host species	Type of graft	Graft site	Results
Bert (1863)	Rabbit	Allo	Abdomen	Failure
Knauer (1896)	Rabbit	Auto	Peritoneum mesentery	Some survived
Griorieff (1897)	Rabbit	Auto	Broad ligament	Pregnancy
Jayle (1897)	Rabbit, guinea pig	Auto/allo	Unknown	Survived
Arendt (1898)	Rabbit	Unknown	Broad ligament	Survived
McCone (1899)	Rabbit	Auto	Mesosalpinx	Failure
	Dog/ rabbit	Allo	Broad ligament/ omentum	Pregnancy
	Sheep	Xeno	Mesosalpinx, omentum	Pregnancy
Föa (1900)	Rabbit	Allo	Broad ligament	Survived
		Fetal	Broad ligament	Survived, pregnancy
Amixo-Roxas (1901)	Rabbit	Auto/allo	Peritoneum	3 month survival

Source: adapted from Nugent *et al.* (1997) [3].

leads to a reduction of the pituitary gonadotropin negative feedback loop, allowing implants to become hyperstimulated in animals. Microsurgical techniques were used to perform heterotopic autotransplant in 1987 by Le Porrier *et al.* [7] in an 18-year-old woman with subdiaphragmatic Hodgkin's disease. The left ovary was moved to the subcutaneous tissue of the arm to avoid irradiation, while the right ovary was transposed to an intraperitoneal site without dividing its vessels. Patency of the anastomoses and vascularization of the ovary moved to the arm were confirmed by angiography. Menstrual cycles were regular and after a year a secondary oocyte was aspirated.

Transplantation of cryopreserved–thawed ovarian tissue: basic research

Ovary and ovarian tissue are suitable for transplantation and grafting since there is a stockpile of primordial follicles in the cortex and these quickly benefit from revascularization. As the transplantation of fragments of cryopreserved ovarian cortex is performed without vascular reanastomosis, perfusion of the tissue depends on the growth of, and invasion by, new blood vessels. Ovarian follicles may be resistant to ischemia, as they normally develop within an avascular epithelium and a relatively hypoxic environment [8]. In addition, the primordial follicle population appears to be more resistant to the effects of ischemia than the growing stages, presumably by virtue of being dormant and having a low metabolic rate. Long-term follow-up of patients who had twisted adnexa and documented ischemic–hemorrhagic ovaries managed by detorsion showed normal follicular development and normal ovarian size, indicating long-term resistance to ischemia [9]. However, the time needed to achieve an adequate perfusion of the grafted ovarian tissue is critical for follicular survival and is related to the functional longevity of the graft.

To date, ovarian tissue has been successfully cryopreserved and transplanted into rodents, sheep, rabbits, and marmoset monkeys [10–12]. Successful fertilization and pregnancy after oocyte collection from fresh transplanted ovarian tissue has been described in a monkey; the grafted tissue functioned without any surgical connection to major blood vessels [13]. In rodents, there is an extensive network of vessels invading the cortex after 48 hours [14]. Functional vessels within rat ovaries transplanted into the muscle of castrated nude mice were detected by magnetic resonance imaging and histology from day 7 onwards [15]. By 2–3 weeks, blood volume was found to be higher in the graft than in adjacent muscles. There is a significant follicular depletion that occurs during an ischemic period and lasts until revascularization. Approximately 50% of the primordial follicle population survive in isologous grafts in mice [16–18]. After orthotopic and heterotopic transplantation of frozen–thawed ovarian cortex in sheep, primordial follicle loss is estimated to be above 60% [19–21]. Experiments in sheep have also shown that the autograft results in a three- to fourfold increase in follicle-stimulating hormone (FSH) during the estrus cycle, possibly through a deficiency in ovarian factors such as inhibin A and anti-Müllerian hormone (AMH) normally produced by the pool of small developing follicles [22].

Transplantation of human ovarian tissue can be evaluated using xenograft recipients, commonly the immunodeficient (with severe combined immunodeficiency [SCID]) mouse model. Abir *et al.* [23] showed

Table 24.2 Selected clinical case reports of ovarian implantation from the early literature

Author (Year)	Country	Graft type	Cases	Specimens	Graft site	Results
Morris (1895)	USA	Allo/auto	2	Slices	Uterus, tubes	Miscarriage
Frank (1896)	Germany	Auto	3	Slices	Tubes	Pregnancy
Dudley-Palmer (1899)	USA	Auto	1	Ovary	Uterine fundus	Menses
Mauclaire (1900–1917)	France	Allo/auto	12	Ovary	Subcutaneous, omentum	Pregnancy
Martin (1903–1908)	USA	Allo/auto	5	Slices	Broad ligament	Miscarriage
Morris (1906)	USA	Allo	1	Slices	Broad ligament	Pregnancies
Cramer (1906–1919)	Germany	Allo/auto	102	Slices	Many sites	Menses
Davidson (1912)	UK	Auto	3	Ovary?	Rectus abdominis	1 success
Tuffier (1921)	France	Allo/auto	230	Slices	Many sites	Good results
Sippel (1923)	Germany	Allo	48	Ovary	Unknown	Pregnancies
Norris (1929)	USA	Unknown	31	Slices	Rectus abdominis	Unknown

Source: adapted from Nugent *et al.* (1997) [3].

that the kidney is a better transplantation site than a subcutaneous site, probably because of its superior vascularization. At least 25% of the primordial follicles are lost as a result of xenografting human cryopreserved ovarian tissue into mice [24,25]. Following transplantation, follicle growth and maturation can be demonstrated. Oktay *et al.* [26] achieved follicular development up to the antral stage, and Gook *et al.* [27,28] obtained oocytes at the metaphase II (MII) stage. Follicles that developed after xenograft transplantation of human ovarian tissue to SCID mice also showed ovulatory capacity, as indicated morphologically with formation of corpora lutea and progesterone production [28,29].

Influence of the site of ovarian transplantation

Transplantation of ovarian tissue has been tested in orthotopic and heterotopic sites. For each site, there are considerable differences in procedure convenience, the ease of visualization of the heterotopic location, vascular bed, and the volume of tissue that can be transplanted. A rich blood supply at the transplantation site provides a better support, thus reducing the ischemic injury. The possibility of future pregnancy either naturally (orthotopic sites only) or using egg collection and in vitro fertilization (IVF) must also be taken into consideration. A large panel of heterotopic sites have been tested, including the rectus muscle, subcutaneous sites (forearm or abdominal), omentum, and uterus [3].

Animal experiments allow comparison of the follicular development potential at the different orthotopic and heterotopic sites after ovarian tissue autograft or xenograft. These studies indicated that ovarian bursa or kidney capsule sites are more favorable than subcutaneous or intraperitoneal sites. In the rat, the subcutaneous site displays fewer primary follicles and corpora lutea than the subperitoneal site. Graft site can also affect the number and quality of oocytes produced from ovarian grafts. A mouse ovarian grafting model to investigate reproductive parameters after transplantation of ovarian tissue to different sites (bursal cavity, kidney capsule, or subcutaneous sites) showed that the number of oocytes found in each graft was lowest in the subcutaneous graft site and the number of 2-cell embryos produced was significantly higher with oocytes from grafts to the bursa [30–33].

Environmental factors with possible effects on transplantation

Several methods have been tested as a means of reducing tissue injury by improving graft revascularization and shortening the ischemic period. Growth factors that are involved in the invasion of the tissue by new vessels have been tested but failed to show beneficial effects on the primate's graft function. Nugent *et al.* [34] investigated the effects of administering an antioxidant, vitamin E, on products of lipid peroxidation and total follicle survival

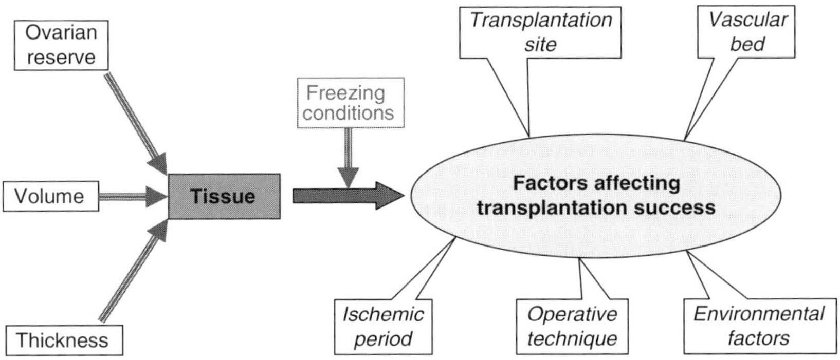

Figure 24.1. Success with ovarian tissue transplantation is related to factors affecting tissue quality at harvesting, freezing conditions, and important environmental and surgical parameters during transplantation.

after transplantation of murine ovarian grafts and human ovarian xenografts in SCID mice. They showed that antioxidant treatment improved the survival of follicles in ovarian grafts by reducing ischaemia–reperfusion injury. Gonadotropin administration, before or after transplantation, upregulates angiogenic factors. Animal studies have shown that gonadotropin stimulation of a recipient, initiated before and continued after grafting, had a positive effect on follicular survival. However, administration of gonadotropin-releasing hormone agonist failed to prevent follicular depletion [35].

Today, there is no accepted well-studied condition that can be recommended for transplantation; hence no conclusions concerning the effects of gonadotropins can be drawn from these animal studies. Consequently, human ovarian tissue transplantation procedures use different approaches. We have administrated estrogen–progesterone tablets during and after transplantation to avoid elevation in gonadotropin levels [36], Oktay *et al.* [37] injected FSH directly into the transplantation site, and Demeestere *et al.* [38] avoided any hormonal treatment during and after transplantation procedure. Transplantation into angiogenic granulation tissue created (at least 24 hours earlier) during wound healing has been proposed to shorten the ischemic interval [39]. This was used clinically by Donnez *et al.* [40] and Demeestere *et al.* [38], who opened the ovary or peritoneal pocket 1 week before the transplantation procedure (two-step laparoscopy). Figure 24.1 indicates the parameters affecting the success of ovarian tissue transplantation.

Current clinical applications for ovarian tissue storage and transplantation

Ovarian cryobanking allows for the storage of abundant primordial follicles containing small, less-differentiated oocytes [41]. However, in order to restore fertility, this technique requires surgical grafting procedures that ideally can restore both the synthesis of sex steroids and the cyclical production of oocytes. The most realizable and pressing need for this procedure appears to be for those women with premature sterility as a result of a variety of medical treatments. Cancer treatment, including high-dose chemotherapy and abdominal irradiation, is associated with ovarian toxicity as a common long-term side effect [42]. For these young cancer patients, the success of treatment with regimens that are toxic to the gonads has made infertility an important problem, which negatively affects their quality of life [43]. Hundreds of patients all over the world have already undergone cryopreservation of ovarian tissue before oncological treatments, hoping later to restore their fertility.

Although ovarian tissue cryopreservation is preferably performed before the initiation of chemotherapy treatment, in some cases patients who have had first-line chemotherapy prior to high-dose chemotherapy request to store their ovarian tissue between the two chemotherapy cycles [44]. For these patients, IVF is not an option to preserve fertility because of the poor quality of the growing follicles, which had been recently exposed to chemotherapy [45,46].

If premature ovarian failure occurs and if complete remission of the disease is confirmed, these women will ask for fertility restoration if they wish to conceive. Transplantation of cryopreserved ovarian tissue is, at present, the only option to achieve this goal. However, currently, new technologies are emerging that enable follicle maturation from cryopreserved ovarian tissue; this may in the future restore fertility via the fertilization of oocytes matured in vitro [47,48].

Storing ovarian tissue in cancer patients

The following text briefly summarizes the clinical and laboratory practice at the Sheba Medical Center, Israel.

Clinical workup

In order to decide when fertility preservation procedures should be considered, the individual patient's risk of ovarian failure should be assessed. The likelihood of permanent sterility and compromised fertility after chemotherapy or radiotherapy varies and depends on several factors that influence ovarian reserve. These factors include patient's age at treatment, with older women having a much higher incidence of complete ovarian failure and permanent infertility compared with younger women; the nature of the drugs administered; treatment protocols (doses and cycles); and previous cancer treatments [49]. Menstrual history, hormonal profile, and antral follicular count provide an indication of ovarian reserve. This is especially important in patients who have had previous chemotherapy treatments and may suffer from ovarian injury. Steps needed to evaluate cancer patients prior to fertility preservation procedure include:

- diagnosis, staging
- sterilization risk: disease, treatment protocol, age
- ovarian reserve: age, endocrine profile, AMH, antral follicle count
- previous exposure to chemotherapy
- medical status
    - surgical and anesthesiology complications
    - blood (anemia, thrombocytopenia)
    - thorax (mass, pressure, effusion)
    - hypercoagulable state
- risk of ovarian involvement: sonography, imaging (computed tomography [CT] and positron emission tomography [PET])
- hematology/oncology: reproductive team consultation
- use of protective agents.

Handling ovarian tissue

Harvested ovarian tissue is transferred promptly in medium to the laboratory and is prepared for cryopreservation: cleaned from the medulla and thinned to 1–2 mm cortical tissue. The cortex is divided into slices that fit the size of the cryodevice, usually large 5 mm × 10 mm × 1 mm strips or smaller fragments [50]. For all patients, an additional smaller cortical tissue is marked and stored in a separate vial for future clinical and safety investigations. This sample allows early thawing prior to transplantation in order to evaluate freezing and storage conditions as well as enables a search for the presence of malignant cells in each patient. Part of the medulla that is removed from the cortex during preparation for freezing is also stored for future evaluation of cancer cells. A small additional fragment of the cortex is fixed, embedded in paraffin wax, and stained with hematoxylin and eosin in order to determine the presence and morphology of primordial follicles as well as to detect possible malignant cells [51,52]. Documentation of follicular morphology and density is especially important in patients previously exposed to chemotherapy. The slow-freezing method is used for ovarian tissue storage [24,53], which results in a high survival rate of primordial follicles (up to 70%).

Evaluation of patients before transplantation

Post-chemotherapy, patients are routinely followed by the oncological/hematological clinics. In addition, reproductive endocrinologists monitor if and when recovery of ovarian function occurs. Ovarian failure is documented by persistent amenorrhea, repeated endocrine studies that indicate high gonadotropin levels, low ovarian steroids, and low AMH levels, as well as an inability to visualize antral follicles by ovarian sonography. These tests are started no less than 3 months post-treatment and are repeated periodically. Some patients maintain very low ovarian reserve post-chemotherapy but do not have complete ovarian failure. These patients present with oligomenorrhea, high gonadotropin levels, and low AMH, but secretion of estradiol is documented. Sonography shows ovarian cysts and active endometrium; bleeding occasionally occurs spontaneously or after progesterone challenge. These patients are frequently infertile but pregnancy is possible with the native ovaries without the need for ovarian tissue transplantation [54].

Before a patient can request autotransplantation of the stored ovarian tissue in an attempt to restore fertility, it is important to receive permission from the oncological team. The risk of relapse in the near future and general health of the patient, with consideration of medical complications caused by cancer treatment, must be taken into account. Institutional review board approval should be obtained, although the indications and approaches for ovarian tissue transplantation are still experimental and remain unclear [55]. Initially, a small fragment of tissue should be thawed. Histological evaluation of the tissue is conducted in order to evaluate freezing conditions and follicle survival and safety tests are performed [37].

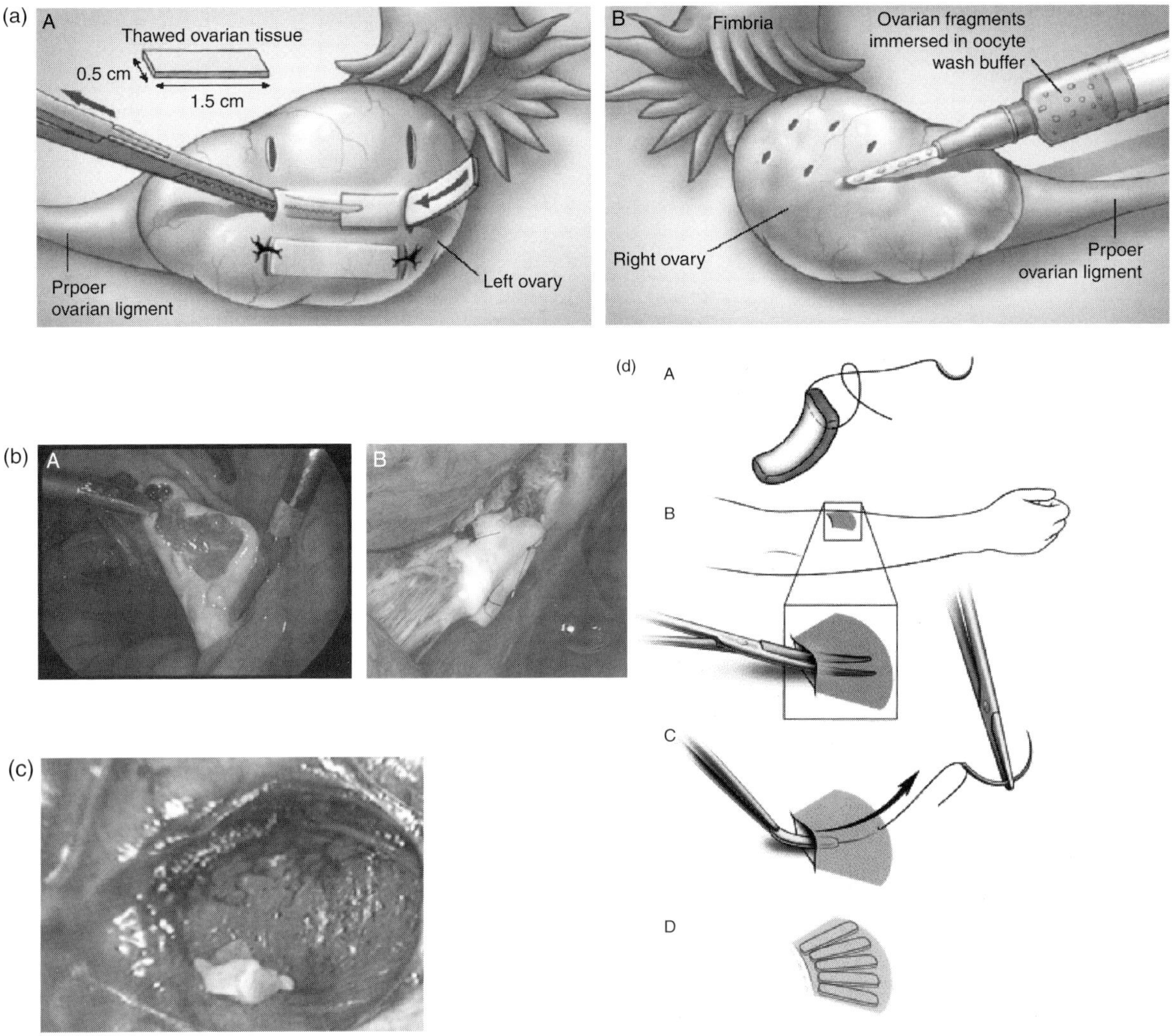

Figure 24.2. Transplantation surgical techniques. (a) Orthotopic transplantation to the ovary. Three pairs of 5 mm transverse incisions were made in the left ovary through the tunica albuginea (A). With blunt dissection, cavities were formed beneath the cortex for each of the three strips. Each piece of thawed ovarian tissue (1.5 cm by 0.5 cm in area and 0.1 cm to 0.2 cm in thickness) was gently placed in a cavity, and the incisions were closed with 4/0 Vicryl sutures. In the smaller, right ovary, tiny ovarian fragments immersed in oocyte wash buffer were injected beneath the cortex (B). (Adapted from Meirow *et al.* [36,61].) (b) Orthotopic transplantation to the ovary. Ovarian cortical tissues measuring 4–5 mm were grafted to the ovary after the cortex of this ovary had been removed. The cortex of the remaining ovary was removed (A). The cortical pieces were sutured with 7-0 stitches (B). (Adapted from Donnez *et al.* [67].) (c) Ovarian tissue transplanted at an orthotopic site, the parietal peritoneum in the pelvis. An initial laparoscopy prepared the transplantation sites for creation of a peritoneal pocket. One week later the cryopreserved ovarian pieces were transplanted to the peritoneal site in a second laproscopy. (Adapted from Demeestere *et al.* [38].) (d) A surgical technique for heterotopic transplantation of ovarian tissue to the forearm shown as four steps (A–D). (Adapted from Oktay *et al.* [37].)

Transplantation: method, place, monitoring

Different orthotopic and heterotopic sites for transplantation of human ovarian tissue have been reported (Figure 24.2). Once the tissue is sited, the ovarian responses must be monitored (Figure 24.3). For each site, clinical considerations such as the possibility of natural conception and the easiness of the surgical procedure (i.e. pelvic adhesions and the presence of one or two ovaries) should be considered. In addition, convenient access for oocyte collection and the volume of tissue planned to be transplanted should be taken into consideration. Orthotopic sites for ovarian tissue transplantation in the ovary include the peritoneum of the pelvic wall and the ovary. Heterotopic sites are easily accessible

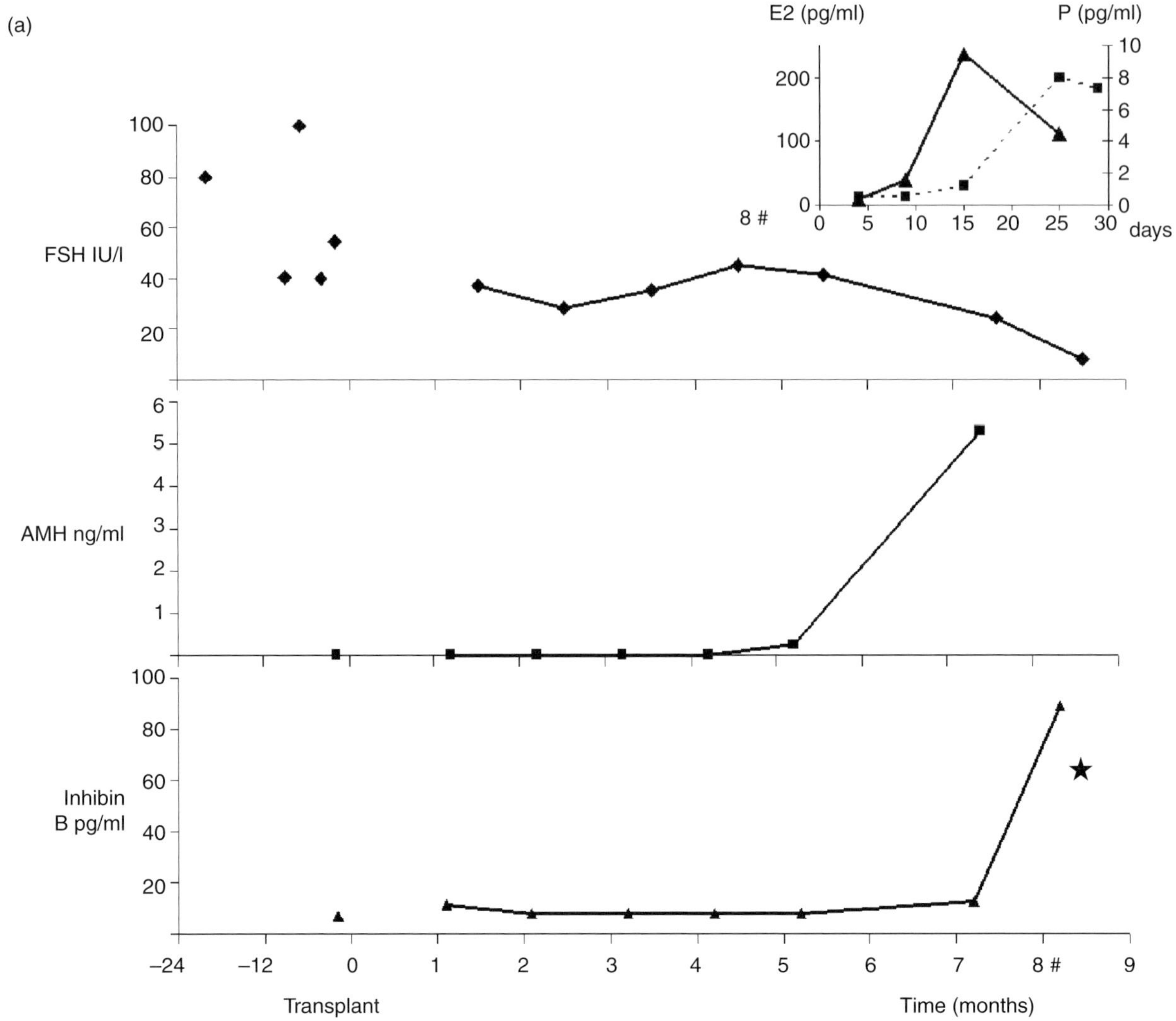

Figure 24.3. Endocrine monitoring post-transplantation of ovarian tissue. (a) Basal blood levels of follicle-stimulating hormone (FSH), anti-Müllerian hormone (AMH), and inhibin B during the months after transplantation. Levels of FSH gradually decreased from the sixth post-transplantation month to normal levels in the ninth month; AMH levels were undetectable until the sixth month hafter transplantation. High levels of AMH were measured in the eighth post-transplantation month, compatible with good ovarian reserve. Basal inhibin B levels were undetectable following transplantation but by the ninth month a high normal basal level of inhibin B was measured. The inset shows estradiol (E2; ▲) and progesterone (P; ■) levels over the eighth month. (b) Levels of E2 (▲) and inhibin B (■) plus follicle diameters are shown for the second, third, eighth, and ninth months after ovarian tissue transplantation. At month eight and month nine, hormone levels are also presented during luteal phase. In month three and month nine, the ovaries were stimulated. Follicles with diameter of 19–22 mm developed in all cycles; however, inhibin B levels were low during the second, third, and eighth months and did not correlate with follicular size. Only in the ninth month were levels of inhibin B high and showed normal pattern of rise and fall during follicle growth. In this cycle, an egg was retrieved, fertilized, and the patient conceived and delivered a healthy baby. (Adapted from Meirow *et al.* [36].)

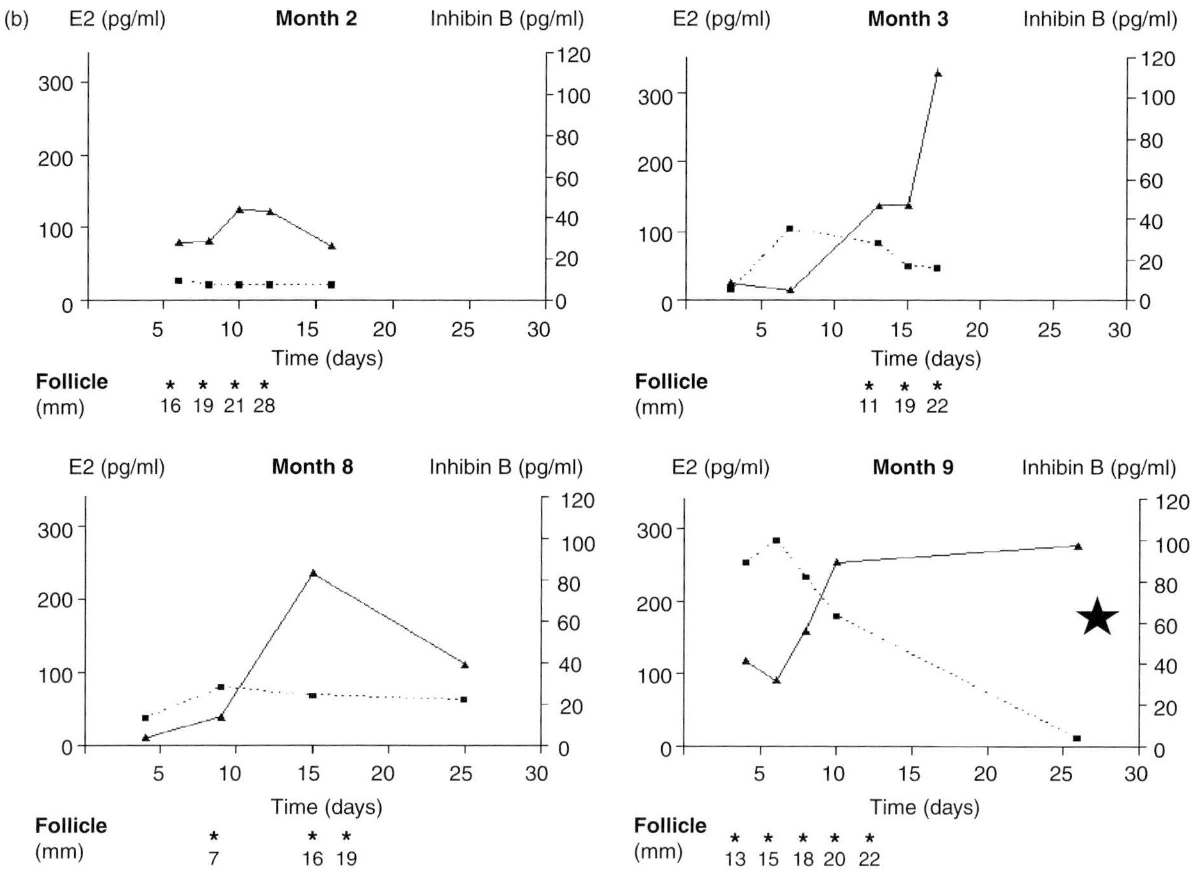

Figure 24.3. (*Cont.*)

and include the subcutaneous site on the abdominal wall, above the pectoralis and rectus abdominal muscles, and the forearm. Heterotopic sites have proved effective in restoring ovarian function, and a recent report has indicated that the ovarian transplants were still functioning after 42 months in one patient and 62 months in another[56]. However, in terms of reproduction, the success with orthotopic sites is superior at present and possibly also allows future natural conception, which is not possible with heterotopic transplantations.

When ovarian tissue was transplanted simultaneously heterotopically to a subcutaneous site and orthotopically to the pelvic peritoneum or to the ovaries, follicles developed more often in ovarian sites than at the peritoneal or subcutaneous sites. Furthermore, follicular development was limited at the heterotopic site (< 15 mm) and oocyte recovery rate and fertilization rate obtained from heterotopic sites were low [38,57]. These results are in agreement with animal studies previously presented. Since ovarian tissue grafts function for only a limited period of time, transplantation is performed only according to fertility indications at the time of the patient's request to conceive, and not for recovery of ovarian steroid secretion.

Transplantation to the ovary

The transplanted tissue should be in close connection with the ovarian vasculature. To achieve this, cavities are formed beneath the cortex using blunt dissection and the strips are gently placed and sutured into the cavity. Attempts to inject small pieces beneath the cortex did not succeed. In reports from other clinics, part of the cortex is removed and the thawed slices are attached to the rough bleeding surface. If the ovary is too small or the vascular bed is poor, transplantation to the peritoneum is preferable. In order to implant the tissue to the peritoneum, a peritoneal window is formed; the ovarian tissue is placed into the cavity and then sutured or covered. There are some reports of laparoscopy being performed a few days prior to implantation to create a peritoneal window in order to induce angiogenesis and neovascularization in the transplant [38,40]. This is also supported by animal studies.

In all cases of birth reported after transplantation, cryopreserved and thawed ovarian tissue was transplanted at the orthotopic site: to the peritoneum in the ovarian fossa [40] or to the remaining ovary [37,57,58]. The location for transplantation of fresh ovarian tissue between healthy monozygotic twins reported by Silber *et al.*, [59,60] was orthotopically directly onto the ovarian medulla of the recipient. Figure 24.2 demonstrates the techniques used for ovarian tissue transplantation in different orthotopic and heterotopic sites.

Monitoring after transplantation of tissue

During the immediate post-transplantation months, patients should be constantly evaluated for ovarian response. Monitoring should include gonadotropin levels, ovarian steroids, and, if possible, AMH and inhibin B levels (Figure 24.3). Sonography is performed to monitor follicle growth and endometrial development. However, frequently, hormone profiles during the recovery of ovarian activity after transplantation do not show classical patterns. Transplantation reports have indicated a period of imbalance between high FSH levels, low AMH levels, follicle development, and adequate secretion of estradiol. These results probably reflect disturbances in stromal activity. In these circumstances, no eggs are retrieved in aspirated follicles ("empty follicles"). This is frequently found to be the case in patients with low ovarian reserve and elevated FSH. A few months (4–6) usually pass before good ovarian response can be documented [61,62].

Restoration of fertility

Up to 2006, a few dozen transplantations of cryopreserved, thawed ovarian tissue have been reported in the literature. The results of some of these transplantations are presented in Table 24.3. [36,40,63–67]. Since then, more studies have been reported [38,58,68–77] and a complete overview of all these studies is given in Appendix I (p. 257). There are no reports in the literature that indicate how many patients worldwide have undergone transplantation of ovarian tissue as they only indicate scientific achievements and success. However, it is clear that many of these patients will not use their stored ovarian tissue for many years after harvesting, if at all. This may be because of recovery of ovarian function and spontaneous pregnancies after chemotherapy, patient death, or because the tissue was harvested from young children many years before restoration of fertility will be requested. A few physicians and health authorities have raised doubts regarding the justification and necessity of providing the facilities for ovarian tissue banking prior to chemotherapy, most likely because of the relatively small number of patients making use of it following completion of treatment and, therefore, the small number of children born as a result of using cryopreserved ovarian tissue [55]. Consultation and proper patient selection, based on research regarding chemotherapy's effects on reproduction is important prior to tissue harvesting. Furthermore, although only a relatively small number of male patients [3–10] return for fertility treatment following chemotherapy, not offering the option to freeze their sperm before treatment is considered malpractice [78]. The same approach is justified with female patients.

Procedure safety

In order to increase the safety of ovarian tissue cryopreservation, implantation procedures, identification of tumor involvement in the ovaries, and detection of small numbers of cancer cells in ovarian tissue is indicated. An algorithm that includes clinical evaluation and laboratory studies was suggested to increase the safety of cryopreservation–implantation procedures [54]. Imaging of the pelvis before tissue harvesting (sonography, CT scan, and/or CT/PET) is important to reveal macroscopic ovarian pathology related to the primary disease and prevent unnecessary operations. A meticulous inspection to look for malignancy in pelvic organs and the abdominal cavity should be performed during tissue harvesting. In addition, histological evaluation of ovarian tissue should be routinely performed to detect possible malignant cells (Figure 24.4).

Specific and sensitive methods for minimal residual disease (MRD) monitoring that are currently used as markers of molecular response to treatment during clinical remission can also be used on ovarian tissue. These methods include specific immunohistochemical stains, polymerase chain reaction (PCR) amplification of fusion transcripts (*BCL–ABL*), rearranged immunoglobulin or T cell receptor genes, and flow cytometric detection of aberrant immunophenotypes. Chromosomal aberrations provide tumor-specific PCR targets for MRD detection that are tumor-specific, reliable estimates of residual malignant cells.

In patients with hematological malignancies, investigation of ovarian tissue for MRD is performed together with diseased tissue (bone marrow or lymph nodes). In one patient with chronic myelocytic leukemia (Figure 24.5), real-time reverse transcriptase PCR was positive in ovarian tissue and implantation was not performed. Although the clinical significance of MRD in stored ovarian tissue needs further investigation, the sensitivity of tumor markers to identify MRD is high. It is essential

Table 24.3. Autotransplantation of cryopreserved–thawed human ovarian tissue

Reference	Age at freezing (years)	Chemotherapy before freezing	Indication	Graft site*	Graft size (mm)	Recovery of ovarian function	Outcome
Oktay & Karlikaya (2000) [63]	29	No	Not cancer	P	8 pc (5 × 10 × 2)	16 weeks	↑ E2; FD after stimulation; ovulation; menses
Radford *et al.* (2001) [64]	36	Yes	Hodgkin's lymphoma	O	2 pc (10 × 5 × 1)	8 months	↓ FSH and LH; ↑ E2; FD; ovulation; menses (1 cycle)
Callejo *et al.* (2001) [65]	47	No	Not cancer	Rectus abdominius muscle	40–45 pc (2–3 mm^3)	3–4 months	↑ E2; FD after stimulation (follicle of 20 mm)
Kim *et al.* (2004) [66]	37	No	Cervical carcinoma (Ib)	Above pectoralis muscle (a) + above rectus abdominus muscle (b)	40 pc (5 × 5 × 1): 20 (a) + 20 (b)	14 weeks	↑ E2; ↓ FSH; FD (follicle of 11–16 mm) only in (b); ovulation
Oktay *et al.* (2004) [67]	30	No	Breast cancer	Subcutaneous abdominal wall	15 pc (5 × 5 × 1 to 15 × 5 × 2)	3 months	FD after gonadotrophin stimulation; OPU; 20 oocytes, 8 IVF-ICSI; 4-cell embryo transfer + 1 aneuploidic embryo
Donnez *et al.* (2004) [40]	25	No	Hodgkin lymphoma	P	1 pc (12 × 4 × 1) + 67 (35 + 32) pc (2 × 2 × 1)	4.5 months	↑ E2; ↓ FSH and LH; FD (follicle of 22 mm); regular cycles (±5 weeks); pregnancy; live birth
Meirow *et al.* (2005) [36]	28	Yes	Non-Hodgkin lymphoma	Ov transplant (a); O injection (b)	3pc (15 × 5 × 1) (a) + tiny fragments (b)	8 months	↓ FSH, ↑ AMH and inhibin B; FD; ovulation; menses; modified natural cycle; OPU; 1 metaphase II oocyte IVF-ICSI; 4-cell embryo transfer; pregnancy and live birth; spontaneous pregnancy miscarriage (30 months after transplant)

pc, pieces; P, pelvic peritoneum; O, remaining ovary; E2, estradiol; FD, follicle development; FSH, follicle-stimulating hormone; LH, luteinizing hormone; AMH, anti-Müllerian hormone; OPU, ovum pick-up; IVF, in vitro fertilization; ICSI, intracytoplasmic sperm injection.

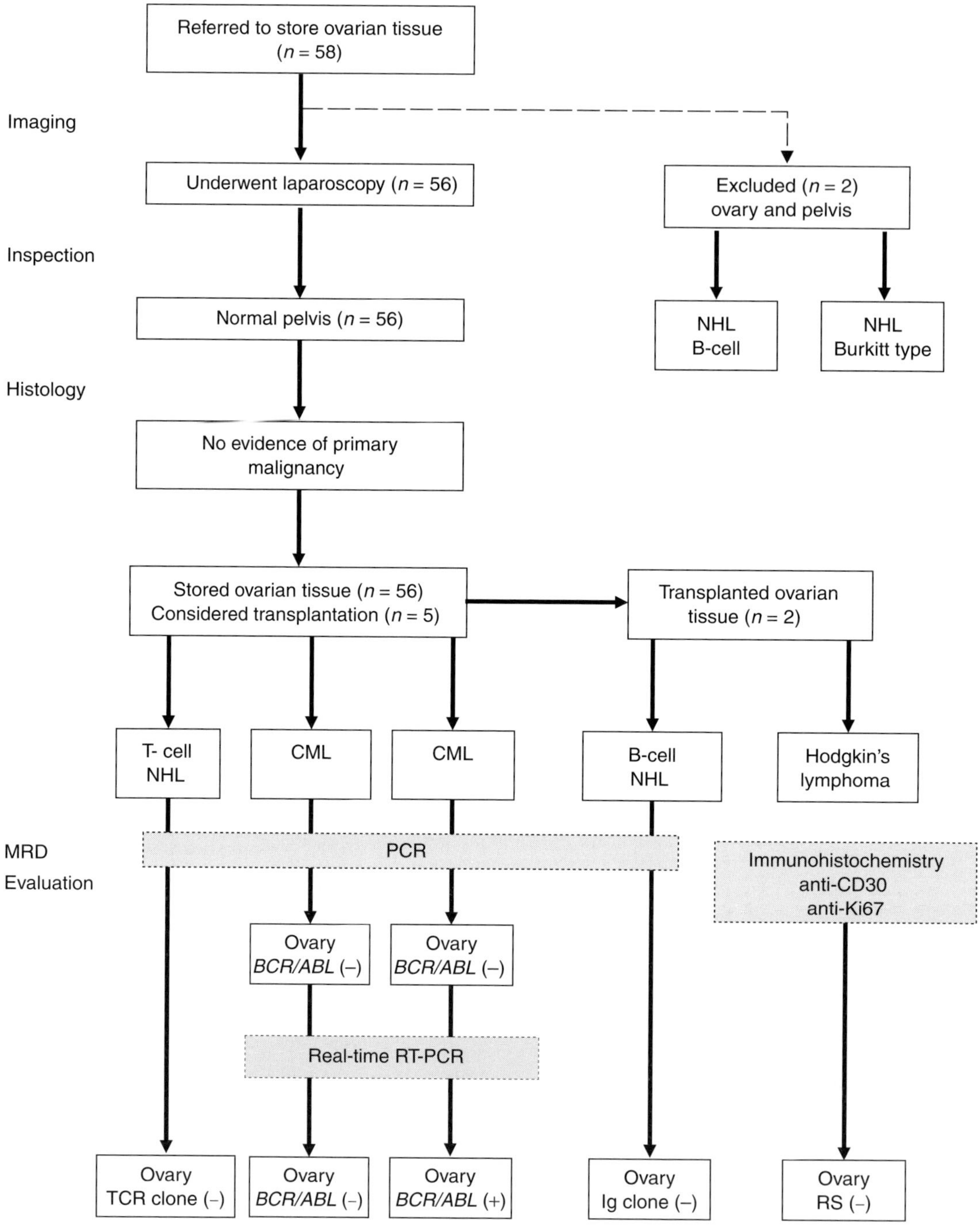

Figure 24.4. The protocol used to detect disease in ovarian tissue stored for fertility preservation in patients with hematological malignancies. Preoperative imaging prevented tissue collection in patients with disease in the ovaries. Ovarian tissue was stored only in patients whose ovaries looked normal at laparoscopy and in whom histology did not disclose malignant cells. Thawed ovarian tissue was evaluated for MRD status in five patients. NHL, non-Hodgkin lymphoma; CML, chronic myelogenous leukemia; TCR, T cell receptor; PCR, polymerase chain reaction; Ig, immunoglobulin; MRD, minimal residual disease; RS, Richter syndrome lymphoma. (Adapted from Meirow *et al.* [52].)

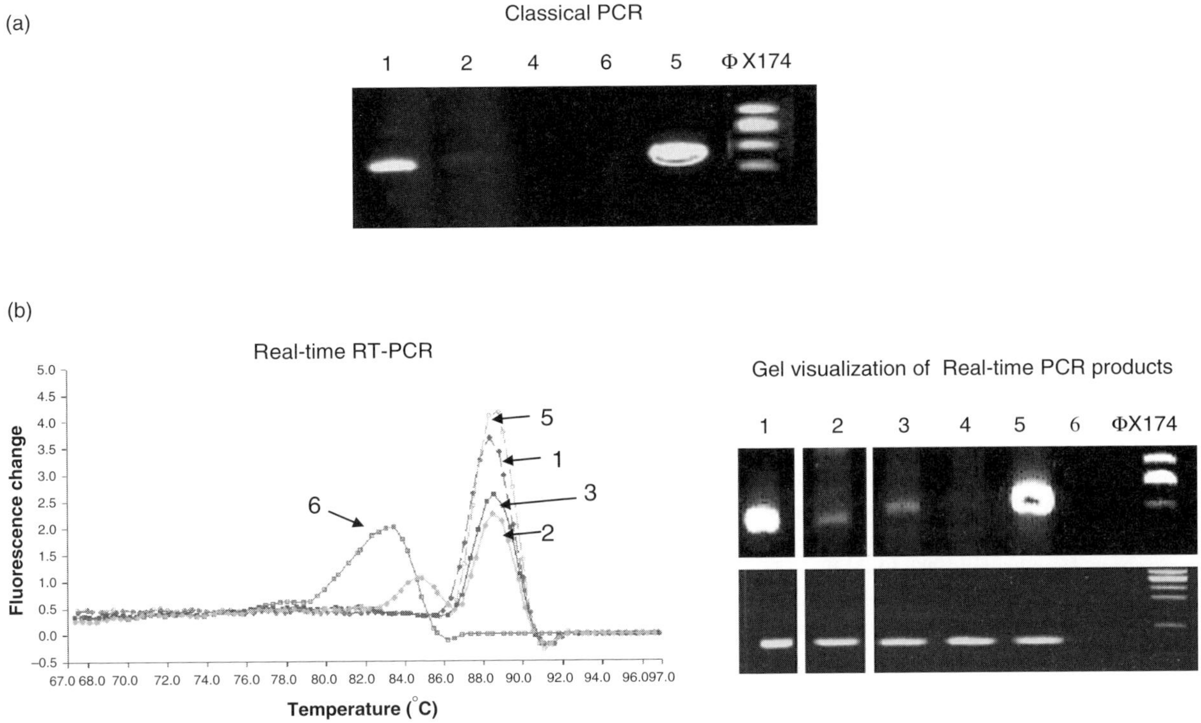

Figure 24.5. Detection of minimal residual disease in frozen thawed ovarian tissue. Use of real-time reverse transcriptase polymerase chain reaction (RT-PCR) for *BCR–ABL* mRNA, indicating the presence of the Philadelphia chromosome, was used as a tumor marker and evaluated in a 20-year-old female diagnosed with chronic myelocytic leukemia in 1999. Ovarian tissue was cryopreserved prior to ablative chemotherapy and allogeneic bone marrow transplantation. Cryopreserved–thawed ovarian tissue and bone marrow stored prior to chemotherapy were evaluated simultaneously. (a) First classical PCR for the *BCR–ABL* transcript was performed shortly after tissue harvesting, when real-time PCR was not available in our laboratory. The results indicate that the bone marrow was involved while there was no evidence of the *BCR–ABL* transcript in the ovarian tissue sent for evaluation. (b) Real-time RT-PCR analysis for the detection of the *BCR–ABL* transcript was performed 5 years after tissue harvesting when the patient asked for an autologous transplant of the stored ovarian tissue. A thawed fragment of ovarian tissue was evaluated for presence of minimal residual disease using this more sensitive technique. The results were positive for *BCR–ABL*, indicating the presence of malignant cells in the tissue. Re-examination of the mRNA products extracted for the first evaluation of ovarian tissue using real-time RT-PCR now gave positive results. 1, bone marrow; 2, ovarian biopsy mRNA prepared in 1999; 3, ovarian biopsy mRNA prepared in 2004; 4, negative sample; 5, positive control cells with b3a2 translocation; 6, without DNA, no template controls; ΦX, *HAE*III-digested DNA size marker. (Adapted from Meirow *et al.* [52].)

to increase procedure safety and to prevent implantation of tissue with malignant cells. In addition, positive control investigation of ovarian tissue for MRD must be performed together with diseased tissue (bone marrow or lymph nodes).

Patients with Hodgkin's lymphoma, a common disease during a woman's reproductive age, rarely have ovarian involvement [79]. Studies using immunohistochemical staining for Reed–Sternberg cells [80] and xenotransplantation into SCID mice [81] of cryopreserved–thawed ovarian tissue from patients suffering from Hodgkin's lymphoma did not disclose the presence of Hodgkin's lymphoma in the ovaries.

Since ovarian tissue is stored for many years, investigation for MRD prior to transplantation is recommended. As MRD evaluation is expensive and laborious, and only a few cancer patients will ask to implant the stored tissue, a separate vial with samples of ovarian tissue should be stored for a final evaluation for MRD just prior to ovarian tissue implantation [54]. Tumor markers do not exist for all malignancies and so in these cases a decision should rely upon clinical judgment, taking into account the type of malignancy, staging, and whether remission was induced prior to ovarian tissue collection.

Conclusions

Live births obtained after transplantation of frozen–thawed ovarian tissue in humans indicate that the procedure appears to be a viable and valuable method for fertility preservation that provides hope to young female cancer patients. Research on both the indications for ovarian tissue transplantation and on technique improvement should continue [82].

Acknowledgements

The authors would like to thank Hannah Biederman for her assistance with the manuscript.

References

1. Gosden RG. Ovary and uterus transplantation. *Reproduction* 2008; **136:** 671–680.
2. Morris RT. The ovarian graft. *N Y Med J* 1895; **62:** 436.
3. Nugent D, Meirow D, Brook PF, Aubard Y, Gosden R. Transplantation in reproductive medicine. *Hum Reprod Update* 1997; **3:** 267–280.
4. Goldman MB. Immunogenetic factors in the survival of ovarian transplants. *Transplantation* 1974; **17:** 518–523.
5. Aubard Y, Piver P, Cognié Y, *et al.* Orthotopic and heterotopic autografts of frozen–thawed ovarian cortex in sheep. *Hum Reprod* 1999; **14:** 2149–2154.
6. Estes WL. A method of implanting ovarian tissue in order to maintain ovarian function. *Pennsylvania Med J* 1909; **13:** 610–613.
7. Le Porrier M, von Theobold, P, Roffe JL, *et al.* A new technique to protect ovarian function before pelvic irrradiation. *Cancer* 1987; **60:** 2201–2204.
8. Gosden RG, Byatt-Smith JG. Oxygen concentration gradient across the ovarian follicle epithelium: model, predictions and implications. *Hum Reprod* 1986; **1:** 65–68.
9. Oelsner G, Bider D, Goldenberg M, Admon D, Mashiach S. Long-term follow-up of the twisted ischemic adnexa managed by detorsion. *Fertil Steril* 1993; **60:** 976–979.
10. Salle B, Demirci B, Franck M, *et al.* Normal pregnancies and live births after autograft of frozen–thawed hemiovaries into ewes. *Fertil Steril* 2002; **77:** 403–408.
11. Almodin CG, Minguetti-Camara VC, Meister H, *et al.* Recovery of fertility after grafting of cryopreserved germinative tissue in female rabbits following radiotherapy. *Hum Reprod* 2004; **19:** 1287–1293.
12. Candy CJ, Wood MJ, Whittingham DG. Follicular development in cryopreserved marmoset ovarian tissue after transplantation. *Hum Reprod* 1995; **10:** 2334–2338.
13. Lee DM, Yeoman RR, Battaglia DE, *et al.* Live birth after ovarian tissue transplant. *Nature* 2004; **428:** 137–138.
14. Dissen GA, Lara HE, Fahrenbach WH, *et al.* Immature rat ovaries become revascularised rapidly after autotransplantation and show a gonadotrophin-dependent increase in angiogenic factor gene expression. *Endocrinology* 1994; **134:** 1146–1154.
15. Israely T, Dafni H, Nevo N, Tsafriri A, Neeman M. Angiogenesis in ectopic xenotransplantation: multiparameter characterization of the neovasculature by dynamic contrast-enhanced MRI. *Magn Reson Med* 2004; **52:** 741–750.
16. Jones EC, Krohn PL. Orthotopic ovarian transplantation in mice. *J Endocrinol* 1960; **20:** 135–146.
17. Felicio LS, Nelson JF, Gosden RG, *et al.* Restoration of ovulatory cycles by young ovarian grafts in aging mice: potentiation by long term ovariectomy decreases with age. *Proc Natl Acad Sci USA* 1983; **80:** 6076–6080.
18. Liu J, Van der Elst J, van den Broecke R, Dhont M. Early massive follicle loss and apoptosis in heterotopically grafted newborn mouse ovaries. *Hum Reprod* 2002; **17:** 605–611.
19. Aubard Y, Piver P, Cognié Y, *et al.* Orthotopic and heterotopic autografts of frozen–thawed ovarian cortex in sheep. *Hum Reprod* 1999; **14:** 2149–2154.
20. Aubard Y. Ovarian tissue xenografting. *Eur J Obstet Gynecol Reprod Biol* 2003; **108:** 14–18.
21. Baird DT, Webb R, Campbell BK, Harkness LM, Gosden RG. Long-term ovarian function in sheep after ovariectomy and transplantation of autografts stored at −196°C. *Endocrinology* 1999; **140:** 462–464.
22. Campbell BK, Telfer EE, Webb R, Baird DT. Ovarian autografts in sheep as a model for studying folliculogenesis. *Mol Cell Endocrinol* 2000; **163:** 131–139.
23. Abir R, Orvieto R, Raanani H, Feldberg D, Nitke S, Fisch B. Parameters affecting successful transplantation of frozen–thawed human fetal ovaries into immunodeficient mice. *Fertil Steril* 2003; **80:** 421–428.
24. Newton H, Aubard Y, Rutherford A, *et al.* Low temperature storage and grafting of human ovarian tissue. *Hum Reprod* 1996; **11:** 1487–1491.
25. Nisolle M, Godin PA, Casanas-Roux F, *et al.* Histological and ultrastructural evaluation of fresh and frozen–thawed human ovarian xenografts in nude mice. *Fertil Steril* 2000; **74:** 122–129.
26. Oktay K, Newton H, Mullan J, Gosden RG. Development of human primordial follicles to antral stages in SCID/hpg mice stimulated with follicle stimulating hormone. *Hum Reprod* 1998; **13:** 1133–1138.
27. Gook DA, Edgar DH, Borg J, *et al.* Oocyte maturation, follicle rupture and luteinization in human cryopreserved ovarian tissue following xenografting. *Hum Reprod* 2003; **18:** 1772–1781.
28. Gook DA, Edgar DH, Borg J, Archer J, McBain JC. Diagnostic assessment of the developmental potential of human cryopreserved ovarian tissue from multiple patients using xenografting. *Hum Reprod* 2005; **20:** 72–78.
29. Kim SS, Soules MR, Battaglia DE. Follicular development, ovulation, and corpus luteum formation in cryopreserved human ovarian tissue after xenotransplantation. *Fertil Steril* 2002; **78:** 77–82.
30. Imthurn B, Cox SL, Jenkin G, Trounson AO, Shaw JM. Gonadotrophin administration can benefit ovarian tissue grafted to the body wall: implications for human ovarian grafting. *Mol Cell Endocrinol* 2000; **163:** 141–146.

31. Callejo J, Vilaseca S, Ordi J, *et al.* Heterotopic ovarian transplantation without vascular pedicle in syngeneic Lewis rats: long-term evaluation of effects on ovarian structure and function. *Fertil Steril* 2002; **77:** 396–402.
32. Risvanli A, Timurkan H, Akpolat N, Gulacti I, Ulakoglu E. A study of ovarian autotransplantation without a vascular pedicle in rats. *J Assist Reprod Genet* 2006; **23:** 401–406.
33. Yang HY, Cox SL, Jenkin G, *et al.* Graft site and gonadotrophin stimulation influences the number and quality of oocytes from murine ovarian tissue grafts *Reproduction* 2006; **131**: 851–859.
34. Nugent D, Newton H, Gallivan L, Gosden RG. Protective effect of vitamin E on ischaemia–reperfusion injury in ovarian grafts. *J Reprod Fertil* 1998; **114:** 341–346.
35. Maltaris T, Beckmann MW, Binder H, *et al.* The effect of a GnRH agonist on cryopreserved human ovarian grafts in severe combined immunodeficient mice. *Reproduction* 2007; **133**: 503–509.
36. Meirow D, Levron J, Eldar-Geva T, *et al.* Pregnancy after transplantation of cryopreserved ovarian tissue in a patient with ovarian failure after chemotherapy. *N Engl J Med* 2005; **353:** 318–321.
37. Oktay K, Buyuk E, Rosenwaks Z, Rucinski JA. Technique for transplantation of ovarian cortical strips to the forearm. *Fertil Steril* 2003; **80:** 193–198.
38. Demeestere I, Simon P, Buxant F, *et al.* Ovarian function and spontaneous pregnancy after combined heterotopic and orthotopic cryopreserved ovarian tissue transplantation in a patient previously treated with bone marrow transplantation. *Hum Reprod* 2006; **21:** 2010–2014.
39. Israely T, Nevo N, Harmelin A, Neeman M, Tsafriri A. Reducing ischaemic damage in rodent ovarian xenografts transplanted into granulation tissue. *Hum Reprod* 2006; **21:** 1368–1379.
40. Donnez J, Dolmans MM, Demylle D, *et al.* Livebirth after orthotopic transplantation of cryopreserved ovarian tissue. *Lancet* 2004; **364:** 1405–1410.
41. Torrents E, Boiso I, Barri PN, Veiga A. Applications of ovarian tissue transplantation in experimental biology and medicine. *Hum Reprod Update* 2003; **9:** 471–481.
42. Falcone T, Bedaiwy MA. Fertility preservation and pregnancy outcome after malignancy. *Curr Opin Obstet Gynecol* 2005; **17:** 21–26.
43. Meirow D. Ovarian injury and modern options to perserve fertility in female cancer patients treated with high dose radio-chemotherapy for hemato-oncological neoplasias and other cancers. *Leuk Lymphoma* 1999; **33:** 65–76.
44. Meirow D. Fertility preservation in cancer patients using stored ovarian tissue: clinical aspects. *Curr Opin Endocrinol Diabetes Obes* 2008; **15:** 536–547.
45. Meirow D, Epstein M, Lewis H. Administration of cyclophosphamide at different stages of follicular maturation in mice: effects on reproductive performance and fetal malformations. *Hum Reprod* 2001; **16:** 632–637.
46. Meirow D, Schiff E. Impact of maternal exposure to chemotherapy on embryos and offspring. *J Nat Can Inst* 2005; **34:** 21–25.
47. Telfer EE, McLaughlin M, Ding C, Thong KJ. A two-step serum-free culture system supports development of human oocytes from primordial follicles in the presence of activin. *Hum Reprod* 2008; **23:** 1151–1158.
48. Xu M, Kreeger PK, Shea LD, Woodruff TK. Tissue-engineered follicles produce live, fertile offspring. *Tissue Eng* 2006; **12**: 2739–46.
49. Meirow D, Dor J. Epidemiology and infertility in cancer patients. In Tulandi T, Gosden R, eds. *Preservation of Fertility*. London: Taylor & Francis, 2004, pp.21–38.
50. Oktay KH, Yih M. Preliminary experience with orthotopic and heterotopic transplantation of ovarian cortical strips. *Semin Reprod Med* 2002; **20:** 63–74.
51. Seshadri T, Gook D, Lade S, *et al.* Lack of evidence of disease contamination in ovarian tissue harvested for cryopreservation from patients with Hodgkin lymphoma and analysis of factors predictive of oocyte yield. *Br J Cancer* 2006; **94:** 1007–1010.
52. Meirow D, Hardan I, Dor J, *et al.* Searching for evidence of disease and malignant cell contamination in ovarian tissue stored from hematologic cancer patients. *Hum Reprod* 2008; **23:** 1007–1013.
53. Gosden RG, Baird DT, Wade JC, Webb R. Restoration of fertility to oophorectomised sheep by ovarian autografts stored at −196°C. *Hum Reprod* 1994; **9:** 597–603.
54. Meirow D, Baum M, Yaron R, *et al.* Ovarian tissue cryopreservation in hematologic malignancy: ten years' experience. *Leuk Lymphoma* 2007; **48:** 1569–1576.
55. Anderson RA, Wallace WHB, Baird DT. Ovarian cryopreservation for fertility preservation: indications and outcomes. *Reproduction* 2008; **136:** 681–689.
56. Oktay K, Oktem O. Ovarian cryopreservation and transplantation for fertility preservation for medical indications: report of an ongoing experience. *Fertil Steril* 2008; epub ahead of print.
57. Demeestere I, Simon P, Emiliani S, Delbaere A, Englert Y. Orthotopic and heterotopic ovarian tissue transplantation.*Hum Reprod Update* 2009; epub ahead of print.
58. Andersen CY, Rosendahl M, Byskov AG, *et al.* Two successful pregnancies following autotransplantation of frozen/thawed ovarian tissue. *Hum Reprod* 2008; **23:** 2266–2272.
59. Silber SJ, Lenahan KM, Levine DJ, *et al.* Ovarian transplantation between monozygotic twins discordant for premature ovarian failure. *N Engl J Med* 2005; **353:** 58–63.

60. Silber SJ, Gosden RG. Ovarian transplantation in a series of monozygotic twins discordant for ovarian failure. *N Engl J Med* 2007; **356:** 1382–1384.
61. Meirow D, Levron J, Eldar-Geva T, *et al.* Monitoring the ovaries after autotransplantation of cryopreserved ovarian tissue: endocrine studies, in vitro fertilization cycles, and live birth. *Fertil Steril* 2007; **87:** 418.e417.
62. Dolmans MM, *et al. Results of Autotransplantation of Cryopreserved Human Ovarian Tissue.* 2008. http://www.isfp-fertility.org/members-only/scientific-articles/fertility-preservation-in-women/cryopreservation-of-ovarian-cortex-reimplantation-of-cryopreserved-ovarian-cortex.
63. Oktay K, Karlikaya G. Ovarian function after transplantation of frozen, banked autologous ovarian tissue. *N Engl J Med* 2000; **342**: 1919.
64. Radford JA, Liebermann BA, Brison D, *et al.* Orthotopic reimplantation of cryopreserved ovarian cortical strips after high-dose chemotherapy for Hodgkin's lymphoma. *Lancet* 2001; **357**: 1172–1175.
65. Callejo J, Salvador C, Miralles A, *et al.* Long-term ovarian function evaluation after autografting by implantation with fresh and frozen-thawed human ovarian tissue. *J Clin Endocrinol Metab* 2001; **86**: 4489–4494.
66. Kim SS, Hwang I-T, Lee H-C. Heterotopic autotransplantation of cryobanked human ovarian tissue as a strategy to restore ovarian function. *Fertil Steril* 2004; **82**: 930–932.
67. Oktay K, Buyuk E, Veeck L, *et al.* Embryo development after heterotopic transplantation of cryopreserved ovarian tissue. *Lancet* 2004; **363**: 837–840.
68. Schmidt KL, Yding Andersen C, Loft A, *et al.* Follow-up of ovarian function post-chemotherapy following ovarian cryopreservation and transplantation. *Hum Reprod* 2005; **20**: 3539–3546.
69. Wolner-Hanssen P, Hagglund L, Ploman F, *et al.* Autotransplantation of cryopreserved ovarian tissue to the right forearm 2005; 4½ years after autologous stem cell transplantation. *Acta Obstet Gynecol Scand* **84:** 695–698.
70. Donnez J, Dolmans MM, Demylle D, *et al.* Restoration of ovarian function after orthotopic (intraovarian and periovarian) transplantation of cryopreserved ovarian tissue in a woman treated by bone marrrow transplantation for sickle cell anaemia: case report. *Hum Reprod* 2006; **21:** 183–188.
71. Oktay K. Spontaneous conceptions and live birth after heterotopic ovarian transplantation: is there a germline stem cell connection? *Hum Reprod* 2006; **21:** 1345–1348.
72. Rosendahl M, Loft A, Byskov AG, *et al.* Biochemical pregnancy after fertilization of an oocyte aspirated from a heterotopic autotransplant of cryopreserved ovarian tissue: case report. *Hum Reprod* 2006; **21:** 2006–2009.
73. Demeestere I, Simon P, Emiliani S, Delbaere A, Englert Y. Fertility preservation: successful transplantation of cryopreserved ovarian tissue in a young patient previously treated for Hodgkin's disease. *Oncologist* 2007; **12:** 1437–1442.
74. Silber SJ, Derosa M, Pineda J, *et al.* A series of monozygotic twins discordant for ovarian failure: ovary transplantation (cortical versus microvascular) and cryopreservation. *Hum Reprod* 2008; **23:** 1531–1537.
75. Donnez J, Squifflet J, Van Eyck A-S, *et al.* Restoration of ovarian function in orthotopically transplanted cryopreserved ovarian tissue: a pilot experience. *RBM online* 2008; **16:** 694–704.
76. Sanchez-Serrano M, Crespo J, Mirabet V, *et al.* Twins born after transplantation of ovarian cortical tissue and oocyte vitrification. *Fertil Steril* 2010; **93:** 268.
77. Piver P, Amiot C, Agnani G, *et al.* Two pregnancies obtained after a new technique of autotransplantation of cryopreserved ovarian tissue. In *Proceedings of the 25th Annual Meeting of ESHRE*, Amsterdam, the Netherlands, June–July, 2009.
78. Lass A, Akagbosu F, Brinsden P. Sperm banking and assisted reproduction treatment for couples following cancer treatment of the male partner. *Hum Reprod Update* 2001; **7:** 370–377.
79. Khan MA, Dahill SW, Stewart KS. Primary Hodgkin's disease of the ovary. *Br J Obstet Gynaecol* 1986; **93:** 1300–1301.
80. Seshadri T, Gook D, Lade S, *et al.* Lack of evidence of disease contamination in ovarian tissue harvested for cryopreservation from patients with Hodgkin lymphoma and analysis of factors predictive of oocyte yield. *Br J Cancer* 2006; **94:** 1007–1010.
81. Kim SS, Radford J, Harris M, *et al.* Ovarian tissue harvested from lymphoma patients to preserve fertility may be safe for autotransplantation. *Hum Reprod* 2001; **16:** 2056–2060.
82. Donnez J, Martinez-Madrid B, Jadoul P, *et al.* Ovarian tissue cryopreservation and transplantation: a review. *Hum Reprod Update* 2006; **12:** 519–535.

Chapter 25

Whole ovary cryopreservation

Jason G. Bromer and Pasquale Patrizio

Introduction

While previous chapters have focused on preservation of oocytes and embryos as well as ovarian tissue cortex, much progress has been made recently in the area of cryopreservation of the whole ovary. Patients who require immediate (within days) gonadotoxic therapy (whether chemo- or radiotherapy, or a combination of both) have few options for fertility preservation: (1) cryopreservation of ovarian tissues as cortical strips; (2) dual cryopreservation of both ovarian cortical tissue with cryopreservation and in vitro maturation of a few immature oocytes extracted from small follicles visible within the ovarian cortex; or (3) cryopreservation of one whole ovary [1–10]. To date, ovarian cryopreservation and subsequent transplantation procedures, whether as heterotopic or orthotopic allografts, have been almost exclusively limited to avascular cortical pieces [8,11,12].

Despite the careful use of cryoprotectants to prevent ice crystal formation at the time of freezing, the main drawback to cryopreservation of ovarian cortical strips is the ischemia that occurs at the time of transplantation. As these small cortical pieces are grafted without any vascular anastomosis, they are completely dependent for their survival on the speed at which neovascularization can be established after grafting. As this process requires a minimum of 7 days [13, 14], the cells in the graft undergo significant ischemic damage, which results in massive loss of primordial follicles [15–19] and, in turn, limits the lifespan of the graft [20, 21]. For a patient who desires long-term reproductive and endocrine function after transplantation, this method of fertility preservation may be suboptimal. Therefore, reducing the ischemic interval between transplantation and revascularization is essential for maintaining the viability and functional lifetime of the graft. To this end, cryopreservation of the whole ovary with an intact pedicle and vascular supply can potentially overcome this problem, as reperfusion will occur immediately upon retransplantation and anastomosis [4,19,22,23]. The cryopreservation of intact, large organs was a breakthrough in medical science, with early reports of canine kidneys showing low toxicity and high longevity [24,25].

Yet progress into whole ovary cryopreservation has been slow as two main issues in whole organ cryopreservation needed to be adequately addressed: the first was related to the feasibility of re-establishing the vascular anastomosis of the organ to be transplanted and the second to the creation of a valid cryopreservation protocol. Wang *et al.* [26] demonstrated that cryopreservation and subsequent transplantation of the reproductive system "en bloc" could be performed in rats. Subsequently, to prove that anastomosis of the ovarian pedicle in large animals and humans was technically feasible, transplantation of whole fresh ovaries has been successfully performed in rats [26,27], rabbits [28], sheep [29,30], dogs [31], monkeys [32], and humans [19,20,33–35].

The second issue, researching a valid cryopreservation protocol for large-sized intact ovaries, has posed greater difficulties and challenges. These include the scarcity of information on the physical changes occurring in ovarian tissues during cooling, the physical constraints related to heat transfer between the core and periphery of the organ, and difficulties with adequate perfusion and diffusion of cryoprotectants [36,37] to prevent intravascular ice formation [19].

Nevertheless, successful cryopreservation and vascular transplantation of intact frozen–thawed ovaries has been reported in both rats and sheep.

This chapter will review the progress in cryopreservation and transplantation of whole ovaries that have been made in both animal and human models. As cryopreservation of whole tissues from small and large animals and humans present different challenges and difficulties, these topics will be addressed separately. As this new and exciting field remains in its infancy, this chapter will focus mainly on a review of the existing literature and what conclusions can be drawn from the initial studies that have been performed.

The rodent model

Wang *et al.* in 2002 [26] first described the feasibility of cryopreservation of whole reproductive organs (ovaries, tubes, and uterus) using a rat model. In this pilot study, ovaries from adult female rats were removed, and the ovarian vessels were dissected to create short cuffs from the aorta and vena cava. Seven such dissections were perfused for 30 minutes at 0.35 ml/min with M2 medium containing 0.1 M fructose and increasing concentrations of dimethyl sulfoxide (DMSO). The organs were then cooled slowly in cryovials. After overnight storage in liquid nitrogen, the vials were rapidly thawed and the cryoprotectant was removed by perfusion with a reversed concentration gradient. In four of seven animals receiving transplanted cryopreserved grafts, the ovaries showed subsequent follicular activity, with corpora lutea indicating recent ovulation, and one animal achieved pregnancy. Importantly, tubal and uterine morphology were indistinguishable from non-operated controls. However, the rats had higher serum follicle-stimulating hormone (FSH) levels, fewer follicles, and lower estradiol levels and uterine weights than controls. These results indicated that ovarian function was compromised by freezing and suggested that advances in freezing techniques could potentially overcome this problem [26].

The same group followed up this work using a similar model to investigate the long-term longevity of these grafts, as well as to assess the effect of ischemia by keeping the organs for 24 hours at 4°C prior to freezing [27]. Graft survival with endocrine function was seen at 60 days and ovulatory response to FSH was seen at 120 days, suggesting long-term graft longevity after cryopreservation and vascular anastomosis. Furthermore, graft function after transplant was also seen in grafts that had been held for 24 hours under ischemic conditions before freezing, although, as expected, the number of surviving follicles was less [27].

The sheep model

The adult female sheep has recently become a standard model to explore intact ovarian cryopreservation. Despite the fact that adult human ovaries are larger in size and have different pedicle anatomy, ovine ovaries are similar to human ovaries in having a dense fibrous stroma and relatively high primordial follicle density in the cortex [38]. Similar to the rat model, the first experiments were carried out to determine the feasibility of transplantation using fresh ovine ovaries. Jeremias *et al.* in 2002 [30] first described a novel method of orthotopic transplantation in an adult sheep with anastomosis of the vascular pedicle. Fresh ovaries were autotransplanted to the abdominal wall via microsurgical anastomosis of the ovarian to the inferior epigastric vessels, and showed resumption of endocrine function post-transplant.

Once a whole ovine ovary transplant was proven feasible, the next step was to repeat the experiments using whole frozen–thawed ovaries. Whole ovary cryopreservation in the sheep has been attempted through both slow-cooling and vitrification methodologies (see Table 25.1, below). The first transplant of an intact frozen–thawed ovary via microvascular anastomosis occurred in 2003 [36]. After laparascopic dissection, the protocol utilized consisted of perfusion via the ovarian artery with heparin, followed by Leibovitz L-15 medium, 10% fetal calf serum (FCS), and 1.5 M DMSO at 1.3 ml/min. Ovaries were cryopreserved with cooling at 2°C/min beginning at 4°C and continuing until ice nucleation occurred at −7°C. The temperature was then reduced at 2°C/min until −35°C and finally by 25°C/min until −140°C was reached; at which point the cryovials were plunged into liquid nitrogen.

The ovaries were thawed by placing the cryovials in a water bath at 37°C and perfusing with Leibovitz L-15 medium and 10% FCS for 20 minutes before they were implanted with vascular connections to the epigastric artery.

Of the 11 ovaries transplanted, immediate and long-term patency were documented in 100% and 27% of grafts, respectively. There were no significant differences in the mean values of apoptosis and follicular viability compared with ovarian cortical strip cryopreservation and autotransplantation. Postoperative FSH levels were much lower in the whole ovary graft group ($p = 0.03$) than in the animals grafted with ovarian cortical strips. Further, the endocrine activity of the whole frozen–thawed and transplanted ovaries was similar to preoperative values in animals with patent vessels [36].

Post-transplanted ovaries responded to stimulation with FSH and produced viable oocytes. Once the ewes were sacrificed, all ovaries showed primordial, primary, secondary, antral, and preovulatory follicles along with fully functional vascularization manifested by the expression of factor VIII, vascular endothelial growth factor, and smooth muscle cell actin [39].

Further experiments by Revel *et al.* [38] have also documented success in cryopreservation with whole ovine ovaries, using sheep aged 8–12 months. In these cases, the ovarian artery was perfused with 4°C University of Wisconsin (UW) solution with 10% DMSO for 3 minutes. The ovary with its pedicle was then placed in a glass freezing tube properly designed to accommodate the whole ovary.

In addition, freezing was performed using a novel device, the Multi-Thermal-Gradient (MTG; IMT Ltd., Ness Ziona, Israel) [38,40]. The peculiarity of this freezing method is the speed at which the temperature gradients are programmed. The freezing tube and ovary were carried at a constant velocity of 0.01 mm/s through the device, and freezing was performed at 0.6°C/min until a seeding temperature was reached, and then at 0.3°C/min until −30°C, after which, the tubes were plunged into liquid nitrogen.

After thawing and removal of the cryoprotectant, grafting was performed 3 to 14 days later by end-to-end anastomosis of the ovarian artery and vein to the contralateral ovarian vascular pedicle of the same sheep via repeat laparotomy. This method confirmed the feasibility of successful reanastomosis of thawed ovaries, which occurred in five of eight sheep. In subsequent follow-up studies, Arav *et al.* [40] showed no significant difference in follicular survival between fresh ovaries and frozen–thawed ovaries, as well as similar histological morphology. Furthermore, they showed normal immunohistochemical expression of factor VIII in frozen–thawed ovaries, suggesting normally functioning vascular pedicles. Six oocytes were also aspirated from two sheep, and subsequent fertilization and embryo development occurred. Two of the sheep continued to show normal hormonal cyclicity by progesterone levels up to 36 months after the transplantation, and follow-up magnetic resonance imaging studies confirmed normal ovarian size and intact vasculature [40].

A third group has also explored whole ovary cryopreservation in a sheep model. Imhof *et al.* [41] first explored cryopreservation by cannulating the ovarian artery from porcine ovaries and flushing with Roswell Park Memorial Institute (RPMI)-1640 solution containing 1.5 M DMSO and 10% human albumin for 30 minutes on ice. The ovaries were transferred to a programmable freezer at a starting temperature of 4°C, and cooled at 2°C/min to 0°C. The temperature was then lowered at 1.5°C/min to −9°C and then at 0.5°C/min to −40°C. Cooling was then continued at 10°C/min to −150°C. The vials were then plunged into liquid nitrogen. Thawing was performed by immersion in a 25°C water bath with removal of cryoprotectant by washing in saline and fresh medium [41].

Light and electron microscopy confirmed histological viability in 84.4% of the primordial follicles in the frozen–thawed ovaries, with 73% of the follicles looking similar to those from the unfrozen contralateral ovary [41].

A follow-up study with ewe ovaries was accompanied by microvascular end-to-end anastomosis of the frozen–thawed ovaries to the contralateral pedicle. Concentrations of FSH reached normal physiologic levels approximately 6 months after transplantation. Two of nine sheep resumed normal ovarian function, and one achieved a spontaneous pregnancy, with delivery of a healthy lamb [42].

While many attempts have been made to cryopreserve whole ovaries by slow-freezing techniques, few have attempted to use vitrification. Vitrification may be particularly appealing to whole organ cryopreservation as it prevents the formation of ice crystals from aqueous cryoprotectant solutions, which could lead to architectural disruption inside whole tissues [43].

Fahy *et al.* [44] have described two vitrification solutions that may be useful for whole ovary cryopreservation: VS1 contains 20.5% (w/v) DMSO, 15.5% (w/v) acetamide, 10% (w/v) propylene glycol, and 6% (w/v) polyethylene glycol in a modified Dulbecco's saline; VS4 contains 2.75 M DMSO, 2.76 M formamide, and 1.97 M propylene glycol diluted in BM1 medium [45].

The two vitrification solutions, VS1 and VS4, have been compared by Courbiere *et al.* [46] in a sheep model of whole ovary cryopreservation using ovaries from lambs aged 5–6 months. Each ovary was perfused via the ovarian artery with heparinized Ringer's solution, followed by either VS1 or VS4 at 0.35 ml/min in a stepwise increase in concentration of cryoprotectant. After perfusion, ovaries were transferred into cryobags and immediately plunged into liquid nitrogen. Thawing was performed rapidly in a 37°C water bath, and the cryoprotectant was removed by a reversed concentration gradient. Follicle viability fell from 75.6 ± 1.1% without vitrification to 68.2 ± 1.9% after vitrification with VS1, and from 68.0 ± 3.8% to 60.7 ± 2.4% after vitrification with VS4. Follicle density remained significantly higher after vitrification with VS4 ($p < 0.05$).

Table 25.1. Summary of whole ovary cryopreservation experiments in sheep

Study	No.	Surgical method	Freezing method	Cryoprotectant	Transplanted?	Outcomes measured	Endocrine function?	Pregnancy achieved
Bedaiwy *et al.* (2003) [36]	11	Laparoscopy	Slow cooling	DMSO	Yes	Blood flow, apoptosis, follicular viability, endocrine function, histology	Yes (3/11)	No
Revel *et al.* (2004) [38]	8	Laparotomy	Slow cooling	Ethylene glycol	Yes	Cyclic progesterone	Yes (3/8)	No
Courbiere *et al.* (2005) [46]	15	Laparotomy	Vitrification	DMSO, acetamide, propylene glycol DMSO, formamide, propylene glycol	No	Follicle viability, histology of ovary and vessels	N/A	N/A
Imhof *et al.* (2006) [42]	9	Laparotomy	Slow cooling	DMSO	Yes	Histology, follicle-stimulating hormone and progesterone	Yes (4/9)	Yes (1/9)
Grazul-Bilska *et al.* (2008) [39]	4	Laparoscopy	Slow cooling	DMSO	Yes	No. follicles, No. fertilized, morphology, vessel viability, cellular proliferation, apoptosis	Yes (2/4)	No
Courbiere *et al.* (2009) [47]	5	Laparotomy	Vitrification	DMSO, formamide, propylene glycol	Yes	Progesterone levels, histology	1/5	No

DMSO, dimethyl sulfide.

Histologically, 25.2 ± 7.0% of follicles appeared normal with VS1 and 53.5 ± 3.2% with VS4. There were also more postvitrification cytoplasmic anomalies with VS4 ($p < 0.05$) and more nuclear and combined anomalies with VS1 ($p < 0.05$). Fractures occurred in vessels during thawing in three of the five ovaries with VS1 and in 8 of 10 with VS4 [46].

A recent follow-up study by Courbiere *et al.* [47] attempted vascular anastomosis to the contralateral pedicle either fresh or after vitrification. While successful microsurgical transplantation was performed in both groups, the median ischemia time was significantly longer in the cryopreservation group. Only one of five ewes recovered endocrine function 6 months after transplantation, and histological evaluation showed total follicle loss.

These experiments suggest that attempts at cryopreservation with vitrification may be unsuccessful, despite technical feasibility. Table 25.1 summarizes the attempts to cryopreserve whole ovaries in sheep.

Whole ovary cryopreservation in humans

Despite the technical challenges which have been discussed, there have been some promising preliminary results, with attempts at whole ovary cryopreservation in humans. The first report of this technique was by Martinez-Madrid *et al.* in 2004 [19]. Ovaries from three premenopausal women undergoing oopohorectomy were resected with the vascular pedicle intact. The ovarian artery was perfused first with heparin, and then with a cryoprotective solution of Leibovitz L-15 medium, 10% DMSO, and 2% human serum albumin. Cooling was performed at a rate of 1°C/min to −80°C, at which time the ovary was plunged into

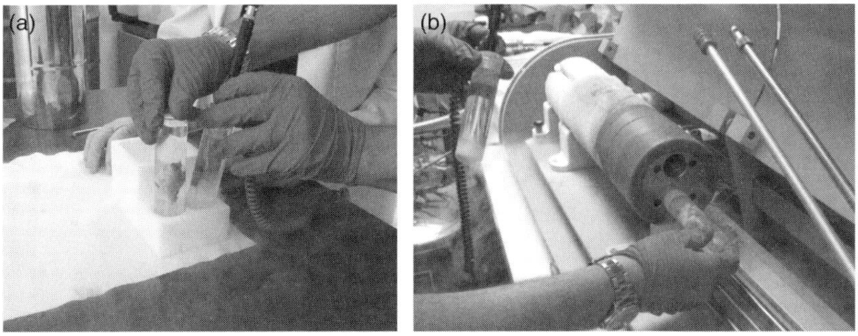

Figure 25.1. Procedure for freezing whole human ovary. (a) Modified cryovial to allow for freezing of whole intact human ovary. (b) Loading of the cryovial into the Multi-Thermal-Gradient (IMT Ltd., Ness Ziona, Israel) for a slow-cooling procedure.

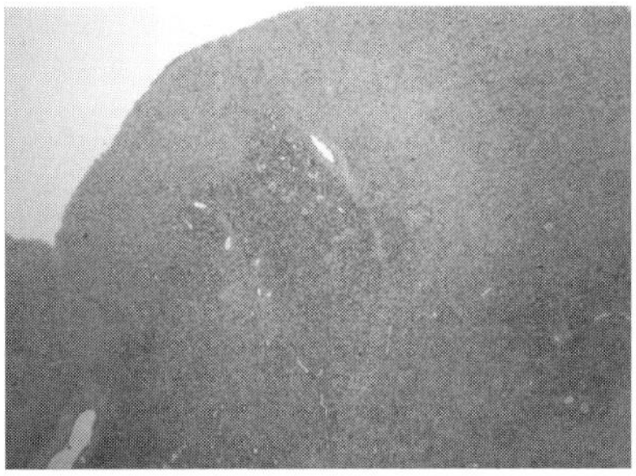

Figure 25.2 After freezing for 48 h, the thawed human ovary shows an intact ovarian cortex, containing multiple follicles with a normal appearance.

liquid nitrogen. Thawing was performed in a water bath at 60°C with removal of cryoprotectant. The percentage of live follicles was found to be 99.4% in fresh tissue, 98.1% after cryoprotectant exposure, and 75.1% after thawing. Live stromal cells and small vessels were also found after thawing. On histological evaluation, the morphology of follicles and cortical and medullar tissue was similar in all three groups. No primordial or primary follicles showed signs of apoptosis by either TUNEL or active caspase-3 assay. Electron microscopy also showed a well-preserved ultrastructure, healthy-appearing primordial and primary follicles, and normal endothelial cells [22]. While this work utilized a much more simplified cryopreservation algorithm than previous studies, and it did not report on vascular endothelial viability [48], it did suggest that a slow-cooling method could be utilized preserving whole human ovaries [19].

The same group has subsequently reported on the optimum conditions for oophorectomy with the intent of whole ovary removal by laparoscopy for cryopreservation [49]. In a recent case series of nine patients, the whole ovary was successfully removed and cryopreserved by arterial catheterization in all patients. Martinez-Madrid *et al.* [49] concluded that, for success, great care must be taken to remove the ovary with a large part (≥ 5 cm) of the infundibulopelvic ligament in order to allow for dissection of the ovarian vessels and perfusion with a cryoprotective medium. Furthermore, they recommended that the period of ischemia between ligation of the ovarian pedicle and ovarian cryopreservation must be as short as possible [49].

Bedaiwy *et al.* [18] have also recently described successful cryopreservation of the human ovary in two premenopausal women. In each case, one ovary was harvested and perfused as described above. However, after perfusion, each ovary was bisected and transferred to smaller cryovials. After thawing, the overall viability of the primordial follicles in the two ovaries was 75 and 78%; there were similar primordial follicle counts, absence of features of necrosis, and mean values of apoptosis compared with control ovaries. While this technique is currently suboptimal as the ovary had to be transected prior to freezing, it could be potentially modified with the use of a larger cryovial to accommodate a whole ovary.

Most recently, Patrizio *et al.* [4,50] have reported on successful whole human ovary cryopreservation with the vascular pedicle utilizing the same Multi-Thermal-Gradient device and a slow-cooling, rapid thawing protocol described earlier for the sheep ovaries (Figure 25.1). With this method, ovaries from premenopausal women undergoing hysterectomy have been successfully cryopreserved for 2–4 days following either laparotomy or laparoscopic/robotic-assisted laparascopic oophorectomy [51]. In all cases, the ovarian artery was successfully cannulated for perfusion of cryoprotectant. The frozen–thawed ovary was histologically indistinguishable from the fresh contralateral ovary, which was used as the control (Figure 25.2). Immunohistochemistry and Western blot assays did show some increase in anti-caspase 3 and p53 phosphoserine expression, suggesting some increased level of apoptosis in the frozen–thawed specimens [51].

In three cases, the ipsilateral fallopian tube was also cryopreserved intact with the associated ovary and

Table 25.2. Summary of whole ovary cryopreservation experiments in humans

	No.	Surgical method	Freezing method	Cryoprotectant	Outcomes measured
Martinez-Madrid *et al.*,2004 [19]	3	Laparoscopy	Slow cooling	DMSO	Follicle, stromal cell, vascular viability, histomorphology
Bedaiwy *et al.*, 2006 [18]	2	Laparoscopy	Slow cooling (ovary bisected)	DMSO	Follicle viability, apoptosis
Martinez-Madrid *et al.*, 2007 [49]	3	Laparoscopy	Slow cooling	DMSO	Apoptosis, ultrastructural assessment
Jadoul *et al.*, 2007 [49]	9	Laparoscopy	Slow cooling	DMSO	Feasibility of oophorectomy and freezing
Patrizio *et al.*, 2008 [50]	11	Laparoscopy, laparotomy	Slow cooling	EG	Apoptosis, histomorphology

DMSO, dimethyl sulfoxide; EG, ethylene glycol.

pedicle. In these cases, the histological architecture was also preserved, suggesting that cryopreservation of the entire adnexa may also be technically feasible [52].

Table 25.2 summarizes the studies on cryopreservation of human ovaries.

Conclusions

Large strides have been taken in the field of whole ovary cryopreservation since it was first described in small rodents in 2002. More successful cryopreservation protocols have made the theoretical problems of ice crystal formation less of a liability, and results to date with histological and cytological architecture, as well as quantification of apoptosis, have been very encouraging. Although the process of vitrification would empirically suggest superiority for large organs, only protocols using slow cooling have showed promise thus far.

Another area of continued refinement in whole organ cryopreservation and subsequent transplantation will be the method of oophorectomy. Laparoscopy has been shown to be successful in resection of the ovary and pedicle, and the advent of robotic surgery will continue to aid in the long dissection of the vascular pedicle that is a prerequisite both for perfusion of the ovarian artery and for a future anastomosis.

While no human studies of whole ovary transplant after cryopreservation have been performed to date, large animal studies have been encouraging, and it is likely that this option for fertility preservation will be a viable treatment option in the future.

References

1. Georgescu ES, Goldberg JM, du Plessis SS, Agarwal A. Present and future fertility preservation strategies for female cancer patients. *Obstet Gynecol Surv* 2008; **63:** 725–732.
2. Demirtas E, Elizur SE, *et al.* Immature oocyte retrieval in the luteal phase to preserve fertility in cancer patients. *Reprod Biomed Online* 2008; **17:** 520–523.
3. Donnez J, Martinez-Madrid B, Jadoul P, *et al.* Ovarian tissue cryopreservation and transplantation: a review. *Hum Reprod Update*. 2006; **12:** 519–535.
4. Bromer JG, Patrizio P. Preservation and postponement of female fertility: an overview and the initial Yale experience. *Placenta* 2008; **29**(Suppl B): 200–205.
5. ACOG Committee. Opinion No. 405: ovarian tissue and oocyte cryopreservation. *Obstet Gynecol* 2008; **111:** 1255–1256.
6. Martin JR, Kodaman P, Oktay K, Taylor HS. Ovarian cryopreservation with transposition of a contralateral ovary: a combined approach for fertility preservation in women receiving pelvic radiation. *Fertil Steril* 2007; **87:** 189.e5–e7.
7. Lee SJ, Schover LR, Partridge AH, *et al.* American Society of Clinical Oncology recommendations on fertility preservation in cancer patients. *J Clin Oncol* 2006; **24:** 2917–2931.
8. Tao T, Del Valle A. Human oocyte and ovarian tissue cryopreservation and its application. *J Assist Reprod Genet* 2008; **25:** 287–296.
9. Oktay K, Sonmezer M. Fertility preservation in gynecologic cancers. *Curr Opin Oncol* 2007; **19:** 506–511.

10. von Wolff M, Strowitzki T, van der Ven H, Montag M. In vitro maturation is an efficient technique to generate oocytes and should be considered in combination with cryopreservation of ovarian tissue for preservation of fertility in women. *J Clin Oncol* 2006; **24:** 5336–5337; author reply 7–8.
11. Donnez J, Squifflet J, Van Eyck AS, *et al.* Restoration of ovarian function in orthotopically transplanted cryopreserved ovarian tissue: a pilot experience. *Reprod Biomed Online* 2008; **16:** 694–704.
12. Oktay K. Spontaneous conceptions and live birth after heterotopic ovarian transplantation: is there a germline stem cell connection? *Hum Reprod* 2006; **21:** 1345–1348.
13. Israely T, Dafni H, Nevo N, Tsafriri A, Neeman M. Angiogenesis in ectopic ovarian xenotransplantation: multiparameter characterization of the neovasculature by dynamic contrast-enhanced MRI. *Magn Reson Med* 2004; **52:** 741–750.
14. Israely T, Nevo N, Harmelin A, Neeman M, Tsafriri A. Reducing ischaemic damage in rodent ovarian xenografts transplanted into granulation tissue. *Hum Reprod* 2006; **21:** 1368–1379.
15. Qi S, Ma A, Xu D, Daloze P, Chen H. Cryopreservation of vascularized ovary: an evaluation of histology and function in rats. *Microsurgery* 2008; **28:** 380–386.
16. Oktay K. Ovarian tissue cryopreservation and transplantation: preliminary findings and implications for cancer patients. *Hum Reprod Update* 2001; **7:** 526–534.
17. Oktay K, Karlikaya G. Ovarian function after transplantation of frozen, banked autologous ovarian tissue. *N Engl J Med* 2000; **342:** 1919.
18. Bedaiwy MA, Hussein MR, Biscotti C, Falcone T. Cryopreservation of intact human ovary with its vascular pedicle. *Hum Reprod* 2006; **21:** 3258–3269.
19. Martinez-Madrid B, Dolmans MM, Van Langendonckt A, Defrere S, Donnez J. Freeze–thawing intact human ovary with its vascular pedicle with a passive cooling device. *Fertil Steril* 2004; **82:** 1390–1394.
20. Silber SJ, DeRosa M, Pineda J, *et al.* A series of monozygotic twins discordant for ovarian failure: ovary transplantation (cortical versus microvascular) and cryopreservation. *Hum Reprod* 2008; **23:** 1531–1537.
21. Gosden RG. Ovary and uterus transplantation. *Reproduction* 2008; **136:** 671–680.
22. Martinez-Madrid B, Camboni A, Dolmans MM, *et al.* Apoptosis and ultrastructural assessment after cryopreservation of whole human ovaries with their vascular pedicle. *Fertil Steril* 2007; **87:** 1153–1165.
23. Falcone T, Attaran M, Bedaiwy MA, Goldberg JM. Ovarian function preservation in the cancer patient. *Fertil Steril* 2004; **81:** 243–257.
24. Guttman FM, Lizin J, Robitaille P, Blanchard H, Turgeon-Knaack C. Survival of canine kidneys after treatment with dimethyl-sulfoxide, freezing at −80 degrees C, and thawing by microwave illumination. *Cryobiology* 1977; **14:** 559–567.
25. Guttman FM, Robitaille P, Lizin J, Blanchard H. Physiologic investigation of frozen–thawed canine kidneys. *Transpl Proc* 1977; **9:** 255–256.
26. Wang X, Chen H, Yin H, *et al.* Fertility after intact ovary transplantation. *Nature* 2002; **415:** 385.
27. Yin H, Wang X, Kim SS, *et al.* Transplantation of intact rat gonads using vascular anastomosis: effects of cryopreservation, ischaemia and genotype. *Hum Reprod* 2003; **18:** 1165–1172.
28. Winston RM, Browne JC. Pregnancy following autograft transplantation of Fallopian tube and ovary in the rabbit. *Lancet* 1974; **ii:** 494–495.
29. Goding JR, McCracken JA, Baird DT. The study of ovarian function in the ewe by means of a vascular autotransplantation technique. *J Endocrinol* 1967; **39:** 37–52.
30. Jeremias E, Bedaiwy MA, Gurunluoglu R, *et al.* Heterotopic autotransplantation of the ovary with microvascular anastomosis: a novel surgical technique. *Fertil Steril* 2002; **77:** 1278–1282.
31. Paldi E, Gal D, Barzilai A, Hampel N, Malberger E. Genital organs. Auto and homotransplantation in forty dogs. *Int J Fertil* 1975; **20:** 5–12.
32. Scott JR, Keye WR, Poulson AM, Reynolds WA. Microsurgical ovarian transplantation in the primate. *Fertil Steril* 1981; **36:** 512–515.
33. Mhatre P, Mhatre J, Magotra R. Ovarian transplant: a new frontier. *Trans Proc* 2005; **37:** 1396–1398.
34. Leporrier M, von Theobald P, Roffe JL, Muller G. A new technique to protect ovarian function before pelvic irradiation. Heterotopic ovarian autotransplantation. *Cancer* 1987; **60:** 2201–2204.
35. Hilders CG, Baranski AG, Peters L, Ramkhelawan A, Trimbos JB. Successful human ovarian autotransplantation to the upper arm. *Cancer* 2004; **101:** 2771–2778.
36. Bedaiwy MA, Jeremias E, Gurunluoglu R, *et al.* Restoration of ovarian function after autotransplantation of intact frozen–thawed sheep ovaries with microvascular anastomosis. *Fertil Steril* 2003; **79:** 594–602.
37. Falcone T, Bedaiwy MA. Cryopreservation of intact ovaries: size is a variable? *Fertil Steril* 2005; **83:** 1587; author reply 8.
38. Revel A, Elami A, Bor A, *et al.* Whole sheep ovary cryopreservation and transplantation. *Fertil Steril* 2004; **82:** 1714–1715.
39. Grazul-Bilska AT, Banerjee J, Yazici I, *et al.* Morphology and function of cryopreserved whole ovine ovaries after heterotopic autotransplantation. *Reprod Biol Endocrinol* 2008; **6:** 16.
40. Arav A, Revel A, Nathan Y, *et al.* Oocyte recovery, embryo development and ovarian function after

cryopreservation and transplantation of whole sheep ovary. *Hum Reprod* 2005; **20:** 3554–3559.

41. Imhof M, Hofstetter G, Bergmeister H, *et al.* Cryopreservation of a whole ovary as a strategy for restoring ovarian function. *J Assist Reprod Genet* 2004; **21:** 459–465.
42. Imhof M, Bergmeister H, Lipovac M. Orthotopic microvascular reanastomosis of whole cryopreserved ovine ovaries resulting in pregnancy and live birth. *Fertil Steril* 2006; **85**(Suppl 1): 1208–1215.
43. Fahy GM, Wowk B, Wu J, *et al.* Cryopreservation of organs by vitrification: perspectives and recent advances. *Cryobiology* 2004; **48:** 157–178.
44. Rall WF, Fahy GM. Ice-free cryopreservation of mouse embryos at −196 degrees C by vitrification. *Nature* 1985; **313:** 573–575.
45. Kheirabadi BS, Fahy GM. Permanent life support by kidneys perfused with a vitrifiable (7.5 molar) cryoprotectant solution. *Transplantation* 2000; **70:** 51–57.
46. Courbiere B, Massardier J, Salle B, *et al.* Follicular viability and histological assessment after cryopreservation of whole sheep ovaries with vascular pedicle by vitrification. *Fertil Steril* 2005; **84**(Suppl 2): 1065–1071.
47. Courbiere B, Caquant L, Mazoyer C, *et al.* Difficulties improving ovarian functional recovery by microvascular transplantation and whole ovary vitrification. *Fertil Steril* 2009; **91**: 2697–2706.
48. Bedaiwy MA, Falcone T. Technical challenges in freeze–thawing of human ovary. *Fertil Steril* 2005; **83:** 1068–1069; author reply 1069–1070.
49. Jadoul P, Donnez J, Dolmans MM, *et al.* Laparoscopic ovariectomy for whole human ovary cryopreservation: technical aspects. *Fertil Steril* 2007; **87:** 971–975.
50. Patrizio P, Gavish Z, Martel M, *et al.* Whole human ovary cryopreservation using a novel multi-gradient freezing device. *Fertil Steril* 2007; **87**(Suppl 1): s355.
51. Patrizio P, Bromer JGJJ, Martel M, Silber S, Arav A. Cryopreservation of eleven whole human ovaries: histology, immunohistochemistry, and technical details. *Fertil Steril* 2008; **88**(Suppl 1): s38.
52. Patrizio P, Arav A, Bromer JG, Martel M, Azodi M, Silber S. Cryopreservation of whole human ovaries together with fallopian tubes. *Fertil Steril* 2008; **88**(Suppl 1): s38.

Chapter 26

Transplantation of whole frozen–thawed ovaries

Amir Arav and Yehudit Natan

Introduction

Transplantation attempts were performed well before people had the knowledge and skill for it to succeed. The Chinese physician Pien Chi'ao (550 BC) reportedly exchanged hearts between a man of strong spirit but weak will with one of a man of weak spirit but strong will in an attempt to achieve balance in each man [1]. In the second century, the Indian surgeon Sushruta used autografted skin transplantation in nose reconstruction rhinoplasty [2], and there are accounts of the third-century saints Damian and Cosmas replacing the gangrenous leg of the Roman deacon Justinian with the leg of a recently deceased Ethiopian [3]. Most accounts have the saints performing the transplant in the fourth century, decades after their deaths; some accounts have them only instructing living surgeons who performed the procedure.

These transplantation attempts were not well documented and so the outcome is in most cases unknown. Today we know that three main factors determine successful transplantation: (1) surgical technique, (2) overcoming rejection, and (3) maintaining the transplant viable.

Alexis Carrel, a French surgeon, was the major pioneer of vascular surgery. He was working in 1902 at the University of Lyons and continued to the University of Chicago and later at the Rockefeller Institute for Medical Research. He performed with Charles Guthrie skillful anastomosis operations and developed new suturing techniques. This laid the groundwork for later transplant surgery and won Carrel the 1912 Nobel Prize for Medicine or Physiology. From 1902, Carrel performed transplant experiments on dogs. He was surgically successful in moving kidneys, hearts, and spleens and was one of the first to identify the problem of rejection, which remained insurmountable for decades.

Carrel in his Nobel Prize lecture of 1912 said the following about organ transplantation, "... Many surgeons before me have had this idea, but they were prevented from applying it, owing to the lack of a method for reestablishing immediately a normal circulation through the transplanted structures" [4].

Rejection has been a major obstacle in transplantation attempts. In 1597, the Italian surgeon Gasparo Tagliacozzi, who had performed successful skin autografts and failing consistently with allografts, offered the first suggestion of rejection as the "force and power of individuality" in his work *De Curtorum Chirurgia per Insitionem Libri Duo.*

In 1933, Dr. YuYu Voronoy in Russia attempted allogeneic transplantation of a human kidney. A kidney was taken from a recently deceased individual and connected to a young woman who was suffering from lead poisoning. No immunosuppression was given. The kidney never functioned [5]. In the late 1940s, Peter Medawar, working for the National Institute for Medical Research, performed experiments that for the first time defined the immunology of transplantation and improved the understanding of rejection. For his pioneering work in transplant immunology, Dr. Medawar received the Nobel Prize in Medicine in 1960 [6]. The development of immunosuppressant drugs and the finding of cyclosporine altered transplants from research surgery to life-saving treatment. Belzer [7] and Collins [8] provided a grounding in organ preservation that enabled organs to be retrieved at one location and transported to the site of the recipient surgery.

The first pioneer of ovarian transplantation was Paul Bert in 1863 in Paris [9]. He had experimented with rabbits and his initial results were disappointing. However, the work was continued by others and in 1895 the first transplantation in a human was reported by Robert Morris, a New York surgeon [10]. One of the major obstacles that needs to be overcome is to establish blood flow to the transplanted ovary. The main

Fertility Cryopreservation, ed. Ri-Cheng Chian and Patrick Quinn. Published by Cambridge University Press.

disadvantage of grafting ovarian tissue over whole ovary is the shorter lifetime of the tissue, which is limited to 3 years. Vascular anastomosis and minimizing ischemia time significantly reduces follicle losses [11].

Some gynecological surgeons took up the challenge, but evidently with limited success, probably because of the tiny ovarian artery. Nevertheless, 1906 was an annus mirabilis for ovarian transplantation, with a live birth of a baby girl to a woman who had undergone an ovarian homograft transplant by Morris [12].

Ovarian slices and ovary freezing overview

Audrey Smith, known as the mother of cryobiology, discovered the cryoprotectant glycerol with Christopher Polge and Alan Parkes [13]. She was the first to try and freeze a whole organ and performed many of the early freezing experiments, trying to freeze different cells, organs, and even an entire animal. In 1951, Smith and Parkes [14] tried freezing large slices of rat ovaries (the ovary was cut into three slices) with 15% glycerol. Good results were only achieved when slow freezing was performed but the slices showed reduced viability after 10 days storage at −79°C. Ovaries minced in serum without protective agents were viable after 9 days at −79°C storage but not after 1 hour at −190°C. Different parameters were evaluated and the best survival was achieved when the ovarian slices were frozen with 15–25% glycerol in rat serum, with a pre-freezing incubation of 5–15 minutes at room temperature, and a slow cooling rate of 1–2°C/min. Other cryoprotectants were evaluated (ethylene glycol, propylene glycol, diethylene glycol) but were not as effective as glycerol. Grafts of frozen–thawed ovarian tissue were transplanted into sterilized irradiated mice, which could be fertilized and give rise to normal offspring [15]. These studies were summarized by Smith [16].

Cryopreservation and transplantation of ovarian tissue has been successfully performed in animals such as rodents, rabbits, dogs, ewes, and marmoset monkeys [17–20]. In addition, cryopreservation of human ovarian slices has been shown to be successful in animal models. Today, women are being offered the option to cryopreserve ovarian tissue slices prior to chemo- or radiotherapy in many centers in the world. However, to date, only two deliveries of babies with this technology [21,22] have been reported. The main problem with ovarian slices is that there is an ischemic period between the transplantation of the graft and revascularization.

Fresh ovarian vascular transplantations have been performed successfully in rabbits [23], sheep [24], dogs [25], monkeys [26], and humans [27].

The first successful cryopreservation and transplantation of an intact ovary was described in 2001 [28,29]. Following this, other groups have reported successful cryopreservation and transplantation of an intact ovary. In 2002, Wang *et al.* [30] reported the cryopreservation and subsequent transplantation of rat ovaries and reproductive tract. Four out of seven rats survived for 60 or more days and the transplants were ovulatory and resulted in one pregnancy. Chen *et al.* [31] have performed transplants of frozen–thawed rabbit ovaries that showed functionality for up to 7 months after microvascular transplantation in 13 out of 15 animals.

However, cryopreservation of organs of large mammals and humans is a much more complicated task. Nevertheless, Arav and colleagues have successfully cryopreserved and transplanted whole ovaries with their vascular pedicle in five sheep, showing functionality in three for 24 to 36 months after the transplantation [32]. Currently, we have shown functionality in two out of the three sheep with successful transplants at 6 years after the transplant [33].

Heat and mass transfers in large tissues

Heat transfer from an organ (cooling) and to an organ (heating) is conventionally by convection (liquid nitrogen vapor, alcohol bath, cold air, water bath). Heat transfer by convection always begins from the outer part of the organ and progresses towards its center. Additionally, heat transfer through gas or liquid material (convection) is slower relatively to solid material (conduction).

Similarly to heat transfer, mass transfers through tissue and organ suffer from the same limitations. In order for organs to be cryopreserved, cryoprotective agents (CPAs) must be introduced into the organ. The best way for doing that is by vascular perfusion. The CPAs used are usually low-molecular-weight molecules that penetrate the cells membrane by diffusion, such as dimethyl sulfoxide (DMSO), glycerol, and ethylene glycol. The perfusion procedure might damage the organ and the CPAs are toxic at the concentrations needed to promote a protective effect during slow freezing. Perfusing a freezing solution for 3 minutes through a sheep ovary is enough to saturate the organ with the CPAs [32].

During the freezing process, water freezes and the concentration of solutes increases; as a result, the cells are exposed to increasing concentrations of the CPAs and this has a detrimental effect on cell viability [34]. The aim in a slow-freezing process is to have a protocol that is slow enough to dehydrate the cells in order to prevent intracellular crystallization and fast enough to minimize osmotic stress to the cells.

In general the type of damage that occurs in large tissues and organs is similar to the damage that occurs to large volumes of cell suspensions, although, the presence of extracellular ice, which may not be problematic with cell suspensions, can be a major problem when freezing tissues/organs [35]. For example, isolated chondrocytes can survive freezing but the same freezing conditions will not allow successful freezing of cartilage tissue [36].

Thermal gradient versus cooling rate

In order to successfully freeze a biological sample, cooling needs to occur at a rate that permits dehydration of the cells down to a level that will form a glass when the solution reaches its glass transition temperature. The cells can be preserved below the glass transition temperature in an amorphous state for long periods. Dehydration occurs because of the increasing solute concentration as the freezing process progress, causing water to flow out of the cells by exosmosis. Cooling too slowly will extend the exposure time of the cells to an increasingly concentrated and toxic solution, whereas cooling too rapidly can allow intracellular crystallization to occur. Most cell suspensions will require slow-cooling rates of around 1°C/min. However, there is evidence that a large tissue or a whole organ will require much slower cooling rates [37]. When trying to freeze a large tissue or a whole organ, one of the major problems is that cooling rates will vary across the sample depending on the geometry (surface, depth, and volume) and the heat conductivity.

Another issue is supercooling; supercooling is a non-equilibrium thermodynamic state in which a solution is cooled below its freezing point without crystallization. It is dependent on time, volume, and viscosity [38]. In certain tissues/organs where the extracellular matrix has small volume and high viscosity, intracellular crystallization can occur owing to the supercooling conditions.

To start the dehydration of cells, ice crystals need to form in the solution. If ice formation does not start at the freezing point temperature (supercooling), there is a risk that ice will form intracellular and will kill the cell. If ice formation is not induced by seeding, ice will form spontaneously when the solution is cooled sufficiently far below its equilibrium melting point. This will cause three kinds of problems. First, since ice formation will occur at random, unpredictable temperatures, the survival rates will be highly variable between repeated trials with the same freezing protocol. Second, when ice does form, the large thermal gradient will cause extremely rapid crystallization, which will damage the cells by inducing mechanical stress through uneven expansion or contraction [39]. Finally, when crystallization starts at low temperatures, water will not leave the cells since dehydration of the cells can only occur within a certain range of subzero temperatures; at lower temperatures, the membrane itself becomes impermeable. Therefore, supercooling must be avoided and crystallization should start at a temperature as close as possible to the freezing point of the solution.

Latent heat

Latent heat is the heat released when crystallization occurs. There are two problems regarding latent heat release. The first problem is that the heat is transferred to colder areas in which the ice has just formed and so it could possibly re-warm the ice and cause local melting. The second problem is that of the isothermal period. When samples of large volume with relatively low surface-to-volume ratios are frozen, the release of latent heat may cause a long isothermal period (or even heating) in the material being frozen. At the same time, the temperature of the cooling mechanism or of the surrounding medium is lowered, thus increasing the temperature difference between the sample and its surroundings. Consequently, when latent heat is no longer released, the temperature of the material being frozen will drop very rapidly to a temperature close to the temperature of the surrounding environment (because the thermal conductivity of water [0–6] is lower than that of ice [1.6]). This might lead to a non-optimal cooling rate and possibly to cellular damage through intracellular crystallization.

Recrystallization

Slow thawing is known to be a major destructive factor. The longer the duration of the thawing period, the greater is the damage that occurs to the cells from the increase in solute effects and the maximal growth of ice crystals. Large crystals have an abrasive action, producing mechanical disruption of cells. Crystal growth is maximal in the range from −40°C to 0°C. Disruptive ultrastructural changes in cells increase by recrystallization [40]. Thawing is most destructive if it is completed so that all of the frozen tissue is thawed, which then exposes the tissue to all the effects of recrystallization. Basically, there are two types of damage during slow thawing; the first is recrystallization, which is the growth of ice that was formed during freezing, and the second is refreezing of the solution, which occurs after complete thawing. It is not necessary to distinguish between the two events since both are destructive and both are the result of too slow a warming rate.

Resolution of heat transfer problems

Freezing of large volume samples

Cryopreservation of samples of large volume (i.e. tissues, organs, or large volumes of semen [41]) is associated with heat and mass transfer problems that are distinct from those associated with an isolated cell model. In a macroscopic sample, there may be a large thermal gradient from the surface to the interior of the system [35,42]. As a result, the cooling rate, which should be precisely controlled [43], is difficult to predict, especially when a very slow cooling rate is required (1°C/min, the optimal cooling rate for most cells). In addition, the existing temperature gradient within the freezing chamber and the unreliability of temperature measurements [44] make it more difficult to achieve an optimal cooling rate.

Directional freezing principles

The multigradient temperature change approach

A new freezing method, the "multigradient directional cooling and warming of biological samples" [45], aims to overcome the problems discussed above and allow cryopreservation of samples of large volume. The technology is based on a series of heat conductive blocks (usually built of brass or aluminum) arranged in a line, with a straight track running through the blocks (Figure 26.1). Along the blocks, different temperatures can be set, thereby imposing a temperature gradient along the blocks. The blocks are separated by a gap and the temperature of the block on one side of the gap is above the freezing point temperature and on the other side of the gap is below the freezing point temperature, thereby imposing a temperature gradient across the gap. Biological samples to be frozen or thawed are placed inside test tubes and are moved along the track

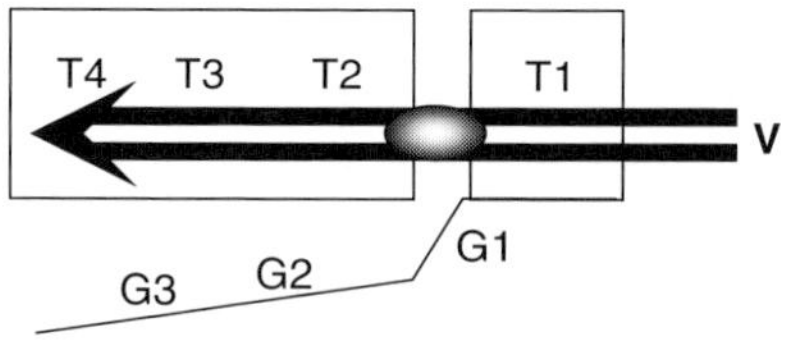

Figure 26.1. Schematic sketch of a directional freezing apparatus. Blocks can be set at different temperatures (T1–T4), thereby imposing a temperature gradient along the blocks (G1–G3).

at a certain velocity. The samples are frozen at rates that are specified in a protocol; the rate of freezing is given by the temperature gradient multiplied by the velocity.

Advantages of the multigradient approach

There are a number of advantages to a set up that allows a gradient of temperatures to be imposed on a sample of large volume.

1. A linear thermal gradient can be generated in an organ/tissue to be cooled. Heat transfer can then be changed in a directional way according to the heat conductivity in the sample (i.e. 0.01–0.06 mm/s; $G_2 = 0.17$ °C/mm). The movement of the organ in the thermal gradient should not exceed this velocity to ensure that heat will remain directional. In this way, heat conductivity will propagate in the tissue in a linear way and thermal history (cooling rate) for each point in the organ will be equally the same.
2. Heat transfer in directional solidification is opposed to the direction of movement. This occurs when the velocity is slower than the speed at which the heat is removed from the center of the sample towards its periphery. This means that latent heat is removed towards the direction of the liquid and towards the conductive material of which the device is built.
3. In directional freezing, ice formation (nucleation) is determined by the solution's freezing point temperature. Therefore, supercooling is avoided completely.
4. The freezing technology is based on directional freezing in which the biological material is transferred through a linear temperature gradient so that the cooling rate and ice front propagation are precisely controlled. Maximizing the survival rate of cells subjected to freezing and thawing requires careful control of the freezing process, here set by the interface velocity. Using cryomicroscopy observations, it has been shown that survival of sperm demonstrates a biphasic curve. At a very slow

velocity, ice will grow in a planer form, which will kill all cells; at a higher velocity, ice crystals form secondary branches and survival will increase. However, at even higher velocities (i.e. 0.3 mm/s), ice will start to form needle-like crystals, which will decrease post-thaw viability. If velocity is increased very high survival is permitted [45] depending on the space between the ice crystals. Finally, at even higher velocities (i.e. > 4 mm/s), directional solidification will not occur and survival will decrease.

Freezing whole ovaries

In experiments where whole sheep ovaries were frozen, the freezing protocol was optimized to 0.1°C/min from −6°C to −35°C. After storage in liquid nitrogen for 1 to 4 weeks, the ovaries were thawed rapidly by using a 66°C water bath and perfusion with University of Wisconsin (UW) solution containing 0.5 M sucrose, following washing with UW. After an initial in vitro study using ovaries from a slaughterhouse, the experiments were extended to include whole ovaries of live animals. Five sheep have undergone successful autotransplantation of the frozen–thawed ovary to the contralateral ovarian pedicle by end-to-end anastomosis, with functioning ovaries in three animals. Functionality includes hormonal cyclicity, presence of follicles, and retrieval of competent oocytes [32]. Two heifers have functioning frozen–thawed and transplanted ovaries out of three trials [46].

Six years follow-up of transplanted ovaries

Six years after successful transplantation of frozen–thawed ovaries into the three sheep, and after inducing superovulation, the sheep were sacrificed and the ovaries analyzed. Two of the three ovaries were of normal size and shape, showing some recent corpora lutea, while the third showed atrophic changes. A total of 36 antral follicles were counted by transillumination (Figure 26.2) and four germinal vesicle oocytes were aspirated and matured in vitro to metaphase II. Serial serum progesterone levels were indicative of ovulatory activity in two of the three sheep. Histological evaluation revealed normal tissue architecture, including follicles at various developmental stages and intact blood vessels.

To date, this is the longest recorded ovarian functional survival of whole sheep ovaries cryopreserved and then transplanted. Cryopreservation of whole ovaries, using the directional freezing technology combined with microvascular anastomosis, is a very promising method for preserving long-term reproductive capacity and endocrine function.

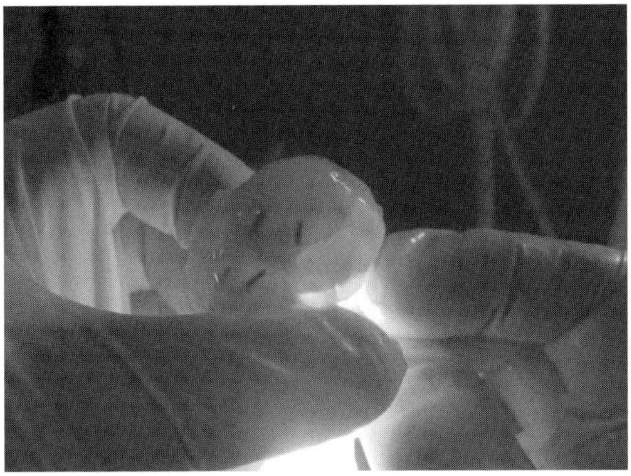

Figure 26.2. Excised ovary (sheep) showing antral follicles by transillumination (also shown are the sutures left of the artery and vein anastomosis).

Freezing other organs

Hearts

Long-term organ preservation for transplantation may allow optimal donor–recipient matching, with potential reduction in the incidence and severity of rejection. Complete cessation of metabolism may be obtained by freezing. Previous attempts to freeze intact mammalian hearts have been limited to a temperature of −3.6°C, which restricted tissue ice content to 34%.

In a study by Elami *et al.* [47], four isolated rat hearts were attached to a Langendorff apparatus. After normothermic perfusion, cold cardioplegia was induced followed by perfusion with a cryoprotecting agent. The hearts were then frozen to −8°C, thawed, and reperfused for 60 minutes. All frozen–thawed hearts regained normal electric activity. At −8°C, ice content was 64%. Mean recovery was to 65.2% (SD, 30.8) of coronary flow and 50.4% (SD, 23.9) of left ventricular developed pressure. The hearts maintained 81.3% viability compared with 69.3% (not significant) in control hearts kept at 0°C for the same duration. The integrity of muscle fibers and intracellular organelles after thawing and reperfusion was demonstrated by electron microscopy [47].

Liver

A study by Gavish *et al.* [48] demonstrates for the first time the feasibility of recovering a functional liver after low temperature storage. This study utilized a newly developed technique to freeze and thaw large organs such as the liver. After freezing and keeping the frozen livers in storage for up to 21 days, the livers were thawed and their viability was tested by means of cellular and tissue integrity and in an auxiliary liver transplantation in pigs. The livers demonstrated viability of over 80% and maintained their structural integrity and bile production ability.

Conclusions

One of the most difficult issues for patients needing organ transplants is the narrow time window needed between the donation and transplantation of the donated organ. The situation is complicated by the logistical challenges of handling these life-giving donations and maintaining organ viability until the time of transplant. With the donation of a human liver, a healthcare provider is restricted to only a few hours of harvest, transport, and transplant time, which precludes optimal pathogen screening and donor–recipient matching between remote locations. Because of these time constraints, matching is limited to blood type and patient size. This creates a risk of immunological mismatches and increases the likelihood of organ rejection. Other types of organs face similar issues, with the clock ticking rapidly when scarce organs become available.

The biggest challenge for research is to prolong the shelf-life of donated organs, allowing more people in more places to be matched with the optimal life-saving organs they desperately need. Improved the ability to match donors and recipients would also help to decrease rejection rates and reduce the intensity of immunosuppression treatments after transplantation. This would be expected to improve patient outcomes while reducing the cost of care.

References

1. Woodford P. Transplantation timeline. *Natl Rev Med* 2004; **1,** No. 2.
2. Dwived G, Dwivedi S. History of medicine. Sushrua: the clinician–teacher par excellence. *Indian J Chest Dis Allied Sci* 2007; **49:** 243–244.
3. Conolly BW, Benanzio M. Cosmas and Damian revisited. In Lanzetta M, Dubernard J-M, Petruzzo P, eds. *Hand Transplantation*. Milan: Springer Milan, 2007, pp.3–10.
4. Lindsten J (ed.) *Nobel Lectures, Physiology or Medicine 1901–1921*. Amsterdam: Elsevier, 1967.
5. Petechuk D. *Organ Transplantation*. Westport, CT: Greenwood Press, 2006, p. 10.
6. Lindsten J (ed.) *Nobel Lectures, Physiology or Medicine 1941–1962*. Amsterdam: Elsevier, 1964.
7. Belzer FO, Ashby BS, Gulyassy PF. Successful seventeen-hour preservation and transplantation of human cadaver kidney. *N Engl J Med* 1968; **278:** 608–610.
8. Collins GM, Bravo-Shugarman M, Terasaki PI. Kidney preservation for transplantation. Initial perfusion and 30 hours' ice storage. *Lancet* 1969; **ii**: 1219–1222.
9. Tuland T, Gosden RG. *Preservation of Fertility*. London: Informa HealthCare, 2004, p. 158.
10. Simmer HH. Robert Tuttle Morris (1857–1945): a pioneer in ovarian transplant. *Obstet Gynecol* 1970; **35:** 314–328.
11. Yin H, Wang X, Kim SS, *et al.* Transplantation of intact rat gonads using vascular anastomosis: effects of cryopreservation. *Hum Reprod* 2003; **18:** 1165–1172.
12. Morris RT. A case of heteroplastic ovarian grafting followed by pregnancy and the delivery of a living child. *Med Rec* 1906; **69:** 697–698.
13. Polge C, Smith AU, Parkes AS. Revival of spermatozoa after vitrification and dehydration at low temperatures. *Nature* 1949; **164:** 666.
14. Smith AU, Parkes AS. Preservation of ovarian tissue at low temperatures. *Lancet* 1951; **ii**: 570–572.
15. Parrott DMV. The fertility of mice with orthotopic ovarian grafts derived from frozen tissue. *J Reprod Fertil* 1960; **1:** 230–241.
16. Smith AU. *Biological Effects of Freezing and Supercooling*. Baltimore, MD: Williams & Wilkins, 1961.
17. Candy J, Wood MJ, Whittingham DG. Follicular development in cryopreserved marmoset ovarian tissue after transplantation. *Hum Reprod* 1995; **10:** 2234–2238.
18. Candy CJ, Wood MJ, Whittingham DG. Restoration of a normal reproductive lifespan after grafting cryopreserved mouse ovaries. *Hum Reprod* 2000; **15:** 1300–1304.
19. Salle B, Demirei B, Franck M, *et al.* Normal pregnancies and live births after autograft of frozen thawed hemi-ovaries into ewes. *Fertil Steril* 2002; **77:** 403–408.
20. Almodin CG, Minguetti-Camara VC, Meister H, *et al.* Recovery of fertility after grafting of cryopreserved germinative tissue in female rabbits following radiotherapy. *Hum Reprod* 2004; **19:** 1287–1293.
21. Donnes J, Dolmans MM, Demylle D, *et al.* Livebirth after orthotopic transplantation of cryopreserved ovarian tissue. *Lancet* 2004; **364:** 1405–1410.
22. Meirow D, Levron J, Eldar-Geva T, *et al.* Pregnancy after transplantation of cryopreserved ovarian tissue in a patient with ovarian failure after chemotherapy. *N Engl J Med* 2005; **353:** 318–321.
23. Winston RM, Browne JC. Pregnancy following autograft of Fallopian tube and ovary in rabbit. Lancet 1974; **ii:** 494–495.
24. Godding JR, McCracken JA, Baird DT. The study of ovarian function in the ewe by means of vascular autotransplantation technique. *J Endocrinol* 1967; **39:** 37–52.

25. Paldi E, Gal D, Barlizai A, Hampel N, Alberger EM. Genital organs: auto and homotransplantation in forty dogs. *Int J Feril* 1974; **20:** 5–12.
26. Scott JR, Keye WR, Poulson AM, Reynolds WA. Microsurgical ovarian transplantation in the primate. *Fertil Steril* 1981; **36:** 512–515.
27. Leporrier M, von Theobald P, Roffe JL, Muller G. A new technique to protect ovarian function before pelvic irradiation. Heterotopic ovarian autotransplantation. *Cancer* 1987; **60:** 2201–2204.
28. Arav A, Elami A, Bor A, *et al.* Successfully whole organ cryopreservation and transplantation. In *Annual Meeting of the American Society of Reproductive Medicine,* Orlando, USA, October 2001.
29. Revel A, Elami A, Bor A, *et al.* Whole ovary cryopreservation and transplantation in sheep. *Fertil Steril* 2001; **76**: S42–S43.
30. Wang X, Chen H, Yin H, *et al.* Fertility after intact ovary transplantation. *Nature* 2002; **415:** 385.
31. Chen C, Chen S, Chang F, *et al.* Autologous heterotopic transplantation of intact rabbit ovary after cryopreservation. *Hum Reprod* 2005; **20**(Suppl 1): i145–i150.
32. Arav A, Revel A, Nathan Y, *et al.* Oocyte recovery, embryo development and ovarian function after cryopreservation and transplantation of whole sheep ovary. *Hum Reprod* 2005; **20:** 3554–3559.
33. Arav A Gavish Z, Elami E, *et al.* Ovarian function 6 years after cryopreservation and transplantation of whole sheep ovaries. *Reprod BioMed Online* 2010; **20:** 48–52.
34. Mazur P. Cryobiology: the freezing of biological systems. *Science* 1970; **168:** 939–949.
35. Karlsson JO, Toner M. Long term storage of tissue by cryopreservation: critical issues. *Biomaterials* 1996; **17:** 243–256.
36. Pegg DE, Wang L, Vaughan D, Hunt CJ. Cryopreservation of articular cartilage. Part 2: mechanisms of cryoinjury. *Cryobiology* 2006; **52:** 347–359.
37. Hubel A, Toner M, Cravalho EG, Yermush ML, Tompkins RG. Intracellular ice formation during the freezing of hepatocytes cultured in double collagen gel. *Biotechnol Prog* 1991; **7:** 554–559.
38. Yavin S, Arav A. Measurements of essential physical properties of vitrification solution. *Theriogenology* 2007; **67:** 81–89.
39. Fahy GM, Saur J, Williams RJ. Physical problems with the vitrification of large biological systems. *Cryobiology* 1990; **27:** 492–510.
40. Forsyth M, MacFarlane DR. Recrystallization revisited. *Cryo Letters* 1986; **7:** 367–378.
41. Gacitua H, Arav A. Successful pregnancies with directional freezing of large volume buck semen. *Theriogenology* 2005; **63:** 931–938.
42. Diller KR. Modeling of bioheat transfer processes at high and low temperatures. In Cho YI, ed. *Advances in Heat Transfer*, Vol. 221: *Bioengineering Heat Transfer.* San Diego, CA: Academic Press, 1992, pp. 157–357.
43. Mazur P. Theoretical and experimental effects of cooling and warming velocity on the survival of frozen and thawed cells. *Cryobiology* 1966; **2:** 181–192.
44. Keobe HG, Werner A, Lange V, Schildberg FW. Temperature gradients in freezing chambers of rate-controlled cooling machines. *Cryobiology* 1993; **30:** 349–352.
45. Arav A, Yavin S, Zeron Y, Natan Y, Dekel I, Gacitua H. New trends in gamete's cryopreservation. *Mol Cell Endocrinol* 2002; **187:** 77–81.
46. Arav A. Large tissue freezing. *J Assist Reprod Genet* 2003; **20:** 351.
47. Elami A, Gavish Z, Korach A, *et al.* Successful restoration of function of frozen and thawed isolated rat hearts. *J Thorac Cardiovasc Surg* 2005; **135:** 666–672.
48. Gavish Z, Ben-Haim M, Arav A. Cryopreservation of whole murine and porcine livers. *Rejuvenation Res* 2008; **11:** 765–772.

Section 6 Chapter 27

Ethical considerations

Ethical considerations in fertility cryopreservation in young cancer patients

Edwin C. Hui

Introduction

This chapter on the ethics of fertility cryopreservation builds on the previous chapters, which have provided the most up-to-date scientific understanding and clinical applications of cryopreservation of human gametes and tissues. The ethical positions represented here are subject to modification and change as new information on the principles and applications of cryobiology becomes available. The discussion excludes approaches to fertility preservation in which freezing–thawing of cells or tissues are not a part (e.g. hormonal gonadoprotection); it includes fertility cryopreservation for pre- and postpubertal male and female adolescents and is written in the context of fertility preservation for cancer patients, although the ethical principles developed here should, in general, apply to more mature men and women seeking fertility preservation for other health issues or for non-therapeutic social reasons (e.g. to postpone having a family).

Cryopreservation of male fertility

Male fertility is highly susceptible to toxic effects of radiation and chemotherapy at all stages of life, and depending on the therapeutic agents used and the duration of treatment, up to 80% of patients may have long-lasting or permanent gonadal dysfunction resulting in oligozoospermia or azoospermia [1,2]. At the same time, it has been shown that 76% of childless cancer survivors, including male and female patients, desire to have children in the future; 80% believe that having had cancer would make them better parents, and 94% feel that they are healthy enough to be good parents [3]. Based on these findings, it seems justified to make it a moral duty of doctors treating young male cancer patients to inform their patients of the risks of post-treatment infertility and the options for fertility cryopreservation available to them, depending on their age and development of sexual organs. The US President's Cancer Panel has endorsed a similar position [4], yet, as many as 40% of male cancer patients do not recall being informed of infertility as a side effect of cancer treatment [5].

Postpubertal males

Cryopreservation of sperm

For postpubertal males, the commonest option is freezing of ejaculated sperm before cancer treatment, followed by artificial insemination, in vitro fertilization (IVF), or intracytoplasmic sperm injection (ICSI) using thawed sperm. The availability of ICSI has greatly enhanced the efficacy of using frozen–thawed sperm, leading to high fertilization and pregnancy rates even when the banked semen samples are not of the best quality because of cancer-related spermatogenic depression. Studies have shown that many oncologists are still unaware of the newer possibilities of assisted reproductive technologies (ART), with the result that young male cancer patients are inadequately informed of their risk of infertility and options available for its reduction [6]. However, as part of the informed consent process, the risks of fertility preservation using frozen–thawed sperm should be clearly explained to the patients prior to banking. These may include possible mutations in the sperm, especially for patients who bank their semen after starting their cancer treatment. But even if semen samples are banked before treatment, cancer patients may have higher aneuploidy rates and increased DNA damage, which may produce long-term adverse genetic effects in their offspring. The possibility of controlling for aneuploidy by preimplantation genetic diagnosis (PGD) may also be suggested to patients, but PGD has both benefits and risks of its own that need to be disclosed (e.g. it is expensive). Some patients may be reluctant to bank sperm because

Fertility Cryopreservation, ed. Ri-Cheng Chian and Patrick Quinn. Published by Cambridge University Press.

of religious or cultural objections to masturbation, which is the most common and least intrusive way to obtain sperm. Such patients should be offered other methods of obtaining sperm, including the non-invasive penile vibratory stimulation. Invasive methods including electroejaculation, which requires a general anesthetic, and surgical retrieval of sperm by either epididymal aspiration or testicular biopsy should not be offered without full disclosure of the invasive nature and the extra risks entailed in these procedures.

When the relevant risks and benefits of fertility preservation have been fully explained to and understood by the patients, prevalent medical ethical norms require that patients be allowed to make a decision to agree or disagree to bank sperm. This is particularly important for adolescent patients since most of them will not be legally empowered to provide consent and parental consent will be required. For sperm banking by an adolescent male cancer patient, there are three possible scenarios: (1) the adolescent assents and the parents give the legal consent; (2) parents consent and the minor does not assent; (3) parents do not consent and minor requests the treatment. The first scenario is fortunately the most common scenario and the attending physician only needs to note two things in particular. First, parents who have just been told of their child's cancer are very anxious, and they are just as vulnerable as the adolescent patients. Since both the adolescent and the parents have to make a major decision in a short time about a procedure with many uncertain ramifications, they must fully understand the purpose of sperm banking and have enough time to weigh the risks and benefits of the procedure in their own personal and socioeconomical contexts. Second, the attending physician should ensure that the adolescent patient is not under undue influence, which can come from two sources, the attending physician and the parents. Doctors, on the one hand, should be aware that they often unintentionally give their offer of medical service to preserve fertility an imperative character – "you may be sorry later if you don't decide to do this now" – and must ensure that this so-called "anticipated decision regret phenomenon" plays no part in the decision-making process. On the other hand, parents of young cancer patients are filled with guilt and they have the tendency to want to take advantage of every available medical option to promote their child's wellbeing; consequently they often are the over-enthusiastic driving force behind the effort to preserve fertility of their child without making an objective assessment of the risks of preserving fertility [7]. These undue influences are coercive in nature and undermine the integrity of the adolescent's assent. An assent made under undue influence or coercion is not an acceptable assent since the requirements of informed assent and informed consent are essentially the same, with the exception that an assent does not authorize physicians to render treatment.

The second and third scenarios are more problematic, at least in jurisdictions where parental authority over minor children is still carefully guarded. In the UK, the second scenario is resolved by the Human Fertilisation and Embryology Act (HFEA), which stipulates that "it is legally impossible for anyone to give consent for storage of gametes on behalf of another. Thus people with parental responsibility cannot give consent on behalf of the child" [9]. Hence, unless the adolescent is judged to be legally competent to consent and gives consent, cryopreservation of sperm will not take place. In the UK, the Family Law Reform Act (1969) also resolves the third scenario, by empowering adolescents 16 years of age and over to consent to medical treatment without parental agreement, provided that they are not incompetent. Adolescents under the age of 16 years may also consent to treatment if in the judgment of the attending physician the adolescent has the mental capacity to make the decision [10]. In the USA, where parents make decisions on the basis of their children's best interest, the parents will have to decide whether the importance of preserving the possibility of having genetically related offspring in the future outweighs the current risk of sperm cryopreservation for the child in the second and third scenarios [8]. This sentiment is shared by many people from cultures that emphasize the importance of family blood lineage such as the Chinese. Physicians providing care for adolescent cancer patients should be sensitive of cultural influences that may bear on parental decisions to favor preservation of fertility.

Prepubertal males

Cryopreservation of testicular tissue

Fertility preservation for prepubertal male cancer patients is technically and ethically more complex than for postpubertal males. The only option for these patients is removal of testicular tissue surgically from the patient prior to cancer treatment and to store the cryopreserved tissue for use in the future to restore fertility through autologous transplantation, xenografting, or in vitro maturation. Since these approaches to use cryopreserved testicular tissues are still considered to be experimental, their employment is regulated by medical research protocols in addition to conventional medical norms. Since most, if not all, prepubertal male patients are of minority age, all the restrictions for postpubertal minors discussed above apply to these patients. In addition, there are additional risks with cryopreservation of testicular tissues. First, testicular biopsy and subsequent re-implantation are considerably more invasive than any form of sperm banking; second, and more importantly, there is a real risk of re-implanting malignant cells together with cryopreserved tissues or cells, especially in adolescent patients with hematological cancers. For an experimental procedure to be applied to a minor adolescent, the local institutional review board (IRB) would require that the experimental intervention can be shown to promote the best interest of the minor patient and that there is a reasonable chance for the patient to gain a net benefit from the procedure. In the USA, cryopreservation of testicular tissue can proceed with parental consent and adolescent assent (assuming that the minor is competent to assent). But if the adolescent patient is too immature to comprehend, the parents are allowed to decide on the basis of the minor's best interest.

Since the cryopreserved testicular tissue may not be used until some time later when the adolescent recovers from his cancer, there is a good chance that the adolescent may either become competent to assent or reach the age of majority for consent. Potentially, at such a time, the adolescent may refuse re-implantation of immature germ cells or in vitro maturation of the germ cells that his parents have previously consented to store. For that matter, an adolescent who has previously assented to cryopreservation of testicular tissue may change his mind and opt for no further treatment. This illustrates the dynamic nature of consent taking in medical decision making, which is always a process rather than an event. To resolve this problem, a two-stage consenting process can be adopted, with the first stage primarily concerned with harvesting and cryostoring of gonadal tissues and the second stage in relation to manipulating and using the tissues to restore fertility. The ownership of the preserved tissue may also be decided in the second stage [11]. The advantage of such a two-stage consenting process becomes evident in the case of an adolescent who is too immature to assent at the time his gonadal tissue is removed, and his parents provide the consent for the first stage on the presumption that such an intervention may be beneficial to their adolescent child; this does not preclude the adolescent from exercising his autonomy in the second stage when he becomes competent enough to take ownership and full control over the use of the tissue to restore fertility. The adolescent may also exercise his right to decide how to dispose of the cryopreserved tissue in the event he decides not to restore fertility or dies. For the two-stage consent process to work, the adolescent will have to acquire mental competence at some point in the period after his tissue has been cryopreserved and before it is used to restore fertility. The two-stage process collapses if, for example, the adolescent becomes permanently incompetent owing to his cancer, disease, or treatment, or if he dies while receiving treatment for his cancer. For this reason, some institutions recommend that parental rights should be limited to the first stage of the consent process and excluded from deciding about the use or disposal of the preserved tissue under all circumstances [7].

In the UK, because of the stipulations of the HFEA about human gametes discussed above, if an adolescent is prepubertal and pre-Tanner stage II (in the six Tanner grades of puberty) [12], then his testicular tissue is unlikely to contain gametes as defined by HFEA as "a cell with a haploid set of chromosomes which is able to take part in fertilization with another of the opposite sex to form a zygote" [9]. This implies that cryopreservation of the testicular tissue can be consented by parents as long as the adolescent assents. However, when the cryopreserved testicular tissue is subsequently manipulated in vitro to create "gametes," then only a competent adolescent is empowered to give consent. This closely resembles the two-stage consent process discussed above except that parents of a prepubertal adolescent who has reached Tanner stage II or beyond would not be allowed to consent to tissue preservation since the adolescent's testicular tissue may contain haploid cells that are defined by HFEA as "gametes." In such a case, only the adolescent can give consent, and only if he is competent to do so.

Cryopreservation of female fertility

Postpubertal females

Cryopreservation of embryos

Like their male counterparts, postpubertal female patients have the advantage of producing mature gametes in their effort to preserve fertility before anti-cancer therapy. However, unlike male gametes, cryopreservation of mature human oocytes results in extensive damage. Hence, at present, the most clinically established approach for fertility cryopreservation in postpubertal females is to fertilize the mature oocytes in vitro and follow this by embryo cryopreservation for future transfer and implantation. In contrast to human oocytes, the human embryo is very resistant to damage caused by cryopreservation, with a post-thaw survival rate anywhere from 35% to 90%. Since the first report of a successful pregnancy using a frozen–thawed embryo in 1983, frozen embryo replacement has become a routine practice in ART [13]. This approach requires the cooperation of the patient's partner, who must be willing to donate sperm and create embryos for future use; alternatively, the patient must be willing to use donor sperm for fertilization. This approach also would not benefit those who for cultural or religious reasons hold the view that human embryos are full human persons with the right to life, since human embryos cannot be frozen for longer than 5 to 10 years, at the end of which they will be destroyed unless they are adopted. At the present time, the number of frozen embryos waiting for adoption far exceeds the number of prospective embryo adopters. Another related concern is the approximately 20% risk of embryo loss as a consequence of freezing and thawing. In addition, the long-term risks to offspring derived from frozen–thawed embryos remains unclear, although significant increases in congenital malformation have not yet been demonstrated.

One of the most significant risks in fertility preservation through embryo banking is the potential delay in cancer treatment, since hormonal stimulation of the ovary is necessary for IVF and that requires 2–5 weeks for just one cycle [13]. Another risk is the potential adverse effect of hormonal stimulation for the patient's primary cancer disease. This is particularly true for women who have hormonally sensitive tumors such as breast carcinoma. There may also be an increased chance of pregnancy complications, including miscarriage, low birthweight infants, or premature infants [5]. For certain cancer patients who need radiotherapy for their primary cancers, in addition to ovarian damage, their uterus may also be adversely affected, leading to uterine growth retardation and impaired vascular supply. This implies that even if embryos are created and cryopreserved, the patients who recover from cancer may have difficulty completing the gestation of a full-term fetus or may give birth to an infant with compromised health [14]. The potential for the recovered cancer patient to relapse as a result of being pregnant should also be considered with seriousness, since pregnancy can theoretically aggravate cancer. It is generally recommended that pregnancy be delayed well after cancer treatment is concluded, although the optimal timing is unknown [23]. For parents acting as the minor adolescent's proxy decision-maker, weighing these risks against their adolescent's best interest is a daunting task. The two-stage consenting method discussed above is less effective for the cryopreservation of embryo since the oocytes have already been used for fertilization and human embryos would have been created after the first stage of consent. Nonetheless, it may be ethically prudent to limit the parental consent to retrieval and fertilization of oocytes, particularly for adolescents using donor sperm, and leave the decision to re-implant or dispose of embryos to the adolescents in the second-stage consent later. In the UK, only the competent minor can consent to use her own mature oocytes for creation of embryos. The HFEA, which governs the use of male gametes as discussed above, applies equally to the retrieval, storage, and uses of the female gametes. Disposal of embryos created in the event the patient dies of cancer is ethically and legally problematic and will be discussed below in a separate section devoted to disposal of frozen embryos, gametes, and reproductive tissues.

Cryopreservation of oocytes

For postpubertal female patients who have moral objections against cryopreservation of embryos, are without a partner to serve as a sperm donor for oocyte fertilization, or are reluctant to use donor sperm from strangers, cryopreservation of mature oocytes is an alternative to embryo banking. Banking of mature oocytes avoids the moral controversy of storing embryos, but like embryo banking it also delays cancer treatment for several weeks because harvesting oocytes requires ovarian stimulation and it exposes the patient to potentially hazardous hormonal stimulation. Human oocytes are also highly sensitive to chilling, and low temperature causes cytoskeletal disorganization and chromosomal and DNA abnormalities, all of which impair the oocyte's developmental competence. Although vitrification and cryoprotective agents may ameliorate the damage caused by freezing and thawing, at the present time cryopreservation of mature oocyte remains the least successful approach and has significant limitations. The overall birth rate per cryopreserved oocyte is approximately 2% and the pregnancy rate is reduced by 25–33% compared with using unfrozen oocytes [15]. This suggests that a large number of oocytes would have to be banked to assure a successful pregnancy, and this potentially entails more than one treatment cycle, which is probably an unacceptable amount of delay for cancer treatment. In addition, the long-term effects on children born from cryopreserved oocytes are unknown.

In view of the low pregnancy rate and high uncertainty about the efficacy, benefit, and safety of oocyte cryopreservation under present technologies, this option for fertility preservation is presently seen as an experimental procedure not recommended for routine use. Parents who act as proxy for a postpubertal minor are not justified in opting for this method of fertility preservation unless other methods are unavailable and even then only as part of an IRB-approved protocol with full disclosure of risks and uncertainty of benefits to the consenting parents and the minor, who must assent [16]. The Practice Committee of the Society for Assisted Reproductive Technology and the Practice Committee of the American Society for Reproductive Medicine have jointly published a guideline enumerating what women considering oocyte cryopreservation must be informed of so that they can make a truly informed decision and give valid consent. The guideline lists 13 "essential elements" of such an informed consent, including the side effects and potential risks of oocyte retrieval; methods and costs of oocyte cryopreservation; thaw-survival rate for oocytes; requirement for, success rate, and cost of ICSI; clinic-specific data and outcome; the high likelihood of natural conception for women below the age of 35 years of age; disposition of unused cryopreserved oocytes and the laws regulating their donation; and the instability of storage facility and the possibility of accidental loss of cryopreserved oocytes in the course of their storage [17]. Some argue that cancer patients, particularly adolescents and very young adults awaiting anti-cancer therapy, are too vulnerable to be appropriate research subjects and that oocyte cryopreservation should not even be offered at all [18].

Prepubertal females

Cryopreservation of ovarian tissue

For prepubertal females and those postpubertal females who either cannot delay treatment to undergo ovarian stimulation or for whatever reason decide not to preserve fertility by cryopreservation of embryos or oocytes, cryopreservation and autotransplantation of ovarian tissues has become a viable but experimental option. Compared with oocyte cryopreservation, this approach has greater fertility potential because the ovarian cortex contains primordial follicles with a much larger number of immature oocytes, which are more resistant to cryoinjury, and the procedure does not delay cancer treatment or expose the patient to hormonal stimulation. But it has its own technical challenges and one of these is the intrusive nature of obtaining ovarian tissues. For older adolescents, laparoscopic biopsy may be possible, although patients should be warned of the possibilities of postoperative bleeding and infection. But for girls younger than 10 years of age, abdominal surgery may be needed to obtain ovarian tissues. This makes fertility preservation in young females ethically sensitive and underscores that such a treatment should be recommended to minor patients only when there is a clear favorable risk–benefit ratio. Another challenge with this procedure is to develop the immature oocytes in ovarian tissue for fertilization after the patient recovers from her cancer; currently, autotransplantation of frozen–thawed ovarian tissue is the only clinically applicable strategy, and both endocrine and gametogenic functions of the cryopreserved ovarian tissues have been demonstrated after autotransplantation. Since transplanted ovarian tissues are susceptible to ischemic injury because of incomplete or failed revascularization, the longevity of ovarian grafts is usually unpredictable, and repeated grafts may be necessary in some cases. These are also risks that minor patients and their parents should be told before they consent to the procedure. So far, no data are available regarding the qualities of oocytes matured *in situ* in transplanted ovarian tissue, and the potential risks of congenital malformations in the resulting offspring remains unknown.

The most crucial ethical issue in the cryopreservation of ovarian tissue is the risk of re-introduction of malignant cells to the recovered patient through the autotransplanted ovarian tissue that was removed before chemotherapy commenced. Although it has been reported that ovarian grafting in patients with lymphoma is safe [19], similar data are unavailable for other malignancies. Hence, this approach of fertility preservation is particularly not indicated for female patients with systematic or disseminated malignancies until reliable cancer screening methods become available. Given the various uncertainties of the efficacy and risks of this mode of fertility preservation, the treatment should only be performed as an experimental procedure under IRB guidelines, with all the risks disclosed. The American Society for Reproductive Medicine has narrowly restricted the indication of this experimental procedure as "an alternative for women who immediately face near term medical therapies that clearly threaten their future fertility" [20]. Similarly, the Edinburgh Criteria limit the procedure for patients with "realistic chance of long-term survival" and "high risk of treatment-induced immediate ovarian failure (estimated > 50%)" [21]. For patients under 18 years, parental consent with patient assent should be obtained, and the two-stage consent process discussed above in relation to cryopreservation of testicular tissue should be used. This applies in the UK also since the HFEA does not regulate storage of immature oocytes in ovarian cortex, where no mature gametes are present, but consent by the patient is required in the process of oocyte maturation either *in situ* or in vitro as gamete formation is under the jurisdiction of the HFEA [21]. In all circumstances in the USA and the UK, if the minor patient refuses to assent and her parents consent, the fertility doctors should withhold both the removal and transplantation of ovarian tissue [22].

Ethical issues common to male and female fertility preservation

The concern of preservation of 'flawed' genetic material

A dilemma in fertility cryopreservation arises from the concern that cancer patients may pass on causative or predisposing factors in their gamete and produce cancerous offspring or offspring with higher risks of cancer. This is particularly true for high-penetrance cancer-predisposition syndromes such as hereditary retinoblastoma and breast cancer; the risks involving low-penetrance cancer susceptibility genes are less certain [10]. The question at to whether cancer patients' offspring may also be exposed to higher health risks because of the cancer treatment that their parents have received or the ART used for their conception has not been definitively answered [10]. Furthermore, the offspring may also have a higher risk of losing a parent in the event that the cancer recurs and kills a parent who was thought to have been cured. Some have suggested that it may be unethical to assist cancer patients with expected shorter lifespan to have offspring [23]. However, it can be argued that to deny cancer patients the right to preserve their fertility amounts to "forced" sterilization, which is ethically unacceptable. On the one hand, cancer patients must make an informed decision about the cancer and other health-related risks in their child-to-be and weigh that against their own desire to have genetically related offspring. Only they have the right to decide that "no life" is better than a life with health risks for their offspring. On the other hand, if fertility cryopreservation leads to the unfortunate result of an offspring developing cancer, it may potentially lead to a "wrongful birth" action from the parents against the doctor and possibly a "wrongful life" from the child with cancer. This underscores the importance of providing detailed explanation of all health-related risks, including the risk of begetting a child who develops cancer, to the cancer patient seeking fertility cryopreservation service before the service is provided.

Ownership and disposition of cryopreserved material

Patients who have cryostored gametes or gonadal tissues may die before they have the chance to put them to their "reproductive" uses. The critical issue is whether these biomaterials are considered as "properties." Considering biomaterials as property gives minor children the right to control the bodily materials. For example, minor children should be able to decide that if they do not survive the cancer, the biomaterials cryopreserved should be destroyed. We have discussed above the two-stage consenting process in which a minor child who survives to majority age should take full control of the disposition of the biomaterials stored and become the sole person entitled to consent either to use of the biomaterials for its original "reproductive" purposes or to dispose of them in one of the several ways. If the minor child does not survive to adulthood, it is recommended that all tissues and gametes should be discarded or donated for research, and, specifically, the parents should not have the right to decide on the reproductive uses of their child's biomaterials posthumously [8]. A single young adult should preferably also indicate in writing what his/her wishes are as to the posthumous disposition of the biomaterials in the event of his/her premature death.

Although the most common disposition for cryopreserved gametes and gonadal tissues is to destroy them posthumously, donation of sperm by a single healthy young adult to others for reproductive purposes is acceptable. For couples, posthumous use of sperm by the surviving partner is acceptable provided there is a prior written instruction by the deceased partner agreeing to this disposition. The fact that the child produced will be born without the biological father is not sufficient reason to deny a couple the use of sperm posthumously. Posthumous oocyte donation to others or spouse is not recommended as the cryopreservation of oocytes is still an experimental procedure and the use of a surrogate mother is involved [8]. These arrangements reflect the sound ethical principle of respecting the donor's autonomy and are generally consistent with the prevalent legal practice that the person's prior wishes about disposition of biomaterials are controlling after death [23].

The disposition of cryopreserved human embryos is more complicated, and the number of cryopreserved embryos is increasing rapidly (400 000 embryos were cryopreserved in the USA alone up to 2002). The couple who have undergone IVF to create embryos should have some prior agreement about the ownership of the embryos in the event of a subsequent divorce and the conservatorship of the embryos in the event of the death of one or both partners. For the disposition of cryopreserved embryos, there are essentially five options to choose from: embryo transfer to achieve pregnancy; donate embryos to other infertile couples for embryo transfer; donate embryos for research; discard embryos; and keep embryos in cryostorage and do nothing. Studies have shown that couples' preferences for embryo disposition are "unstable" and subject to changes as they gain new information and experiences, including the experience of going through IVF to create the embryos. These findings support the two-stage consent approach: the first query of the couples' dispositional preferences at the time of creation of embryos and cryostorage, and the second query before thawing of the embryos for use. This implies that the first stage of the consent (sometimes called "pre-freeze agreement") should not be made binding for the couple. In fact, to require a couple to make a comprehensive decision regarding the disposition of embryos before IVF, embryo transfer, pregnancy or pregnancy loss, and other life events occurring with the passage of time is an uninformed decision since these significant life events can be expected to have profound effects on the couples' view on the moral status of embryos and their proper uses [24].

Of the five options of embryo disposition, the least problematic option is for the owner-couples to transfer the cryopreserved embryos to obtain a pregnancy. As long as they are fully informed of the risks of embryo cryopreservation discussed above, the benefit of having a child fulfills the couple's original intention to create the embryos. Donating embryos to infertile "recipients" is also uncomplicated, but certain guidelines would have to be followed. The American Society for Reproductive Medicine has published detailed guidelines regarding embryo donation [25] and some of the most ethically relevant items include prohibiting monetary compensation for the donors except reimbursement for specific expenses, for example mandatory blood tests related to donation, screening of embryo donors for viruses and other transmissible diseases, executing a written informed consent for embryo donation that, among other things, specifically relinquishes their rights to the embryos and any child or children resulting from their transfer, and receiving appropriate counseling as donors and for the recipients. Embryo recipients must agree to take full responsibility for the embryos and any child or children resulting from their transfer; they must also release the donors from any and all liability from complications of the embryo donation and pregnancies resulting from their transfer, including the birthing of infants with congenital abnormalities or diseases. Some IVF facilities may have guidelines that decline to transfer donated embryos to "single women" or lesbian couples or recipients who are deemed unsuitable to be parents by the institution.

Donation of embryos for research is more complex, and different studies have found a remarkable ambivalence among couples about embryo donation for research. In some studies, few couples are interested in this option, and in the USA, only 2.8% of embryos are targeted for research purposes [24]. Research on infertility and embryonic stem cells are the two main areas that attract donation of embryos. An Australian study involving 509 couples with cryostored embryos has reported that only 10% of couples indicate it probable and 34% possible that they would donate their embryos for research. The study has shown that couples agree that to destroy the surplus embryos is a waste and to donate them for research is to advance scientific and medical knowledge: both are positive factors that incline them to donate their surplus embryos for research. Factors that disincline donation include seeing the surplus embryos as potential children rather than experimental "specimens" and a perceived lack of control over the type of research that is to be carried out on the donated embryos [26]. Destruction of embryos for the harvesting of embryonic stem cells also dampens couples' desires to donate embryos for research. In this regard, guidelines developed by the American Society for Reproductive Medicine require that embryo donors must be informed of the differences between embryonic stem cell research and other types of research, including the inevitable destruction of the embryo in the process of harvesting the stem cells and the fact that embryonic stem cell lines can be used for many years and have potential commercial value that donors would not share [27].

The last two options for disposing of embryos are discarding embryos and keeping embryos in cryostorage indefinitely and doing nothing. Both options are ethically controversial and may reflect embryo-owners' belief about the moral values of embryos. Couples who believe that the embryo is nothing more than a mere cluster of cells would readily discard surplus embryos for which they have no use. Such a low view of embryonic life is not shared by the majority of people. At the other extreme, there are couples who view the embryo as a person with the moral right to life and they would consider discarding embryos as an act of murder. However, these people are also the most likely to be those who leave their embryos in cryostorage indefinitely. In Italy, where the Catholic Church defends the moral rights of the human embryo, a study has reported that as many as 25% of couples have failed to designate what to do with their surplus embryos and "simply 'let' their embryos be discarded without assuming the responsibility of signing a definitive 'act of disposal'" [28]. One author has opined that such a relinquishment of responsibility probably represents the embryo-owners' inability to cope with the ethical dilemma of either discarding or donating the embryo, and not to designate a preference may well represent the wish that the storage facility or the authority would make the decision for them [29], as the British Government did in 1996 when it ordered British clinics to destroy over 3300 embryos that had been cryopreserved for longer than 5 years. These findings of embryo-donors' ambivalence underscore the difficulties associated with the unsettled moral status of the human embryo that practitioners of fertility preservation should be aware of lest they find themselves unwittingly caught in a similar controversy.

References

1. Chung K, Irani J, Knee G, *et al.* Sperm cryopreservation for male patients with cancer: an epidemiological analysis at the University of Pennsylvania. *Eur J Obstet Gynecol Reprod Biol* 2004; **113**(Suppl 1): S7–S11.
2. Revel A, Revel-Vilk S. Pediatric fertility preservation: is it time to offer testicular tissue cryopreservation? *Mol Cell Endocrinol* 2008; **282**: 143–149.
3. Schover LR, Brey K, Lichtin A, *et al.* Knowledge and experience regarding cancer, infertility, and sperm banking in younger male survivors. *J Clin Oncol* 2002; **20:** 1880–1889.
4. President's Cancer Panel. *Annual Report 2003–2004.* Bethesda, MD: National Cancer Institute, 2004.
5. Schover LR, Rybicki LA, Martin BA, *et al.* Having children after cancer: a pilot survey of survivors' attitude and experiences. *Cancer* 1999; **86:** 697–709.
6. Tournaye H, Goossens E, Verheyen G, *et al.* Preserving the reproductive potential of men and boys with cancer: current concepts and future prospects. *Hum Reprod Update* 2004; **10:** 525–532.
7. Bahadur G, Chatterjee R, Ralph D. Case report: testicular tissue cryopreservation in boys. Ethical and legal issues. *Hum Reprod* 2000; **15:** 1416–1420.
8. ESHIRE Task Force on Ethics and Law. Taskforce 7: ethical considerations for the cryopreservation of gametes and reproductive tissues for self use. *Hum Reprod* 2004; **19**: 460–462.
9. Human Fertilisation and Embryology Act. London: HMSO, 1990.
10. Grundy R, Gosden RG, Hewitt M, *et al.* Fertility preservation for children treated for cancer (1): scientific advances and research dilemmas. *Arch Dis Child* 2001; **84:** 355–359.
11. Grundy R, Larcher V, Gosden RG, *et al.* Fertility preservation for children treated for cancer (2): ethics of consent for gamete storage and experimentation. *Arch Dis Child* 2001; **84:** 360–362.
12. Tanner JM. *Foetus into Man: Physical Growth from Conception to Maturity,* 2nd edn. Ware, UK: Castlemead, 1989.
13. Michelmann HW, Nayudu P. Cryopreservation of human embryos. *Cell Tissue Banking* 2006; **7:** 135–141.
14. Pacey AA. Fertility issues in survivors from adolescent cancers. *Canc Treat Rev* 2007; **33:** 646–655.
15. Ambrosini G, Andrisani A, Porcu E, *et al.* Oocytes cryopreservation: state of art. *Reprod Toxicol* 2006; **22:** 250–262.
16. Jain JK, Paulson RJ. Oocyte cryopreservation. *Fertil Steril* 2006; **86**(Suppl 4): S1037–S1046.
17. Practice Committees of the Society for Assisted Reproductive Technology and the American Society of Reproductive Medicine. Essential elements of informal consent for elective oocyte cryopreservation: a Practice Committee opinion. *Fertil Steril* 2007; **88**: 1495–1496.
18. Melo-Martin I, Cholst IN. Researching human oocyte cryopreservation: ethical issues. *Fertil Steril* 2008; **89**: 523–528.

19. Kim SS. Fertility preservation in female cancer patients: current developments and future directions. *Fertil Steril* 2006; **85**: 1–11.
20. Practice Committees of the American Society of Reproductive Medicine and the Society for Assisted Reproductive Technology. Ovarian tissue and oocyte cryopreservation. *Fertil Steril* 2006; **86**(Suppl 1): S142–S147.
21. Wallace WHB, Anderson RA, Irvine DS. Fertility preservation for young patients with cancer: who is at risk and what can be offered? *Lancet Oncol* 2005; **6**: 209–218.
22. Dudzinski DM. Ethical issues in fertility preservation for adolescent cancer survivors: oocyte and ovarian tissue cryopreservation. *J Pediatr Adolesc Gynecol* 2004; **17**: 97–102.
23. Ethics Committee of the American Society for Reproductive Medicine. Fertility preservation and reproduction in cancer patients. *Fertil Steril* 2005; **83**: 1622–1628.
24. Bankowski BJ, Lyerly AD, Faden RR, *et al.* The social implications of embryo cryopreservation. *Fertil Steril* 2005; **84**: 823–832.
25. American Society for Reproductive Medicine. Guidelines for cryopreserved embryo donation. *Fertil Steril* 2004; **82**(Suppl 1): S16–S17.
26. McMahon CA, Gibson FL, Leslie GI, *et al.* Embryo donation for medical research: attitudes and concerns of potential donors. *Hum Reprod* 2003; **18**: 871–877.
27. Ethics Committee of the American Society for Reproductive Medicine. Donating spare embryos for embryonic stem cell research. *Fertil Steril* 2009; **91**: 667–670.
28. Cattoli M, Borini A, Bonu MA. Fate of stored embryos: our 10 years' experience. *Eur J Obstet Gynecol Reprod Biol* 2004; **115**(Suppl 1): S16–S18.
29. Dawson KJ. The storage of human embryos. *Hum Reprod* 1997; **12**: 6.

Appendix 1 Autotransplantation of cryopreserved thawed human ovarian tissue

Study	Age at freezing (years)	Chemotherapy before freezing	Indication	Graft site	Recovery of ovarian function	Outcome
Oktay and Karlikaya (2000)	29	No	Not cancer	P	16 wk	↑E2, ovulation, menses
Radford *et al.* (2001)	36	Yes	HL	O	8 mo	↓FSH, ↑E2, ovulation, menses (1 cycle)
Callejo *et al.* (2001)	47	No	Not cancer	Rectus abdominism.	3–4 mo	↑E2, follicles
Kim *et al.* (2004)	37	No	Cervical carcinoma (Ib)	Above pectoralis m. (a) + above rectus m. (b)	14 wk	↑ E2, ↓FSH, ovulation (in b)
Oktay *et al.* (2004)	30	No	Breast cancer	Subcutaneous abdominal wall	3 mo	30 follicles, 20 oocytes (IVF) embryo transfer
Donnez *et al.* (2004)	25	No	HL	P	4.5 mo	↑E2, ↓FSH, follicles, menses, live birth
Meirow *et al.* (2005)	28	Yes	NHL	O transplant (a), O injection (b)	8 mo	↓FSH, ↑AMH, ↑inhibin B, follicles, menses, oocyte (IVF), embryo, live birth, spontaneous pregnancy miscarriage (30 mo post-transplant)
Schmidt *et al.* (2005)	28	No	HL	O + P + A	19/22 wk	↑E2, ↓FSH, follicles, menses
	25	No	HL	O + P + A	18/25 wk	↑E2, ↓FSH, follicles, menses, 2 oocytes (IVF), 2-cell embryo
	32	No	NHL	O	8/14 wk	↑E2,↓FSH, follicles, menses, 2 oocytes (IVF), mature and GV 4-cell embryo
Wolner-Hanssen *et al.* (2005)	30	No	Pure red cell aplasia + BMT	Forearm, sc	18 wk	Follicles poststimulation
Donnez *et al.* (2006)	21	No	SCA + BMT	O + P	4.5 mo	↑E2, ↓FSH,↓LH, FD (follicle of 20 mm), menses

Table (*Cont.*)

Study	Age at freezing (years)	Chemotherapy before freezing	Indication	Graft site	Recovery of ovarian function	Outcome
Oktay (2006)	29	Yes	HL	Abdominal wall, sc	2 mo	↑E2, ovulation, pregnancies: 1 miscarriage, 1 live birth from native ovary
Demeestere *et al.* (2006)	24	Yes	HL	O + P + abdominal wall, sc	4 mo	↑E2, ↑inhibin B, ↓FSH, follicles in all sites, ovulations, natural conception, pregnancy, miscarriage (7 wk) (aneuploidy)
Rosendahl *et al.* (2006)	28	No	HL	O + P + A	19/22 wk	↑E2, ↓FSH, follicles, menses, oocytes (IVF), embryo development, biochemical pregnancy
Demeestere *et al.* (2007)	24	Yes	HL	O + abdominal wall, sc		Menses, follicles in orthotopic only, natural conception, live birth
Silber *et al.* (2008)	25	No	Not cancer	O	4–5 mo	First spontaneous cycle: live birth
Donnez *et al.* (2008)	21 (Donnez *et al.* (2006)	No	SCA +BMT	O + P	4.5 mo	↑E2, ↓FSH, menses, follicles, live birth
	23	Yes	HL + BMT	O	5 mo	↑E2, ↓FSH, menses, follicles
	28	Yes	NHL + BMT	O bilateral	6.5 mo	↑E2, ↓FSH, menses, follicles
	22	No	WG	O bilateral	4.5 mo	↑ E2,↓ FSH, menses, Follicles
Andersen *et al.* (2008)	A: 32	No	NHL	O	19/22 wk	3 IVF cycles, 2 mature oocytes, transfer of one embryo
	B: 28	No	HL	O + P + A	18/25 wk	Biochemical pregnancy
	C: 25	Yes	HL	O + P + A	16/20 wk?	Clinical pregnancy, miscarriage 7 wk (site O)

Study	Age at freezing (years)	Chemotherapy before freezing	Indication	Graft site	Recovery of ovarian function	Outcome
	D: 26	Yes	HL	O	20 wk, NA	Birth of healthy boy
	E: 27	No	Ewing sarcoma	O	15 wk	Birth of healthy girl
	F: 36	No	Breast cancer	O	21 wk?	Follicles, menses, no oocytes
Sánchez-Serrano et.al. (2010)	36	No	Breast cancer	O	9 wk	4 IVF cycles, 16 oocytes, egg vitrification, birth of healthy twins
Piver *et al.* (2009)		No	Periarteritis nodosa	O + P	4 mo	Ectopic pregnancy
	.	No	SCA	O + P	4 mo	Birth of healthy child

A, abdominal wall, subperitoneal; AMH, anti-Müllerian hormone; BMT, bone marrow transplantation; E2, estradiol; FD, follicular development; FSH, follicle-stimulating hormone; GV, germinal vesicle; HL, Hodgkin's lymphoma; IVF, in vitro fertilization; m., muscle; mo, month; NA, not available; NHL, non-Hodgkin's lymphoma; O, remaining ovary; P, pelvic peritoneum; sc, subcutaneous; SCA, sickle cell anemia; WG, Wegener granulomatosis; wk, week.

Sources:

Callejo J, Salvador C, Miralles A, *et al.* Long-term ovarian function evaluation after autografting by implantation with fresh and frozen-thawed human ovarian tissue. *J Clin Endocrinol Metab* 2001; **86**: 4489–4494.

Demeestere I, Simon P, Emiliani S, Delbaere A, Englert Y. Fertility preservation: successful transplantation of cryopreserved ovarian tissue in a young patient previously treated for Hodgkin's disease. *Oncologist* 2007; **12**: 1437–1442.

Donnez J, Dolmans MM, Demylle D, *et al.* Livebirth after orthotopic transplantation of cryopreserved ovarian tissue. *Lancet* 2004; **364:** 1405–1410.

Donnez J, Dolmans MM, Demylle D, *et al.* Restoration of ovarian function after orthotopic (intraovarian and periovarian) transplantation of cryopreserved ovarian tissue in a woman treated by bone marrrow transplantation for sickle cell anaemia: case report. *Hum Reprod* 2006; **21**: 183–188.

Donnez J, Squifflet J, Van Eyck A-S, *et al.* Restoration of ovarian function in orthotopically transplanted cryopreserved ovarian tissue: a pilot experience. *RBM online* 2008; **16**: 694–704.

Kim SS, Hwang I-T, Lee H-C. Heterotopic autotransplantation of cryobanked human ovarian tissue as a strategy to restore ovarian function. *Fertil Steril* 2004; **82**: 930–932.

Meirow D, Levron J, Eldar-Geva T, *et al.* Pregnancy after transplantation of cryopreserved ovarian tissue in a patient with ovarian failure after chemotherapy. *N Engl J Med* 2005; **353:** 318–321.

Oktay K. Spontaneous conceptions and live birth after heterotopic ovarian transplantation: is there a germline stem cell connection? *Hum Reprod* 2006; **21**: 1345–1348.

Oktay K, Karlikaya G. Ovarian function after transplantation of frozen, banked autologous ovarian tissue. *N Engl J Med* 2000; **342**: 1919.

Oktay K, Buyuk E, Veeck L, *et al.* Embryo development after heterotopic transplantation of cryopreserved ovarian tissue. *Lancet* 2004; **363**: 837–840.

Piver P, Amiot C, Agnani G, *et al.* Two pregnancies obtained after a new technique of autotransplantation of cryopreserved ovarian tissue. In *Proceedings of the 25th Annual Meeting of ESHRE*, Amsterdam, the Netherlands, June–July, 2009.

Radford JA, Liebermann BA, Brison D, *et al.* Orthotopic reimplantation of cryopreserved ovarian cortical strips after high-dose chemotherapy for Hodgkin's lymphoma. *Lancet* 2001; **357**: 1172–1175.

Rosendahl M, Loft A, Byskov AG, *et al.* Biochemical pregnancy after fertilization of an oocyte aspirated from a heterotopic autotransplant of cryopreserved ovarian tissue: case report. *Hum Reprod* 2006; **21**: 2006–2009.

Sanchez-Serrano M, Crespo J, Mirabet V, *et al.* Twins born after transplantation of ovarian cortical tissue and oocyte vitrification. *Fertil Steril* 2010; **93**: 268.

Schmidt KL, Yding Andersen C, Loft A, *et al.* Follow-up of ovarian function post-chemotherapy following ovarian cryopreservation and transplantation. *Hum Reprod* 2005; **20**: 3539–3546.

Silber SJ, Derosa M, Pineda J, *et al.* A series of monozygotic twins discordant for ovarian failure: ovary transplantation (cortical versus microvascular) and cryopreservation. *Hum Reprod* 2008; **23**: 1531–1537.

Wolner-Hanssen P, Hagglund L, Ploman F, *et al.* Autotransplantation of cryopreserved ovarian tissue to the right forearm 2005; 4½ years after autologous stem cell transplantation. *Acta Obstet Gynecol Scand* **84**: 695–698.

Index

abdominal ionizing radiation, *see* radiotherapy
abnormalities, children's health outcomes, *see* congenital abnormalities
acetamide, 26–27, 18, 19–20
acquired immunodeficiency syndrome (AIDS), 46
activin A, 205, 208
addonitol, 27–28
adolescents with cancer, 63–69, 195–196
AID (artificial insemination by donor), 46, 48
alcohols, 27
alkylating agents, 57–58, 189
amide cryoprotectants, *see* acetamide; formamide; methanamide
anejaculation, 48–49
angiogenesis, transplantation and, 191, 225
angiogenic granulation tissue, 221
animal breeding
  electroejaculation use, 48
  sperm cryopreservation, 39–40, 41
animal studies
  follicle culture, 200, 204
  McGill Cryoleaf efficacy, 148
  ovarian grafts, 219
  ovarian tissue grafts, 218
  whole ovary cryopreservation, 233–234, 242, 245–248
anonymity, sperm donors, 46–47
anti-Müllerian hormone
  folliculogenesis, 200–201, 205, 207
  ovarian tissue transplantation, 224, 226
antioxidant treatment, 220
antral follicles
  in vitro development, 208
  puncture, 213, 214
apoptosis, culture conditions, 206–207
aquaporins, 17
  aquaporin 3, 18
    early embryos (mouse), 20
    morulae (mouse), 19, 20
    oocytes (mouse), 17–18
aqueous solutions, 3
arabinose, non-penetrating CPAs, 29
Arrhenius activation energy, 17
ART (assisted reproductive technology)
  CPA use, 25, 33
  embryo cryopreservation, 67
  ice crystal prevention, 12
  outcomes, 178–182, 179
    adverse effects, 182
    after oocyte cryopreservation, 178
    babies' neonatal development, 182
    multiple pregnancy, 67–68
  sperm cryopreservation, 40
  vitrification roles, 131
artificial insemination by donor (AID), 46, 48
artificial shrinkage, blastocele, 99–100, 101
aseptic vitrification, 158–159, 165
  blastocysts, 106–107, 109–112, 163–164
    applications, 108–109
    outcomes, 110
    protocols, 109
  cooling speed, 106–107
  embryo carrier devices, 107
    hermetically sealed, 106–107
    illustrated, 158, 159
  GV oocytes, *see* germinal vesicle oocytes
  outcomes, 109
  protocols, 108, 159
  solutions, 108
  vs. non-aseptic vitrification, 108–109
assisted reproductive technology, *see* ART
asthenozoospermia, 48
autoimmune diseases, 40, 151–152, 190
autotransplantation, *see* transplantation
azoospermia, 57–58
  sperm retrieval, 51, 52–53

bacterial agents, risk, 139
basal culture conditions, 204
basic fibroblast growth factor, 205
biochemical pregnancies, 178
biological carriers, sperm cryopreservation, 53–54
biomaterials, ownership and disposition, 253–254
biopsy
  blastocysts, 102
  embryos, 70, 81, 90
biospectroscopy, 123
Biot–Fourier equation, 159
blastoceles, 95–96
  shrinkage, 99–100, 101, 111
blastocyst aseptic vitrification, 106–107, 109–112, 163–164
  applications for, 108–109
  in vitro development for, 109–110
  outcomes, 110
  protocols, 108, 109
blastocyst cryopreservation, 95
  methods, 97–99
  optimal stage for, 82, 96
  pregnancy outcomes, 95
  selection, 72
  slow freezing, 99
  water/CPA movement, 21
blastocyst vitrification, 99
  carrier devices, 107
    Cryoloop, 98
    Cryotop, 98, 100, 102
    electron microscopy grid, 97
  culture methods, 96–97
  in vitro development, 108–109, 162
  optimal stage for, 100–101, 102, 164
  pregnancy rates, 160
  protocol, 69
  rapid freezing, 157–158
  selection for, 70, 77, 111
  structural features, 95–96
  two-step treatment, 21
blastocysts
  after thawing, 101
  bovine, 31
  cooling rate and outcomes, 89
  cryodamage, 71
  for transfer, 100–101

advantages, 97, 157
disadvantages, 96, 97
murine, 17, 18
blastomeres, 95
cryodamage to, 71
in embryo selection, 91, 93
in oocyte quality, 123
bone morphogenetic proteins, 200–201, 205
boys
cancer, 58
prepubertal, 59–61
BRC–ABL detection, 229
breast cancer, 151, 190
1,3 butanediol (butylene glycol), 27
butylene glycol (1,3 butanediol), 27

cancer patients, xi
adolescents, 63–69, 195–196
ART outcome, 184
embryo cryobanking, 68, 251
evaluation for fertility preservation, 223
fertility preservation, 190–191
female, 68
fertility preservation options, 62–63, 190–191
gonadotoxic therapies, 189–190
oocyte cryopreservation, 150–153, 251
ovarian stimulation, 144–145
ovarian tissue cryobanking, 189, 190, 213, 218, 221
evaluation for transplantation, 228
histological analysis, 215–216
indications for, 190
safety of, 226–229
storage protocol, 221–222
pregnancy complications after treatment, 251
pre-transplantation evaluation, 222
primordial follicle cryopreservation, 200
recurrence risk
ovarian tissue autotransplantation, 252
SSC contamination, 62
whole ovary transplantation, 195
sperm cryobanking, 40, 46, 51
SSC transplantation, 59–61
treatment delay, 251
treatment planning, 58–59
young patients, 59, 63–68, 248, 252–253
cancer susceptibility genes, 253
carrier devices, 133, 146
oocyte vitrification, 132–135, 133
effectiveness, 134–135
safety, 138–139
sperm cryopreservation, 53–54
see also embryo carrier devices; McGill Cryoleaf
cell membrane permeability, 4, 10–11, 16
cryobiological property, 16
cryoinjury and, 10–11
developmental changes, 21
measurement, 16–17
penetrating CPAs, 25
transport channels, 4, 10–11, 17
cell membranes, integrity, 161
cells
cryoinjury, 1–2, 4
permeability, 4
proliferation in vitro, 207
channel diffusion, 16, 17
early embryos, 20
morulae, 16–22, 19, 20
oocytes and morulae, 17
chemotherapy, *see* gonadotoxic chemotherapy
childhood cancer, 57, 63–68, 248
ovarian tissue cryopreservation, 189, 252–253
sperm cryopreservation, 58–59
testicular tissue cryopreservation, 59
children, from oocyte cryopreservation, 127–128, 132
chilling, cryobiological property, 16
China, donor sperm cryopreservation, 46–48
choline-based freezing media
MII spindle maintenance, 124–125
oocyte cryopreservation, 116, 122–123
chromatin abnormalities, 163
chromosomal abnormalities, 180–181
classic technique
slow-freezing oocytes, 115, 116
sperm cryopreservation, 41
cleavage stage embryo cryopreservation, 68–69, 70
comparative studies, 81–82, 96
vs. blastocyst, 102
vs. pronuclear, 82
cryodamage, 71
day 2, 81–82, 89, 90
day 3, 89, 90
selection for, 71–72, 77
clinical assisted reproduction, *see* ART (assisted reproductive technology)
co-culture, blastocyst cryopreservation, 95
colligative properties, 4
concentration, in CPA toxicity, 31–32
congenital abnormalities
ART and, 179–181, 180
oocyte cryopreservation and, 127–128, 183–184
consent, *see* informed consent
contamination risk, in vitrification, 84, 98–99, 158
cooling rate
and ice formation, 11
aseptic vitrification, 106–107, 160
carrier devices and, 135–137
danger zones, 13
developmental stage and outcomes, 89
donor egg bank protocol, 172–173
minimum volume cooling protocol, 172–173
phase diagram for CPAs, 12–14
slow-cooling cryopreservation, 77, 121
vitrification, 14, 92, 134, 137–138
whole ovary cryopreservation, 243
cortical tissue, *see* ovarian cortical tissue
CPAs (cryoprotectants), 24, 25, 33
animal model studies, 148
aseptic vitrification, 106–107, 110–112, 158
blastocyst cryopreservation, 99
aseptic vitrification, 110–111
slow-freezing, 99
vitrification, 99
cell permeability to, 12
combination, 13–14
concentrations of, 14, 137 172
cryodamage reduction, 31
embryo cryopreservation, 68–69, 76, 91
vitrification, 84
history of, 4–5
hypothetical solution, 13
introduction, 24
mechanism of action, 5, 8
movement pathway, 18
oocyte cryopreservation
slow cooling, 10, 121, 122
vitrification, 134, 139, 140 , 145
ovarian tissue cryopreservation, 191
ovary (whole) cryopreservation, 242–243
permeability, 16–17, 20, 21
phase diagram for, 12–14, 13
selection of, 16
slow-freezing cryopreservation, 99, 191
sperm cryopreservation, 41

CPAs (cryoprotectants) (*cont.*)
  structures, 6
  toxicity, 7
    assessment issues, 31
    cryobiological property, 16
    factors in, 7, 31–32
    risk reduction, 13–14, 32, 134, 145
  vitrification, 99, 148, 160
    concentration in, 14, 84
    without CPAs, 41
  zona pellucida manipulation, 102
  see also non-penetrating cryoprotectants; penetrating cryoprotectants
cryobanking, 213–214
  disease transmission risk, 139
  donor eggs, 175
  long-term, 72
  ovarian stem cells, 213–214
  ovarian tissue, 213–214
  pronuclear stage embryos, 77
  safety considerations, 72, 84
  sperm, 46
  storage containers, 90
  transportation to, 213
cryobiology, 1–4, 7–8
  cryodamage, 16
  in cryopreservation protocols, 24
  in developmental stages, 21–22
cryodamage, 4, 24
  and outcomes, 90
  blastocysts, 71, 99–100
  cryobiology of, 16
  egg banks and, 169–170
  embryos, 16, 70–71
  membrane permeability and, 10–11
  oocytes, 16, 120–121
  testing for, 79–80
Cryoleaf, 132, 134
Cryolock, 132, 134, 172–173
  in thawing protocol, 173
Cryoloop, 92, 106, 132, 133
  blastocyst vitrification, 98
  cooling/warming rates, 135–137
  oocyte vitrification, 133
  sperm vitrification, 48
cryopreservation, 8
  cooling rate and danger zones, 13
  indications for, 1, 24, 78–80
  in nature, 1
  options for, 190–191
  outcomes, 90
  slow cooling, history, 10
  stress of, 79–80
  timing in, 77
  toxicity avoidance, 32
  water/CPA movement pathways, 20–21
cryopreservation straws, 133, 135–137
  see also cut standard straws (CSS)
cryoprotectants *see* CPAs
cryostability evaluation, 158
cryostorage, *see* cryobanking
Cryotip, 98, 132, 133
Cryotop, 106, 132, 133
  blastocyst vitrification, 98, 100, 102
  cooling/warming rates, 135–137
  MII spindle maintenance, 124–125
  oocyte vitrification, 134
  outcomes, 102
crystal formation, 4
cultural issues in cryopreservation, 174–175, 251
culture containers, in vitro follicle culture, 204
culture duration, clinical efficacy, 127
culture media, 204–206, 205, 208
culture system
  blastocysts, 96–97
  follicles, 204–206, 206–207
cumulus–oocyte complexes, 146
cut standard straws (CSS), 158, 165
  blastocysts, 163–164
  cooling/warming rates, 135–137
  development of, 158–159
  illustrated, 158, 159
cyclophosphamide, 189, 190
cytoplasm, fluorescent staining, 206
cytotoxic chemotherapy, *see* gonadotoxic chemotherapy

danger zones, cooling rate and, 13
dehydration, 1–2, 122
  intracellular, 12
  role of CPAs, 121
  slow-cooling method, 121, 122
  in whole organ cryopreservation, 243
developmental ability, zygote initial score, 162
developmental delay, ART babies, 182
developmental stages
  choice for cryopreservation, 90, 96
  cryopreservation procedures, 16
  for embryo transfer, 96
  permeability changes, 16–22, 18, 20, 21
dextran, 30
diffusion (facilitated), *see* channel diffusion
diffusion (simple), 16, 17
  early embryos (mouse), 20
  oocytes (mouse), 18, 20
dilution procedure, 141
dimethyl sulfoxide (DMSO), 19–20, 25–26
  aquaporin 3 transport, 18
  aseptic vitrification, 158
  blastocyst cryopreservation, 163–164
  combined CPAs, 13–14, 139
  cooling/warming rates, 89, 157
  embryo cryopreservation, 68, 76, 139
  oocyte cryopreservation, 139, 145, 160
  properties of, 5–6
  structure, 6
  toxicity, 31
  vitrification, 139, 160, 163–164
directional freezing, 244–245
disaccharides, 28, 29
disease transmission risk, vitrification, 138–139
DMSO, *see* dimethyl sulfoxide
DNA integrity
  follicle viability, 206–207
  sperm cryopreservation, 48, 54
doctors, influence of, 249
donor programs
  donation defined, 175
  egg donation, 171
  oocyte vitrification, 169–170, 174, 175–176
    egg bank, 172
    protocol, 172–173
  restrictions on, 175
  semen cryopreservation, 48
  sperm cryopreservation, 46
donor–recipient synchronization, 169
donor selection, 170
  criteria, 47, 170
  for recipient, 173
  medical tests, 171
double fertility preservation, 213

early embryo cryopreservation, 20–21
  see also cleavage stage embryo cryopreservation
early-stage follicle culture, 205–206
ectopic pregnancy, 179, 183
EG, *see* ethylene glycol
egg banks
  cryopreservation, 169–170
  donations, 174, 175
egg donation, *see* oocyte donation
egg yolk-citrate buffer, 41
ejaculation, induced, 53
  see also masturbation
ejaculatory dysfunction, electroejaculation therapy, 48–49
electroejaculation, 48–49, 53
electron microscopy grids, 132, 133

blastocyst vitrification, 97
cooling/warming rates, 135–137
embryo vitrification, 106
oocyte vitrification, 133, 134
embryo biopsy, *see* biopsy, embryos
embryo carrier devices, 106, 132–135, 133
aseptic vitrification, 107
effectiveness, 134–135
hermetically sealed, 106–107
non-aseptic, 107
see also Cryoleaf; Cryolock; Cryoloop; Cryotop; cut standard straws; electron microscopy grids; Vitrisafe
embryo cryopreservation, 70, 72, 76
see also cleavage stage embryo cryopreservation; pronuclear stage embryo cryopreservation
cooling rate, 77
CPAs in, 16–17, 20–21, 26, 139
cryodamage, 16
day 3 and day 4, 90–92
ethical issues, 144, 250–252
evaluation, 158
gonadotoxic chemotherapy, 68, 190–191
treatment delay, 190–191, 251
in ART, 67–68, 89, 93, 102
legal issues, 114
methodology, 68–69
outcomes, 69–72, 79–80, 90, 163
embryo survival, 68
prognostic factors, 163
religious objections, 114
slow-freezing technique, 92
volume change measurement, 17
vs. fresh embryos, 102
vs. oocyte cryopreservation, 114, 128
water movement in, 16–17, 20–21
embryo cryopreservation (animals), 76
non-penetrating CPAs, 29, 30
penetrating CPAs, 28
embryo cryostorage, indefinite, 255
embryo donation, 89, 109, 254–255
embryo selection
for cryopreservation, 69–70, 90, 91
for transfer, 70, 71–72, 93
developmental stages, 90, 93
endometrial receptivity, 111
grading, 147–148
oocyte numbers thawed, 126
oocyte quality, 123
embryo transfer (ET)
biopsied embryos, 81
cleavage stage vs. blastocysts, 96, 102
day 6 stage blastocysts, 100–101
fresh vs. cryopreserved, 80, 102
in vitro fertilization and, 67, 102
oocytes GV stage vs. mature, 116, 147–148
pronuclear stage, 80–81
pronuclear vs. blastocysts, 81–82, 96
pronuclear vs. early cleavage stages, 82
embryonic stem cells, 62, 254–255
embryos
cleavage rate, 54
disposal, 254
embryonic stem cell harvesting, 254–255
implantation, 81
ownership, 254–255
permeability changes, 21
embryos (rodent)
1-cell, 17, 20
2-cell, 16, 17, 20
4-cell, 17
CPA permeability, 18, 20
non-penetrating CPAs, 30–31
penetrating CPAs, 26–27, 26
water movement pathway, 17–18
endocrine activity, *see* hormone levels
endometrial preparation, 109
for blastocyst transfer, 101, 109, 111
for embryo transfer, 81, 173
ovarian tissue transplantation, 226
endometriosis, 152, 190
environmental contamination, vitrification risk, 138–139
environmental factors, in transplantation results, 220
enzymatic digestion, follicular isolation, 195, 196, 201–204
epidermal growth factor, 205
epididymal sperm, 52, 54
equilibration, 7
cooling rate and, 137
donor egg bank protocol, 172–173
in pre-freeze stage, 76–77
slow-freezing technique, 91
vitrification, 92, 100
oocytes, 137 146
equilibration solution (ES), 140 , 146
estradiol, 207, 226
estrogen levels, 207, 224
estrogen–progesterone administration, 221
ethanamide, *see* acetamide
1,2 ethandiol, *see* ethylene glycol (EG)
ethanol, 28
ethical issues
embryo donation, 254
fertility cryopreservation, 248–253, 253–255
long-term cryostorage, 72, 255
ovarian transplantation, 195–196
sperm cryopreservation, 43
testicular tissue cryopreservation, 62
young cancer patients, 62–63, 248, 249–250
ethylene glycol (EG), 27
aseptic vitrification, 158
blastocyst vitrification, 160, 164
combined CPAs, 13–14, 139
embryo cryopreservation, 139
mechanism, 18, 19
oocyte cryopreservation, 139, 145
vitrification, 139, 146, 160
properties of, 6–7
structure, 6
toxicity, 7, 122
exposure time, CPA toxicity, 31–32
extracellular ice formation, 12, 120–121
extracellular matrix, 204

facilitated channel diffusion, *see* channel diffusion
fallopian tube cryopreservation, 237–238
families, future effects of donor programs, 175
Family Law Reform Act (1969) UK, 249
family lineage preservation, 249
female age, *see* maternal age
fertility impairment, xi
fertility preservation, xi
fertility restoration
future possibilities, 62
ovarian tissue transplantation, 223–225, 226
SSC transplantation, 59–61
fertilization
cryopreservation complications, 42–43
frozen–thawed oocytes, 126, 147
frozen–thawed sperm, 54
fetal hearts, assessment, 126
fetal ovaries, follicle culture, 201, 207, 208
fetal sacs, assessment, 126
fibroblast growth factor (bFGF), 205
Ficoll, 30
fluorescent microscopy, 206
follicle-stimulating hormone (FSH)
after ovarian tissue graft, 193, 224, 226
in culture media, 205

follicles
  apoptosis in culture, 206–207
  ischemic loss in transplantation, 194
  isolation techniques
    enzymatic digestion, 195, 196, 201–204
    mechanical, 201–204
  ovarian tissue sources, 201, 206
  ultrastructure, 206
follicular culture, 208–209
  difficulties, 195, 208–209
  evaluation methods, 206–207
  hormone production, 207
  outcomes, 207–208
  publications on, 202–213
follicular development
  assessment, 206
  ischemia and, 219–220
  ovarian tissue grafts, 194, 226
    sites, 191, 220, 225
  ovarian transplantation, 245
follicular viability
  determination, 206
  whole ovary cryopreservation, 195, 235–236, 237
  whole ovary transplantation, 234
folliculogenesis
  after ovarian tissue graft, 193
  control of, 200–201
forearm, graft sites, 223–225
formamide, 26
fragmentation, in embryos, 163
freeze–thaw damage, *see* cryodamage
freezing devices, programmable, 235, 237
freezing point, CPAs in lowering, 5
freezing rate, *see* cooling rate
freezing, cell damage in, 1–2
fresh vs. frozen embryo transfer, 80, 102
friend/relative, gamete donation, 169
FSH, *see* follicle-stimulating hormone
functional evaluation
  follicular growth, 207
  of oocytes, 123
functional lifespan
  ovarian tissue transplantation, 233, 241–242
  ovary (whole) cryopreservation, 245
fungi, cryostorage risk, 139

galactose, 28
gamete donation, program options, 169
  see also embryo donation; oocyte donation; sperm donation
gamete donors
  genetic screening, 47
  health screening, 139
gametes
  cryobank storage, 213–214
  informed consent for minors, 250
  ownership and disposition,253–254
gene expression, cultured follicular growth, 207
genetic abnormalities
  continuation, 253
  oocyte donation needed, 169
genetic screening, *see* pre-implantation genetic diagnosis (PGD)
genital surgery, 40
genitourinary health checks, 47–48
germ cells, 59
germinal vesicle (GV) oocytes, 116–117, 160, 213
  aseptic vitrification, 160, 213
  cryopreservation
  difficulties, 144
  immature oocyte, 116–117
  transportation to cryobank, 213
  vitrification, 117, 148, 160
glass state, 11, 13–14
glass transition temperature *(Tg)*, 2–3
glial cell-derived growth factor, 61
glucose, 28
glycerol, 27
  embryo cryopreservation, 76, 139
  gamete cryopreservation, 139
  in water movement pathway, 18–19
  oocyte cryopreservation, 145
  properties of, 5
  sperm cryopreservation, 41
  structure, 6
  toxicity, 31–32
gonadal dysgenesis, 169
gonadal tissue cryopreservation, 253–254
gonadotoxic chemotherapy
  autoimmune disorders, 151–152
  embryo cryopreservation, 68
  in childhood, 57–58
  sperm cryobanking, 40, 46, 51
  toxicity of individual agents, 189, 190
  treatment planning, 40, 58–59, 233
gonadotoxic radiotherapy, *see* radiotherapy
gonadotropin, 221, 226
grafted ovarian tissue, 218
growth differentiation factor, 200–201, 207
growth factor-supplemented media, 204, 207
GV oocytes, *see* germinal vesicle (GV) oocytes
gynecological malignancy, 190
health outcomes, children of fertility preservation, 127–128, 253
heart cryopreservation, 245
heart malformations, babies of fertility preservation, 180, 183
heat transfer
  ultra-rapid warming, 159
  whole ovary, 242–243, 244–245
hematological disease
  malignant, 151, 190, 226–229
  non-malignant, 190
hemi-straw embryo carrier, 107, 132
  cooling/warming rates, 135–137
hepatitis A/B/C, 42, 84
HEPES-buffered media, 139
heterotopic transplantation
  ovarian tissue, 193–194, 218–219, 223
  sites, 220, 223–225
histological analysis
  follicular development, 206
  ovarian tissue, 215, 226
Hodgkin's lymphoma
  oocyte vitrification, 151
  ovarian tissue cryobanking, 192, 229
homosexual couples, 174–175
hormone levels
  after ovarian tissue graft, 192, 193, 194, 219, 224
    monitoring, 224, 226
    sites, 218–219
  after whole ovary transplantation, 234
  in vitro follicle growth, 207
hormone stimulation, oocyte harvesting, 171, 184
hormone therapy, endometrial preparation, 101, 109, 147 , 173
Human Fertilisation and Embryology Act (HFEA) UK, 249, 250, 253
human immunodeficiency virus (HIV), 42, 47, 84
hyaluronan, 31
hydraulic conductivity (or coefficient), 10
hydrostatic pressure, polyvinyl alcohol and, 13
hypothalamic gonadotropin-releasing hormone pulse generator, 200–201

ice formation, 1–2, 10–11
  extracellular, 12, 120–121
  intracellular, 7, 12, 24–25, 120–121
  optical differences, 12
  prevention by CPAs, 24–25, 28, 120–121

solubility and, 4
temperature change rate, 11, 120–121
ice, nature of, 2
ICSI, *see* intracytoplasmic sperm injection
imaging, cancer patients, 228
imide CPAs, *see* formamide; methanamide
implantation rates
after embryo cryopreservation, 71–72
after oocyte cryopreservation, 126, 127
day 6 stage blastocysts, 100–101
success prediction, 71–72, 162
in vitro culture
follicles, 201–204, 207–209, 212–213
ovarian cortical tissue, 201–204
ovarian tissue, 214, 215–216
SSC expansion, 61
zygote post-thawing integrity and, 161
in vitro fertilization (IVF)
blastocyst cryopreservation, 95
congenital abnormality, 179–181
cryopreservation in, 24
embryo transfer, 67
embryo selection, 70
outcomes vs. ICSI, 80–81
embryos, 89
donation, 254
multigestation pregnancy reduction, 67–68, 76
ownership, 254
oocyte cryopreservation, 120, 125
outcomes, 102, 125
ovarian hyperstimulation syndrome risk, 78–79
sperm donation, 48
sperm harvesting, 49, 51
surfactants, 30
in vitro maturation (IVM)
blastocyst vitrification, 108–110, 111
follicules, 206
GM stage oocytes, 148
GV stage oocytes, 116–117, 144–145, 213
oocyte vitrification, 148–150 , 151
primordial follicles, 200–201, 195
infectious disease/infective agents
cryostored embryos, 72
embryo vitrification, 84
oocyte vitrification, 138–139
sperm cryopreservation, 42
sperm donor screening, 47–48
see also aseptic vitrification
infertility,
embryo donation, 254
IVF patients, 108–109
treatment, 72
young boys, 63–58, xi
see also cancer patients; gonadotoxic chemotherapy; premature ovarian failure
informed consent
donor egg programs, 175
donor sperm, 47
embryo cryopreservation, 72, 251
long-term cryostorage, 72
oocyte cryopreservation, 252
ovarian cryopreservation, 195–196
ovarian tissue cryopreservation, 252–253
parental consent, 251
sperm cryobanking, 43, 248–249
two-stage process, 250
validity, 72
young patients, 62, 250, 252–253
inhibin B levels, 224, 226
insect breeding, sperm cryopreservation, 39–40
insulin, 205
insulin-like growth factor (IGF), 205
intracellular dehydration, 12
intracellular ice formation, 7, 12, 24–25, 120–121
intracytoplasmic sperm injection (ICSI)
congenital abnormality, 179–181
donor program, 173
oocyte cryopreservation, 116
semen samples for, 58
sperm cryopreservation, 48, 53–54
sperm retrieval, 51
testicular sperm, 54
testicular tissue, germ cells from, 58, 59
vs. IVF in outcomes, 80–81
intrauterine insemination, 40, 42
ipsigeneic germ cell transplantation, 59
ischemia
follicular development following, 219–220
ovarian tissue transplantation, 233, 241–242
ovary transplantation, 194
ovary vitrification, 236
isolated follicles
early-stage, culture, 205–206
enzymatic digestion, 195, 196
primordial, in vitro maturation, 195
IUI (intrauterine insemination), 40, 42
IVF, *see* in vitro fertilization
IVM, *see* in vitro maturation

Kit ligand, 201, 205

laboratory fertilization, risks in, 184
lactose, non-penetrating CPA, 29
large volume samples, freezing, 244–245
late pregnancy loss, 179, 183
latent heat release, 243
legal aspects
embryo cryopreservation, 72, 78
posthumous disposal of biomaterials, 253–254
sperm cryopreservation, 43
liquid nitrogen (LN_2), 41
contact with, 106, 134, 158
contamination risk, 98–99, 106, 138–139
osmotic stress reduction, 12
storage in, 146–147
tissue destruction by, 1
liver cryopreservation, 245–246
LN_2, *see* liquid nitrogen
long-term storage
ART outcome, 184
ethical issues, 251
low birthweight, ART and, 184
luteinizing hormone (LH), 200–201

macromolecules, CPAs, 30–31
magnetic separation immunoassay analysis, 207
malignancy, *see* cancer patients
malignancy residual disease, *see* minimal residual disease (MRD)
maltose, 29
mannose, 29
masturbation, 41, 58, 248–249
maternal age
ART outcomes, 80, 125–126, 178
late pregnancy loss, 179
oocyte donation needed, 169
maternal ill-health, ART outcomes, 184
McGill Cryoleaf
efficacy of, 148, 148–150
illustrated, 146, 147
oocyte thawing, 147–148
oocyte vitrification, 144–145
vitrification, 146
McGill protocols, 147–148, 150–153
mechanical isolation, of follicles, 201–204
medical practitioners, influence of, 249
meiotic spindle, 145, 148, 172

membranes, *see* cell membranes
menstrual cycle, natural, 101
mental competence, in consent, 250, 251, 252–253
MESA (microsurgical epididymal sperm aspiration), 41, 42–43, 52
metaphase II, *see* MII
methanamide, 26
methanol, 27
methyl sulfoxide, *see* dimethyl sulfoxide
microbial contamination risk, in vitrification, 158
microdissection for testicular sperm extraction (Micro-TESE), 53
microscopy
  frozen–thawed oocytes, 123–124
  MII spindle maintenance, 125
microsurgical epididymal sperm aspiration (MESA), 41, 42–43, 52
microtubule depolimerization, 172
microvacuolization, 124
MII oocytes
  ovarian tissue autotransplantation, 194
  rapid freezing, 157–158
  spindle damage, 122, 124–125
MII oocytes (mouse)
  aquaporin 3 expression, 17–18
  CPA permeability, 18–20
  water movement pathway, 17
minimal residual disease (MRD)
  monitoring, 226 , 228
  risk
    ovarian tissue grafts, 252
    testicular tissue cryopreservation, 250
    use of SSCs, 62
    whole ovary grafts, 195
minimum volume cooling protocol, 172–173
miscarriage, 178–179, 182
molality, 3
molarity, 3
monoethylene glycol (MEG), *see* ethylene glycol
monosaccharides, 28–29
MOPS-buffered media, 139
moral objections
  to egg donation, 175
  to embryo cryopreservation, 251
morulae (mouse)
  CPA permeability, 18, 19, 20
  cryopreservation procedures, 16
  water movement pathways, 17, 18
morulae cryopreservation, 21
motherhood postponed, 153
  oocyte cryopreservation, 114, 131–132, 174–175, 178
  oocyte vitrification, 142
mother-to-daughter oocyte donation, 152–153
mouse developmental stages, 16–22
MRD, *see* minimal residual disease
multigestation pregnancies, 67, 181, 184
  avoidance, 67–68, 89
  legal restrictions on, 76
  rates of, 181
Multi-Thermal-Gradient (MTG) device, 235, 237, 244–245
musculoskeletal abnormalities, 180, 183

neonatal outcomes, ART babies, 149–150, 182, 184
neovasculation, ovarian tissue grafts, 233
nitrogen
  see also liquid nitrogen
  slush device, 132–134
non alkylating agents, 57–58
non-aseptic vitrification, 108–109, 160
non-biological carriers, 54
non-malignant systemic diseases, 40
non-penetrating cryoprotectants, 26, 28–31, 76
  in thawing, 78
  slow-cooling cryopreservation, 121, 122
  vitrification, 140
non-penetrating polymer, 13
non-vitrifying solutions, 108, 109–110
nucleation, ice formation, 2
nucleoli, zygote quality, 161

obstetric outcomes
  oocyte cryopreservation, 132, 178, 184
  singleton pregnancies, 181–182
OHSS, *see* ovarian hyperstimulation syndrome
oligoathenoteratozoopermia, 42
oligozoospermia, 48, 57–58
oncology, *see* cancer patients
oocyte cryopreservation, 69, 114–115, 117, 128
  advantages of, 144
  cell membrane permeability, 16–17
  concerns about, 120
  cooling rate, 77
  CPA permeability, 20–21, 30, 139
  damage during, 16, 31–32
  developmental stage, 116–117
  history, 114–115, 121–122, 132
  indications for, 120, 131–132, 157–158
  legal issues, 251–252
  new developments, 122–123
  outcomes
    effectiveness, 125, 191
    implantation rate, 126
    in cancer patients, 251–252
    perinatal risks, 178, 184
    pregnancy, 182–184, 185
  ownership and disposition, 253–254
  publications, 126
  quality, 123, 124–125
    MII spindle in, 125
    ovarian tissue graft sites, 220
    pronuclei in, 158
  safety, 127–128, 184
  slow cooling, 10, 115–116, 120–121, 172
  slow cooling vs. vitrification, 145, 148
  social and cultural effects, 174–175
  treatment delay in cancer patients, 251
  unfertilized, 69–70
  volume change measurement, 17
  water movement, 20–21
  young patients, 251–252
  see also oocyte vitrification
oocyte donation, 114, 169–170, 174
  donor selection, 170–171
  donor stimulation, 171
  mother-to-daughter, 152–153
  oocyte vitrification, 172
  restrictions on, 175
oocyte retrieval
  in unstimulated menstrual cycle, 144–145
  McGill Cryoleaf protocol, 148–150 , 151
  transvaginal follicular aspiration, 171
oocyte thawing
  in donor program, 173
  McGill Cryoleaf protocol, 147
oocyte vitrification, 115, 116, 131–132, 142, 153
  advantages/disadvantages, 146, 172
  at GV stage, 160
  breast cancer patients, 151
  cooling rate, 134
  CPAs in, 84, 145
  developments in, 144–145
  donor programs, 169–170, 171, 172, 175–176
    advantages, 172
    outcomes, 174
  history, 145

McGill Cryoleaf protocol, 144–145, 146
outcomes, 175
neonatal, 149–150
protocols compared, 127
risks, 178
success rates, 137
principles of, 145
solutions for, 139–141
oocyte-derived factors, 200–201
oocytes
evaluation of, 123–124, 161, 206
folliculogenesis, 200–201, 208–209
in vitro aging, 127
membrane permeability, 10–11, 21
nucleus counting, 206
numbers thawed, 126
reserve, 189
see also germinal vesicle oocytes
oocytes (animal)
polymer CPAs, 30
sugars as CPAs, 29
oocytes (mouse)
CPA permeability, 18–20, 26–27
non-penetrating CPAs, 30
water movement pathway, 17
oophorectomy, for ovary cryopreservation, 237, 238
open pulled straw (OPS), 132, 133
cooling/warming rates, 135–137
in CSS development, 158
oocyte vitrification, 133
organ transplantation, 241
orthotopic transplantation
ovarian tissue, 192–193, 218–219
surgical techniques, 223
sites for, 220, 223–225
osmosis, 4
osmotic pressure, extracellular, 4
osmotic shock, prevention, 28
osmotic shrinkage, 16
osmotic stress, 12, 162–163
osmotic swelling, cryodamage, 16
outcomes,
aseptic vitrification, 109
classic technique, 115, 116
embryo cryopreservation
developmental stages at, 81–82, 91–92
live birth rates, 72, 81–82
embryos
implantation, 81
transfer, 80–81
GV stage oocyte cryopreservation, 116–117
in vitro culture post-thawing, 161
McGill Cryoleaf vitrification protocol, 148, 148–150
obstetric, adverse, 182
oocyte cryopreservation, 115–116, 125, 132
protocols compared, 127
oocyte vitrification, 116, 137, 175
in donor program, 174
ovarian tissue transplantation, 193
slow-freezing technique, 83, 91–92, 115–116
sperm donation, 48
success rates
embryo transfer, 80–82
oocyte vitrification, 137
sucrose in slow-freezing solutions, 115–116
vitrified vs. slow-freezing technique, 83
see also pregnancy outcomes
ovarian cortex, 200, 206, 213
ovarian cortical tissue
culture, 206
primordial follicle activation, 207
two-step system, 205–206
follicles from, 201
handling, 222
in vitro culture, 201–204
ovarian function, 200–201
ovarian hyperstimulation syndrome (OHSS)
embryo cryopreservation need, 68, 78–79, 89
risk in stimulation protocols, 79, 144–145, 175
ovarian neoplasm, 151
ovarian stem cells, 213–214
ovarian stimulation, 67, 171, 184
in breast cancer, 151
outcomes, 81–82
ovarian tissue, 201, 208, 252
ovarian tissue cryobanking, 213–214
indications for, 221–222
outcomes, 214–216
procedure safety, 226–229
storage protocol, 221–222, 226
transportation, 213
ovarian tissue cryopreservation, 189, 196, 242
cancer patients, 191, 252–253
disadvantages, 144
for transplantation, 219–220
histological analysis, 216
in vitro culture, 214
indications for, 190
minimal residual disease risk, 144, 229
ownership and disposition, 253–254
protocol, 191, 214–216, 222
young patients, 252–253
ovarian tissue transplantation, 191–195, 218, 219–220
autotransplantation, 191–195, 227
clinical cases, 227
cortical pieces, 192
endocrine monitoring, 224
functional lifespan, 225, 233, 241–242
heterotopic, 193–194
history, 218–219, 220
indications for, 218, 221–222
ischemia, 241–242
orthotopic, 192–193
patient evaluation, 222
patient monitoring, 226
protocols/procedures, 223
publications, 218
sites for, 218–220, 220, 223
success factors
surgical techniques, 223
xenografting, 191
ovarian vasculature, graft sites, 225
ovary (whole)
as graft site, 223
culture, 204
heat transfer, 242–243
ovary (whole) cryopreservation, 233–234, 238, 242
animal models, 234–236, 245–248
directional freezing, 244–245
follicular viability, 237
heat transfer difficulties, 242–243, 244–245
human studies, 238
pregnancies after, 215
protocols, 195, 236–238
recent developments, 242
ovary (whole) transplantation, 194–195, 220, 241, 245
ovary (whole) with vascular pedicle
cryopreservation, 234–236
advantages in, 233
animal models, 233–236
CPA perfusion, 194
transplantation, 194–195, 234

parental consent
embryo cryopreservation, 251
oocyte cryopreservation, 252
ovarian tissue cryopreservation, 252–253
sperm banking, 249
patient evaluation, pre-transplant, 222

patient monitoring, post-transplant, 226
pelvic imaging, 226
pelvic peritoneum, graft sites, 223–225
penetrating cryoprotectants, 4–7, 24–28
  embryo cryopreservation, 76, 139
  oocyte cryopreservation, 121, 139, 145
  oocyte vitrification, 140
percutaneous epididymal sperm aspiration (PESA), 41, 52
permeability, *see* cell membrane permeability
PG, *see* 1,2-propanediol
pH difference, physiological solutions, 139
phase diagram for CPAs, 12–14
phosphate-buffered saline (PBS), 123, 139
physiological solutions, in vitrification, 139
plasma membranes, *see* cell membranes
polarized light microscopy, 125
Polscope, 125
polycystic ovary syndrome (PCOS), 109, 144–145, 179
polyethylene glycol (PEG), 30
polymerase chain reaction, real-time 207, 227
polymers, 13, 30–31, 145
polyols, 27–28
polysaccharides, 28, 29–30
polyvinyl alcohol, 31
polyvinylpyrrolidone, 30–31
posthumous disposal of biomaterials, 253–254
posthumous sperm retrieval, 51
post-insemination time, embryo transfer outcomes, 80
postpubertal females, 250–252
postpubertal males, 248–249
pre-antral follicles, 204, 207–208
pre-freeze stage, 76–77
pregnancy outcomes
  embryo cryopreservation, 89, 90, 95
  embryo implantation and, 81
  hormone replacement for support, 147
  oocyte cryopreservation, 182–184, 185
  ovarian cryopreservation, 215
  ovarian tissue cryobanking, 214–216
  ovarian tissue transplantation, 192–193, 220
pregnancy rates
  blastocyst stages, 160, 164
  cryopreservation complications, 42–43
  embryo stages, 81–82, 83
  oocyte cryopreservation, 127
  oocytes, 251–252
  pronuclear integrity and, 163
  testicular sperm, 54
  vitrification protocols, 83, 148–150 , 160
pre-implantation genetic diagnosis (PGD), 79, 89, 102
  blastocyst cryopreservation, 102
  embryo biopsy, 82
  pronuclear stage cryopreservation, 79
pre-implantation stage, embryo cryopreservation protocol, 69
premature ovarian failure (POF)
  chemotherapy-induced, 189, 196
  oocyte donation needed, 169
  ovarian cryobanking need, 221
  ovarian tissue cryobanking need, 190, 218
  radiotherapy-induced, 189–190
prepubertal boys, 59–61, 249–250
prepubertal girls, 252–253
prepubertal ovaries, follicle source, 201
preterm delivery, ART and, 184
primordial follicles
  activation of, 204–205
  assessment, 222
  in vitro culture, 195, 200, 204–205, 207, 208
  in vivo development, 200–201
progesterone, 207
PROH, *see* 1,2-propanediol
pronuclear integrity, 161, 163
pronuclear membranes, 161
pronuclear stage embryo cryopreservation, 69–70, 76–78, 157–158
  comparative studies, 81–82, 96
  cooling rate, 77
  cryodamage, 70
  developmental stage and outcomes, 81–82
  freezing stage, 77, 78
  indications for, 78–80
  morphological evaluation, 161–163
  scoring system and outcome, 161, 162, 163
  selection for, 77
  thawing, 77
  timing in, 77
  vitrification, 82–84
pronuclear vs. early cleavage stages, embryo transfer, 82
pronuclear zygotes, *see* pronuclear stage embryo cryopreservation
pronuclei, oocyte and embryo evaluation, 158
1,2-propanediol (PROH, propylene glycol), 18, 27
  combined CPAs, 13–14, 139
  embryo cryopreservation, 68–69, 76, 139
  oocyte cryopreservation, 122, 145
  oocyte vitrification, 139
  properties of, 7
  structure, 6
  toxicity, 31–32, 122
  vitrification solutions, 139, 146
  in water movement pathways, 20
propylene glycol, *see* 1,2-propanediol
protein macromolecules/polymers, 30, 33
psychogenic anejaculation, 48–49
publications
  on carrier devices, 134–135
  on in vitro follicular culture, 202–213
  on oocyte cryopreservation, 126, 132
  on vitrification, 131

quality of life
  cancer survivors, xi
  cancer treatment planning, 58–59
  childhood cancer management, 58

radioimmunoassay, 207
radiotherapy, gonadotoxicity, 40, 189–190
raffinose, 29
rapid freezing,157–158, 173
  see also ultra-rapid cooling; vitrification
real-time polymerase chain reaction, 207, 227
recipient preparation, *see* endometrial preparation
recrystallization, in thawing period, 243–244
rehydration, during warming, 121
rejection, of graft, 241
religious issues, embryo disposal, 255
research, embryo donation for, 254–255
retrograde ejaculation, semen collection, 49
revascularization, grafted ovarian tissue, 191, 219

safety
carrier devices, 138–139
embryo cryopreservation, 72
embryo vitrification, 84
oocyte cryopreservation, 132
ovarian tissue cryobanking, 226–229
ovarian transplantation, 195–196
Sage IVF Vitrification Warming Kit, 141
secondary follicle culture, 200
semen cryopreservation
boys, 58–59
donor program, 47, 48
seminiferous tubules
sperm retrieval from, 52–53
spermatogenesis in, 60
SSC transplantation, 59–61
semipermeable membranes, water transportation, 4
sequential culture, for blastocysts, 96–97
Sertoli cells, 60, 61
serum in culture media, 204
sexually transmitted infections, 47
shared egg donation, 169
shrinkage (artificial), of blastocele, 99–100, 101
simple diffusion, *see* diffusion (simple)
single embryo transfer (SET), 67, 68
single women, 174–175
single-phase culture, 96–97
singleton pregnancies, 181
slow-freezing cryopreservation, 10, 157
blastocysts, 69, 97, 99
CPA phase diagram, 12–14
donor program, 48
embryos, 69
cleavage stage, 70
days 3/4, 91–92
pronuclear stage, 76–77, 83
thawing, 92
Multi-Thermal-Gradient system, 244–245
oocytes, 115–116, 120–121, 127
osmotic stress reduction, 12
ovarian tissue, 191, 215
solutions for, 115–116
sperm, 42, 41
testicular tissue, 59
time factors, 131
vitrification compared, 83, 99, 102, 127
whole organs, 243
whole ovary, 237, 242–243
whole ovary with vascular pedicle, 234–236
social effects, oocyte crypreservation, 174–175
social reasons for fertility preservation
sperm cryopreservation, 39, 40
see also motherhood postponed
sodium-free freezing media, 126
classic technique, 116
MII spindle maintenance, 124–125
slow-freezing protocols, 122–123
solubility, 3–4
solutes
concentration in cryoinjury, 4
in aqueous solutions, 3
membrane permeability to, 10–11
solution effects, in cryopreservation, 12, 122–123
solutions, in vitrification, 134, 146
solvents, 3–4
sperm
abnormal, 42
collection, 41
informed consent for, 248–249
techniques, 51–53, 54, 58
morphology, 42
motility, 42
sperm (animal) cryopreservation
breeding programs, 39–40
CPAs, 26
damage by, 32
non-penetrating
monosaccharides, 29, 28
polymers, 31
sugars, 28–30
penetrating
alcohols, 27, 28
formamide, 26
sperm cryobanking
ethical considerations, 248–249
in China, 46–48
sperm cryobanks
sperm cryopreservation, 40, 43, 62–63
adverse effects, 42–43
boys with cancer, 58–59
clinical applications, 40
complications, 42–43
contraindications, 42
donor programs, 46, 48
history, 39, 95
ownership and disposition, 253–254
protocols, 40–41
quality of sperm, 42, 48, 54
quantity of sperm, 42
retrieval techniques, 51–53
electroejaculation, 48–49
surgically retrieved, 51, 53
viability, 42
vitrification, 41, 84
sperm donation
cryopreservation in, 46, 48
follow-up results, 48
sperm donors, selection/screening, 46–48
spermatids, in ICSI, 58
spermatocytes, in ICSI, 58
spermatogenesis
restoration, 61–62
SSCs in, 60
spermatogonial stem cells, *see* SSC
spermatozoa, vitrification, 160
spinal cord injury, 48–49, 53
spindle malformation, 144, 145
SSC (spermatogonial stem cells), 59, 62–63
in spermatogenesis, 60
in vitro culture, 61
isolation and purification, 61–62
testicular tissue cryopreservation, 61–62
transplantation, 59–61
stage-specific markers, follicular growth, 206–207
stem cells,
ovarian, 213
see also embryonic stem cells; SSC spermatogonial stem cells
stimulation protocols, oocyte donation, 171
storage, *see* cryobanking
straws, *see* cryopreservation straws; cut standard straws (CSS)
subcutaneous sites, for grafts, 223–225
subfertility, male, 42
sucrose, 29, 140
blastocyst vitrification, 164
clinical efficacy, 124, 126–127
concentrations, 122
embryo cryopreservation, 68
in CPA mixture, 139
MII spindle maintenance, 124–125
oocyte cryopreservation, 115–116, 122, 123, 145
oocyte vitrification, 140
osmotic stress reduction, 12
slow-freezing solutions, 12, 115–116, 122
sodium-free freezing media, 123
sugars, 28–30
sulfoxide cryoprotectant, *see* dimethyl sulfoxide
supercooling, 2–3, 99, 243
supplements to culture media, 204–206
surgery
on male genitalia, 40
ovarian tissue grafts, 223

surgically retrieved sperm, 41, 51, 53
survival rates
  childhood malignancies, 57
  cryopreserved oocytes, 127, 147, 174
systemic autoimmune rheumatic diseases, 151–152
systemic lupus erythematosus, 151–152
SYTOX dye, 206–207

temperature
  and equilibration time, 7
  in CPA permeability, 12
  in CPA toxicity, 7, 31–32
  measurement, 2
  nature of water and, 2
  solubility and, 3–4
  transportation to cryobank, 213
  water movement pathways, 16, 17
temperature gradient
  cooling rate, 243
  cooling rate and ice formation, 11
  directional freezing, 244–245
  glass transition *(Tg)*, 2–3
  in cooling and warming, 12
  in slow-cooling method, 121
  ultra-rapid warming, 159
testicular sperm, 52–53, 54
testicular sperm aspiration (TESA), 52
testicular sperm extraction (TESE), 52–53
testicular tissue
  ownership and disposition, 253–254
  sperm retrieval from, 52–53
  SSC numbers, 61–62
testicular tissue (animals), 60–61
testicular tissue cryopreservation, 63–58
  ethical issues, 62, 249–250
  for prepubertal boys, 40, 59, 249–250
  problems with, 61–62
  SSC transplantation, 59–61
Tg (glass transition temperature), 2–3
thawing
  aseptic vitrification and, 110
  blastocysts, 100, 101, 108
  donor program, 173, 174
  embryos, 77–78, 91–92
  non-aseptic vs. aseptic cooling, 108
  oocytes, 126, 147–148, 174
  recrystallization in, 243–244
  slow-freezing technique, 91
  vitrification and, 100, 174
  whole ovary with vascular pedicle, 234, 235
thawing medium, 147
thermal gradient, *see* temperature gradient
tissue handling, ovarian cryopreservation, 222
tools, *see* embryo carrier devices
toxicity, *see* CPAs, toxicity
transforming growth factor-β superfamily, 200–201
transmission electron microscopy, 206
transplantation
  environmental factors in results, 220
  history, 241
  see also heterotopic transplantation; orthotopic transplantation; ovarian tissue transplantation; ovary (whole) transplantation
transportation, 84, 213
transvaginal follicular aspiration, 171
treatment delay, cancer patients, 251
trehalose, 29
TUNEL labeling, 206
Turner syndrome, 152–153, 169
two-stage consenting process, 250
two-step culture system, 205–206, 208
two-step vitrification, 21

UK
  consent for minors, 249, 250
  oocyte cryopreservation, 253
  sperm donor anonymity, 47
ultra-rapid cooling, 106, 108, 111
ultra-rapid warming, 159
urinary tract inflammations, 49
urine alkalinization, 49
urogenital reconstructive surgery, 51
USA
  consent for minors, 249, 250
  oocyte cryopreservation, 252
  sperm donor screening/testing, 47
uterine dysfunction, after radiotherapy, 189

vacuolization
  of embryos, 163
  of oocytes, 174
vascular pedicle, intact ovary and, 194–195, 216
vascular surgery, development of, 241
vascular transplantation, whole ovary, 194–195
Vero cells, co-culture, 95
vibratory stimulation, 53
viral agents, in cryostorage, 139
viscosity, 14
vitamin E, antioxidant treatment, 220
Vitmaster, 132–134
vitreous state, 11
vitrification, 131
  advantages, 11, 146
  aneuploidy, 148
  aseptic, 106–107
  blastocysts, 95, 97–99
    aseptic, 106–107
    CPAs, 21, 99
    slow-freezing compared, 99
    water movement, 21
  closed systems, 84
  CPA damage, 12–14
  CPA movement, 20–21
  developments in, 157–158
  disadvantages, 146
  embryos, 69
    CPAs, 20–21
    day 3 and day 4, 92
    pronuclear stage, 77, 82–84
    water movement, 20–21
  equilibration in, 7
  GV stage oocytes, 117
  ice crystal prevention, 11
  McGill Cryoleaf procedure, 146
  morulae, 21
  one-step treatment, 21
  oocytes, 115, 116, 127
  ovarian tissue, 215
  probability of, 11, 131
  process of, 2, 3
  pronuclear stage embryos, 69–70, 83
  publications on, 131
  relationship of conditions for, 14
  sperm, 41
    for donor program, 48
  two-step treatment, 21
  variables influencing effectiveness, 11
  vs. ice crystals, optical differences, 12
  vs. slow freezing, 102
  water movement, 20–21
  whole ovary with vascular pedicle, 234–236, 235, 131
  see also embryo carrier devices; vitrification carrier devices
vitrification carrier devices, 92, 131, 146
  blastocysts, 97, 100
  oocytes, 132–135
vitrification solutions
  for oocytes, 139–141
  McGill Cryoleaf protocol, 146–147
  McGill Cryoleaf vitrification, 146
  scientific disclosure, 140
vitriplug hemi-straw embryo carrier, 107
Vitrisafe, 107, 110
volume changes, measurement, 16

warming
  after slow cooling, 121
  aseptic vitrification, 159, 160
  carrier devices and, 135–137
  phase diagram for CPAs, 12–14
  Sage IVF Vitrification Warming Kit, 141
  vitrification protocols, 92
    conditions for, 14
    effectiveness, 137–138
    solutions, 140–141
water
  glass transition, 2–3
  intracellular, 1
    reduction by CPAs, 26
  nature of, 2
  properties in cryopreservation, 24
water movement pathways, *see* channel diffusion; diffusion (simple); osmosis
water permeability, 10–11, 16, 21
whole ovary cryopreservation, *see* ovary (whole) cryopreservation

xenogeneic germ cell transplantation, 59
xenografting, 191, 219–220

young boys, fertility cryopreservation, 58, 249–250
young cancer patients, *see* cancer patients, young patients
young men, SSC transplantation, 59–61

zona pellucida
  breach, 138, 164
  hardening, 174
  manipulation, 80–81, 102
zygotes
  cryodamage, 70
  initial score, 162
  selection, 71